Lecture Notes in Computer Science 4046

Commenced Publication in 1973
Founding and Former Series Editors:
Gerhard Goos, Juris Hartmanis, and Jan van Leeuwen

Susan M. Astley   Michael Brady
Chris Rose   Reyer Zwiggelaar (Eds.)

Digital
Mammography

8th International Workshop, IWDM 2006
Manchester, UK, June 18-21, 2006
Proceedings

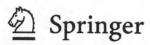 Springer

Volume Editors

Susan M. Astley
Chris Rose
University of Manchester
Imaging Science and Biomedical Engineering, Stopford Medical Building
Oxford Road, Manchester M13 9PT, UK
E-mail: sue.astley@manchester.ac.uk chris.rose@man.ac.uk

Michael Brady
Oxford University
Department of Engineering Science
Parks Road, Oxford OX1 3PJ, UK
E-mail: jmb@robots.ox.ac.uk

Reyer Zwiggelaar
University of Wales
Department of Computer Science
Aberystwyth, Ceredigion, SY23 3DB, Wales, UK
E-mail: rrz@aber.ac.uk

Library of Congress Control Number: 2006927811

CR Subject Classification (1998): I.4, I.5, H.3, J.3

LNCS Sublibrary: SL 6 – Image Processing, Computer Vision, Pattern Recognition, and Graphics

ISSN   0302-9743
ISBN-10   3-540-35625-8 Springer Berlin Heidelberg New York
ISBN-13   978-3-540-35625-7 Springer Berlin Heidelberg New York

Springer is a part of Springer Science+Business Media

springer.com

© Springer-Verlag Berlin Heidelberg 2006

Typesetting: Camera-ready by author, data conversion by Scientific Publishing Services, Chennai, India
Printed on acid-free paper   SPIN: 11783237   06/3142   5 4 3 2 1 0

Preface

This volume of Springer's *Lecture Notes in Computer Science* series records the proceedings of the 8th International Workshop on Digital Mammography (IWDM), which was held in Manchester, UK, June 18–21, 2006. The meetings bring together a diverse set of researchers (physicists, mathematicians, computer scientists, engineers), clinicians (radiologists, surgeons) and representatives of industry, who are jointly committed to developing technology, not just for its own sake, but to support clinicians in the early detection and subsequent patient management of breast cancer. The conference series was initiated at a 1993 meeting of the SPIE in San Jose, with subsequent meetings hosted every two years by researchers around the world. Previous meetings were held in York, Chicago, Nijmegen, Toronto, Bremen, and North Carolina.

It is interesting to reflect on the changes that have occurred during the past 13 years. Then, the dominant technology was film-screen mammography; now it is full-field digital mammography. Then, there were few screening programmes world-wide; now there are many. Then, there was the hope that computer-aided detection (CAD) of early signs of cancer might be possible; now CAD is not only a reality but (more importantly) a commercially led clinical reality. Then, algorithms were almost entirely heuristic with little clinical support; now there is a requirement for substantial clinical support for any algorithm that is developed and published. However, upon reflection, could we have predicted with absolute certainty what would be the key questions to be addressed over the subsequent (say) six years? No! That is the nature, joy, and frustration of research. There are more blind alleys to explore than there are rich veins that bring gold (in all senses of that analogy!).

What are the current preoccupations? What are currently the ideas that we believe will bear handsome fruit over the next 20 years? These are reflected in the programme, and in the choice of invited speakers. However, it is first important to realize that what have been identified as the major challenges over the past 13 years continue to be challenges: robust, reliable, efficient algorithms for CAD, segmentation, registration, and texture analysis await definitive solution, as they do in image analysis generally (and mammography poses additional challenges). Second, the challenges of delivering the technology effectively to end-users remain unmet: what are the optimal prompts? How do you deliver CAD in large rural areas? How do you deliver mammographic image analysis over the emerging Grid? How do you integrate film-screen mammography with full-field digital? How do you fuse mammography with other imaging modalities, such as MRI, ultrasound, and PET. . . These observations explain about half of the sessions, as they did at previous meetings (though we all believe we have made progress)!

Like great music, however, for all the increasingly understood and recurrent themes there are some newer ones that press for attention! Among these we can clearly identify tomosynthesis—subject of an invited address by Prof. Dan Kopans at UNC in 2004 and now increasingly a commercial and clinical reality—and the estimation and analysis of breast density—again, the subject of an invited address by Prof. Norman Boyd at UNC in 2004. However, with the exquisite hindsight of reflection on the past we will—six years hence—be able to identify a number of other emergent themes, although not only are we not able to see them clearly but would probably reject them as marginal! These might be fusion of mammography with other modalities and x-ray imaging techniques that currently seem *avant garde*.

A successful conference is a blend of inspired organization, financial support, scientific insight; but, ultimately, the quality of the papers that were submitted. Two of us (Sue, Mike) were charged by the IWDM Scientific Committee to organize a meeting in the UK. We invited four-page outline papers, as opposed to the paragraphs that had previously been submitted. We believe that this simultaneously increased the quality and decreased the number of submissions. Each four-page abstract was assessed independently by at least two, often three, members of the Scientific Committee, and the final eight-page submissions were assessed independently by at least two members. We believe that the final proceedings, which you have in your hand, constitute a state-of-the-art statement of mammographic image analysis, its underlying physics, and clinical pull-through. The invited addresses by Julietta Patnick—director of the UK national breast screening programme—and Profs. Andrew Maidment—digital mammography and tomosynthesis—and Etta Pisano—author *inter alia* of the influential DMIST trial—were not included in the published proceedings; but their influence on the future of the research of the community, and its pull-through into practice, cannot be over-emphasized.

Finally, in keeping with the multi-disciplinary nature of the meeting, the meeting was supported by sponsors and there was an excellent industrial exposition, pulled together by Reyer Zwiggelaar. The timely and efficient production of the reviews, final versions, arrangements, etc. depended fundamentally on Dr. Chris Rose and the remarkable CAWS website at Manchester.

Table of Contents

Breast Density

CAD

Clinical Practice

Tomosynthesis

Registration and Multiple View Mammography

Physics Models

Poster Session

Wavelet Methods

Full-Field Digital Mammography

Segmentation

A New Step-Wedge for the Volumetric Measurement of Mammographic Density

Jennifer Diffey[1], Alan Hufton[1], and Susan Astley[2]

[1] North Western Medical Physics, Christie Hospital, Withington, Manchester M20 4BX
jenny.diffey@physics.cr.man.ac.uk
alan.hufton@physics.cr.man.ac.uk
[2] Division of Imaging Science and Biomedical Engineering, Stopford Building,
University of Manchester, Oxford Road, Manchester M13 9PT
sue.astley@manchester.ac.uk

Abstract. The volume of dense breast tissue can be calculated from an x-ray mammogram by imaging a calibrated step-wedge alongside the breast and determining the compressed breast thickness. Previously published work used a step-wedge made of PTFE with a maximum height of 35mm, length 175mm and width 15mm. Although fulfilling all theoretical requirements, it can be difficult to find space on the film for a large step-wedge when examining bigger breasts. Furthermore, the step-wedge is lead-lined, making it heavy and difficult to attach to the bucky. A more compact aluminium step-wedge has been designed to overcome these limitations, and experiments have been carried out on a prototype to evaluate its performance. Initial results show that the maximum and minimum heights of the prototype step-wedge are inadequate to sufficiently cover the range of optical densities within a breast image at the higher and lower exposures required for 6cm and 2cm Perspex (>200mAs and < 40mAs respectively). However, the step increment appears to be satisfactory. Analysis of the mean pixel value and standard deviation within Regions of Interest of varying size and position indicates an optimum step length of 3mm. A new step-wedge has been constructed with an improved specification informed by the evaluation of the prototype.

1 Background

Increased breast density is associated with a higher risk of developing cancer [1, 2, 3, 4]. Various techniques exist for estimating or measuring dense tissue [5, 6, 7, 8, 9, 10]. One such method involving the use of a calibrated step-wedge has been used previously to study women at increased risk of developing cancer [11, 12]. This method, however, suffers from a number of limitations, and we now examine in detail the design considerations for a step-wedge, using a new aluminium prototype for evaluation purposes, and hence develop a specification for a wedge suitable for use in routine clinical practice.

In order to quantify dense breast tissue, a calibrated step-wedge can be imaged alongside the breast, with radio-opaque magnification markers on the compression paddle to enable determination of breast thickness at a series of points. The density at

Susan M. Astley et al. (Eds.): IWDM 2006, LNCS 4046, pp. 1–9, 2006.

each pixel in the resulting mammogram is then matched to the equivalent density in the calibrated step-wedge. The corresponding thickness of the step-wedge at this point, combined with breast thickness measurement, allows composition to be uniquely determined at each pixel.

The original step-wedge [13] was constructed of PTFE (polytetrafluoroethylene / *Teflon*). It had 25 steps, each of height 1mm and length 5mm, giving a maximum height of 25mm and a total length of 125mm. The width of all steps was 12mm. It was necessary to shield the sides of the wedge with lead to ensure that only those parts of each step where x-rays have travelled through the whole thickness of the wedge are imaged. The wedge is positioned at the top left-hand corner of the breast support platform (bucky) and is therefore exposed to x-rays traveling at an oblique angle. Without lead shielding the image becomes blurred by x-rays that only pass through part of the wedge, causing the grey level to vary across each step.

It was found that at the higher exposure factors required for greater breast thickness and density, the optical density of the step-wedge on the image increased to the extent that the 25mm step-wedge did not adequately cover the range of optical densities expected within the breast [12]. An additional 10 steps were added increasing the overall height to 35mm and the length to 175mm. A further limitation was that when placed near the edge of a 24×30cm breast support platform, the distance from the point directly below the x-ray source increased, causing the x-rays pass through the step-wedge at a more oblique angle and reducing the usable width. The width of the 35mm step-wedge was therefore increased to 15mm, giving a usable width of 4mm at height 35mm.

Despite fulfilling the theoretical requirements to enable calibration, in practice the 35mm step-wedge was sometimes too big to fit alongside larger breasts and the lead lining made it a relatively heavy, unwieldy device that could not easily be attached to the bucky [14]. A further limitation of the PTFE wedge was that analysis required accurate identification of step positions in the digital image. Typically, one end of the wedge was overexposed and the other underexposed, so finding the ends accurately was non-trivial.

2 Method

In order to optimize the specification for a new step-wedge that will overcome the limitations shown by the PTFE wedge, a prototype wedge made of aluminium has been constructed and evaluated.

2.1 Step-Wedge Material

PTFE was used previously because it has a similar mass attenuation coefficient to breast tissue, but a higher density than most plastics, allowing a larger range of attenuation to be achieved without requiring too great a thickness. PTFE would also minimise beam hardening effects, which could have been significant in the original analysis method. However, the calibration method is now much less sensitive to these effects and enables higher atomic number materials to be considered.

Aluminium was initially proposed as an alternative material, despite concerns that the increment in step height required would be too small to be machined with any degree of accuracy. However, it is possible to machine a step-wedge from a single block of aluminium using 0.2mm increments in step height. Compounds were rejected to avoid problems with inhomogeneity. Magnesium was also considered as it has a slightly lower density and mass attenuation coefficient than aluminium. However, magnesium was discounted for safety reasons as it is classed as a severe irritant and is also highly flammable.

2.2 Step-Wedge Dimensions

A 28kV molybdenum spectrum with 0.03mm molybdenum filtration was generated using specialist software [15]. Although the mean photon energy of the spectrum was 16.3keV, photon attenuation by a number of materials was considered at 20keV. The corresponding thickness of aluminium required to give the same photon attenuation as a range of thicknesses of adipose tissue, fibroglandular tissue and PTFE was calculated. Equations were solved using the density and mass attenuation coefficient [16] of each material, with the only unknown in the equation being the thickness of aluminium. This yielded results of 1mm and 8mm for minimum and maximum step height respectively, with step increments of 0.2mm.

2.3 Construction of a Prototype Aluminium Wedge

For evaluation purposes a prototype aluminium step-wedge was constructed, in which the step length was varied to enable investigation of the optimum length. Ideally the step-wedge should be as compact as possible, but each step must allow the sampling region to be large enough to ensure that any variations due to inhomogeneity in the material are averaged out, giving an accurate greyscale value.

Lead lining is not necessary as the smaller dimensions of the wedge have reduced the problem of shadowing. The usable width of each step is greater for the same reason. Notches were introduced every third step on the prototype step-wedge to aid with step identification on the digitized x-ray image. A comparison of the aluminium prototype and the PTFE step-wedge is shown in Figure 1.

2.4 Evaluation of Step-Wedge

Evaluation of the prototype step-wedge has been carried out in order to determine if the dimensions are adequate. In the initial experiments, the prototype aluminium step-wedge was imaged alongside 2, 4, 6 and 7cm of Perspex on a Lorad M-IV mammography unit. The Autofilter mode which is used in clinical practice was used in this study, so that a wide range of exposure factors was covered. Measurements were made using the 18×24 and 24×30cm buckies. The same exposures were repeated using the 35mm PTFE step-wedge placed in the same location on the bucky. The optical density of each step on the aluminium and PTFE step-wedge images was measured using a Parry Transmission Densitometer DT1105 with a 1.0mm aperture.

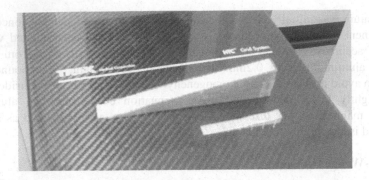

Fig. 1. Comparison of PTFE step-wedge (rear) with prototype aluminium step-wedge (front)

The films were digitized using a Kodak LS85 digitizer at a pixel size of 50 µm and a pixel depth of 12 bits (4096 grey levels). The grey level is linearly related to optical density (OD) in the range 0.03-4.1 OD [17]. This particular digitizer produces images with grey level 0 (corresponding to an OD of zero) displayed as white and grey level 4096 (corresponding to the maximum OD value) displayed as black. The pixel depth was reduced to 8 bits (256 grey levels) after digitizing, using a window based on the maximum and minimum OD present in the image. This was to reduce file sizes of the stored images. The images were analysed using *ImageJ* [18], a Java-based software application.

3 Results

Step-height increment was assessed by comparing the PTFE and aluminium step-wedges imaged alongside 4cm Perspex under identical exposure conditions (25kV, molybdenum target and filter, 135mAs). The incremental change in optical density in the aluminium step-wedge was equal to or less than that in the PTFE step-wedge, suggesting that a step increment of 0.2mm is satisfactory. Under these conditions, the image of the prototype aluminium step-wedge was acceptable (Figure 2) with the inclusion of a range of optical densities from 0.25 to 3.70 being covered.

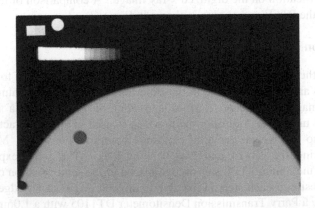

Fig. 2. Aluminium prototype step-wedge imaged alongside 4cm Perspex

However, at the higher exposure factors required to expose 6cm Perspex in Autofilter mode (29kV, rhodium target, 241mAs), the lowest optical density was 1.0, suggesting that the maximum height is insufficient. Conversely, for the lower exposure factors required to expose 2cm Perspex (24kV, molybdenum target, 32mAs), the highest optical density was 2.1, suggesting that the minimum height is too great. Therefore the current height dimensions of the prototype step-wedge are likely to be inadequate to sufficiently cover the range of optical densities within a breast image over the full range of exposures (Figure 3).

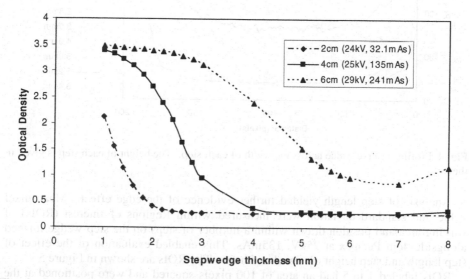

Fig. 3. Optical densities on the step-wedge for three films using different thicknesses of Perspex

The unexpected upturn in the curves at the maximum step-wedge thickness of 8 mm has been observed in previous work [19]. It is thought to be an artifact, attributed to the fact that on the image, only a very small area of the last step is visible for which the x-rays have passed through the whole step-wedge thickness, with the remainder of the step appearing as heavily shadowed.

Step width was assessed by analyzing line profiles of mean pixel value across the width of each step within the step-wedge exposed alongside 4cm Perspex at 25kV, 135mAs. Although step width was 200 pixels, all profiles covered a distance of 183 pixels (Figure 4). Step edges were difficult to differentiate from the background and care was taken with the positioning of the line profile to avoid the inclusion of background pixels.

Within each step, there is a relatively uniform region where fluctuation in pixel value is low. However, it can be seen that there is an "edge effect" which becomes more significant as step height increases. Step width is currently 10mm. Figure 4 suggests that only the central 5mm (pixel distance 50 – 150) can be used to determine the true mean pixel value within the step.

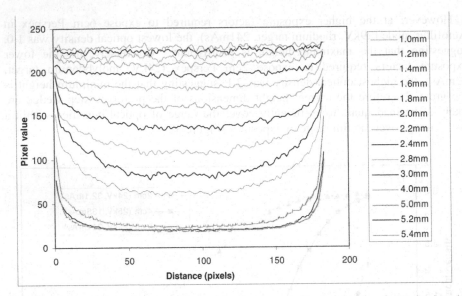

Fig. 4. Profiles of pixel value across the width of each step. The height of each step is given in the key.

Analysis of step length yielded further evidence of the edge effect. Mean pixel value and standard deviation were measured within Regions of Interest (ROIs) of varying area and position drawn within a number of steps on the step-wedge imaged alongside 4cm Perspex at 25kV, 135mAs. This enabled evaluation of the effect of step length and step height on signal and noise. The ROIs are shown in Figure 5.

ROIs labeled 1 to 5 had an area of 100 pixels squared and were positioned at the centre and four corners of each step. The area of ROIs labeled (a) and (b) remained constant over all steps but the area of ROI (c) was varied according to step length and

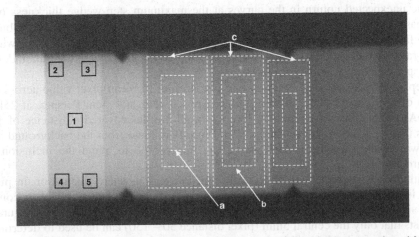

Fig. 5. Regions of Interest (ROIs) used to determine the effect of ROI area and position on mean pixel value and standard deviation

Table 1. The effect of step height and ROI area on mean pixel value and standard deviation (s.d). (a) Inner ROI = 800 pixels squared; (b) Middle ROI = 3300 pixels squared; (c) Outer ROI = 7500 pixels squared (3mm step length), 11900 pixels squared (4mm step length), 15300 pixels squared (5mm step length).

Step height (mm)	Step length (mm)	(a) Inner ROI Mean Pixel Value	s.d	(b) Middle ROI Mean Pixel Value	s.d	(c) Outer ROI Mean Pixel Value	s.d
1.0	3	227.4	2.08	227.5	2.20	227.6	2.29
1.2	4	223.9	2.18	224.0	2.15	224.1	2.38
1.4	5	217.1	2.53	217.2	2.43	217.9	2.66
1.6	3	208.7	1.96	208.8	2.03	209.3	2.33
1.8	4	196.4	1.79	196.7	1.94	198.1	3.05
2.0	5	181.5	1.52	182.0	1.85	184.0	3.65
2.2	3	159.9	2.33	161.0	2.82	163.5	5.02
2.4	4	137.8	2.14	138.8	2.94	143.4	8.17
2.6	5	109.1	2.64	110.9	3.82	118.1	11.38
2.8	3	82.9	2.69	84.8	4.49	90.0	10.12
3.0	4	63.2	2.35	64.9	3.81	73.2	13.71
4.0	5	24.3	0.83	25.2	1.72	30.3	8.66
5.0	3	20.0	0.39	20.3	0.70	21.6	2.62
5.2	4	19.5	0.50	19.8	0.72	22.3	4.77

was chosen to cover as much of the step as possible without including background pixels or overlapping another step.

The results for mean pixel value within ROI 1 (Figure 5) were very similar to those quoted in Table 1 with standard deviation being comparable to or lower than the values for the inner ROI (a). The standard deviation for the corner ROIs 2 – 5 was significantly greater, particularly as step height increased, thus providing further evidence of the edge effect. As a result, the mean pixel values differed considerably from those at the centre.

4 Discussion

Results show that mean pixel value remains almost constant regardless of the area of the region of interest (ROI), provided that the region does not include pixels close to the edge of the step. In addition, the standard deviation decreases with decreasing area suggesting that quantum noise and impurities within the image are not limiting factors and there is no need for a large ROI to 'average out' these effects. The step lengths within the prototype are 3, 4 and 5mm. Given that the step-wedge should be as compact as possible, a step length of 3mm is therefore considered to be the optimum.

Although shadowing of the edge pixels is not apparent on visual inspection, it is demonstrated by the line profiles across the width of each step. Further evidence is given by the fact that the small ROIs (100 pixels squared) positioned at the corners of each step exhibit a much greater standard deviation than a ROI positioned at the centre. Similarly, the standard deviation within the outer ROIs was greater than that within the inner and middle ROIs, particularly at the larger step heights. The "edge effect" becomes increasingly significant as step height increases, to the extent that the usable step width is reduced to approximately 5mm.

The major drawback with using a PTFE step-wedge was that in order to encompass the range of densities encountered in clinical practice, all three dimensions were too great. In addition, the radiographers found the lead lining made the step-wedge heavy and difficult to attach to the bucky. Our initial results using aluminium indicate that this should prove to be more acceptable.

Because aluminium has a higher effective atomic number than breast tissue ($Z=13$ compared with $Z_{eff}\sim7$), beam hardening effects imply that equal pixel values under the step wedge and breast will not represent equal photon or energy fluences. However, in the calibration method used such effects should not be significant. Essentially, the breast tissue transmission is calibrated against a phantom consisting of various thicknesses of epoxy resin based tissue substitutes AP6 and WT1 to simulate fat and dense tissue respectively [20]. The step wedge merely provides a practical intermediate step, since the tissue equivalent phantoms would be too large to include alongside the breast. In other words, it is not essential for the step wedge to provide the same absolute transmission as the breast or phantom, as long as the relative values are the same. However, this will only hold true as long as the calibration x-ray spectrum and clinical x-ray spectrum are the same. It may therefore be necessary to generate separate calibration curves for different spectra, although previous work with a PTFE step wedge ($Z_{eff}=8.5$) showed no measurable difference between a wide range of x-ray beam qualities [19].

In principle, the method described can be used for quantifying dense breast tissue from digitally acquired mammograms. However, it may be possible to simplify the procedure. By analysing the raw pixel values one can take advantage of the known wide dynamic range and linearity of digital detectors, thereby avoiding the complex non-linear, film processing dependent relation between film density and exposure. A much simpler step-wedge consisting of only a very few steps may suffice. In fact, Kaufhold et al [21] have shown that it may be possible to eliminate the need for a step-wedge entirely by normalising the mammograms and calibration data to a fixed mAs.

References

1. Wolfe, J. N.: Breast patterns as an index of risk for developing breast cancer. Am. J. Roentgenol. 126(6) (1976) 1130-1137
2. Boyd, N. F., O'Sullivan, B., Campbell, J. E., Fishell, E., Simor, I., Cooke, G., Germanson, T.: Mammographic signs as risk factors for breast cancer. Br. J. Cancer 45(2) (1982) 185-193
3. Boyd, N. F., Byng, J. W., Jong, R. A., Fishell, E. K., Little, L. E., Miller, A. B., Lockwood, G. A., Tritchler, D. L., Yaffe, M. J.: Quantitative classification of mammographic densities and breast cancer risk: results from the Canadian National Breast Screening Study. J. Natl. Cancer Inst. 87(9) (1995) 670-675

4. Byng, J. W., Yaffe, M. J, Lockwood, G. A., Little, L. E., Tritchler, D. L., Boyd, N. F.: Automated analysis of mammographic densities and breast carcinoma risk. Cancer 80(1) (1997) 66-74
5. Byng, J. W., Boyd, N. F., Fishell, E., Jong, R. A., Yaffe, M. J.: Automated analysis of mammographic densities. Phys. Med. Biol. 41(5) (1996) 909-923
6. Byng, J. W., Boyd, N. F., Fishell, E., Jong, R. A., Yaffe, M. J.: The quantitative analysis of mammographic densities. Phys. Med. Biol. 39(10) (1994) 1629-1638
7. Zhou, C., Chan H. P., Petrick, N., Helvie, M. A., Goodsitt, M. M., Sahiner, B., Hadjiiski, L. M.: Computerized image analysis: estimation of breast density on mammograms. Med. Phys. 28(6) (2001) 1056-1069
8. Pawluczyk, O., Augustine, B. J., Yaffe, M. J., Rico, D., Yang, J., Mawdsley, G. E., Boyd, N. F.: A volumetric method for estimation of breast density on digitized screen-film mammograms. Med. Phys. 30(3) (2003) 352-364
9. Highnam, R. P., Brady, M., Shepstone, B. J.: A representation for mammographic image processing. Med. Image. Anal. 1(1) (1996) 1-18
10. Highnam, R. P., Brady, M., Shepstone, B. J.: Mammographic image analysis. Eur. J. Radiol. 24(1) (1997) 20-32
11. Patel, H.G., Astley, S. M., Hufton, A. P., Harvie, M., Hagan, K., Marchant, T. E., Hillier, V., Howell, A.: Automated breast tissue measurement of women at increased risk of breast cancer, Proceedings of the 7th International Workshop on Digital Mammography, Ed. Etta Pisano, June 18-21, 2004, Durham, North Carolina (2006)
12. Hufton, A. P., Astley, S. M., Marchant, T. E., Patel, H. G.: A method for the quantification of dense breast tissue from digitised mammograms, Proceedings of the 7th International Workshop on Digital Mammography, Ed. Etta Pisano, June 18-21, (2006) Manchester, England
13. Smith, J. H., Astley, S. M., Graham, J., Hufton, A.P.: The calibration of grey levels in mammograms. 3rd International Workshop on Digital Mammography, June 1996, Chicago, published in, 'Digital Mammography '96', ed. Doi K, Giger ML, Nishikawa RM and Schmidt RA (1996) 195-200 (Elsevier, New York)
14. Berks, M., Diffey, J., Hufton, A., Astley, S.: Feasibility and acceptability of stepwedge-based density measurement. Proceedings of the 8th International Workshop on Digital Mammography, June 18-21 (2006) Manchester, England
15. Reilly, A. J., Sutton, D.: Report 78 Spectrum Processor. Institute of Physics and Engineering in Medicine (1997)
16. http://www.physics.nist.gov/PhysRefData/XrayMassCoef/cover.html
17. Kodak.: Kodak LS85 film digitizer product specifications. Eastman Kodak Company, Rochester, NY. Cat. No. 165 2908 (2001)
18. http://rsb.info.nih.gov/ij/
19. Marchant, T. E.: Calibrating densities in mammography. MSc thesis, Department of Imaging Science and Biomedical Engineering, University of Manchester, UK (2002)
20. ICRU Report 44.: Tissue Substitutes in Radiation Dosimetry and Measurement. International Commission on Radiation Units and Measurements (1989)
21. Kaufhold, J., Thomas, J. A., Eberhard, J. W., Galbo, C. E., Gonzalez Trotter, D. E.: A calibration approach to glandular tissue composition estimation in digital mammography. Med Phys. 29(8) (2002) 1867-80

Assessing Ground Truth of Glandular Tissue

Christina Olsén and Fredrik Georgsson

Department of Computing Science,
Umeå University, SE-901 87 Umeå Sweden
{colsen, fredrikg}@cs.umu.se

Abstract. In medical image analysis a ground truth to compare results against is of vital importance. This ground truth is often obtained from human experts. The aim of this paper is to discuss the problem related to the use of markings made by an expert panel. As a partial solution, we propose a method to relate markings to each other in order to establish levels of agreement. By using this method we can assess the performance of, for instance, segmentation algorithms.

1 Background

Performance evaluation is essential for providing a scientific basis for image analysis in general and for medical image analysis in particular. In order to evaluate the performance of an image analysis system the output of the system has to be correlated to a true value. This true value is often referred to as ground truth, golden truth, golden standard, etc. In some cases it can be difficult and highly controversial for a layman to assess the true value that the image analysis system is supposed to achieve. In these cases the solution often involve human domain experts who define the true value.

Several researchers in image analysis have studied the evaluation of segmentation algorithms based on ground truth obtained from a group of experts. Many of them emphasize the importance of an objective ground truth. Zou et al. [13] presented systematic approaches to validate the accuracy of automated image segmentation. Based on the Expectation-Maximization algorithm for computing a probability estimate of the ground truth segmentation from a group of expert segmentations presented in [12], the authors modeled the probabilistic segmentation results using a mixture of two beta distributions with different shape parameters for the interpretation of the tumor class. Furthermore, Warfield et al. [12] present a simultaneous measure of the quality of each expert, which enables the assessment of an automated image segmentation algorithm, and direct comparison of expert and algorithm performance. Smyth [11] and Bromiley et al. [3] have also addressed the problems related to algorithm evaluation based on uncertain ground truth. Olsén and Georgsson [9] and Olsén [8] addressed these problems in relation to segmentation methods concerning mammography.

The aim of this paper is to discuss the problem of assessing ground truth and to provide a novel method of estimating ground truth in the case of binary markings in $\mathbb{Z}^n$.

Susan M. Astley et al. (Eds.): IWDM 2006, LNCS 4046, pp. 10–17, 2006.

2   Theoretical Background

We assume that we have K different domain experts who all marked some properties p regarding anatomical landmarks depicted in L images. A measure of agreement can be defined as

$$\Lambda_i^p = \frac{\mu(A_1^p \cap A_2^p \cap \ldots \cap A_K^p)}{\mu(A_1^p \cup A_2^p \cup \ldots \cup A_K^p)}. \tag{1}$$

where $i = 1, 2, \ldots, L$ and $\mu(\cdot)$ is a measure of the set (i.e. the numbers of points if A is discrete).

In the general case, a ground truth can be any subset $A_i \subset \mathbb{Z}^n$, where n is the spatial dimensionality of the media, i.e. $n = 1$ for a signal, $n = 2$ for an image, $n = 3$ for a volume etc. In passing, it is noted that the dimensionality of the set A_i may be lower than n. Examples of this are; marking a line in an image, a point in a volume etc.

We define the distance from a point $\mathbf{p}$ to a set $S \subset \mathbb{Z}^n$ to be $D(\mathbf{p}, S) = \inf\{d(\mathbf{p}, \mathbf{q}) \mid \mathbf{q} \in S\}$, where $d(\cdot, \cdot)$ is some metric defined on $\mathbb{Z}^n$. We note that $D(\mathbf{p}, S) = 0$ if $\mathbf{p} \in S$. The distance can be estimated efficiently by using a distance transformation [1].

A distance between two discrete sets S and U can then be defined as

$$\mathcal{D}(S, U) = \sum_{\mathbf{p} \in S} D(\mathbf{p}, U) + \sum_{\mathbf{q} \in U} D(\mathbf{q}, S). \tag{2}$$

The distance between a set S and an ensemble of sets $\mathbf{\Lambda} = \{A_1, \ldots, A_K\}$ is given by

$$\mathbf{D_A}(S) = \sum_{A_i \in \mathbf{A}} \mathcal{D}(S, A_i). \tag{3}$$

It is easily seen that if we have different overlapping sets S_i, then the set with the smallest measure contained in the intersection of the sets (i.e. the set marking the smallest *area* if the underlying dimensionality of S_i is 2) is likely to minimize $\mathbf{D_A}(S_i)$. This property makes a distance measure such as the one defined in Eq. 3 unsuitable for comparing a marking to that of a set of experts. It can be said that the distance defined in Eq. 3 penalizes sets that fill the plane and thus we need to add a measure of how well a set S "fills" the ensemble $\mathbf{A}$. In order to construct such a measure we define an occurrence operator

$$\phi_S(\mathbf{p}) = \begin{cases} 1 & \text{if } \mathbf{p} \in S \\ 0 & \text{otherwise} \end{cases}$$

for every set S of points. By using $\phi(\cdot)$ the ensemble $\mathbf{A}$ now gives rise to a measure of the subsets S of $\mathbb{Z}^n$, which is defined by

$$\mathbf{M_A}(S) = \sum_{A_i \in \mathbf{A}} \sum_{\mathbf{p} \in S} \phi_{A_i}(\mathbf{p}). \tag{4}$$

Given an ensemble of ground truths $\mathbf{A}$, any set S that maximizes $\mathbf{M_A}(S)$ whilst simultaneously minimizing $\mathbf{D_A}(S)$ is said to be in good agreement with the ensemble.

For a set S and the ensemble $\mathbf{A}$ shown in Figure 1(a), $r = \mathbf{M_A}(S)$ and $s = \mathbf{D_A}(S)$ are calculated using Eq. 3 and 4, see Figure 1(b)-1(g) and Figure 1(h). By projecting the vector $(r, s)^T$ onto a base vector $(a, b)^T$ an estimate of the agreement between the set S and the ensemble $\mathbf{A}$ is obtained (Figure 1(i)). The values of the components of the base vector $(a, b)^T$ are obtained as follows. For a, a positive value is chosen because a a corresponds to r, which is to be maximized. Similarly, a negative value is chosen for b as s is to be minimized. The relative size of $|a|$ and $|b|$ determines the weight we put on the measures. Typically they get the same weight, and thus the two elements of the vector should be the same value but of opposite sign. The actual numerical value chosen, only scales the subspace and is not important as long as it is positive. We used $a = 1$ and $b = -1$.

The agreement of a set S with an ensemble $\mathbf{A}$ can thus be expressed as

$$\alpha(S, \mathbf{A}) = (r, s)(1, -1)^T = \mathbf{M_A}(S) - \mathbf{D_A}(S). \tag{5}$$

The scaling of the function α is rather arbitrary and depends on the measures of the involved sets etc. Thus it only makes sense to compare different sets S_i with an ensemble $\mathbf{A}$ and to say that the S_i that maximizes $\alpha(S_i, \mathbf{A})$ is most in agreement with the ensemble $\mathbf{A}$. Furthermore, it is possible to use α in the following way. Suppose we have a set S (for example a proposed segmentation of the glandular tissue) and an ensemble $\mathbf{A}$ (expert markings of the glandular tissue). First we let $A_{K+1} = S$ and define $\mathbf{A}' = \{A_1, \ldots, A_K, A_{K+1}\}$. Then we calculate

$$\alpha_k = \alpha(A_k, \mathbf{B}) \tag{6}$$

where $\mathbf{B}$ is $\mathbf{A}'$ minus A_k and $k \in \{1, \ldots, K+1\}$. The value α_k describes how member k of the ensemble $\mathbf{A}'$ fit in with the rest of the members. Let k_{min} be the k that minimizes α_k. If $k_{min} \neq K+1$ then we can say that the proposed set S mixes in with the ensemble. When using ensembles, the values r_i and s_i are normalised to zero mean and unit variance prior to projection. The is done to ensure that we have a proper scaling of the values.

3   Results

3.1   Data Set

In order to gather data about the way in which human experts assess the ground truth in mammograms, we developed a questionnaire[1]. It forms the basis for a study in which we asked three radiologists and two groups of several radiographs to evaluate 200 randomly selected mammograms (cases) from two different standard databases, i.e. the Digital Database for Screening Mammography (DDSM) and Mammographic Image Analysis Society Database (MIAS). The experts were asked to mark/outline anatomical features as well as answer questions concerning their decision making. The utility of gathering the markings of anatomical landmarks is to determine diagnostic quality of mammograms, see Olsén [10].

---

[1] http://www.cs.umu.se/~colsen/study.html

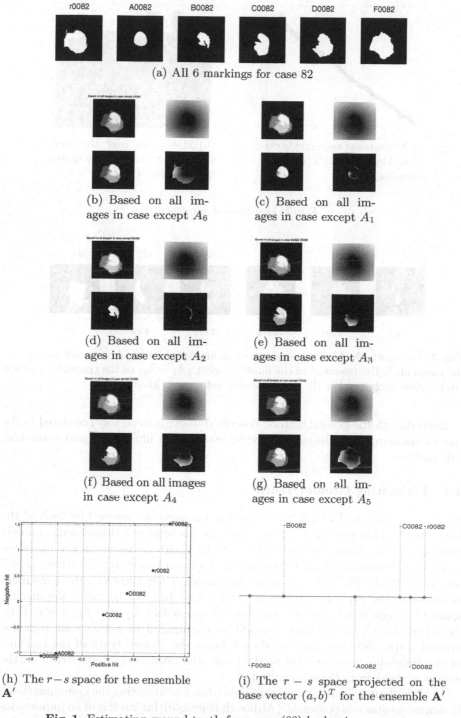

(a) All 6 markings for case 82

(b) Based on all images in case except A_6

(c) Based on all images in case except A_1

(d) Based on all images in case except A_2

(e) Based on all images in case except A_3

(f) Based on all images in case except A_4

(g) Based on all images in case except A_5

(h) The $r - s$ space for the ensemble $\mathbf{A}'$

(i) The $r - s$ space projected on the base vector $(a, b)^T$ for the ensemble $\mathbf{A}'$

Fig. 1. Estimating ground truth for a case (82) by leaving one out

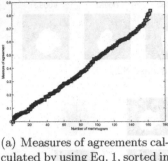

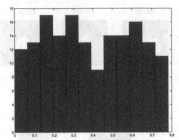

(a) Measures of agreements calculated by using Eq. 1, sorted in
ascending order.

(b) Histogram over the measures of agreements calculated
by using Eq. 1.

Fig. 2. Measures of agreement

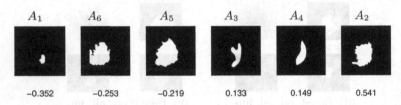

A_1	A_6	A_5	A_3	A_4	A_2
−0.352	−0.253	−0.219	0.133	0.149	0.541

Fig. 3. The ensemble $\mathbf{A}'$ with respect to α_k in increasing order. Above each member of the ensemble is the reference to the human expert ($A_1 - A_5$) or the computer method (A_6). Below each member the corresponding value α_k is given.

Even though the general method described above is in no way restricted to the case of mammograms, the study provides material for illustrating and evaluating this method.

3.2   Estimating Ground Truth

We have compiled all of the 200 cases of mammograms assessed by each of the five experts. This gives us 1000 markings for the anatomical landmark, namely glandular tissue. Based on the outlines of the glandular tissue on the questionnaire we have estimated the agreement among them based on Eq. 1 where $K = 5$ and $L = 200$. In Fig. 2(a) it is seen that amongst the 200 cases the agreement as calculated by Eq. 1 is in the range $0.05 - 0.85$. In fact, the values are linearly spaced between these extremes and thus we can safely say that Eq. 1 is of little use to us. This indicates that it would be meaningful to work on an objective ground truth. However, since we do not know the ground truth of the marking of the glandular tissue we still need to base the estimated ground truth on the expert answers from the data collected.

In Mukhdoomi [7], a segmentation algorithm for extracting the glandular tissue in mammograms was proposed. (Although the algorithm itself is of no importance here, let us mention that it is divided into two main phases. In the first phase, an optimal threshold value is calculated that gives a preliminary glandular tissue segmentation. Such an optimal threshold is found through the LLBP approach described in [2, 5, 6], that is based on the principle of minimizing cross-entropy values between an image and its thresholded version over a certain range of threshold values.) We have evaluated the algorithm using our method. The marking resulting from that algorithm is here denoted A_6. Let us consider the markings produced by the five experts in a typical case $(A_1 - A_5)$. Following the method proposed in Section 2, the value α_k was calculated for each marking of the ensemble using Eq. 6. As can be seen in Fig. 3 human expert A_1 is the one that is in least agreement with the rest of the experts, whilst expert A_2 is in best agreement with the ensemble in this particular case. In this case, the segmentation done by the proposed automatic segmentation algorithm A_6 mixes in with the human experts.

Table 1. The rank sum given by Eq. 7. Rank 1 corresponds to the best agreement and rank 6 to the least agreement.

(a) Rank sum, were A_6 is a marking from the system.

Rank sum	Expert
1	359	A_4
2	365	A_2
3	434	A_5
4	436	A_3
5	480	A_6
6	488	A_1

(b) Rank sum, were A_6' is a marking from a random case.

Rank sum	Expert
1	330	A_5
2	354	A_4
3	356	A_2
4	428	A_3
5	481	A_1
6	634	A_6'

Table 2. Histogram over the rank values. Rank 1 corresponds to the best agreement and rank 6 to the least agreement.

(a) Histogram over the rank values, were A_6 is a marking from the system.

Expert	1	2	3	4	5	6
A_1	5	21	21	22	28	25
A_2	31	25	19	20	15	12
A_3	12	16	35	26	15	18
A_4	29	29	20	20	12	12
A_5	22	18	15	21	29	17
A_6	23	13	12	13	23	38

(b) Histogram over the rank values. A_6' is a markings from a random case.

Expert	1	2	3	4	5	6
A_1	8	14	25	28	30	18
A_2	20	37	30	15	14	7
A_3	7	30	28	27	17	14
A_4	26	31	26	19	14	7
A_5	57	9	12	18	15	12
A_6'	5	2	2	16	33	65

If we run the test on all expert cases, case A_6 still mixes in with the human experts (A_6 in Table 1(a)) and if we had to choose one expert to represent the ensemble it would be A_4. If we instead randomly pick a marking from any other different case from the database (A'_6 in Table 1(b)) it is, as expected, on average the one that is considerably in least agreement with the rest of the experts.

The rank sum for i is:

$$RankSum_i = \sum_j E_{ij} \cdot j, \tag{7}$$

where $i = 1, \ldots, 6$, $j = 1, \ldots, 6$ and E_{ij} is a histogram over the rank values for each of the markings. An example of a histogram is given in Table 2.

4 Discussion

As mentioned earlier, several researchers in image analysis have studied the evaluation of segmentation algorithms based on using a group of experts as ground truth. This experience made many of them emphasize the importance of an objective ground truth. The reason for the importance of an objective ground truth is due to the large variation among the markings done by the group of experts. For example, a large variation among human experts in radiology is very common, see e.g. Gual-Arnau et al. [4]. During discussions several experts have communicated that this is actually the case in practice as well. They also realize the problems this involve, especially while developing objective computer aided tools. Therefore, the aim of this paper has been to discuss the problem of assessing ground truth with large inter-variation and to propose a novel method of estimating ground truth in the case of binary markings in $\mathbb{Z}^n$.

Even though the proposed method for estimating ground truth still needs to be evaluated further, it can be used for assess the agreement amongst domain experts. The fact that a random segmentation "stands out" from the rest of the markings in the sense that it is given the lowest value α_k (on average) indicates a minimum level of soundness of the proposed method. It is, however, hard to assess the performance of the method. One way would be to study how an initially agreeable marking becomes less agreeable if it is transformed in different ways. This is subject to future work.

5 Conclusions

We have shown that the classical measure of agreement (Eq. 1) is of no use if the variance amongst the domain expert is high. We have also proposed a method for assessing agreements amongst domain experts and show how this method can be used to assess the performance of segmentation methods.

Bibliography

[1] G. Borgefors. Distance transformations in digital images. *Comput. Vision, Graphics, Image Processing*, 34:344–371, 1986.

[2] A. D. Brink and N. E. Pendock. Minimum Cross-Entropy Threshold Selection. *Pattern Recognition*, 29(1):179–188, 1996.

[3] P. A. Bromiley, P. Courtney, and N. A. Thacker. A case study in the use of ROC curves for algorithm design. *The British Machine Vision Conference (BMVC)*, 2001.

[4] X. Gual-Arnau, M.V. Ibáñez-Gual, F. Lliso, and S. Roldán. Organ contouring for prostate cancer: Interobserver and internal organ motion variability. *Computerized Medical Imaging and Graphics*, 29:639647, 2005.

[5] C. H. Li and C. K. Lee. Minimum Cross-Entropy Thresholding. *Pattern Recognition*, 26(4):617–625, 1993.

[6] M. Masek. *Hierarchical Segmentation Of Mammograms Based On Pixel Intensity*. PhD thesis, Centre for Intelligent Processing Systems, School of Electrical, Electronic, and Computer Engineering, The University of Western Australia, February 2004.

[7] A. Mukhdoomi. On the problem of segementing fibro-glandular tissue in mammograms. Master's thesis, UMNAD 619/06 Umeå University, Department of Computing Science, 2006.

[8] C. Olsén. Automatic breast border extraction. In J. M. Fitzpatrick and J. M. Reinhardt, editors, *Image Processing*, volume 5747, 2005. To appear in proceedings of the International Society for Optical Engineering (SPIE) Medical Imaging 2005.

[9] C. Olsén and F. Georgsson. Problems related to automatic nipple extraction. In *Scandinavian Conference on Image Analysis (SCIA) 2005*, Lecture Notes in Computer Science, pages 470–480. Springer Verlag, 2005.

[10] O. Olsén. *Automatic Assessment of Mammogram Adequacy*. Licentitate Thesis, Umeå University, Department of Computing Science, 2005.

[11] P. Smyth. Bounds on the mean classification error rate of multiple experts. *Pattern Recognition Letters*, 17:1253–1257, 1996.

[12] S. K. Warfield, K. H. Zou, and W. M. Wells. Validation of image segmentation and expert quality with an expectation-maximization algorithm. In *Fifth International Conference on Medical Image Computing and Computer-Assisted Intervention*, pages 298–306. Springer Verlag, Heidelbarg, Germany, 2002.

[13] K. H. Zou, W. M. Wells, R. Kikinis, and S. K. Warfield. Three validation metrics for automated probablistic image segmentation of brain tumours. *Statistics in Medicine*, 23:1259–1282, 2004.

Volumetric Breast Density Estimation on Mammograms Using Breast Tissue Equivalent Phantoms – An Update

Bindu J. Augustine[1], Gordon E. Mawdsley[1], Norman F. Boyd[2], and Martin J. Yaffe[1]

[1] Imaging Research, Sunnybrook Health Sciences Centre and Department of Medical Biophysics, University of Toronto
Room S657, 2075 Bayview Avenue, Toronto, ON, Can M4N 3M5
martin.yaffe@swri.ca
[2] Division of Epidemiology and Statistics, Ontario Cancer Institute,
610 University Avenue, Toronto, Ontario M4G 1K9, Canada
boyd@uhnres.utoronto.ca

Abstract. Methods for improving the accuracy of a technique for estimating volumetric breast density are described. A breast tissue-equivalent phantom encompassing a range of thicknesses and compositions of tissue is used to evaluate the sources of error in the technique. The image acquisition parameters that can affect the accuracy of calibration are considered, and sensitivity to these factors is evaluated. The robustness of the technique was tested by obtaining calibration images on 24 mammography machines, at 18 different sites, over a period of 3 years. The ability to use a single calibration on all machines of a given model type was assessed by comparing effective linear attenuation coefficients of fat and fibroglandular tissues, derived from the calibration phantom images obtained from various machines.

1 Introduction

Mammographic density has been proven to be strongly associated with breast cancer risk. Various quantitative methods for measuring breast density have been developed, based on the assessment of the fractional area of the breast occupied by fibroglandular tissue [1], [2]. These methods are subjective and results may vary, depending on the imaging conditions (tube potential, tube current and anode/filter materials) as well as the type film used. Furthermore, the effect of breast thickness may confound the determination of tissue composition. A more accurate and relevant measure of the amount of dense breast tissue is likely to be achieved using volumetric quantification of breast density. Highnam and Brady [3] approached this problem by estimating the primary energy at the receptor by mathematically removing the scattered radiation and glare. Their method is limited by the accuracy of the reported attenuation coefficients from the literature, variability of the film response to exposure and the uncertainty in breast thickness estimation [4].

Our volumetric technique involves the direct calibration of mammography units using a plastic step phantom composed of breast tissue equivalent materials [5].

Susan M. Astley et al. (Eds.): IWDM 2006, LNCS 4046, pp. 18–25, 2006.

2 Method

Calibration was accomplished by imaging a plastic phantom composed of steps providing 8 different thickness and 5 different breast tissue-equivalent compositions ranging from 100% fat to 100% fibroglandular tissue. Calibration images were obtained for all possible kV and anode-filter combinations that are used clinically. An aluminum step wedge, placed at the distal corner of the image receptor was imaged at the same time as the calibration phantom, and also as part of every clinical mammogram.

The aluminum step wedge was placed to track any subsequent variations in optical density that might be caused by variations in the mAs, film-processing, film-emulsion, as well as by scattering, beam hardening and reciprocity law failure of the film-screen systems. X-ray field non-uniformities were corrected by obtaining images of a plastic annular spherical phantom. Optical sensitometry data were used to convert the image pixel intensities to log relative exposure (LRE) values, which is a representation of the transmitted x-ray intensity plus contributions from scatter and glare. A surface relating the percent density, total thickness, and LRE was then constructed from the plastic step phantom for each kV and anode-filter combination and each image receptor size of the mammography unit used clinically. A 'useful thickness range' was selected for each tissue type calibration curve taken from the step phantom. This is where the signal values fall on the 'straight line' part of the sensitometric curve. The very short dynamic range of the film-screen systems made the polyenergetic approximation of the calibration surface almost impossible and, therefore, a monoenergetic approximation was made in the useful thickness range for each exposure technique. A 'linearised' three-dimensional surface relating the log relative exposure, breast composition and thickness was then generated.

From the exposure parameters for the mammogram, the compressed breast thickness and the image signal value at each pixel location, the fraction of the path through the breast that is composed of fibroglandular tissue can be extrapolated from the calibration surface, obtained for the same kV and anode-filter combination on the same machine and image receptor size. The total breast volume and the volume of fibroglandular tissue in the entire breast can also be calculated to yield the volumetric breast density (VBD).

The robustness of the VBD technique was tested by obtaining calibration images at six-month intervals from 24 mammography machines at 18 different sites over a period of 3 years. Calibration images included a set of slab phantoms made of breast tissue equivalent material on which the VBD measurements were calculated. The processed films were digitized using a Lumisys 85 digital laser film scanner, at 12 bits and a pixel size of 260 μm. Optical sensitometry was performed using the same mammographic film and processing employed for clinical use from each site on the same day as calibration images were obtained. The resulting calibration curves were then compared to test the ability of the aluminum step wedge to capture all of the inherent variations. The various parameters that could affect the accuracy of VBD values were studied during this period of time, including a) design of the aluminum stepwedge, b) variations in exposure, c) variations in film processing and film-screen combinations, d) shift in the kVp and tube replacement, and e) beam hardening and scatter.

2.1   Design of a New Aluminum Step Wedge

The aluminum wedge described in our previous paper [5] consisted of 7 steps, each of dimension 6 x 13 mm x 1.5 mm thick. With this step wedge, occasionally no step provided a measurement lying in the straight-line portion of the sensitometric curve. Therefore, a new aluminum wedge with 8 steps, increasing from 1.5mm (~3 HVL) in 0.5 mm increments to a maximum of 5 mm to cover a broader range of transmission was designed. One important goal for designing this thinner stepwedge was to ensure that at least two steps provided optical densities within the "straight-line" portion of the film characteristic curve.

2.2   Variations in Exposure

The exposure (mAs and kVp) used for initial imaging of the calibration phantom is based on the factors that would be used by the automatic exposure control (AEC) for imaging a breast of a particular thickness and composition. For individual clinical images, where the mAs may differ, the calibration surface (for the appropriate kV and target/filter) is then shifted to match the actual mAs, using the image of the Al step wedge as a reference. Because the AEC selects the exposure values based on the compressed breast thickness and composition, a lower mAs value will be used to image the thinner steps of the plastic step phantom and a higher mAs will be used for properly exposing the thicker regions at a given kVp. To test whether a calibration image acquired at a given kVp and single mAs value is sufficient to correct for exposure variations, three calibration images with different mAs values for a given kVp were obtained. A shift in the transmitted energies from the medium exposure to the lower and higher exposure values was then calculated from a step of the aluminum wedge which gave LRE values in the "straight-line" portion of the sensitometric curve (Al_shift).

By doing a logarithmic subtraction of the transmitted energies, the shift required to correct for the exposure can be estimated by taking the logarithm of the ratio of mAs values used (Fig. 1).

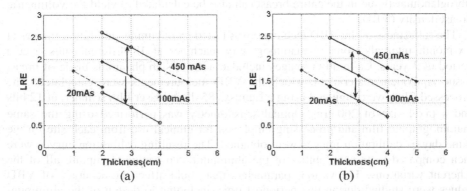

Fig. 1. (a) Calibration curve (Fibroglandular) obtained at 100 mAs is linearly shifted up or down to correct for exposure differences (20 mAs and 450 mAs) using Al_shift. b) Shift using the log of mAs ratio does not make calibration lines match.

For a simple change of exposure, with no change in kVp, the Scatter to Primary ratio is constant for the same thickness. When the thickness of the object is changed at the same time as the exposure is changed, beam hardening and scatter to Primary ratio will affect the simple exposure correction, since the x-ray beam is polyenergetic.

According to the reciprocity law, the response of the film to radiation exposure of a given spectral quality will remain unchanged if technique factors (mA, time, distance, grid) are adjusted so that mAs remains constant. Failure of this law was verified by taking three images of an aluminum stepwedge at 40 kVp, keeping mAs constant and varying the mA and time (Figure 2). The reciprocity law failure will result in a loss of optical density on the film for long exposure times and therefore a simple exposure correction will not be sufficient.

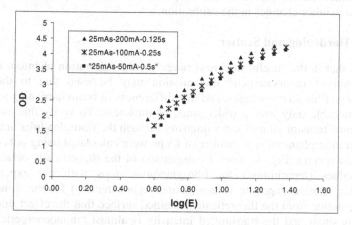

Fig. 2. The response of the film to exposure changes when mAs is kept constant, changing the mA and time (Reciprocity law failure)

2.3 Variations in Film Processing

Film sensitometry can vary on a day-to-day basis due to changes in emulsion, changes in the processing chemistry or replenishment, or changes in the developer temperature and time. By monitoring the daily sensitometric variations over a three-year time period, it was found that the film speed and contrast values could vary by more than ±0.15 OD units from the values obtained on the calibration day. We have developed a model to simulate the daily sensitometry curve from three parameters: D_{max} (the maximum signal value on the film), contrast (the density difference on the straight line portion of the sensitometric curve), and speed (OD at the mid-point of the sensitometric curve), that are all measured in the daily QC program at each clinical site. Using these parameters, the sensitometric curve on the day on which any mammogram is taken can be reproduced.

If there is a major variation in the speed or contrast due to the changes in the film screen system, or due to other processor related problems, the sensitometric curve for that specific day can be produced using Eqn 1,

$$D = ((\frac{\tanh(\alpha * (LRE - \beta))}{\pi}) + 0.5) * D_{max} \tag{1}$$

where D is the predicted optical density, α is related to the contrast, β is the LRE corresponding to the speed point.

2.4 kV Shift and Tube Replacement

For some mammography units, a slight shift in kV was noted after the acquisition of the initial set of calibration images. At two other sites, x-ray tube replacements took place after the acquisition of the initial set of calibration images. The calibration images obtained before and after the kVp shift and tube replacement were then compared to monitor changes in the calibration.

2.5 Beam Hardening and Scatter

We assume that in the "useful thickness range" of the calibration phantom image, an approximation of monoenergetic transmission may be used due to the limited dynamic range film-screen images, and that differences in beam hardening and scatter become noticeable only over a wider range of thickness. To verify this assumption, the logarithmic transmission of x-ray intensity through the fibroglandular and fat steps of the calibration phantom at a number of kVps were calculated using poly-energetic Molybdenum spectra. Fig. 3 shows a comparison of the theoretically obtained x-ray intensity values (logarithmic) for fibroglandular steps with the experimentally measured log relative exposure values (screen light intensity) for the same steps at 25kVp. We notice from the theoretically-obtained surface that the effect due to beam hardening is small and the transmitted intensity is almost "monoenergetic". This is because the absorber itself acts as a filter and absorbs most of the low energy photons from the already filtered incoming spectra. To further study the robustness of our volumetric technique, effective "attenuation" coefficients calculated from the slope values (at the "useful thickness range") of the experimentally measured fat and fibroglandular calibration curves were compared on several mammography units.

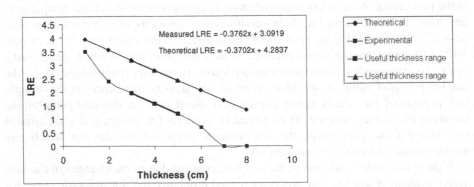

Fig. 3. A comparison of the theoretical and experimental log relative intensity values for fibroglandular tissue. Note that the slopes on both curves match for the "useful thickness range".

3 Results and Discussions

Calibration images acquired for 3 different exposure values (low, medium and high) for each kVp verified that mAs variations can be properly corrected with the aluminum stepwedge, provided that a step yielding an optical density in the linear region of the characteristic curve was used to shift the calibration surface. The calibration images taken at different times over a three-year period were tested against a set of 'baseline' calibration images to verify that the aluminum stepwedge data adequately corrects for the combined variations in optical density caused by exposure differences, film processing, film emulsion, changes in the film-screen combinations, mAs, reciprocity law failure, scatter and glare etc.

Table 1. Error in VBD estimate when there is a change in the film characteristic curve due to variations in the film processing/emulsion or film screen combination. The results also show that a simple correction using mAs ratio only is inadequate.

Error in VBD	Speed+0.1 Cnt+0.1	Speed+0.2 Cnt+0.2	Speed+0.4 Cnt+0.4	Speed+0.6 Cnt+0.6
Al_shift	<3%	<3%	~4%	~5%
mAs ratio	5%	9%	20%	30%

The Aluminum shift method is found to correct for the widest expected variations in film processing (±0.2 OD). Our experimental results indicate that if there is a larger change in the film characteristic curve, *e.g.* due to a change in the film processing or film-screen combination, a new film response curve should be modelled using Eqn. 1.

The calibration images obtained before and after a shift in kV and a tube replacement were tested and only very slight variations in the calibration surface were observed due to these changes. The results are summarized in Table 2.

Table 2. Accuracy of VBD calculations made on the breast tissue equivalent phantoms before and after the replacement of an x-ray tube and kV shift (~0.5 kV) is shown. The tube replacement did not cause any change in the x-ray spectra.

Error in VBD	30 % tissue	50% tissue	70% tissue
Before the kV shift and Tube replacement	<2%	<2%	<2%
After the Tube replacement	<2%	<2%	<2%
After the kV shift	<3%	<3%	<3%

A monoenergetic approximation is found to be appropriate for the limited dynamic range of an individual film-screen image. The slope of the each calibration surface obtained for different target/filter/kV combinations is analogous to a measurement of the effective linear attenuation coefficients of the breast tissues. These were compared for the values obtained from machines of a common model type and also to the theoretically obtained attenuation coefficients using the polyenergetic Mo spectra at a given kVp. They were found to match closely. The results are summarized in Table 3. A good match was also found between the calculated attenuation coefficients of fat and fibroglandular tissues and reported values in the literature measured at the K-edge energy of molybdenum [6].

Table 3. μ values calculated using the calibration data from 3 types of machines at various sites. The measured μ values closely match values calculated from the theoretical model.

Machine	Units	100% Fibroglandular		100% Fatty	
		Mean(μ)	Stdev	Mean(μ)	Stdev
Lorad MIV	7	0.88	0.03	0.58	0.03
GE 800T	4	0.86	0.03	0.56	0.02
Siemens	4	0.87	0.01	0.58	0.01
Theoretical		0.87		0.56	

4 Conclusions

We have studied the dependence of volumetric breast density measurements made from digitized mammograms on various parameters including exposure, film processing, changes in the film-screen combinations, tube replacements and kVp shifts. Methods for improving the accuracy of the technique were discussed. We found that exposure variations and other system changes can be tracked by measuring a step on the image of the Al wedge which falls in the straight-line portion of the sensitometric curve. The wedge was also found to be very useful in successfully capturing film reciprocity law failure. The effective linear attenuation coefficients derived from the calibration phantom and the theoretical measurements matched very well on a number of units suggesting that a single calibration per machine may be sufficient in future.

To further improve the accuracy of the technique, attempts to remove the effects of scatter and glare will be made by comparing the experimentally-obtained and theoretically-modelled log intensity values from the calibration phantom. In addition, reciprocity law failure will be characterized more thoroughly.

References

1. Wolfe, J.N.: Risk for Breast Cancer Development Determined by Mammographic Parenchymal Pattern. Cancer. Vol. 37 (1976) 2486-2492
2. Boyd, N.F., Byng, J.W., Yaffe, M.J.: Quantitative Classification of Mammographic Densities and Breast Cancer Risk: Results From the Canadian National Breast Screening Study. Journal of the National Cancer Institute. Vol. 87 (1995) 670-675
3. Highnam, R., Brady, M., Shepstone, B.: A Representation for Mammographic Image Processing. Medical Image Analysis. Vol. 1 (1996) 1-18
4. Blot, L. Zwiggelaar, R.: A volumetric approach to glandularity estimation in mammography: a feasibility study. Physics in Medicine and Biology. Vol. 50 (2005) 695-708

5. Pawluczyk, O., Augustine, B.J., Yaffe, M.J., Mawdsley G.E.: A volumetric method for estimation of breast density on digitized screen-film mammograms. Medical Physics. Vol. 30 (2003) 352-364
6. Johns, P.C., Yaffe, M.J.: X-ray Characterisation of normal and neoplastic breast tissues. Physics in Medicine and Biology. Vol. 32 (1987) 675-695

An Alternative Approach to Measuring Volumetric Mammographic Breast Density

Christopher Tromans and Michael Brady

Wolfson Medical Vision Laboratory, Department of Engineering Science,
University of Oxford, Parks Road, Oxford, UK, OX1 3PJ
cet@robots.ox.ac.uk

Abstract. The effect on the measurement of volumetric breast density of variations in physical and chemical properties of adipose and fibroglandular tissue reported in a number of studies is investigated using the authors' model of mammographic image formation. This model is developed specifically for the measurement of breast density. The effect of varying stromal composition, a popular histopathological explanation of mammographic density, is also discussed. Given the uncertainties in tissue attenuation highlighted by this study, as well as noise, and acquisition model error, the validity of this measurement is discussed, together with alternative measurement scales. Several issues are considered, including the effect of beam quality on normalisation accuracy, and the measurement failure which can occur when clinical data falls outside the limited range defined by 100% adipose to 100% fibroglandular tissue.

1 Introduction

The correlation between radiological features of the breast and the likelihood of the breast containing, or subsequently developing, a malignant lesion, is termed breast density. Work in this area was pioneered by Wolfe in 1969 [1] who proposed a four category classification for assessing mammographic parenchymal patterns: in particular this considered the prominence of ductal patterns and the occurrence of connective tissue hyperplasia. Wolfe presented findings showing that each of the four groups, from lowest to highest density, had an incidence of developing breast cancer of 0.1, 0.4, 1.7 and 2.2 [2]. Boyd et al [3] defined a six category classification (SCC) system which focuses on mammographic hyperplasia. Both these measures suffer from reader subjectivity, which caused Byng et al [4] to develop a interactive thresholding technique to segment, and thereby quantify, mammographic hyperplasia. Such measures are termed "area measurements" since they ignore the third dimension, and treat the projected image as entirely representative.

To take account of the three-dimensional breast, "volumetric measurements" of breast density have been developed. Such measures approximate the quantities of fibroglandular and adipose tissue present in the cone between a detector pixel, and the x-ray focal spot, using the likely x-ray attenuation coefficients of these tissues.

In 1996 Highnam and Brady proposed [5] the h_{int} representation which measures volumetric density. They developed a model of image formation considering the path of x-ray photons from point of emission in the x-ray tube, to absorption at the detector.

Susan M. Astley et al. (Eds.): IWDM 2006, LNCS 4046, pp. 26–33, 2006.

Several alternative techniques of measurement have been subsequently proposed, for example Kaufhold et al [6], which approximates a transfer function describing imaging formation gleaned from tissue equivalent phantom images.

Inspired by Highnam and Brady's work [7], a second generation of their model has been developed [8]. The extra power made available by modern computers has enabled the removal of many of their simplifying assumptions. Features of the enhanced model include: a ray tracing architecture, removing the parallel beam approximation; consideration of self-filtration within the tube target to model spatial inhomogenity of the x-ray beam; a theoretical scatter model removing the need for interpolation from empirical data; and an enhanced detector calibration procedure. Our findings are presented here, using our enhanced model, concerning the significant impact on density readings of the likely variation in x-ray attenuation of fibroglandular and adipose tissues within the population, and also consider the impact of the various sources of error present within the model.

2 The Histopathology of Mammographic Density

The most common form of breast cancer is a carcinoma, a tumour arising from epithelial malignancies. It has therefore been suggested that epithelial hyperplasia results in high mammographic density. In this case, a large number of cells exist, increasing the likelihood of mutation, and hence risk. Several studies however, including that of Alowami et al [9], have found no correlation between density of ductal units and areas of high mammographic density. Alowami et al did however report that such areas showed significantly higher collagen density and extent of fibrosis within the stroma. The stroma is a major tissue fraction, orders of magnitude larger than that of the epithelium, and so its composition is likely to have a discernable effect on the x-ray attenuation of the breast. The key question concerns the link, should it exist, between cancer development and stromal composition.

3 The Difficulty of Measuring Tissue Composition

The ratio of fibroglandular to adipose tissue may be approximately measured using a model of image formation by varying the tissue ratio in the modelled breast at each pixel until such a value is reached that the simulated pixel intensity matches that in the acquired image. Errors in the model, both systematic and random, will inevitably result in the incorrect ratio of tissues being calculated. Consideration in this paper is given to two such sources of uncertainty. The first is that which arises from inconsistencies between the various components of the image formation model, and their counterparts in reality. A certain level of uncertainty is expected due to effects such as stochastic noise and engineering tolerances in the manufacture of components. Whilst every effort may be made to limit the resulting errors, perfection will never be achieved, and a compromise has to be struck at a acceptable level of uncertainty. Inaccuracies within the model of image formation are dependant on a number of factors, such as beam quality; thickness of the item under investigation; exposure time; and the portion of the image receptor transfer characteristics in which the image is recorded. The second source of uncertainty considered is that which arises from errors in the attenuation coefficients of adipose and fibroglandular tissue occurring due to natural variation within the population.

3.1 Errors in the Model of Image Acquisition

Experimental validation is performed through the comparison of simulated images with those acquired using a GE Senographe 2000D in current clinical use. The model is configured to match the design of the 2000D, and the x-ray tube and image receptor are calibrated to match the specific machine according to the procedure described in [8]. Tissue equivalent resins, manufactured by CIRS (which are designed using the compositions reported by Hammerstein et al [10]), are used for the phantom material in order that the results are as close as possible to those likely in human tissue. In order that both the attenuation and scattering properties are investigated, a series of images were acquired employing the beam stop method: a method which provides a measure of the primary beam, together with an indirect measurement of scattering characteristics. A series of lead apertures of varying diameters are placed on top of the phantom, which itself sits on the breast table. The sides of the phantom are shielded using lead to prevent any radiation reaching the image receptor which has not passed through the aperture. The diameter of the aperture governs the volume of scattering material contributing to the energy incident upon the small group of detector pixels at the centre of the aperture shadow. The scattering characteristics of the material dictate the magnitude of the energy contributed by each infinitesimally small scattering point, and thus measuring the pixel intensities at the centre of the shadow provides an indirect measure of the characteristics, together with the attenuation between the scatter origination point and the image receptor. The median pixel intensity for a circle of pixels covering an area of approximately 1mm is used as the aforementioned measurement in order to provide a degree of robustness to noise. The primary component is measured through the use of a magnification tower which holds the phantom, with the smallest diameter aperture upon it, as close to the tube window as possible (around 450mm above the breast table on the 2000D). The pixel intensity is measured in an identical fashion, through averaging across a 1mm diameter circular area in the centre of the aperture shadow. Due to the magnifying effect of the large distance between the scatter originator and the image receptor only photons scattered over a very limited range of angles will be present, and so the measurement will consist almost solely of the primary component. Table 1 summarises the experimental results for 60mm adipose and fibroglandular phantoms, exposed at 29kVp, Mo-Mo, 100mAs. The '%Uncertainty' values are the relative magnitude, expressed as a percentage of the energy experimentally measured, of twice the standard deviation of the pixel intensities within the 1mm circular area at the centre of the aperture shadow (that from which measurements are taken). The '%Error' is that between the experimental and simulated values. A graph visualising the simulated and measured values for both tissue equivalent phantoms is included as Figure 1.

Inspection of Figure 1 and Table 1 suggests a good agreement between the simulated and measured imparted energies. The variation in relative error with aperture diameter is approximately constant, and the error is of a similar magnitude to that

Table 1. The results of the experimental model validation

		Primary	2	5	10	15
Adipose	%Uncertainty	2.55	2.90	2.71	2.30	2.21
	%Error	12.34	10.99	11.16	11.37	11.63
		20	25	30	35	40
	%Uncertainty	2.27	2.28	2.69	2.00	2.19
	%Error	12.13	12.09	12.57	12.90	13.42
Fibroglandular		Primary	2	5	10	15
	%Uncertainty	5.41	6.20	4.72	4.65	4.90
	%Error	9.40	9.49	8.68	8.28	7.46
		20	25	30	35	40
	%Uncertainty	3.66	4.19	4.13	4.13	4.00
	%Error	7.32	7.26	7.24	7.96	8.67

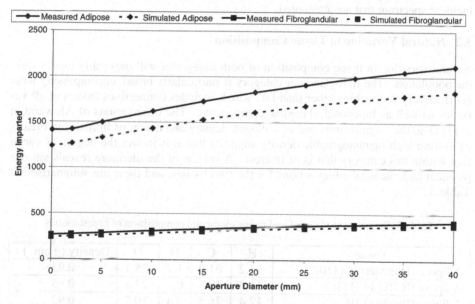

Fig. 1. The relationship between aperture diameter and energy imparted to the image receptor

seen in the primary component alone; which suggests the scatter model is performing well. The error in the primary component is likely to be due to errors in the modelled attenuation of the incident beam by the phantom, although inaccuracies within the calibration of the image receptor transfer characteristics may also contribute. The attenuation characteristics of the phantom materials are dependant on x-ray photon energy, and although the total energy of the incident beam is calibrated, the energy spectrum is calculated by modelling [8]. Error from this source may be quantified through the use of normalised attenuation curves. The primary component of the x-ray beam traversing PMMA phantoms varying in thickness between 30mm and 45mm in steps of 5mm were measured and simulated under identical exposure conditions. The attenuation ratio of each thickness relative to the 30mm thickness were calculated, and the results are presented in Table 2.

Table 2. Normalised errors in primary beam attenuation in PMMA exposed at 28kVp, Mo-Mo

Thickness (mm)	Measured Ratio	Simulated Ratio	%Error
30	1.0	1.0	0
35	0.679	0.667	1.27
40	0.465	0.450	1.58
45	0.319	0.307	1.19

The magnitude of the error in energy imparted to the image receptor due to errors in attenuation characteristics such as those apparent in Table 2 depends upon the exposure, since they are discrepancies in the proportion of the x-ray photons within the incident spectrum that are attenuated.

3.2 Natural Variation in Tissue Composition

Natural variation in tissue composition of both categories will inevitably exist within the population. The fibroglandular category is particularly broad, encompassing what is effectively "everything other than fat" which includes connectives tissues of all varieties as well as functional glandular components. The observations of Alowami et al [9] as to the "significantly higher collagen density and extent of fibrosis" in breasts exhibiting high mammographic density suggests that it is in fact the degree of variation within this category that is of interest. A review of the literature reveals various physical and chemical compositions for the two tissues, and these are summarised in Table 3.

Table 3. Summary of physical and major elemental composition of breast tissues

Tissue	H	C	N	O	Density (g cm^{-3})
Adipose (Hammerstein [10])	11.2	61.9	1.7	25.1	0.93
Adipose (ICRU 44 [11])	11.4	59.8	0.7	27.8	0.95
Adipose (Poletti [12])	12.4	76.5	0.4	10.7	0.92
Fibroglandular (Hammerstein [10])	10.2	18.4	3.2	67.7	1.04
Fibroglandular (ICRU 44 [11])	10.6	33.2	3.0	52.7	1.02
Fibroglandular (Poletti [12])	9.3	18.4	4.4	67.9	1.04

Inspection of Table 3 suggests significant variation in the results of the various studies. The ICRU44 study takes results from the work of Woodard [13], who noted widely varying compositions, for example lipid proportions in adipose tissue varying between 61.4% and 87.3%. The purity of the samples of each type must also be considered. Poletti et al [12] pack their samples into a "cylindrical container with 8mm diameter", however adipocytes have a diameter of up to 100µm, and histological sections can be approximately 5µm in thickness. Orders of difference in magnitude in sample sizes therefore exist between histological work like that of Alowami et al, and physical property measurement.

To investigate the effect of the variation seen in Table 3, Table 4 and Figure 2 show the variation in energy imparted, calculated using the model of image formation configured and calibrated to match the GE Senographe 2000D, with tube voltage (and hence beam quality) for the varying definitions of tissue composition. The simulation was configured to mimic the experimental technique to measure the primary beam using a small aperture and magnification tower described previously. The phantom used was a 60mm thickness of homogenous material and the exposure conditions were Mo-Mo, 100mAs.

Table 4. The relative difference in simulated energy imparted for Poletti and ICRU44 tissue compositions compared to that of Hammerstein

Tube Voltage (kVp)	Poletti		ICRU 44	
	Adipose	Fibroglandular	Adipose	Fibroglandular
25	74.62%	12.94%	-19.89%	60.00%
28	68.46%	12.62%	-18.85%	55.34%
32	59.19%	9.94%	-16.90%	42.59%

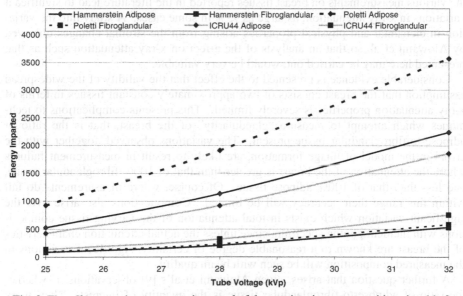

Fig. 2. The effect on primary energy imparted of the varying tissue compositions in table 2

Inspection of Table 4 and Figure 2 reveals significant differences in the x-ray characteristics of what are various measurements of tissue compositions which are generally assumed constant in work in breast density. For example, the discrepancy between Poletti et al's measurements and those of Hammerstein in both Oxygen (10.7% to 25.1%) and Carbon (76.5% to 61.9%) in adipose tissue produces a difference in imparted energy of between 59.2% and 74.6% depending upon beam quality. Likewise, in the fibroglandular case the discrepancy between the ICRU measurements and those of Hammerstein in both Oxygen (66.7% to 52.7%) and Carbon (18.4% to 33.2%) result in a difference in energy imparted of between 60.0% and 42.6%, again depending on beam quality.

4 Discussion

The results in Figure 1 show a good agreement between the experimental readings ascertained on the GE Senographe 2000D and the simulated values using the CIRS tissue equivalent phantoms. Given the results presented here, and further studies not presented due to limitations of space [8], an upper bound of 15% may be placed on the magnitude of the error within the model. The error in many cases is likely to be smaller than this, depending on a number of factors, such as beam quality; thickness of the item under investigation; exposure time; and the portion of the image receptor transfer characteristics in which the image is recorded. Errors in the tube spectrum have been found to be significant through comparison of simulated and measured attenuation curves.

The variations in the elemental compositions and specific gravity found amongst the various measurements on breast tissues reported in the literature lead to significant variations in x-ray attenuation; as large as 75% in some cases. A study into the variation in elemental and physical properties arising from the stromal changes observed by Alowami et al, so that an analysis of the effect on x-ray attenuation such as that presented here may be carried out, would be very valuable.

Considerable evidence is presented to the effect that the validity of the widespread assumption that the breast consists of two approximately constant tissues in terms of x-ray attenuation properties is severely limited. This presents complications to techniques which attempt to measure "glandularity" of the breast, that is the ratio of adipose-to-fibroglandular tissue present. The variations observed, together with the errors in the model of image formation, are likely to result in measurement failures where the attenuation of the breast is greater than that of 100% fibroglandular tissue, and less than that of 100% adipose tissue. Of course, where measurements do fall within this range their accuracy will be limited. Complications also arise over the significant variation which exists in total attenuation of the varying tissue compositions with incident photon spectrum, since unless the actual attenuation characteristics of the breast are known to a reasonable degree of certainty, significant variations in the measured composition will be seen with beam quality.

A further question that arises, given Alowami et al's [9] observations, is whether the ratio of adipose-to-fibroglandular tissue is the quantity of interest. Their work suggests a technique for measuring the variation in fibroglandular (stromal) composition is the more useful. Quantifying such an effect from a single image is limited to measuring the attenuation per unit traversal distance of the breast at each pixel. Since a polyenergetic spectrum is used the complication here comes from the attenuation varying with energy, but no feasible technique existing for separating individual energies. A possible solution is to measure the attenuation relative to that of some known material. However said material is required to mimic as closely as possible the attenuation characteristics of the breast across all photon energies present in the mammographic spectra in clinical use. The limitation of the use of a single image is that breasts exhibiting high attenuation may be possessing either a higher proportion of fibroglandular tissue than that of adipose, or a higher density of collagen within the connective stroma giving rise to a higher attenuating form of fibroglandular tissue. The results in Table 4 suggest it may be feasible to distinguish between these cases if two images are acquired at different beam qualities since a variation in attenuating characteristics with both tissue type and composition is observed under these conditions.

A number of issues in this paper have been raised which require multi-disciplinary study in order to resolve. The importance of constantly considering the underlying biological and physical phenomena, and the accuracy in which they can be measured using mammography is clearly apparent.

References

[1] J. N. Wolfe, "The prominent duct pattern as an indicator of cancer risk," *Oncology*, vol. 23, pp. 149-58, 1969.

[2] J. N. Wolfe, "Risk for breast cancer development determined by mammographic parenchymal pattern," *Cancer*, vol. 37, pp. 2486-92, 1976.

[3] N. F. Boyd, B. O'Sullivan, J. E. Campbell, E. Fishell, I. Simor, G. Cooke, and T. Germanson, "Mammographic signs as risk factors for breast cancer," *Br J Cancer*, vol. 45, pp. 185-93, 1982.

[4] J. W. Byng, N. F. Boyd, E. Fishell, R. A. Jong, and M. J. Yaffe, "The quantitative analysis of mammographic densities," *Phys Med Biol*, vol. 39, pp. 1629-38, 1994.

[5] R. Highnam, M. Brady, and B. Shepstone, "A representation for mammographic image processing," *Med Image Anal*, vol. 1, pp. 1-18, 1996.

[6] J. Kaufhold, J. A. Thomas, J. W. Eberhard, C. E. Galbo, and D. E. Trotter, "A calibration approach to glandular tissue composition estimation in digital mammography," *Med Phys*, vol. 29, pp. 1867-80, 2002.

[7] R. Highnam and M. Brady, *Mammographic image analysis*. Dordrecht; London: Kluwer Academic, 1999.

[8] C. Tromans, "DPhil Thesis: Measuring Breast Density from X-Ray Mammograms," in *Engineering Science*: Oxford University, to be submitted.

[9] S. Alowami, S. Troup, S. Al-Haddad, I. Kirkpatrick, and P. H. Watson, "Mammographic density is related to stroma and stromal proteoglycan expression," *Breast Cancer Res*, vol. 5, pp. R129-35, 2003.

[10] G. R. Hammerstein, D. W. Miller, D. R. White, M. E. Masterson, H. Q. Woodard, and J. S. Laughlin, "Absorbed radiation dose in mammography," *Radiology*, vol. 130, pp. 485-91, 1979.

[11] "Tissue substitutes in radiation dosimetry and measurement. ICRU Report 44," International Commission on Radiation Units and Measurements 1989.

[12] M. E. Poletti, D. Goncalves, and I. Mazzaro, "X-ray scattering from human breast tissues and breast-equivalent materials," *Phys Med Biol*, vol. 47, pp. 47-63, 2002.

[13] H. Q. Woodard and D. R. White, "The composition of body tissues," *Br J Radiol*, vol. 59, pp. 1209-18, 1986.

Breast Density Dependent Computer Aided Detection

Styliani Petroudi and Michael Brady

Wolfson Medical Vision Laboratory, Oxford University,
Oxford, OX2 7DD, United Kingdom
{styliani, jmb}@robots.ox.ac.uk

Abstract. This paper describes initial steps towards the development of a Computer Aided Detection (CAD) system based on breast density pattern classes. We present evidence that the sensitivity and specificity of such a system will improve if it is developed for, and applied to, specific breast density classes.

1 Introduction

Mammographic CAD systems are increasingly used clinically to support radiologists in their evaluation of mammograms. Modifications to the UK National Breast Screening Programme, such as requirements for an additional mammogram view, extension of the age range of women invited to screening, combined with the demographic increase resulting from the baby boom generation entering the screening programme are resulting in a huge increase in film reading [2] at a time when it is increasingly difficult to recruit and train skilled mammogram readers. The additional workload necessitates the introduction of alternative strategies for film screening, such as computer-aided detection systems. Possible solutions to this problem include the use of CAD systems to detect and prompt for abnormalities in mammograms, the introduction of pre-screening [4] and the use of image enhancement methods to facilitate viewing, such as the Standard Mammogram Form [6] and texture classification [8].

Pre-screening involves automatic classification into either normal or suspicious categories, followed by viewing of the suspicious cases by the radiologist along with a small sample of the other images for case control [3]. Sensitivity and specificity are two of the figures of merit used to evaluate the performance of such systems. In pre-screening, the overall sensitivity of sorting normal and suspicious categories is limited by the sensitivity of the system. It may be possible, however, to pre-screen a more limited set of films, such as those that are predominantly fat with greater success [4]. This is one area in which breast pattern density classification is potentially useful.

The Breast Imaging Reporting and Data System (BIRADS) breast density categorization provides a means for such a classification. The American College of Radiologists suggests that breast composition should be reported in all patients using the BIRADS classification [1]. The classification categories are:

Susan M. Astley et al. (Eds.): IWDM 2006, LNCS 4046, pp. 34–38, 2006.

1. The breast is almost entirely fat.
2. There are scattered fibroglandular densities.
3. The breast tissue is heterogeneously dense. This may lower the sensitivity of mammography.
4. The breast tissue is extremely dense, which could obscure a lesion on mammography.

Breast pattern classification algorithms [9] may be used, for example, to select mammograms belonging to the first BIRADS category in order that they can be evaluated by pre-screening. Of course, this is the category of image that human film readers can also dismiss most easily. However, a majority of women in the screening programme belong to the age group 50-69 years of age, for whom a large proportion have predominantly fatty breasts. It follows that the benefits of pre-screening this group of mammograms, if only in terms of radiologist time, are potentially significant.

2   Method

We have investigated the performance of a mammographic image analysis system developed recently by [7] by evaluating the performance of the algorithm on different breast density classes. The aim is to evaluate how the specificity and sensitivity of CAD systems can be affected when these systems are used only for the assessment of mammograms that belong a specific BIRADS category.

The algorithm developed in [7] proposes a segmentation method for delineating regions of interest (ROIs) in mammograms. A topographic representation, called the iso-level contour map is used, in which a salient region forms a dense quasiconcentric pattern of contours. The topological and geometrical structure of the image is analysed using an inclusion tree that is a hierarchical representation of the enclosure relationships between contours. The "saliency" of a region is measured topologically as the minimum nesting depth (Figure 1). The algorithm was developed for prompting suspicious regions independent of the density class the mammogram belonged to.

The results of the algorithm, along with the minimum nesting depth for detection, were available for the suggested assessment. They were based on a set of 400 mammograms with masses varying in size and subtlety selected from various pathological categories in the digital database for screening mammography (DDSM) database [5]. Since the aim of [7] was mass detection and breast segmentation, unfortunately, no normal cases were included in the available evaluations.

The mammograms are first classified into one of the four BIRADS classes. The detected regions, according to minimum depth, are used to create ROC (True Positive Fraction versus False Positive Fraction) curves in order to evaluate the performance of the algorithm under different breast pattern density scenarios.

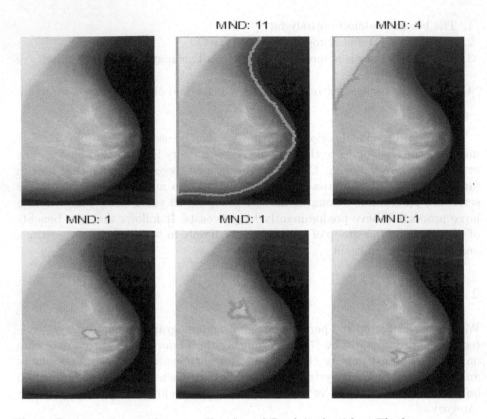

Fig. 1. Segmentation results using Hong's and Brady's algorithm. The base contours and their minimum nesting depth measure.

3   Results-Discussion

Figure 2 shows the ROC curve for the evaluation of the algorithm applied separately to each breast pattern class. The detection system clearly performs better if applied to breasts belonging either the first or second BIRADS classes. The results show that the detection algorithm (despite the fact that it was created without taking density into account) has better sensitivity and specificity and sensitivity.

The results suggest that taking breast density information into account for the development and application of CAD systems can significantly improve their performance. Despite the fact that the developed methods will not be applicable to all mammograms, they can still result in a reduction of the increasingly heavy demand on radiologists and radiographers that are currently being overwhelmed by the masses of mammograms that need evaluation. Breast density classification may provide an important stepping stone for the development of CAD systems with better sensitivity and specificity for at least a certain number of different breast pattern classes.

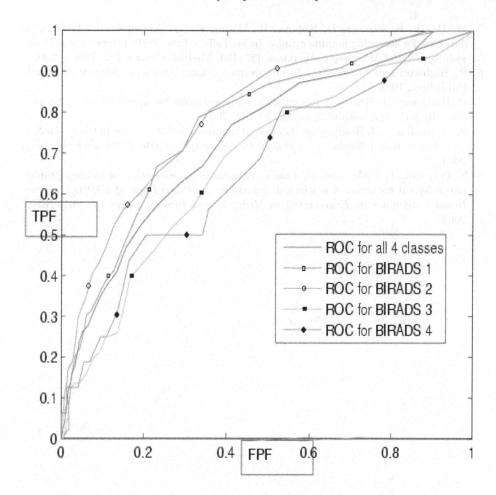

Fig. 2. The set of ROC curves of the detection system for each BI-RADS class separately along with the ROC curve of the system applied to mammograms in general, independently of breast pattern, for comparison

References

1. *Illustrated Breast Imaging Reporting and Data System (BI-RADS)*. American College of Radiology, third edition, 1998.
2. S. Astley. Computer-based detection and prompting of mammographic abnormalities. *British Journal of Radiology*, 77:194–200, 2004.
3. S. Astley and F. Gilbert. Computer-aided detection in mammography. *Clinical Radiology*, 59:390–399, 2004.
4. S. Astley, T. Mistry, C. Boggis, and V. Hiller. Should we use humans or a machine to pre-screen mammograms? In H.-O. Peitgen, editor, *Sixth International Workshop in Digital Mammography*, pages 476–480. Springer, 2002.

5. M. Heath, K. Bowyer, D. Kopans, R. Moore, and P. Kegelmeyer. The digital database for screening mammography. In M. Yaffe, editor, *Fifth International Workshop on Digital Mammography*, pages 457–460. Medical Physics Publishing, 2000.
6. R. Highnam and M. Brady. *Mammographic Image Analysis*. Kluwer Academic Publishers, 1999.
7. B. Hong and M. Brady. A topographic representation for mammogram segmentation. In *MICCAI*, volume 2, pages 730–737, 2003.
8. S. Petroudi and M. Brady. Classification of mammographic texture patterns. In *Seventh International Workshop on Digital Mammography*. Medical Physics Publishing, 2004.
9. S. Petroudi, T. Kadir, and M. Brady. Automatic classification of mammographic parenchymal patterns: A statistical approach. In *Proceedings of EMBC, International Conference on Engineering in Medicine and Biology*, pages 798–801. IEEE, 2003.

Evaluation of Effects of HRT on Breast Density

Styliani Petroudi[1], Kostantinos Marias[2], and Michael Brady[1]

[1] Wolfson Medical Vision Laboratory, Oxford University, Oxford,
OX2 7DD, United Kingdom
{styliani, jmb}@robots.ox.ac.uk
[2] Institute of Computer Science, Foundation for Research and Technology - Hellas

Abstract. Breast density segmentation and classification methods are combined to enable the automatic and quantitative comparison of temporal mammograms of women using Hormone Replacement Therapy (HRT). The results are based on registration and density quantification, so that potentially the clinician may be informed about substantial localised breast density changes. The measures use texture based density segmentation as well as a normalized representation of mammograms.

1   Introduction

Hormone Replacement Therapy (HRT) replaces the hormones a woman's body ceases to produce after the menopause. However, the use of HRT in post-menopausal women has created controversy, not least, because its effects are difficult to characterise and quantify. According to the Million Women Study in the UK [1], HRT use is associated with increased incidence and risk of breast cancer mortality, especially so for combined oestrogen-progesterone therapy. The risk increases with the duration of use and decreases after cessation. It seems that this may be due to *localised* increases in breast density, a known risk factor for breast cancer [2].

The response to HRT is specific to the individual. The changes due to HRT are neither necessarily homogeneous nor global, rather, they depend on the hormonal receptivity of the epithelial elements. Therefore, HRT use may result in density increases both locally, or in the breast pattern, globally. The changes can be characterised as:

- Tissue regeneration: increase in breast density over time.
- No change: no obvious change in breast density.
- Involution: decrease in breast density over time.

The type and degree of change depends on the receptivity of the hormones by the individual, and on the combination of hormones used. Localised tissue changes visible in a mammogram may signal the development of a new cancer, especially if breast cell proliferation occurs in high risk areas such as the Upper Outer Quadrant of the breast. For all of these reasons, there is broad consensus that women taking HRT should be monitored more carefully and more frequently

Susan M. Astley et al. (Eds.): IWDM 2006, LNCS 4046, pp. 39–45, 2006.
© Springer-Verlag Berlin Heidelberg 2006

for breast cancer. Density segmentation, mammogram registration and local tissue density quantification can be incorporated into a clinical framework to assess the general effects of exogenous factors such as HRT.

The Standard Mammogram Form (SMF) representation of interesting tissue introduced by Highnam and Brady [3] is a method to normalise mammograms by calculating anatomical information from the mammogram image. In the resulting SMF image, each pixel represents the thickness of 'interesting' (non-fat) tissue of the compressed breast above that pixel. This effectively provides objective quantitative information about the breast anatomy. Changes of fatty to glandular tissue are precisely changes in non-fatty *i.e.* 'interesting' tissue. This information, combined with the information obtained using the texture-based approaches, can potentially provide both local and global quantitative information about density changes.

This paper describes how texture-based breast parenchymal density classification [4] and SMF may be combined with breast registration to enable automatic and quantitative comparison of temporal mammograms of women using HRT.

2   Method

Initially, the method needs to evaluate whether tissue density has changed due to use of HRT. To this end, two measures, one based on a texture-based segmented representation, the other based on the SMF representation are computed. For the texture based representation each pixel in the mammogram is replaced by the texton (texture primitive element) in the texton dictionary which lies closest to it in the texture feature space [5]. The texton value is achieved following texture classification as presented in [6]. The texton dictionary is obtained by clustering mammogram filter responses with the MR8 filter bank [6] using the following procedure: all filtered responses are aggregated over all the randomly selected training images and the k-means algorithm [7] is used to compute n cluster centres. The training test included mammograms of women using HRT and women who were not using HRT. As usual, the cases of mammograms in this training set were excluded from the test set of mammograms for which the results are presented. The measure using breast density analysis, *mean texture based difference*,

$$\Delta T_\mu = T_\mu(current) - T_\mu(previous)$$

is based on evaluating the difference between the mean texton values T_μ representing the breast area in each of the temporal mammograms. The different density classes are assigned numbers/labels T_l from 1 to n, the total number of textons used to segment the mammograms,according to the energy of the texton they represent. The mean texture based density value is given by:

$$T_\mu = \frac{1}{N_b} \sum_{i=1}^{N_b} T_l(i) \tag{1}$$

where N_b is the total number of pixels in the breast area. The second measure, *difference sum of interesting tissue*,

$$\Delta S_{int} = (S_{int}(current) - S_{int}(previous))/(S_{int}(previous))$$

is based on the normalised difference in the sum of interesting tissue S_{int} [8] in the SMF representation of the corresponding temporal pairs of mammograms:

$$S_{int} = \sum_{i=1}^{N_b} h_{int}(p_i) \qquad (2)$$

where p_i corresponds to pixel i in the breast area. (Of course, the texture segmentation algorithm could also be directly applied to SMF images.) These difference measures can be used to evaluate a global increase or decrease in breast density due to use of HRT in order to recommend further investigation. The density changes are evaluated globally as either regeneration or involution, as shown in Table 1. Although "no change" in breast density is not as important as tissue regeneration, it is included in the same classification.

Table 1. Rules to assess global mammographic density changes due to HRT between temporal mammogram sequences

Difference Measures	Corresponding Change in Breast Density
$\Delta T_\mu > 0$ or $\Delta S_{int} > 0$	Tissue Regeneration or No Change
$\Delta T_\mu < 0$ and $\Delta S_{int} < 0$	Involution

To achieve this, a two-step registration algorithm using internal landmarks and Thin Plate Splines is applied to register the SMF images and the texture segmented mammograms [9]. The resulting difference images combine registration with normalisation, and can in turn show where the changes occur and how significant they are, providing the clinician with local change information. If there is an apparent increase in breast density, the issue will need to be investigated further and monitored closely.

3 Results and Discussion

The algorithm was evaluated on a pilot dataset of 15 pairs of temporal mammograms (with a three year time interval) of women taking HRT belonging to the Screen Database collected in Oxford [10]. The ground truth was defined by a radiologist who examined the original mammogram pairs and classified global and local density changes. Seven mammograms were judged to exhibit involution, six mammograms were judged to exhibit tissue regeneration, and two mammograms were judged to exhibit "no change". The global density change evaluation results are presented in Table 2. It must be noted that there was enough tissue regeneration to result in a global breast pattern class change in only two of the included regeneration pairs. Global density classification is followed by registration in order to evaluate local difference changes.

Table 2. Results on the agreement of the evaluation of global density changes with clinician's ground truth

Density change measure	ΔT_μ	ΔS_{int}	ΔT_μ and ΔS_{int}
Agreement in regeneration and no change pairs	88%	62%	88 %
Agreement in Involution pairs	71%	85%	85%

a. Target mammogram   b. Source mammogram   c. Registered mammogram

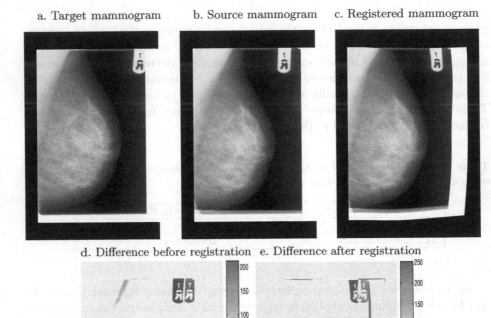

d. Difference before registration   e. Difference after registration

Fig. 1. A pair of right temporal mammograms of a woman on HRT exhibiting involution. Registration and differences on the original mammograms.

The example that follows corresponds to a woman who had been using HRT for a period of 4 years exhibiting tissue involution. Figures 1, 2 and 3 show the right temporal pair of mammograms of the woman exhibiting involution. As can be seen from the colour difference images after registration, the target image exhibits lower density (Figure 2 (e)) as well as lower height of non-fat tissue (Figure 3 (e)). This is especially obvious in the upper outer quadrant of the

a. Texture target image   b. Texture source image   c. Texture registered image

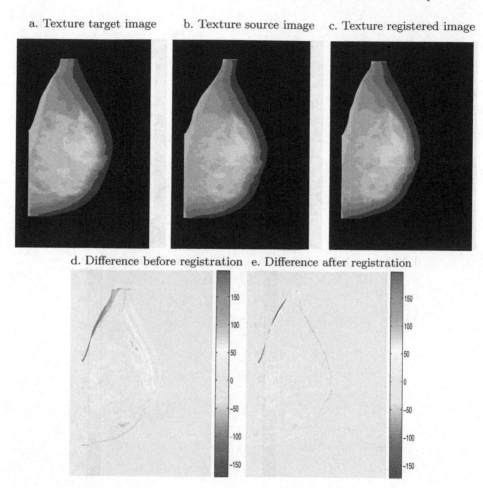

d. Difference before registration   e. Difference after registration

Fig. 2. The pair of right temporal texture segmented mammograms of the same woman on HRT exhibiting involution. Registration and differences on the texture segmented representation.

breast. The texture difference image shows where the involution takes place and how it is distributed throughout the breast region.

4   Conclusions

The method shows that there are ways to evaluate density changes quantitatively, and enables close monitoring of any changes. The performance was evaluated by assessing the agreement with the radiologist's assessment. The results suggest how the use of texture based segmentation and density based classification may have a role to play in the clinical framework of mammographic image analysis. They are also encouraging for developing computer tools that automatically monitor changes in mammographic density between successive scans.

a. SMF target image   b. SMF source image   c. SMF registered image

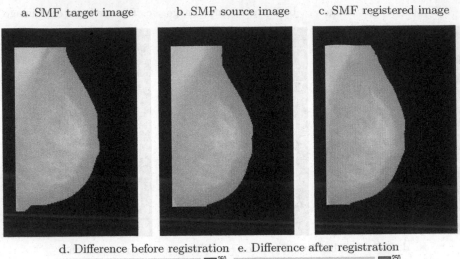

d. Difference before registration   e. Difference after registration

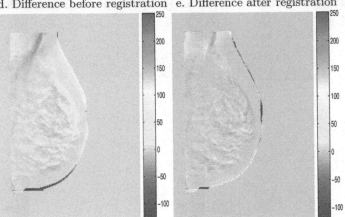

Fig. 3. The pair of right temporal SMF images of the same woman on HRT exhibiting involution. Registration and differences on the texture segmented representation.

References

1. Breast cancer and hormone replacement therapy in the million women study. *Lancet*, 362:419–427, 2003.
2. K. Marias, C.P. Behrenbruch, R.P. Highnam, J.M. Brady, S. Parbhoo, and A. Seifalian. Assessing the role of quantitative analysis of mammograms in describing breast density changes in women using hrt. In *International Workshop on Digital Mammography*, pages 547–551, 2002.
3. R. Highnam and M. Brady. *Mammographic Image Analysis*. Kluwer Academic Publishers, 1999.
4. S. Petroudi, T. Kadir, and M. Brady. Automatic classification of mammographic parenchymal patterns: A statistical approach. In *Proceedings of EMBC, International Conference on Engineering in Medicine and Biology*, pages 798–801. IEEE, 2003.

5. Styliani Petroudi. *Texture in Mammographic Image Analysis*. PhD thesis, University of Oxford, 2005.
6. M. Varma and A. Zisserman. Classifying images of materials: Achieving viewpoint and illumination independence. In *Proceedings of the European Conference on Computer Vision, Copenhagen, Denmark*, pages 255–271, 2002.
7. R. O. Duda and P.E. Hart. *Pattern Classificaton and Scene Analysis*. Wiley, 1973.
8. S. Petroudi, K. Marias, R. English, R. Adams, and M. Brady. Classification of mammogram patterns using area measurements and the standard mammogram form (SMF). In *Medical Imaging Understanding and Analysis*, pages 197–200, 2002.
9. S. Petroudi and M. Brady. Textons contours and regions for improved mammogram registration. In *Seventh International Workshop on Digital Mammography*. Medical Physics Publishing, 2004.
10. C.J.G. Evertsz, A. Bodicker, S. Bohnenkamp, D. Dechow, C. Beck, H.-O. Peitgen, L. Berger, U. Weber, H. Jurgens, C.L. Hendriks, N. Karssemeijer, and M. Brady. Soft-copy reading environment for screening mammography - screen. In M. Yaffe, editor, *Fifth International Workshop in Digital Mammogrphy*, pages 566–572, 2000.

Modeling the Effect of Computer-Aided Detection on the Sensitivity of Screening Mammography

Robert M. Nishikawa

Department of Radiology and Committee on Medical Physics, University of Chicago
5841 S Maryland Ave., MC-2026. Chicago, IL 60637, USA
r-nishikawa@uchicago.edu

Abstract. We have developed a Monte Carlo model to examine the cancer detection rate in screening mammography. We simulated the situation where screening was implemented for 9 years and then CADe was implemented for an additional 9 years. We investigated the effectiveness of two different methods for measuring changes in cancer detection rate. The first method was a sequential method in which the radiologist first reads without CADe and then immediately reads with CADe. The second method is temporal comparison where the cancer detection rates for two periods of time are compared: one without the use of CADe and one when CADe is in use. The model predictions have important implications for clinical studies of CADe. The temporal method is unlikely to measure a real affect, because the effect is small. A sequential method can measure an increase in the number of cancers detected because of CADe, but it cannot measure an overall increase in the cancer detection rate of the screening program.

1 Introduction

Computer-aided detection (CADe) has been proposed as a method for reducing the number of missed cancers. There have been six clinical studies of CADe published to date. The first by Freer and Ulisseys showed a 19.5% increase in the number of cancers detected with an increase in the recall rate from 6.5% to 7.7% when CADe was used [2]. Gur *et al.* reported that when CADe was used, the cancer detection rate increased from 3.49 to 3.55 with virtually no change in the recall rate [3]. Feig *et al.* performed a subanalysis of the Gur study and found that the low volume readers had a 19.7% increase in cancer detection rate, while the high volume readers had a 3.2% *decrease* [4]. Birdwell *et al.* measured a 7% increase in cancers detected due to CADe with 8% increase in recall rate [5]. Cupples *et al.* found a 16% increase in cancer detection rate with an 11% increase in recall rate [1]. Helvie *et al.* found a 10% increase in both number of cancers detected and recall rate, although it was a relatively small study [6]. Khoo *et al.* found a 1.7% increase in the number of cancers detected with a 6% increase in the recall rate [7]. This study was done in the context of double reading. None of the differences in any of the studies reach statistical significance.

On the surface, these studies seem to be contradictory, however, different methods were used to measure the effectiveness of CADe. The Freer, Helvie, Birdwell, and

Susan M. Astley et al. (Eds.): IWDM 2006, LNCS 4046, pp. 46–53, 2006.

Khoo studies used a sequential method. In this method, the radiologist first reads the mammograms without any computer assistance and he or she renders an interpretation. Immediately after, the radiologist reviews the computer analysis of the mammograms and renders another interpretation. By comparing the number of cancers detected in each of the two reading conditions, the impact of CADe was measured. The Gur and the Cupples studies used a temporal method based on historical comparisons. In this method, clinical data is collected retrospectively from two time periods. The first time period is from mammograms read without using CADe and the second time period is from mammograms read using CADe. A comparison of the cancer detection rates in the two time periods is a measure of the effectiveness of CADe.

The goal of the present study is to use a computer model of CADe in screening mammography to understand how these two methods can lead to different conclusions. We will show that the results of the clinical studies are not unexpected.

2 Method

An outline of the model is given in Figure 1. The model was implemented in Excel (Microsoft Corporation, Redmond, WA). Each decision outlined in the flowchart was implemented using a random number and comparing it to the probability of an event

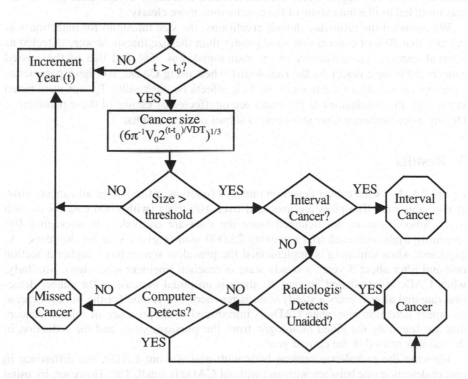

Fig. 1. Schematic of model. t_0 is the time the cancer starts to grow. This process is performed once for each cancer in the simulation.

occurring. Each cancer was followed from the time it was initiated until it was detected. It was also assumed that 125 cancers developed every year for 30 years at equal intervals between cancer initiations. In total, 100 runs consisting of 4000 cancer cases each were averaged. We assumed the tumor grew by doubling in volume at a given fixed rate. Although the first cancer started growing at year 0, screening did not start until year 11 and CADe was implemented starting in year 20.

In our model, cancers could be detected either in the interval between mammography screening (interval cancers), by the radiologist unaided, or by the radiologist using CADe to find a cancer that they initially overlooked. If the cancer grew undetected to larger than 5 cm in diameter, it was assumed to be detected as an interval cancer. Cancers could be missed by the radiologist unaided or by the radiologist using CADe. The cancer detection rate (number of cancers detected per 1000 women screened) was measured for without and with CADe being implemented.

We modeled the cancer as growing at a fixed rate using two different assumptions. The first is that all cancers had the same growth rate, with a volume doubling time of 157 days. The second is that the cancers had different growth rates. The growth rates were generated by randomly selecting from a normal distribution of mean of 147 days and a standard deviation of 90 days, except negative growth rates were not allowed. This resulted in the population having both fast growing and slow growing cancers (median value=157 days), which is more realistic clinically. A universal growth rate was modeled to illustrate some of the conclusions more clearly.

We assumed the following default conditions: the size threshold for detection was 0.5 cm, that 20% of cancers that were greater than the size threshold were detected as interval cancers, the sensitivity of the radiologist was 75% and that of the missed cancers 50% were detect by the radiologist when using CADe. All these parameters were systematically varied to examine their affects on our results. Except were noted in the text, the conclusions of this paper are unaffected by choice of these parameters. Due to space limitations, we show only a subset of these results.

3 Results

Figure 2A shows the cancer detection rate as a function of time when all cancers grow at the same rate. The plots are averaged over 100 trials (with 4000 cancers in each trial). Smooth curves are obtained since the data are equivalent to averaging 100 screening trials with each trial screening 25,000 women every year for 30 years. As expected, when screening is implemented the prevalent screen has a higher detection rate and after about 3 years a steady state is reached (incident screening). Similarly, when CADe is introduced, in year 20, there is an initial increase in the cancer detection rate and after 2 years a steady-state is reached. The reason for the initial increase in cancer detection rate when CADe is introduced is the presence of missed cancers that are found by the aided radiologist from the previous years and the reduction in the number missed in the current year.

Ignoring the prevalence screens both with and without CADe, the difference in cancer detection rate between with and without CADe is small, 4%. However, by using CADe the radiologist is able to detect 14 more cancers (17% increase) (lower curve in the Fig. 2A). Since these cancers are no longer available for detection in subsequent years, the unaided cancer detection rate actually decreases when CADe is used.

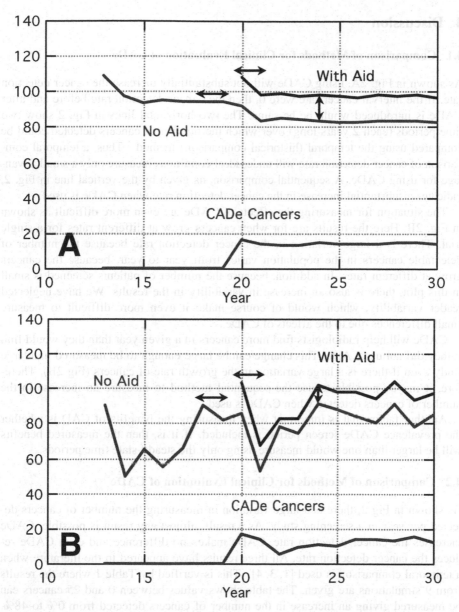

Fig. 2. The number of cancers detected per year in a screening population as a function of time. CADe is introduced in year 20. (A) All cancers grow with the same doubling time and the curves are averaged over 100 trials. (B) A single trial result is shown and the cancers have a distribution of doubling times. The lower curve in each plot, labeled CADe Cancers, is the number of cancers found because the radiologist used CADe. The horizontal lines with arrowheads indicate two time periods to compare the benefits of CADe for the historical comparison method and the vertical line indicates the difference in the radiologist's cancer detection with and without computer aid.

4 Discussion

4.1 Comparison of Methods for Clinical Evaluation of CADe

As shown in Fig. 2A, using CADe will not substantially increase the cancer detection rate. If the interval cancer rate were 0, then the cancer detection rate before and after CADe is introduced would be he same. The two horizontal lines in Fig. 2 show two time periods (each 2 years long) over which the number of cancers detected could be compared using the temporal (historical comparison) method. Thus, a temporal comparison of cancer detection rate will under ideal conditions measure only a small advantage for using CADe. A sequential comparison, as given by the vertical line in Fig. 2, indicates a substantial increase in the cancer detection rate when CADe is used.

The situation for measuring the effects of CADe are even more difficult as shown in Fig. 2B. Here the results are for when cancers grow at different rates for a single trial. There is a large variation in the cancer detection rate because the number of detectable cancers in the population varies from year to year, because the cancers grow at different rates. In addition, because the number of patients screened is small in this plot, there is also an increase in variability in the results. We have neglected reader variability, which would of course make it even more difficult to measure small differences due to the affects of CADe.

CADe will help radiologists find more cancers in a given year than they would find if they did not use CADe. This change can be large enough to be measured in a large study even if there is a large variation in the growth rate of cancers (Fig 2B). Therefore, it maybe possible to use the sequential method to measure an increase in the number of cancers detected when CADe is used.

Another factor that is important when measuring the benefits of CAD is whether the prevalence CADe screen period is included. If it is, then the measured benefits will be larger than one would measure using only the steady-state time periods.

4.2 Comparison of Methods for Clinical Evaluation of CADe

As shown in Fig 2, there is a large variation in measuring the number of cancers detected per year in a screening study. As a result, almost any result is possible: CADe increases the cancer detection rate, CADe makes no difference and even CADe reduces the cancer detection rate. All three results have appeared in the literature when a temporal comparison is used [1, 3, 4]. This is verified by Table 1 where the results from 9 simulations are given. The table shows values between 0 and 25 cancers can be measured giving an increase in the number of cancers detected from 0% to 48%. The average value in the table is 11.9, which is a 23% increase in cancers detected when using CADe.

In Table 1, two different time periods are reported. The values for a period of 1 year (i.e., a 1-yr period in which the number of cancers detected without CADe is measured and compared to a 1-yr period when CADe is used) are higher than the 2-year period. This is because the 1-year period only includes the CADe prevalence screen (the peak at year 20 in Fig. 2) and thus is higher than subsequent years. All clinical CADe studies include the CADe prevalence screen and therefore are optimistically biased. Even the Cupples study, which used a 2-year period to measure the cancer detection rate, is biased by the CADe prevalence screen. In that study, the average time between screens was 21 months with a median time of 14 months. Thus most of the women who were screened in the CADe time period were having their first mammogram where CADe was used.

All published studies using the sequential method measure at least a 10% increase in the number of cancers radiologists detected when using CADe. The exception is the Khoo. However, in their study double reading was used and the screening interval was three years. Our model does not include double reading and we only modeled annual screening. Thus we cannot make reliable predictions of the Khoo study.

Table 1. A comparison of the number of cancers detected per year with and without CADe as measured using a temporal comparison. The time period refers to the number of years measurements are made without and then with CADe. Ten different realizations are shown. It is assumed that 67 new cancers begin growing each year, but each cancer grows at a different rate. On average, 52 of those cancers are detected per year by mammography. This about the size of the Cupples [1] and Freer [2] studies.

Method	Time Period	Trial Number								
		1	2	3	4	5	6	7	8	9
Temporal	1 yr	16	15	9	20	2	25	10	8	18
Temporal	2 yrs	7.5	14	9.5	11	6.5	17	0	12	13

4.3 Assumptions and Limitations of This Study

We made a number of assumptions in our current model: the radiologist's sensitivity (75%), CADe sensitivity (75%), size threshold for detection (0.5 cm), and the interval cancer rate (15%), cancer volume doubling time (157 days). To study the effects of these parameters, we systematically varied them to span the full parameter space. An example is shown in Figure 3. The major conclusions of this study are unaffected of the exact choice of these parameters.

We also assumed that if the computer detected a cancer that the radiologist missed unaided, then the radiologist would always recognized that the computer detected a missed cancer. This not true clinically and we will incorporate this into future studies. In addition, we have not addressed the issue of computer false detections and radiologists' recall rate. This is the topic of an ongoing study.

There are also assumptions made because we have at present only a simple model. We do not use a Gompertzian model of tumor growth [8], we assume patients are screened at exactly 1 year intervals, technically all on the same day, and all women begin screening in the same year. How these assumptions affect the results and conclusions of our study are unknown. A sophisticated model is required to study these factors and we are currently developing such a model.

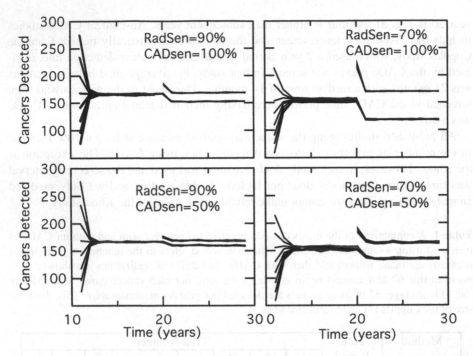

Fig. 3. An example of plots used to study the effects of changing the radiologist's sensitivity (RadSen), the computer's sensitivity (CADsen), and the threshold size for detection. In each plot there are 8 curves for thresholds of 0.5 cm (top curve) to 1.2 cm (lowest curve) in 0.1 cm increments. Except for the prevalence screens (years 11-13) all curves overlap indicating that the size threshold does not affect the number of cancers detected. Although the difference between the upper sets of curves and the lower sets of curves (years 20-29) change depending on the radiologists and CADe sensitivities, the differences between without CADe (years 11-19) and with CADe (years 20-29) remain the same. Therefore, the conclusions of our study are valid over a range of radiologist and CADe sensitivities and size thresholds.

4 Conclusions

In summary, our model can explain differences in reported clinical performances of CADe. It appears that to measure the effects of CADe the sequential method is more likely to be successful than the temporal comparison. There are, however, significant potential biases with this method that are difficult to control [3, 5]. Further, even though an individual radiologist will find more cancers when he or she uses CADe, the overall cancer detection rate will not be greatly increased.

The reported clinical studies are probably not measuring the best endpoint. The usefulness of CADe is not to increase the cancer detection rate, but to detect the cancers at an earlier time point in screening. Measuring the stage or size of cancers may be a more appropriate. We will model this in the future. Ultimately the affect on mortality is real endpoint, but this is not practical to measure in real life.

References

1. Cupples TE, Cunningham JE and Reynolds JC: Impact of computer-aided detection in a regional screening mammography program. American Journal of Roentgenology 185:944-950 (2005).
2. Freer TW and Ulissey MJ: Screening mammography with computer-aided detection: prospective study of 12,860 patients in a community breast center. Radiology 220:781-786 (2001).
3. Gur D, Sumkin JH, Rockette HE, Ganott M, Hakim C, et al.: Changes in breast cancer detection and mammography recall rates after the introduction of a computer-aided detection system. Journal of the National Cancer Institute 96:185-190 (2004).
4. Feig SA, Sickles EA, Evans WP and Linver MN: Re: Changes in breast cancer detection and mammography recall rates after the introduction of a computer-aided detection system. Journal of the National Cancer Institute 96:1260-1261 (2004).
5. Birdwell RL, Bandodkar P and Ikeda DM: Computer-aided detection with screening mammography in a university hospital setting. Radiology 236:451-457 (2005).
6. Helvie MA, Hadjiiski L, Makariou E, Chan HP, Petrick N, et al.: Sensitivity of noncommercial computer-aided detection system for mammographic breast cancer detection: pilot clinical trial. Radiology 231:208-214 (2004).
7. Khoo LA, Taylor P and Given-Wilson RM: Computer-aided detection in the United Kingdom National Breast Screening Programme: prospective study. Radiology 237:444-449 (2005).
8. Norton L: A Gompertzian model of human breast cancer growth. Cancer Res 48:7067-7071 (1988).

Use of Prompt Magnitude in Computer Aided Detection of Masses in Mammograms

Nico Karssemeijer

Radboud University Nijmegen Medical Centre
Department of Radiology
The Netherlands

Abstract. Systems for computer aided detection of masses may be used more effectively when they are used for interpretation of suspect abnormalities, instead of solely using them as a prompting aid to avoid oversights. To use CAD algorithms for detection of masses as a decision aid it may be helpful to display suspiciousness of regions computed by CAD. In this paper the quality of probabilities computed for masses by a commercial CAD system is studied in two ways: 1) by comparing standalone performance of the system to that of experienced screening radiologists, and 2) by determining results of independent double reading with CAD. The study involves results of 15 readers who each read 500 mammograms, and two releases of the CAD algorithm. Independent double reading results are obtained by combining probabilities of the CAD system with the reader assessment for each localized finding reported by the reader, and by computing the fraction of cancers localized correctly as a function of false positive referrals. It was found that standalone performance of CAD is less than that of any reader in the study. Nevertheless, it was found that performance improves significantly with independent CAD reading, and that use of an improved CAD algorithm lead to significantly better results of the combined reader with CAD.

1 Introduction

In computer aided detection (CAD) systems prompts are displayed on regions identified by a computer as suspicious for breast cancer, after the reader has inspected the mammogram without CAD. These prompts may help radiologists to find cancers that initially were overlooked. Results of some prospective studies confirm that screening results are improved when CAD is used [1],[2]. However, considering the high sensitivity of CAD systems, it is also felt that the technology is less effective than expected, particularly for masses, architectural distortion and asymmetry. The reason for this is that it frequently occurs that radiologists do not act on prompts that later appear to be true positives. This suggest that these cancers were not missed by oversight but misinterpreted. Also in experimental studies evidence is found that the majority of screening errors related to masses may be due to misinterpretation rather than oversight [3], [4].

In a previous study it was found that radiologist may be able to use CAD prompting systems to help with interpretation of masses. The use of the system should be radically different though from what is currently recommended.

Susan M. Astley et al. (Eds.): IWDM 2006, LNCS 4046, pp. 54–60, 2006.
© Springer-Verlag Berlin Heidelberg 2006

Instead of ignoring prompts on regions already inspected, the reader should reconsider decisions with respect to these regions with the use of CAD. On the other hand, prompts of the computer on regions not identified as potential abnormalities might better be ignored, unless it is a clear abnormality that was overlooked. In this paper this way of using CAD mass prompts explored further. First, a comparison is made of the standalone performance of a CAD system with that of experienced screening radiologists. This comparison shows that probabilities, or suspiciousness levels, of prompted regions computed by the CAD system correlate well with radiologists' findings. Second, we conduct an experiment with two versions of a CAD system, of which the most recent one has higher detection performance. It is investigated if the higher performance of CAD leads to better detection results if probabilities of the CAD system are independently combined with human reader assessments, focusing on areas identified by the readers as potential abnormalities.

By comparing ratings of suspiciousness of CAD and human readers it may be understood better how CAD can assist readers with interpretation. Because of the large number of false positives, in practice readers do not have much confidence in CAD as a decision aid. By showing that performance of a CAD system is in fact close to that of a human reader it may be more easy for a radiologist to recognize it as a system that can truly help with screening.

2 Observer Data and CAD System

In this study we make use of data from an observer study, which has been described in detail previously [3]. Fifteen experienced screening radiologists from different countries were involved in this study of which five can be regarded as leading experts in the area of breast cancer screening. In the study they read 500 mammograms of which 250 were priors of cancer cases. It turned out that in 142 cases a visible lesion could be seen in the prior. In 116 of these cases a mass, architectural distortion or an asymmetry was the major sign. These were selected as the true lesions in this investigation.

In the observer study radiologists had been asked to mark and rate all regions that attracted their attention, also those that they would normally not recall. For their ratings they used a scale of suspiciousness ranging from 0 to 100%. They read the mammograms with priors, as is common in screening. So in fact in the study the priors and former priors of the cancer cases were presented, randomly mixed with the 250 normal cases, which also consisted of two subsequent screenings. In total, the 15 readers marked 7173 findings in the selected sample of cases.

In this study we use mass detection results of the R2 ImageChecker. Two versions of the system were used, with software releases from 2001 and 2004. Each mass prompt of the system had a measure indicating importance of the prompt, which is intended to be used in combination with a threshold to select prompts to be displayed.

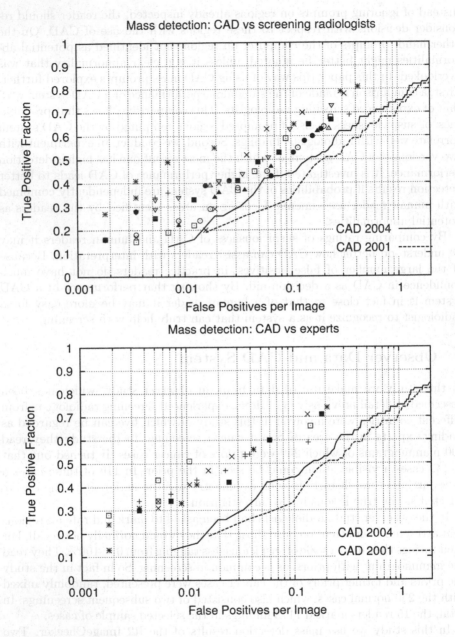

Fig. 1. Mass detection performance of CAD and 10 experienced screening radiologists (upper) and 5 experts (lower). Each point represents an operating point of a radiologist. The solid and dashed lines show CAD results of two software versions. In practice, operating points in European screening programs are in the range of 0.005 - 0.02 FP/image.

3   FROC Performance of the Readers

It is common practice to report CAD performance by FROC curves, while observer performance is usually determined by one operating point or by ROC analysis. However, the observer data collected in our study allowed computation of both ROC and FROC results for the readers, as they marked locations of abnormalities. Using FROC analysis, a direct comparison between radiologists and CAD could be made. True positive detections were determined by a distance criterion. If a CAD mark or an annotation of a radiologist was close enough to a true cancer location a true positive was counted. For the radiologists we used a distance of 2.5 cm. For CAD a smaller distance criterion of 1.5 cm was used. These thresholds were chosen taking into account 1) the inaccuracy of the radiologists' annotations (which were drawn on small paper printouts of the mammograms) and 2) the fact that there were many CAD marks, making the risk of erroneously counting a true positive CAD mark due to a nearby false positive relatively high. Case based FROC curves were computed, i.e. a true positive was counted if a cancer is found in either the CC or the MLO view.

The false positive rate was determined based on findings in the 250 normal cases. For the radiologists only lesion based findings were available, i.e. if a lesion was visible in two views this was scored as one finding. Therefore, to construct FROC curves of the radiologists two false positives were counted per finding if both the MLO and CC view were present (actually the majority of the cases only had the MLO view).

Results are shown in figure 1. The points indicate operating points of the radiologists determined by varying the detection threshold. Results of the five experts are displayed in a separate figure. The lines shows the CAD results.

4   Effect of Improved CAD Performance on Independent Combination of Readers with CAD

To independently combine observer scores with CAD the scale of importance of CAD marks was converted a standardized level of normality L, using the normal cases in the set. L indicates how often a false positive CAD mark would occur if the threshold was set to the level corresponding with L. For a given reader, the level of suspiciousness of an observed finding combined with CAD was computed by $S_{R+CAD} = S_R + f(L)$ with L the level of normality of the region and S_R the reader score for the finding. It is noted that the reader read the cases without CAD. Only locations where the reader marked a finding are evaluated in this scheme, so CAD marks on areas not marked by the reader are not taken into account. The weight function $f(L)$ was chosen to be linear with $log(L)$ and was the same for all 15 readers. Parameters were optimized separately for the two CAD software versions, which resulted in higher weights for the latest software version.

In mammograms were both CC and MLO views were available and CAD hit the region in both views the level of the mass marker with the lowest value of L was assigned to the finding. When CAD did not hit the region the finding

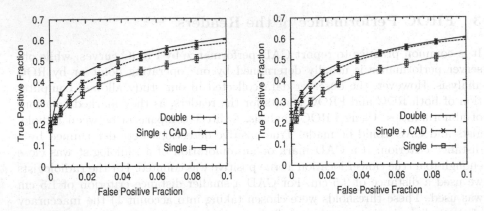

Fig. 2. Mean sensitivity for visible masses on prior mammograms, obtained by single reading, independent double reading, and independent interpretation with CAD, as a function of the false positive fraction. In the left figure results with the software version from 2001 are shown. The right figure shows the results with the newer version of 2004.

Table 1. Mean sensitivity in the range of false positive fractions less than 0.1, for reading without CAD and for reading with CAD using the two different software versions

Radiologist	Without CAD	CAD V2001	CAD V2004
1	42.6	52.4	51.7
2	45.5	57.9	57.2
3	55.9	58.9	57.0
4	35.1	42.3	46.1
5	37.8	48.4	49.5
6	34.3	39.8	43.2
7	40.2	43.6	44.4
8	40.3	46.9	54.5
9	34.2	45.7	47.3
10	41.1	48.8	51.9
11	48.0	50.6	50.0
12	49.9	51.3	51.8
13	47.7	54.5	56.8
14	53.3	54.8	57.6
15	43.1	44.3	46.9
Average	43.3	49.3	51.1

was given the highest level of normality, thus maximally degrading the reader's score. To determine if a mass marker corresponded with a finding of a reader we used the distance between the center of mass of the area drawn by the reader and the location of the mass marker. If this distance was smaller than 1.5 cm a hit was counted, otherwise the marker was regarded as unrelated to the finding.

By varying a detection threshold applied to the level of suspiciousness "localized response" (LROC) curves were constructed that show the fraction of correctly localized lesions (sensitivity) as a function of the false positive fraction [5]. A false positive was counted when a case had at least one false positive finding that exceeded the detection threshold. LROC results are shown in figure 2. Also mean results of independent double reading are displayed. These were obtained by combining each reader with all other readers, and simply averaging their scores to obtain a mean level of suspiciousness for the pooled set of findings of each reader pair. In this way fifteen curves were obtained for each reader, which were subsequently averaged. Table 1 shows the result form each individual reader. Mean sensitivity in the range of false positive fractions less than 0.1 was taken as performance indicator. The improvement obtained when using the newer CAD algorithm was statistically significant (p=0.014, paired t-test).

5   Discussion

As expected, the performance of CAD is lower than that of any radiologist in the study. However, the difference with the performance of the screening radiologists is not very large. It may be expected that the gap will be bridged in the near future when new CAD algorithms become available. It is also noted that all radiologist in the study were very experienced and motivated. The average performance of radiologists in practice may be lower than what we found. Results also show that the difference between the five expert radiologists and CAD is relatively large, almost a ten-fold reduction in false positives of CAD would be needed to reach the level of performance of the experts.

FROC results show that the perception that some radiologists have that CAD is extremely poor on masses is not justified, because the difference between CAD and the human readers is not that large. Negative perception of CAD may be due to the operating point used in the clinical sites: radiologists only see the prompts and have no access to the probabilities of the CAD marks. They cannot easily relate CAD results to their own performance, because they operate at a much lower false positive rate. Moreover, in a screening situation most of what they see are the false positives, because the number of cancers in the population is low. The problem of relating the CAD system to their own level of performance will be worse in sites where the recall is low, like in Europe. For instance, when a radiologists operates at a four percent recall rate his number of false positives per image is about 20 times lower than the setting of the CAD system (around 0.02 FP/image).

Results of independent combination of CAD with observer data demonstrate that CAD can be used in practice as an interpretation aid, i.e. to help deciding which cases should be recalled. This way of using CAD may be greatly facilitated if probabilities computed by CAD were made available for the reader. Further study is needed to determine how these probabilities, which can be seen as prompt magnitude, should best be displayed. For instance, a color scale or marker size could be employed.

It was found that improvement of the CAD algorithm lead to improved combined performance, which is what one would expect. This improvement was statistically significant. Independent reading with CAD almost reached the level of performance of independent double reading of two experience radiologists. The weight given to CAD, optimized over the whole set of observers, was also larger with the improved algorithm, which is consistent with the larger benefit it gave. If CAD keeps improving and reaches the level of a single reading by a radiologist double reading with CAD is expected to become as effective as true double reading.

References

1. T. W. Freer and M. J. Ulissey. Screening mammography with computer-aided detection: prospective study of 12,860 patients in a community breast center. *Radiology*, 220(3):781–6, 2001.
2. T. E. Cupples, J. E. Cunningham, and J. C. Reynolds. Impact of computer-aided detection in a regional screening mammography program. *AJR Am J Roentgenol*, 185(4):944–950, 2005.
3. N. Karssemeijer, J. D. Otten, A. L. Verbeek, J. H. Groenewoud, H. J. de Koning, J. H. Hendriks, and R. Holland. Computer-aided detection versus independent double reading of masses on mammograms. *Radiology*, 227(1):192–200, 2003.
4. D Manning, S Ethell, and T Donovan. Categories of observer error from eye-tracking and afroc data. *SPIE Medical Imaging*, 5372:90–99, 2004.
5. R. G. Swensson. Unified measurement of observer performance in detecting and localizing target objects on images. *Med Phys*, 23(10):1709–25, 1996.

Current Screening Practice: Implications for the Introduction of CAD

Lucy Tomlinson[1], Nathalie Hurley[1], Caroline Boggis[2], Julie Morris[3],
Emma Hurley[2], and Sue Astley[4]

[1] School of Medicine, University of Manchester, Manchester M13 9PT, England
[2] Nightingale Breast Centre, South Manchester University Hospitals Trust
[3] Department of Medical Statistics, South Manchester University Hospitals Trust
[4] Imaging Science and Biomedical Engineering, University of Manchester,
Stopford Building, Oxford Road, Manchester M13 9PT
Sue.Astley@manchester.ac.uk

Abstract. The UK National Health Service Breast Screening Programme
(NHSBSP) provides free mammographic screening for all women between the
ages of 50 and 69. This paper examines in detail the way in which the programme is implemented in one of the busiest breast screening centres, discussing the implications of current practice for the introduction of computer aided
detection systems. The paper also investigates the different types of abnormality
that arise in older and younger women within the screening age group, and discusses how this is likely to affect prompting systems.

1 Breast Cancer Screening

The National Health Service Breast Screening Programme (NHSBSP) was established
in England and Wales in 1988 [1] and achieved national coverage in 1995. Initially,
women between 50 and 64 were invited for screening every three years, with two
view mammography at their first visit and single view mammography thereafter.
Recently, the programme has been extended to include women up to the age of 69,
with two view mammography at every visit [2]. The gold standard for film reading is
double reading with arbitration by a third reader [3]. All screening centres in the UK
are carefully monitored to ensure that the standard of screening offered to women is
consistently high, but within the programme there is considerable variation in local
practice.

The screening process involves two view mammography, carried out either in a
mobile unit or at a hospital base. Women with a normal screening outcome are notified within two weeks. If a significant abnormality is detected, the woman is recalled
for further assessment combining clinical examination with further imaging (mammography and ultrasound) and proceeding to needle biopsy where indicated. It is
predicted that the programme will save 1250 lives per year by 2010 [2].

Quality assurance and monitoring play an important role in maintaining the effectiveness of screening. A number of factors including cancer detection rates and positive predictive values are recorded for each Breast Screening Unit. Both regional and

Susan M. Astley et al. (Eds.): IWDM 2006, LNCS 4046, pp. 61–67, 2006.

national systems are involved in monitoring these criteria and in taking action if required. Although the NHSBSP criteria are based on single reading only, double reading of mammograms is a well-established practice in the UK; by 2003, more than three quarters of mammograms were being double read [4]. Reading regimes vary from centre to centre, with the final decision to recall made by consensus, by arbitration, or if either reader recommends it.

The national programme has responded positively but cautiously to the advent of new technology such as digital acquisition, soft copy reading and CAD. In this paper we examine the way in which a busy screening centre within the NHSBSP operates in practice, and discuss the implications of our findings for the introduction of new technology such as computer-aided detection (CAD).

2 Current Practice

2.1 The Film Reading Process

The current practice in one busy breast screening centre is, where possible, double reading by a radiologist and a radiographer trained in film reading. At this stage the readers score cases, with 1 being a recommendation for return to routine screening, and a score of 2 or more requiring a discussion with the other reader (consensus). Following this, a decision is made to either return the woman to routine screening, refer the case for arbitration, request previous films, request a technical recall, or recall the woman for further assessment.

Analysis of 1174 screening mammograms read in the screening centre over 15 consecutive working days showed that 98.5% of those were double read by a consultant radiologist and a radiographer trained in film reading. Of these, 218 women were recommended for a consensus discussion by one or both readers. Overall, radiographers identified 155 of these cases and radiologists 141, with an overlap of 78 cases recommended by both readers. This difference between radiologists and radiographers was not significant (p=0.272) but radiographers were more likely to request a recall on technical grounds.

Of the 218 sets of films that were subject to consensus discussion by the radiographer and radiologist, 154 (70.6%) were identified as requiring: further assessment, arbitration, technical recall or requests for previous films. The remaining 64 women were returned to routine screening.

During the consensus discussion, of the 33 women recommended for recall by radiographers but not radiologists, 5 women (15.2%) went to arbitration, but of the 32 women recommended for recall by the radiologist but not the radiographer 18 women (56.3%) actually went to arbitration indicating that the radiologists were more influential in the consensus process. Of the 33 sets of mammograms that went to arbitration following consensus 11 (33%) were recalled for further assessment, whilst the remaining 22 were returned to routine screening.

2.2 Implications for the Introduction of CAD

CAD systems are used to aid image interpretation; they are intended to draw the reader's attention to suspicious regions that have been identified by detection algorithms and might otherwise have been overlooked. The way in which they are used in practice depends on existing national and local strategies. In the case of the screening centre discussed above, the film reading process involves a series of stages: independent reading, consensus and arbitration. If a CAD system is introduced, the initial reading stage could be undertaken either by radiographers using CAD or by radiologists using CAD. Research is currently underway to determine whether these are equivalent in terms of cancer detection and recall rate. A key objective will be to replace double reading with single reading using CAD, but this can only be achieved if the two regimes are equivalent. A recent retrospective trial conducted in the UK found that single reading with CAD increased the pick-up of early cancers, but at the expense of an increased rate of recall of normal women [5].

With CAD, a reader will first look at the mammograms without any prompting, then access the prompts and look again. The unprompted review corresponds to independent reading in the existing regime. Currently, readers have the option of referring cases for consensus with the other reader. When single reading with CAD, all the available evidence will have been taken into account during the second prompted look at the images.

The option of discussing cases with another reader after reading with CAD would be a valuable reassurance and safety net. In a recent study, the detection of early cancers was increased at a screening centre employing this method, but again, the rate of recall of normal women was also increased [6]. One possibility is that all cases identified as suspicious by the single reader with CAD are discussed with a second reader. This is neither consensus in the original sense (since the second reader is reading *only* cases believed by the first reader to require additional expertise) nor arbitration (since only a single reader has been involved up to that point). Neither is it arbitration between the human and machine, as the first reader has the opportunity to discard prompts, and cases referred to the second reader may be unprompted.

Currently, 12-13% of cases are recommended for consensus. If these are referred to a second reader, this represents a significant proportion of all cases that will, in effect, be double read with CAD. The implications of this must be taken into account in analysis of the cost-effectiveness of the process, particularly since the reading procedure with CAD is more time consuming than unprompted reading. The proportion could, however, be reduced by excluding technical recalls and unequivocally abnormal cases. For cases which are double read with CAD, the arbitration process could be retained.

3 Types of Cancer

The performance of CAD systems depend on a variety of factors including breast density, size and type of abnormality. The effectiveness of CAD prompting may thus vary depending on the age of the woman at the time of screening, the screening interval, and whether it is a prevalent or incident screening round. We have analysed screening mammograms from women in two age groups (55-59 and 65-69) to determine whether the cancers detected in these two groups were, in fact, similar.

3.1 Type of Cancer *vs* Age

In 2004, 28,855 women were screened in the centre described above. Of these, 57% had been screened routinely in the last 5 years, and 23% had not attended since a previous routine screen more than five years before. 13% were attending for the first time, and the remainder were either self-referrals, women who had missed their first screen or women recalled less than three years after a previous screen.

A total of 208 women (0.7%) were diagnosed as having breast cancer. 24% of these were aged between 55 and 59, and 29% were between 65 and 69. In these two age groups, the older women presented with more masses (60% vs 36%) whereas the younger group had more asymmetries and stromal deformities (28% vs 15%). There was no significant difference between the groups in terms of types of cancer (ductal, lobular, DCIS etc.), grade of tumour or tumour size. Figure 1 shows the types of cancer found in the two groups, and figure 2 shows the proportion of different mammographic abnormalities.

Both groups of women had already been in the screening programme for at least five years, so would be expected to have had a previous screen within that period. However, the number of years since previous mammography was significantly higher (p<0.001) for the women in the older group, with a median of 5 (range 1-9) in comparison with a median of 3 (range 2-7) in the younger group. Overall, 62% of the older women had an interval of greater than the recommended three years, whereas only 26% of the younger women exceeded this duration. Despite this, there was no evidence that these women presented with a larger tumour size than women in the younger group.

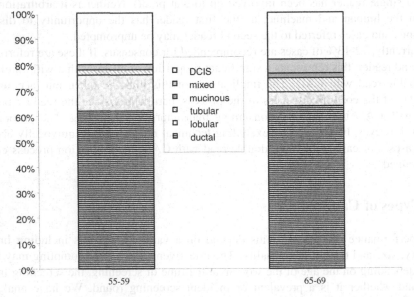

Fig. 1. Proportions of cancer types found in mammograms of women in different age groups

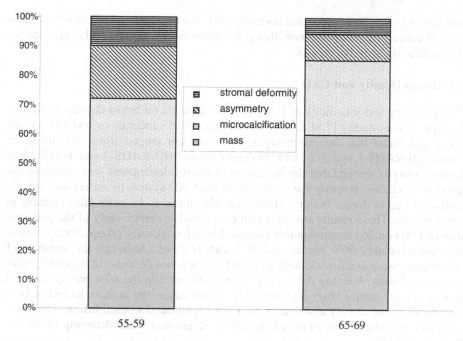

Fig. 2. Proportions of different mammographic abnormalities found in the two age groups

3.2 Type of Abnormality and CAD

CAD systems usually prompt lesions within a given size range. For microcalcifications, systems use rules to establish whether particles are clustered, and how many particles constitute a significant cluster. Since clustering rules are generally based only on a single view and often require as few as three particles, it is possible for false clusters to be prompted, although where two views are available, these should be easily dismissed. The largest masses encountered in screening are very obvious, either because of locally increased density or by virtue of asymmetry between the right and left breasts. Provided that the reader is aware of any cut-off in size of lesions prompted, this is not a problem. For smaller masses, sensitivity of CAD is high; one study reported a sensitivity of 92% for lesions less than 5 mm in size [14].

Different types of breast cancer present in different ways; in one study of 94 invasive lobular carcinoma lesions, 60% presented as masses, of which 71% were spiculated, and 21% as architectural distortions. The remainder appeared as asymmetries or calcifications [15]. Another study measured CAD sensitivity for different pathologies, and found that CAD was particularly sensitive in the detection of ductal carcinoma in situ and lobular carcinoma [16] The performance of CAD depends on appearance rather than diagnosis, with microcalcification clusters generally the most successfully prompted., followed by masses. One study of the performance of CAD on cancers missed at screening show that 70% of these are masses, and that CAD could prompt 73% of these correctly [17].

Asymmetries and stromal deformities are more difficult to detect automatically than masses. In a study of the performance of two commercial CAD systems, fewer than 40% of cases were prompted correctly [18]. For younger women in whom these signs of cancer are more common, this is compounded by the relatively high density of glandular tissue in the breasts.

3.3 Breast Density and CAD

The sensitivity and specificity of CAD systems depends on breast density as well as the type of abnormality [7,8]. One study examined 906 cancer cases and 147 normal cases, and found that the prompting rate for cancers ranged from 90% in fattier breasts (BI-RADS 1 and 2) to 88% in denser breasts (BI-RADS 3 and 4) [8]. More detailed analysis showed that the prompting of microcalcifications was similar in the two density classes, however the sensitivity of the CAD system to masses was significantly reduced in denser breasts. There were also found to be more false prompts in dense breasts. These results are supported by a smaller, earlier study of the performance of CAD on 264 mammograms classified into four density groups, each containing approximately 60% normal and 40% cancer cases. Although the numbers of cancer cases were smaller, the authors found a significant decrease in sensitivity with increasing density, but they did not report any difference in the false prompt rate. In another recent smaller study involving 127 cancer cases, the authors looked at both the overall breast density and that of the local background to each lesion. They also concluded that the effects of breast density were greatest when detecting masses in dense breasts [10].

Increased breast density is associated with an increase in the risk of developing cancer [11, 12], but it has also been reported to increase the risk of having a false positive mammogram [13]. Given that CAD specificity may be reduced in dense breasts [8], and that readers tend to have higher recall rates with CAD [5], the detection of masses in dense breasts should clearly be a key area of focus for future CAD research.

References

1. Forrest APM 1986 Breast Cancer Screening: Report to the Health Ministers of England, Wales, Scotland and Northern Ireland. HMSO London 1986
2. http://www.cancerscreening.nhs.uk/breastscreen/ accessed 10.02.06
3. Blanks RG, Wallis MG, Moss SM: A comparison of cancer detection rates achieved by breast cancer screening programmes by number of readers, for one and two view mammography: results from the UK National Health Service breast screening Programme. Journal of Medical screening 1998 5: 195-201
4. Liston JC, Dall BJG: Can the NHS Breast Screening Programme afford not to double read screening mammograms? Clinical Radiology. 2003; 58:474-477
5. Gilbert FJ, Astley SM, McGee MA, Gillan MGC, Boggis CRM, Griffiths PM and Duffy SW. Comparison of double reading and single reading with CAD in the UK NHS Breast Screening Program: Computer Aided Detection Evaluation Trial. (CADET). *Radiology* (In press)
6. Astley SM, Duffy SW, Boggis CRM , Wilson M, et al Mammography reading with computer-aided detection (CAD): performance of different readers. In: Proceedings of the 8th International Workshop on Digital Mammography, Springer 2006

7. Malich A, Sauner DC et al: Influence of breast lesion size and histologic findings on tumour detection rate of a computer-aided diagnosis system. Radiology 2003; 228(3) 851-856
8. Brem RF, Hoffmeister JW et al: Impact of breast density on computer-aided detection for breast cancer. Am J Roentgenol. 2005 184(2):439-444
9. Ho WT, Lam PWT. Clinical Performance of Computer-Aided Detection (CAD) System in Detecting Carcinoma in Breasts of Different Densities. Clinical Radiology 2003, 58:133-136
10. Malich A, Fischer DR, Facius M, Petrovitch A, BoettcheJ Digit Imaging. 2005 Sep;18(3):227-33r J, Marx C, Hansch A, Kaiser WA. Effect of breast density on computer aided detection.
11. Wolfe JN. Breast patterns as an index of risk for developing breast cancer. American Journal of Roentgenology 1976 Jun 1: 26(6)1130-7
12. Saftlas AF, Szklo M. Mammographic parenchymal patterns and breast cancer risk. Epidemiol Rev 1987: 9:146-74
13. Lehman CD, White E, Peacock S, Drucker MJ, Urban N. Effect of age and breast density on screening mammograms with false-positive findings. AJR Am J Roentgenol. 1999 Dec;173(6):1651-5
14. Brem RF, Hoffmeister JW, Zisman G, DeSimio MP and Rogers SK. A Computer-Aided Detection System for the Evaluation of Breast Cancer by Mammographic Appearance and Lesion Size. American Journal of Roentenology. 184:893-6, 2205 March.
15. Evans WP, Warren Burhennc LJ Laurie L, O'Shaughnessy KF and Castellino RA Invasive Lobular Carcinoma of the Breast: Mammographic Characteristics and Computer-aided Detection. Radiology. 225:182-9, 2002 Oct
16. Brem RF, Rapelyea JA, Zisman G, Hoffmeister JW, DeSimio MP. Evaluation of breast cancer with a computer-aided detection system by mammographic appearance and histopathology. Cancer. 104:931-5, 2005 Sep
17. Birdwell RL, Ikeda DM. O'Shaughnessy KF and Sickles EA Mammographic Characteristics of 115 Missed Cancers Later Detected with Screening Mammography and the Potential Utility of Computer-aided Detection.Radiology. 219:192-202, 2001 April.
18. Baker JA, Rosen EL ct al: CAD in screening mammography: sensitivity of commercial CAD systems for detecting architectural distortion. Am J Roentgenol. 2003 181(4): 1083-1088

Mammographic Mass Detection Using Unsupervised Clustering in Synergy with a Parcimonious Supervised Rule-Based Classifier

Michel Bruynooghe

University Louis Pasteur of Strasbourg,
Yorckstrasse 49, 76185 Karlsruhe, Germany
Michel.Bruynooghe@t-online.de

Abstract. We develop a novel CAD detection system that can help a radiologist to detect masses in mammograms. The proposed algorithm concurrently detects the breast boundary and the pectoral muscle. Then, a clustering and morphology based segmentation algorithm is applied to the enhanced mammography image to separate the mass from the normal breast tissues. This technique outlines the shape of candidate masses in mammograms. To maximize detection specificity, we develop a two-stage hybrid classification network. First, an unsupervised classifier is used to classify suspicious opacities as suspect or not. Then, a few supervised interpretation rules are applied to further reduce the number of false detections. Using a private mammography database and the publicly available USF/DDSM database, experimental results demonstrate that a sensitivity of 94% (resp. 80%) can be achieved at a specificity level of 1.02 (resp. 0.69) false positives per image. Even in dense mammograms, the CAD algorithm can still correctly detect subtle masses.

1   Introduction

Classical computer-assisted detection of masses in mammographic images generally requires a multistage algorithm that includes detection of candidate masses, pattern recognition techniques to classify the candidate objects, and a method to eliminate false detections and to determine if a mass exists. Wavelet or morphological techniques are generally used to enhance the mammography image. Supervised classifiers such as neural networks, fuzzy neural classifiers, bayesian classifiers or rule-based classifiers are applied to discriminate between normal and suspicious objects. These classical supervised classifiers generally require the learning of a rather large number of parameters.

Specificity levels of automatic mass detection methods in mammography are generally rather low. To improve detection scores, te-Brake, Karssemeijer and Hendriks [4] have introduced features that are related to image characteristics that radiologists use to discriminate real lesions from normal tissue. Approximately 75% of all cancers were detected in at least one view at a specificity level of 1.0 false positive per image.

Susan M. Astley et al. (Eds.): IWDM 2006, LNCS 4046, pp. 68–75, 2006.

Yates, Evans and Brady [22] have proposed a pre-processing step for improving te-Brake's mass-detection algorithm. Their method, that is based on wavelets and phase congruency, removes the locally linear fine detail structure, whilst retaining the larger underlying mass structure. The resulting ROC curve has shown that this removal technique improves the mass detection rate. Hong and Brady [11] have proposed a segmentation method for delineating regions of interest in mammograms. Their algorithm concurrently detects the breast boundary, the pectoral muscle, and dense regions that include candidate masses. A topographic representation called the iso-level contour map has been used to estimate the saliency of each suspicious region. This method has achieved a satisfactory performance as a prompt system for mass detection.

An adaptive, multiscale method for mass detection using a circular ring template and a nonparametric test has been presented by Khan et al. [12]. Training data corresponding to the local background intensity level is extracted from the outer ring of the template while test data for mass detection is obtained from the inner disk. Experimental results show a sensitivity of 1.0 and a false positive rate of 1.40 per image on 30 images. Detection algorithms often fail to detect masses with a partial loss of region, that are located on the edge of the film. To overcome this problem, Hatanaka et al. [8] have proposed to identify partial loss masses by their similarity to a sector-form model in the template matching process. The true-positive fraction is 0.97 (resp. 0.84) when the number of false positives (FP) is 1.20 (resp. 1.49) per mammogram on 335 (resp. 1075) digitized mammograms. Petrick et al. [18] have designed an object-based region-growing technique to improve mass segmentation. As a preprocessing step, this segmentation method utilizes the density-weighted contrast enhancement (DWCE) filter to adaptively enhance the contrast between the breast structures and the background. Each suspicious opacity is classified as a mass or normal tissue based on morphological and texture features. This segmentation scheme detected 90% (resp. 80%) of 253 biopsy-proven breast masses at a specificity level of 4.2 (resp. 2.0) false positive per image.

Cheng and Muyi-Cui [6] have recently presented a novel fuzzy neural network approach to detect malignant mass on mammograms. They analyzed 670 ROIs from mammograms of the DDSM database. The true-positive fraction is 0.92 when the number of FPs is 1.33 per mammogram. But, this FP score is underestimated because only a few ROIs have been analyzed per mammogram instead of full mammograms. Hence, it cannot be compared to other specificity scores. Heath et al. [10] have introduced a mass detection algorithm by relative image intensity that estimates the degree to which a surrounding region of a point decreases in intensity. This algorithm requires neither the training of parameters nor the normalization of images. Detection performances and FROC curves have been estimated using datasets from the MIAS and DDSM databases. Experimental results show a sensitivity of 0.65 (resp. 0.70) and a false positive rate of 1.75 (resp. 1.60) per image on 246 MIAS images (resp. 160 USF images).

Performances of other recently published CAD algorithms for mass detection are presented in figure 3. Published detection scores show that the simultaneous achievement of a high sensitivity (more than 0.95) and an acceptable specificity (less than 1 false positive per image) has not yet been achieved by published CAD algorithms. The objective of this paper is to get better detection scores using either an unsupervised classification approach or an hybrid algorithm. Performance evaluation of these two CAD algorithms will be carried out using image data from two mammography databases.

2 Methods

This paper focuses on a methodological approach that (i) removes the locally linear fine detail structure using a morphological algorithm based on successive geodesic openings by linear structuring elements of various orientations, and (ii) eliminates false positives using an unsupervised classifier in synergy with a parcimonious supervised classifier based on a few interpretation rules.

2.1 Detection of Breast Boundary and Pectoral Muscle

The first step of our approach is a pre-processing step that detects the breast boundary and the pectoral muscle using a novel approach based on image segmentation by multidimensional clustering of pixels, on optimized thresholding to get an initial breast segmentation and on an object-based region-growing technique to improve breast segmentation. The region-growing technique uses gray-scale and gradient information to adjust the initial breast borders and to avoid merging between the breast and adjacent background bright markings.

2.2 Computer Perception of Suspicious Opacities

The second step of our approach is to perform the computer perception of objects of interest, i.e. of suspicious opacities. First, we remove the locally linear fine detail structure using morphological algorithms and we filter the mammographic image using anisotropic diffusion. Then, dense regions that include candidate masses are localized and a clustering and morphology based segmentation algorithm is applied to the smoothed mammography image to outline the shape of candidate masses in mammograms. Finally, candidate masses are characterized using standard shape features as well as photometric features that are invariant to monotone transformations of the grey-level scale. The aim of such an invariant representation is to efficiently process mammograms acquired and digitized by various mammography devices.

2.3 Computer Classification of Suspicious Opacities

The third step is to perform the computer classification of objects of interest and to decide if a suspicious opacity is a normal structure or a mass object. We use an hybrid classification approach that integrates an initial unsupervised clustering and a parcimonious supervised classification. In our unsupervised CAD algorithm, suspicious opacities are classified as suspect or not by using clustering algorithms [3] and unsupervised semantic rules that allow to quickly eliminate the overwhelming majority of non-mass objects in a mammogram from any further consideration. Then, our hybrid CAD algorithm integrates the unsupervised CAD algorithm and a supervised classifier, in which a few expert supervised interpretation rules are applied to further reduce the number of false detections and to determine at each location in the mammogram if a mass object is present or not.

3   Experiments

3.1   Data

First database: In this work, we have used a first set of 100 mammograms to test the performance of the detection method. These mammograms came from a private database. This dataset included spiculated, circumscribed, low-contrasted and subtle masses. All mammograms have been digitized at $50\mu m$ and then subsampled to $200\mu m$.

Second database: The second data set used in our experiments is the Digital Database for Screening Mammography (DDSM) (Heath et al. [9]). Thirty nine cases representing 156 images were selected and analyzed, each digitized on a Howtek MultiRAD scanner and having at least one confirmed malignant mass. The spatial resolution of the USF/DDSM images is 43.5 microns, with 12 bits per pixel. Mammography images were subsampled to $174\mu m$ for computer detection of masses. The image difficulty is characterized by American College of Radiology (ACR) breast density ratings and a subtlety rating ranging from obvious (scale 5) to very subtle (scale 1).

3.2   Results

Hybrid detection of supra and infracentimetric masses: Our CAD algorithm has been first applied to the analysis of 100 mammograms from the first database containing 45 masses, divided into 5 training mammograms and 95 testing mammograms. Our hybrid detection algorithm has achieved a sensitivity of 95% at a specificity level of 1.07 false positive per image. Even in dense mammograms, the proposed CAD algorithm can still correctly detect subtle masses. Furthermore, our mass segmentation algorithm correctly delineates 95.6% of the lesions, without any oversegmentation. In comparison, the radial gradient index and probabilistic segmentation algorithms proposed by Kupinski and Giger [13] correctly delineates 92% and 96% of the lesions in their own database.

Unsupervised detection of supracentimetric masses: The detection of supracentimetric masses has been performed using our unsupervised CAD algorithm. Experimental results show a sensitivity of 93.9% (resp. 79.6%) at a false positive rate of 1.02 (resp. 0.69) per image on 100 (resp. 156) images from the private (resp. USF/DDSM) database. Hence, there are less false positives with USF images, but more missed detections. This is because the USF database contains more difficult cases, with less contrasted or barely perceptible masses.

Radiologists make errors that can be categorized into three types [7] : search, detection and interpretation. Most errors are found to be the interpretative ones. It is also true for our unsupervised CAD algorithm : masses that are initially correctly detected may then be missed during classification of candidate masses, and false positives are not enough eliminated. Nevertheless, remaining obvious false positives should be easily eliminated using a statistical supervised classifier in synergy with our unsupervised CAD algorithm.

Number of images	Total number of masses	Number of supracentimetric masses	Number of detected masses	True positive rate	False positives per image
100	44	33	31	93.9%	1.02

Fig. 1. Detection scores of our unsupervised CAD algorithm for 100 images of the first database when applied to the detection of supracentimetric masses

Subtlety level (1 to 5)	Number of images	Total number of masses	Number of supracentimetric masses	Number of detected masses	True positive rate	False positives per image
1	20	10	3	2	66.6%	0.65
2	28	14	7	4	57.1%	0.61
3	28	16	12	9	75.0%	0.54
4	36	19	11	8	72.7%	0.67
5	44	22	16	16	100.0%	0.89
1 to 5	156	91	49	39	79.6%	0.69

Fig. 2. Detection scores of our unsupervised CAD algorithm for 156 images of the USF/DDSM database when applied to the detection of supracentimetric masses of various subtlety levels varying from very subtle (level 1) to very obvious (level 5)

4   Discussion

4.1   Segmentation of Objects of Interest

Segmentation of objects of interest is one of the most difficult and common challenges facing CAD systems, as pointed out by Allen et al. [1] who proposed a normalized active contour technique to perform breast delineation or mass segmentation. Their segmentation method uses a level-set implementation of active contours and mimimizes an energy function. Each of the four energy terms competes with the others and their relative strengths are determined by four parameters whose optimal values may vary from one database to another one. This is also true for the dynamic programming algorithm proposed by Timp et al. [20] that minimizes a composite cost function. In contrast to these algorithms, our segmentation algorithm does not require the estimation of such weighting

Authors	Publication Date	Sensitivity Score	False Positives per image	Nb. of testing images	Database
Campanini et al. [5]	2004	80%	1.10		USF
Khan et al. [12]	2002	100%	1.40	30	
Paquerault et al. [14]	2002	73%	1.00	338	
Hatanaka et al. [8]	2001	97%	1.20	335	
		84%	1.49	1075	
Sahiner et al. [19]	2001	80%	1.50		
Mudigonda et al. [17]	2001	85%	2.45	56	MIAS
Lihua-Li et al. [16]	2001	68%	3.72	79	
Petrick et al. [18]	2001	89%	2.00	253	
Heath et al. [10]	2000	65%	1.75	246	MIAS
		70%	1.60	160	USF
Bin-Zheng et al. [2]	1999	80%	0.76	433	
te Brake et al. [4]	1999	75%	1.00	132	
Our hybrid algorithm	2006	95%	1.07	95	Private
Our unsupervised	2006	93.9%	1.02	100	Private
CAD algorithm		79.6%	0.69	156	USF

Fig. 3. Performances of our two CAD algorithms compared to published detection scores. Our detection specificity is better than by Campanini et al. [5] and Heath et al. [10] who also used the USF/DDSM database.

parameters. Visual observation of segmented breasts and masses shows that it generally produces acceptable segmentations. But, such a visual observation is a subjective one and we project to later realize a performance evaluation of our segmentation algorithm including a comparison to well known methods of breast or mass segmentation.

4.2   Improvement of Detection Specificity and Sensitivity

Improving detection specificity without decreasing sensitivity is another difficult challenge facing CAD systems. Most researchers detect masses using supervised classification. False positives are eliminated using a supervised statistical classifier, such as a neural network or a nearest neighbour classifier for example. In this paper, we introduced a different approach based on unsupervised or hybrid classification. Experimental results have demonstrated the potential of such an approach to improve specificity scores. We will later introduce texture features, add a second resolution level and use a complementary supervised classifier to improve detection sensitivity without decreasing detection specificity.

4.3   Comparing Performances of Different CAD Algorithms

Our hybrid CAD algorithm has detected 95% of all supra and infracentimetric masses using the private database. With our unsupervised CAD algorithm, 93.9% (resp. 79.6%) of all supracentimetric masses were detected at a specificity level of 1.02 (resp. 0.69) false positive per image for mammograms of the private and of the USF/DDSM databases. These detection performances are comparable or slightly better than most of published scores. Furthermore, our detection specificity is better than by Campanini et al. [5] and Heath et al. [10] who also used the USF/DDSM database. Nevertheless, performances of various CAD algorithms vary from one database to another one, as shown by published scores as well as by our results. Comparing performances of different CAD algorithms is generally problematic. This is because researchers almost always use their own image database for evaluation [21]. The consequence is that it is difficult to demonstrate that a new CAD algorithm makes a practical advance in the state-of-art. To allow such a comparison, a large scale evaluation of our CAD algorithm will be later performed using several publicly available databases.

References

1. Allen, B. H.; Oxley, M. E.; Collins M. J. A universal segmentation platform for computer-aided detection. 6th International Workshop on Digital Mammography. June 22-25, 2002, Bremen, Germany. Edited by Heinz-Otto Peitgen. Springer 2003; pp. 164-168
2. Bin-Zheng; Yuan-Hsiang-Chang; Xiao-Hui-Wang; Good,W.F.; Gur,D. Application of a Bayesian belief network in a computer-assisted diagnosis scheme for mass detection. Medical Imaging 1999: Image Processing. 22-25 Feb. 1999 San Diego, CA, USA Proceedings of the SPIE. The International Society for Optical Engineering. 1999; 3661 pt. 1-2: 1553-61
3. Bruynooghe, M. Maximal Theoretical Complexity of Fast Hierarchical Clustering Algorithms Based on the Reducibility Property. International Journal of Pattern Recognition and Artificial Intelligence, 7(3), pp. 541-571, 1993.
4. te-Brake,G.M.; Karssemeijer, N.; Hendriks,J. An automatic method to discriminate malignant masses from normal tissue in digital mammograms. Physics-in-Medicine-and-Biology. Oct. 2000; 45(10): 2843-57
5. Campanini,R.; Dongiovanni,D.; Iampieri,E.; Lanconelli,N.; Masotti, M.; Palermo,G.; Riccardi,A.; Roffilli,M. A novel featureless approach to mass detection in digital mammograms based on support vector machines. Physics-in-Medicine-and-Biology. 21 March 2004; 49(6): 961-75
6. Cheng,H.D.; Muyi Cui. Mass lesion detection with a fuzzy neural network. Pattern-Recognition. June 2004; 37(6): 1189-200
7. Gale, A.; Mugglestone, M.; Cowley, H.; Wooding, D. Human factors considerations for CAD implementation in breast screening. 5th International Workshop on Digital Mammography, pp. 461-467, Toronto, Canada, June 11-14 2000.
8. Hatanaka,Y.; Hara,T.; Fujita,H.; Kasai,S.; Endo,T.; Iwase,T. Development of an automated method for detecting mammographic masses with a partial loss of region. IEEE-Transactions-on-Medical-Imaging. Dec. 2001; 20(12): 1209-14
9. Heath M.; Bowyer, K.; Kopans, D.; Moore, R.; Kegelmeyer, P. The Digital Database for Screening Mammography. 5th International Workshop on Digital Mammography, pp. 212-218, Toronto, Canada, June 11-14 2000.
10. Heath M.; Bowyer, K. Mass detection by relative image intensity. 5th International Workshop on Digital Mammography, pp. 219-225, Toronto, Canada, June 11-14 2000.

11. Hong, B. W.; Brady,M. A topographic representation for mammogram segmentation. Medical Image Computing and Computer Assisted Intervention MICCAI-2003. 6th International Conference. Proceedings. Part-II- Lecture Notes in Comput. Sci. Vol. 2879. 2003: 730-7.

12. Khan,F.; Sarma,A.; Ying-Sun; Tufts,D. Mass detection using tolerance intervals and a rank detector. IEEE International Symposium on Biomedical Imaging. 7-10 July 2002 Washington, DC, USA

13. Kupinski,M.A.; Giger,M.L. Automated seeded lesion segmentation on digital mammograms. IEEE-Transactions-on-Medical-Imaging. Aug. 1998; 17(4): 510-17

14. Paquerault,S.; Petrick,N.; Heang-Ping-Chan; Sahiner,B.; Helvie,M.A. Improvement of computerized mass detection on mammograms: Fusion of two-view information. Medical-Physics. Feb. 2002; 29(2): 238-47

15. Lei-Zheng; Chan,A.K.; McCord,G.; Wu,S.; Liu,J.S. Detection of cancerous masses for screening mammography using discrete wavelet transform-based multiresolution Markov random field. Journal-of-Digital-Imaging. May 1999; 12(2): 18-23

16. Lihua-Li; Yang-Zheng; Lei-Zhang; Clark,R.A. False-positive reduction in CAD mass detection using a competitive classification strategy. Medical-Physics. Feb. 2001; 28(2): 250-8

17. Mudigonda,N.R.; Rangayyan,R.M.; Leo-Desautels,J.E. Detection of breast masses in mammograms by density slicing and texture flow-field analysis. IEEE-Transactions-on-Medical-Imaging. Dec. 2001; 20(12): 1215-27

18. Petrick,N.; Heang-Ping-Chan; Sahiner,B.; Helvie,M.A. Combined adaptive enhancement and region-growing segmentation of breast masses on digitized mammograms. Medical-Physics. Aug. 1999; 26(8): 1642-54

19. Sahiner,B.; Petrick,N.; Heang-ping-Chan; Paquerault,S.; Helvie,M. A.; Hadji-iski,L.M. Recognition of lesion correspondence on two mammographic views-a new method of false-positive reduction for computerized mass detection. Medical Imaging 2001: Image Processing. 19-22 Feb. 2001 San Diego, CA, USA. Proceedings of the SPIE. The International Society for Optical Engineering. 2001; 4322 pt. 1-3: 649-55

20. Timp, S.; Karssemeijer, N.; Hendricks, J. Comparison of three different mass segmentation methods. 6th International Workshop on Digital Mammography. June 22-25, 2002, Bremen, Germany. Edited by Heinz-Otto Peitgen. Springer 2003; pp. 218-222

21. Yarlagadda, N.; Bowyer, K.; Li, R. Baseline Comparison of Microcalcification Detection Algorithms. 5th International Workshop on Digital Mammography, pp. 414-420, Toronto, Canada, June 11-14 2000.

22. Yates, K.; Evans, C.; Brady, M. Improving the Brake's mammographic mass-detection algorithm using phase congruency. Proceedings of the Sixth Digital Image Computing Techniques and Applications. Dicta 2002. 2002: 179-83.

Computerized Classification Can Reduce Unnecessary Biopsies in BI-RADS Category 4A Lesions

Leichter Isaac[1,2], Lederman Richard[3], Buchbinder Shalom[4], Srour Yossi[1],
Bamberger Philippe[1], and Sperber Fanny[5]

[1] Siemens Computer Aided Diagnosis, PO Box 45202, Jerusalem 91450, Israel
{isaac.leichter, yossi.srour, philippe.bamberger}@siemens.com
[2] Department of Medical Engineering, Jerusalem College of Technology,
JCT PO Box 16031, Jerusalem 91160, Israel
[3] Department of Radiology, Hadassah University Hospital, P.O. Box 54202,
Jerusalem 91540, Israel
rlederman@hadassah.org.il
[4] Department of Radiology, Staten Island University Hospital Staten Island, 475 Seaview,
Staten Island, New York 10305-3498
sbuchbinder@siuh.edu
[5] Department of Radiology, Tel Aviv Sourasky Medical Center, 6 Weizman St.,
Tel Aviv 64239, Israel
sperber@tasmc.health.gov.il

Abstract. The objective of the study was to assess the potential of a CAD device with computer aided classification capabilities to reduce interventional procedures for BI-RADS category 4A lesions. 113 such lesions (17 masses, 96 clusters), forwarded for biopsy (103 benign) were analyzed retrospectively by a CAD device that generated descriptors. The device extracted quantitative features characterizing the lesions by shape, margins, size and distribution. Descriptors taken from the BI-RADS lexicon for the appearance of the lesion were generated based on the values of the quantitative features. A paradigm based on the computer generated descriptors was developed to assist in assigning a level of suspicion. The paradigm deemed malignant, all 10 malignant cases of the study (100% sensitivity) and correctly classified 38 of the 103 benign lesions. The CAD-generated descriptors, thus, eliminated 36.9% of unnecessary biopsies without decreasing the sensitivity.

1 Introduction

Computer Aided Diagnosis (CAD) in mammography [1] has received FDA approval and entered the mainstream of clinical practice. Its exact role, however, has yet to be defined [2,3], and its widespread implementation is hindered by the relatively large number of false marks [4]. Also, the current generation of CAD systems serves only as a second reader, designed to avoid missed lesions [5], without offering the radiologist a second opinion regarding the nature of the finding. As with all screening tests, mammography is subject to a lack of specificity, which leads to further evaluation of suspicious findings [6]. The need for breast biopsy, frequently with benign results

Susan M. Astley et al. (Eds.): IWDM 2006, LNCS 4046, pp. 76–83, 2006.

[7,8], has both a financial and psychological cost, which can be cut by increasing the specificity of diagnosis in mammography.

The addition of classification capabilities could potentially improve the efficacy of such systems by calculating the level of suspicion of any finding either detected by the first tier of the system, or considered suspicious by the radiologist. Several machine learning methods based on neural networks and Support Vector Machines have been applied for the classification of mammographic lesions [9,10]. It was found that for microcalcifications, a classifier based on kernel-based methods, such as Support Vector Machines and Kernel Fisher Discriminant, yielded a significantly better performance than neural network [11].

In this study a classification scheme, based on Kernel Fisher Discriminant, is described, and its use is tested in a subdivision of BI-RADS category 4 cases with both benign and malignant pathologies. BI-RADS category 4 includes findings that do not have the classic appearance of malignancy but have a wide range of probability of malignancy. It is the most problematic and subjective category resulting in a high percentage of benign biopsies. Category 4A is a subdivision, which includes findings with the lowest level of suspicion, for which interventional procedures are nevertheless still recommended. It has been shown that the BI-RADS descriptor categories stratify suspicious micro-calcifications appropriately into intermediate and higher probability of malignancy groups [12]. In this study, an attempt was made to further refine which lesions in this BI-RADS category, in fact, should be sent for biopsy, by the use of computerized descriptors reflecting the appearance of the lesions in the mammogram. The descriptors generated by the CAD device are similar to those used by the BI-RADS lexicon and are familiar to the radiologist.

2   Methods and Material

One hundred and nine cases with 113 lesions (17 masses, 96 clusters) were retrospectively culled from the archives of a university affiliated facility. All the cases had been prospectively assigned BI-RADS 4A and forwarded for stereo-tactic biopsy. The mean age of the patients was 54.1 ± 8.6 years (range 33–72). The Institutional Review Board at the institution approved the use of these cases for the study, and did not require informed consent because the study was retrospective and patient anonymity was strictly enforced in all aspects of the study. Of the 113 BI-RADS category 4A lesions, 15 masses and 88 clusters proved to be benign at pathology.

The mammograms of the 109 cases were digitized at high resolution (600 dpi, 12 bit) by a prototype CAD device developed by Siemens CAD, Israel [13,14] and the digital images were displayed on the computer screen for further analysis. All 113 lesions were analyzed retrospectively by a radiologist using the CAD device with classification capabilities. The radiologist interactively defined an ellipse encompassing the lesion, on the digital image, and activated the classification algorithm.

For mass lesions the CAD device automatically extracted quantitative features that characterized the mass encompassed by the ellipse. These features characterized the masses by their shape, definition of margins and speculation. Speculation was considered to be a structure composed of lines radiating from a centroid, rather than a saw-tooth border of a lesion with a distinct margin. Therefore, this analysis could also be applied to areas of architectural distortion, to focal asymmetries, to masses that appeared smoothly marginated, and to masses in which the margins were partially obscured.

For clusters of micro-calcifications, the CAD device automatically highlighted, in the first stage, an initial selection of potential micro-calcifications within the ellipse encompassing the cluster. The algorithm then allowed the radiologist to alter target selection, by modifying two detection filters in order to include only appropriate bright spots, which represent calcifications. The new selection of targets was updated in real time on the computer screen, and once the radiologist was satisfied with the selection of targets, the algorithm proceeded with automated extraction of features that characterize the cluster encompassed by the ellipse. For clusters two groups of features are automatically extracted by the computer as described in detail elsewhere [15]. The features in the first group reflect the shape, size and brightness of the individual micro-calcifications and those in the second group reflect the distribution of the calcifications within the cluster and cluster geometry.

Based on the extracted quantitative features, the classification algorithm, in the second stage, automatically generates descriptors taken from the BI-RADS lexicon, reflecting the appearance of the lesions in the mammogram. Descriptors that illustrate the appearance of a benign lesion are generated when low numerical values are obtained for the extracted features and descriptors that illustrate malignant lesions are generated when high values are obtained for the extracted features. The cut-point values for defining high and low numerical values for each of the extracted features were determined by the use of a separate training database with proven pathology results, which did not include any of the 109 cases described in the present study. The training database consisted of 500 cases of mammographically detected lesions with proven pathology, that were retrospectively collected from the archives of four other university-affiliated facilities, not including the facility from which the study cases were obtained. This database consisted of 289 mass lesions (161 malignant, 128 benign) and 211 clusters of micro-calcifications (94 malignant, 117 benign).

Figure 1 displays the descriptors that are generated by the classification algorithm for mass lesions based on their shape, margins and spiculation. The descriptors highlighted in white are generated for features with low values and describe the appearance of benign masses, while those highlighted in grey are generated for features with high values and describe the appearance of malignant masses.

The CAD-generated BI-RAD descriptors are displayed to the user for further assessment of the finding, as displayed in the example of a malignant mass in Figure 2.

For clusters, two sets of descriptors are generated by the CAD device. Figure 3 describes the first set of descriptors that are generated by the classification algorithm based on the appearance of individual calcifications in the lesion. Figure 4 describes the second set of descriptors that are based on the distribution of the calcifications within the cluster. The descriptors highlighted in white are generated for features with low values and describe the appearance of benign clusters, while those highlighted in grey are generated for features with high values and describe malignant masses.

A lesion is often assigned a combination of descriptors, some reflecting a benign appearance and some reflecting a malignant appearance, and then the resulting course of action is still to be defined. A paradigm was developed to assist the radiologist in assigning a level of suspicion, based on the computer generated descriptors. According to the paradigm a mass was considered benign if there was no evidence of

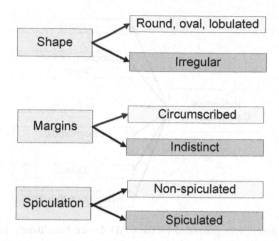

Fig. 1. BI-RADS descriptors generated by the CAD device for masses, based on their shape, margins and spiculation

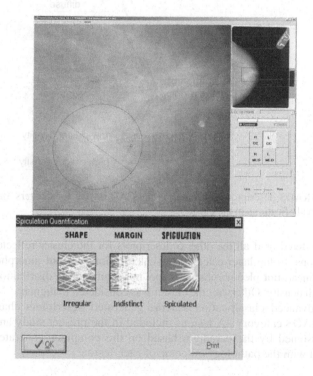

Fig. 2. The CAD-generated BI-RAD descriptors displayed to the user for a malignant mass

spiculation or if the mass was rounded and well circumscribed. Otherwise the mass was assigned a high level of suspicion and considered malignant. According to the paradigm developed for clusters, a cluster was considered benign, if the calcifications were not

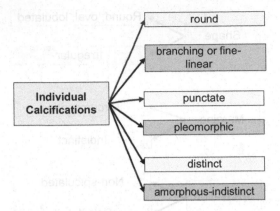

Fig. 3. BI-RADS descriptors generated by the CAD device for clusters, based on the appearance of individual calcifications

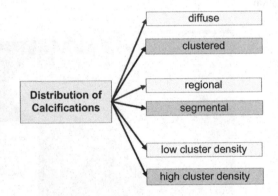

Fig. 4. BI-RADS descriptors generated by the CAD device for clusters, based on the distribution of the calcifications in the cluster

tightly clustered or if all the other 5 descriptors for the cluster reflected typically benign calcifications. In the latter category the calcifications are **not** amorphous, **not** branching **nor** fine-linear, **not** pleomorphic in shape, **not** segmental in distribution and the cluster is **not** of high density. Otherwise the cluster was considered malignant.

The advanced classification scheme generated descriptors characterizing all the 113 BI-RADS category 4A lesions included in the present study and the level of suspicion assigned by the paradigm based on the computer generated descriptors was compared with the pathology outcome of each lesion.

3 Results

According ACR BI-RADS suggestions, in all Category 4A lesions, biopsy should be considered, and the patient and her physician should make an informed decision on the ultimate course of action. All the BI-RADS Category 4A lesions, in this study were forwarded for biopsy. Table 1 displays the results of the conventional interpretation versus the pathology outcome. As can be realized from Table 1, the conventional interpretation resulted for BI-RADS Category 4A lesions, in a Sensitivity of 100%, a Specificity of 0%, a Positive Predictive Value (PPV) of 8.8% and an overall accuracy of 8.8%.

Table 1. Results of the conventional interpretation of the BI-RADS Category 4A lesions

		Conventional Interpretation		
		+	-	Total
Pathology Results	+	10	0	10
	-	103	0	103
	Total	113	0	113

Table 2 displays the results of the computerized analysis, based on the CAD-generated descriptors, versus the pathology outcome. The paradigm, based on the CAD-generated BI-RADS descriptors, deemed malignant, all the 10 malignant BI-RADS Category 4A lesions, included in the study, yielding a sensitivity of 100% for that category. Of the 103 benign lesions, the computerized descriptors correctly classified 38 benign cases, yielding a specificity of 36.9% for BI-RADS Category 4A lesions. Of the 15 benign masses in the BI-RADS 4A Category, the paradigm deemed 12 masses benign, yielding a specificity of 80% for masses. Of the 88 benign clusters in the BI-RADS 4A Category, the paradigm deemed 26 clusters benign, yielding a specificity of 30% for clusters. The paradigm, based on the CAD-generated BI-RADS descriptors, yielded a Positive Predictive Value (PPV) of 13.3% and an overall accuracy of 42.5%, for the BI-RADS 4A Category lesions.

Figure 5 displays the performance of the paradigm based on the BI-RADS descriptors derived from the computer extracted quantitative features, compared to the results of the conventional assessment. This figure demonstrates the increase in the PPV and in the accuracy of diagnosis, caused by the use of the classification scheme, without any loss of sensitivity.

Table 2. Results of the computerized analysis, based on the CAD-generated descriptors, versus the pathology outcome. In this analysis the lesions were considered benign or malignant according to the outcome of the paradigm, using the BI-RADS descriptors.

		Computerized analysis based on CAD-generated descriptors		
		+	-	Total
Pathology Results	+	10	0	10
	-	65	38	103
	Total	75	38	113

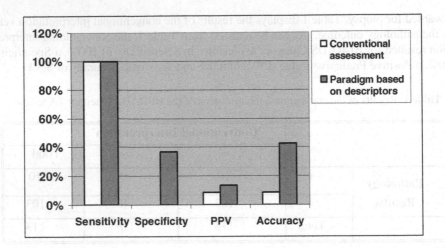

Fig. 5. The performance of the computerized analysis, compared to the conventional assessment

4 Conclusion

BI-RADS category 4A includes findings with the lowest level of suspicion, for which interventional procedures are, nevertheless still recommended. A very high percentage of biopsies performed in this category, results in a benign outcome. This study was performed to explore the hypothesis that computerized classification of the lesions in this category can reduce the number of unnecessary biopsies without affecting the sensitivity of diagnosis.

The use of a computerized analysis, based on BI-RADS descriptors generated by the CAD device, for BI-RADS 4A lesions, significantly increased the accuracy of diagnosis, from 8.8% to 42.5%, compared to conventional interpretation. The paradigm developed to assist the radiologist in establishing a course of action, based on the computer generated descriptors, eliminated 36.9% of unnecessary biopsies without decreasing the sensitivity. The paradigm for interpreting a finding based on these descriptors may well assist the radiologist in the complex task of assessing BI-RADS category 4A lesions.

References

1. Warren-Burhenne, L.L., Wood, S.A., D'Orsi, C.A., Feig, S.A., Kopans, D.B., O'Shaughnessy, K.F., Sickles, E.A., Tabar, L., Vyborny C.J. and Castellino, R.A.: Potential contribution of computer-aided detection to the sensitivity of screening mammography. Radiology (2000) 215:554-562.
2. Ikeda, D.M., Birdwell, R.L., O'Shaughnessy, K.F., Sickles E.A. and Brenner R.J.: Computer-aided detection output on 172 subtle findings on normal mammograms previously obtained in women with breast cancer detected at follow-up screening mammography. Radiology, (2004) 230:811-819.

3. Roque, A.C. and Andre, T.C.: Mammography and computerized decision systems: a review. Ann. NY Acad. Sci. (2002) 980:83-94
4. Gur, D., Sumkin, J.H., Rockette, H.E., Ganott, M., Hakim, C., Hardesty, L., Poller, W.R., Shah, R. and Wallace. L.: Changes in breast cancer detection and mammography recall rates after the introduction of a computer-aided detection system. J. Natl. Cancer Inst. (2004) 96:185-190.
5. Doi, K., MacMahon, H., Katswragawa, S.,. Nishikawa, R.M, and Jiang, W.: Computer-aided diagnosis in radiology: potential and pitfalls. Eur. J. Radiol. (1999) 31:97-109
6. Lederman, R., Leichter, I., Novak, B., Bamberger, P., Fields, S., Buchbinder, S.: Stratification of mammographic cases by BIRADS category with the assistance of a CAD system. European Radiology. 13: (2003) 347-353.
7. Sickles, E.A.: Mammographic features of "early" breast cancer. Am J. Roengenol. (1984) 143:461-464 .
8. Kopans, D.B.: The positive predictive value of mammography. Am J. Roengenol. (1992) 158:521-526.
9. Fu, J.C., Lee, S.K., Wong, S.T. , Yeh, J.Y., Wang, A.H., Wu, H.K.: Image segmentation feature selection and pattern classification for mammographic microcalcifications. Comput Med Imaging Graph. (2005) 9:419-29.
10. Papadopoulos A., Fotiadis, D.I. , Likas, A.: Characterization of clustered microcalcifications in digitized mammograms using neural networks and support vector machines. Artif Intell Med. (2005) 34:141-50.
11. Wei, L., Yang, Y., Nishikawa, R.M., Jiang, Y.: A Study on Several Machine-Learning Methods for Classification of Malignant and Benign microcalcifications. IEEE Trans Med Imaging. (2005) 24:371-380
12. Burnside E.S., Sisney, G.A., Rubin, D.L., Ochsner, J.E., Fowler, K.: The Ability of Microcalcification Descriptors in the BI-RADS 4th Edition to Stratify the Risk of Malignancy. In: Proc. of 91th RSNA, November 27, 2005, Chicago, U.S.A.
13. Fields, S., Lederman, R., Buchbinder, S., Novak, B., Sklair, M., Bamberger, P., Leichter, I.: Improved mammographic accuracy with CAD assisted ranking of lesions. In: Proc. of the 6th IWDM, June 2002, Bremen, Germany
14. Fields, S., Leichter, I., Lederman, R., Buchbinder, S., Novak, B,, Sklair Levy, M., Sperber F., Bamberger, P.: Improving the Performance of Mammographic Assessment by the use of an Advanced Two- tiered CAD/CAC System.. In: Proc. of the 7th IWDM, June 2004, Charlotte, NC, U.S.A.
15. Leichter, I., Lederman, R., Bamberger, P., Novak, B., Fields, S., Buchbinder, S.: The use of an interactive software program for quantitative characterization of microcalcifications on digitized film-screen mammograms. Invest. Radiol. (1999) 34:394-400.

Addressing Image Variability While Learning Classifiers for Detecting Clusters of Micro-calcifications

Glenn Fung[1], Balaji Krishnapuram[1], Nicolas Merlet[2], Eli Ratner[2], Philippe Bamberger[2], Jonathan Stoeckel[3], and R. Bharat Rao[1]

[1] Computer Aided Diagnosis & Therapy group, Siemens Medical Solutions USA, Inc., 51 Valley Stream Pkwy, Malvern, PA-19355, USA
[2] Siemens Computer Aided Diagnosis, 8 Hartoum St, Beck building, Jerusalem 91450, Israel
[3] Siemens Information Systems Ltd, 84 Keonics, Hosur Road, Bangalore 590100, India

Abstract. Computer aided detection systems for mammography typically use standard classification algorithms from machine learning for detecting lesions. However, these general purpose learning algorithms make implicit assumptions that are commonly violated in CAD problems. We propose a new ensemble algorithm that explicitly accounts for the small fraction of outlier images which tend to produce a large number of false positives. A bootstrapping procedure is used to ensure that the candidates from these outlier images do not skew the statistical properties of the training samples. Experimental studies on the detection of clusters of micro-calcifications indicate that the proposed method significantly outperforms a state-of-the-art general purpose method for designing classifiers (SVM), in terms of FROC curves on a hold out test set.

1 Introduction

In *computer aided diagnosis* (CAD) applications the goal is to detect structures of interest to physicians in medical images: *e.g.* to identify potentially malignant lesions in mammography. In an almost universal paradigm, this problem is addressed by a 3 stage system: identification of potentially unhealthy candidate *regions of interest* (ROI) from a medical image, computation of descriptive features for each candidate, and classification of each candidate (*e.g.* normal or diseased) based on its features.

This paper focusses on automatic algorithms for designing (*i.e.* learning) pattern classifiers for the third stage. Automatic learning algorithms are an important part of the modern methodology for efficiently designing computer aided diagnostic products. Besides improving the diagnostic accuracy, these technologies greatly reduce the time required to develop algorithms that act as "second readers".

In the context of computer aided mammography, many standard algorithms (*e.g.* support vector machines, Back-propagation for Neural Nets, Kernel Fisher Discriminants) have been used to learn classifiers for detecting malignant lesions in computer aided mammography [1, 2, 3]. However, these general purpose learning methods make implicit assumptions that are commonly violated in CAD applications, often resulting in sub-optimal prediction accuracy for the classifiers that they learn. For example, these methods almost universally assume that the training samples are *independently* drawn from an *identical*—albeit unobservable—underlying distribution (i.i.d. assumption).

Susan M. Astley et al. (Eds.): IWDM 2006, LNCS 4046, pp. 84–91, 2006.

We propose a new ensemble algorithm that is designed to improve the classification accuracy. This algorithm explicitly accounts for the fact that a set of outlier images tend to produce a large number of false (true) positives in the training set used to learn classifiers, whereas many other images only contribute relatively few positive (negative) samples each. A bootstrapping procedure is used to ensure that the candidates from these outlier images do not skew the statistical properties of the training set.

When we learnt a classifier using a standard state-of-the-art method—support vector machine (SVM)—for detecting clusters of micro-calcs, the resulting system performed (generalized) poorly on a hold out set of test samples, in terms of per-image sensitivity & per-patient sensitivity. By contrast, the proposed methods significantly improved the ROC curves, especially in the operating region of interest (around 0.2 FP per image).

The rest of the paper is organized as follows. Section 2 highlights some of the assumptions that underly almost all algorithms for learning pattern classifiers, and indicates why some of them may be inappropriate for CAD. Based on this analysis, Section 3 develops a novel method for learning classifiers that detect clusters of microcalcifications. Experimental results are provided in Section 4. We conclude with a discussion of the broader applicability of the proposed algorithm and some ideas for future extensions in Section 5.

2 Common Assumptions While Learning Pattern Classifiers

2.1 Creation of the Training Data

During the design of a CAD system, considerable human intervention and domain knowledge engineering is employed in the first two stages of a CAD system for (a) candidate generation (CG): identifying all potentially suspicious regions in a candidate generation stage with very high sensitivity, and (b) feature-extraction: description of each such region quantitatively using a set of medically relevant features. For example quantitative measurements based on texture, shape, intensity and contrast and other such characteristics may be used to characterize any region of interest (ROI). Subsequently, for learning the classifier to be used in the third stage, a training dataset is created by obtaining features which describe each candidate ROI in the training images, and class labels are assigned to them based upon the overlap and/or distance from any radiologist-marked (diseased) region.

2.2 Characteristic Properties of the Data

A few important characteristics of the data are relevant for designing classifiers that generalize well. First, there is a form of stochastic dependence between the labeling errors of a group of candidates, all of which are spatially proximate to the same radiologist mark. Further, the features used to describe spatially adjacent or overlapping samples are also highly correlated. As a result, both the labels and the features for the training samples from an image tend to be highly correlated: the inter sample correlation is particularly high for spatially adjacent candidates.

Second, some types of biological or image structures tend to be identified much more often by CG algorithms in the form of many spatially adjacent candidates. This introduces a sampling bias in the training dataset: *i.e.* the CG algorithm tends to have varying levels of sensitivity to different type of structures. Also, some training images tend to contain far more false positive candidates as compared to the rest of the training database, due to noise or various imaging artifacts present in them.

2.3 Shortcomings in Standard Classification Algorithms

In the CAD literature, many machine learning algorithms—such as *neural networks, support vector machines* (SVM), and *Fisher's linear discriminant*—have been employed to train classifiers. However, almost all the standard methods for classifier design explicitly make certain assumptions that are violated by the somewhat special characteristics of the data as discussed above.

In particular, most of the algorithms assume that the training samples or instances are drawn *identically* and *independently* from an underlying (unknown) distribution. However, as mentioned above, due to spatial adjacency of the regions identified by a candidate generator, both the features and the class labels of several adjacent training candidates are highly correlated.

Further, the standard methods for classifier design implicitly assume that the appropriate measure for evaluating the classifier is based only on the accuracy of the system on a per-lesion basis. In other words, these algorithms try to most correctly classify each candidate from the CG algorithm; they do not account for the sampling bias introduced by the common tendency of CG algorithms to produce more candidates corresponding to certain types of structures and fewer candidates corresponding to others.

The appropriate measure of accuracy for evaluating a CAD system is different from the standard measures that are optimized by conventional classifiers. In particular, even if one of the candidates that refers to the underlying malignant structure is correctly highlighted to the radiologist, the *lesion* is detected. Thus, correct classification of every candidate instance is not as important as the ability to detect *at least one* candidate that points to a malignant lesion. At another level, in many CAD problems it is even more relevant to measure the accuracy in terms of FROC curves plotting the per-patient sensitivity—the fraction of diseased patients correctly identified by the system—versus the rate of false positives per patient.

These considerations motivated the development of a novel algorithm for learning ensemble classifiers in an effort to adjust for the sampling bias of the CG algorithm and the correlations between subsets of samples for the same image or patient.

3   Learning Ensemble Classifiers for CAD Using Bagging

Instead of learning a single classifier, we learn a set (ensemble) of k classifiers. The final prediction of the ensemble is obtained by weighted voting, *i.e.* the final prediction is obtained by averaging the predictions of the classifiers in the ensemble. Furthermore, in order to promote diversity in the ensemble, we use the technique known as bagging [4], where each classifier is trained on a random redistribution of the training set. In our case, each classifier's training set is generated by randomly drawing, without replacement, N^+ positive examples and N^- negative examples from the original training set.

Most machine learning algorithms tend to be biased toward the majority class when provided with a very unbalanced training set, *i.e.* the number of negatives samples (false positive candidates) is much larger that the number of positive samples. In order to address this issue and to reduce computational complexity, for each of the classifiers in the ensemble we chose N^- to be a relatively smaller number ($N^- = 1000$ was chosen by tuning in our experiments). The number of positives N^+ was chosen as a function of the number of positive images in the training set. For each positive image in the training set only i positive samples were randomly chosen from all the positive candidates in the image.

Each one of the linear classifiers in the ensemble is obtained using the Relevance Vector Machine algorithm (RVM) [5]. RVM is a Bayesian formulation for learning logistic regression classifiers. It relies on a form of automatic relevance determination (ARD) to select a small subset of diagnostically useful features while simultaneously learning a linear classifier. Enforcing each member of the ensemble to depend on a small number of features also promotes diversity of the ensemble since each classifier tends to make predictions based on different features.

Next, we present our proposed algorithm to learn an ensemble classifier for detecting clusters of micro-calcifications from digital mammograms:

Algorithm 1. *BuildEnsemble* **return:** $W = \begin{bmatrix} w^1, \ldots, w^{nc} \end{bmatrix}$:

0. Given
  - *the number nc that defines the number of classifiers in the ensemble.*
  - *The* training set *comprised of a matrix $A \in R^{m \times n}$ (m is the number of points and n is the number of input features and the vector $l \in \{1, -1\}^m$ containing the labels.*
  - *The number of positive points N^+ and negative points N^- to be randomly selected to train each one of the nc classifiers members of the ensemble.*

1. initialize $k = 0$
2. If $k = nc$, stop, return the matrix $W \in R^{n \times nc}$ hyperplane coefficients $W = \begin{bmatrix} w^1, \ldots, w^{nc} \end{bmatrix}$
3. otherwise, generate training set for classifier k by randomly drawing, without replacement, N^+ positive examples and N^- negative examples from the original training set.
4. Obtain the coefficients w^k for classifier k using a general purpose RVM classifier.
5. do $k = k + 1$; go to step 2.

Given an unseen sample (column vector) $x \in R^n$, the final ensemble classifier prediction is given by:

$$pred(x) = \frac{1}{nc} \sum_{k=1}^{nc} \frac{1}{1 + \exp(-x^T w^k)}.$$

4 Experiments

Our numerical experiments were performed in a dataset consisting of 37098 microcalcification clusters candidates extracted from 1891 digitized film-screen mammography (FSM) images belonging to 621 cases (242 Malignant and 379 normals). Each candidate consists of a vector of 1051 descriptors or features that were extracted from the microcalcification clusters candidates based on shape, texture, density , etc. The images of all the cases were digitized at high resolution (600 dpi, 12 bit) by a prototype CAD device developed by Siemens CAD, Israel. In order to validate the generalization performance of the proposed system, the available 621 cases were randomly divided into two subsets:

- A *training set* comprised of 945 images from 311 cases (190 normals and 121 malignants). 744 of the The 945 images belong to the normal cases (normal images) and the remaining 201 images belong to the malign cases. The total number of candidates (generated by the CG algorithm) in the training set is 18459, only 443 of these candidates are real microcalcification clusters, the remaining 18016 are false positives.
- A *testing* or *validation set* comprised of 946 images from 310 cases (189 normals and 121 malignants). 754 of the The 946 images belong to the normal cases (normal images) and the remaining 192 images belong to the malign cases. The total number of candidates in the training set is 18639; 462 of these candidates are real microcalcification clusters, the remaining 18177 are false positives.

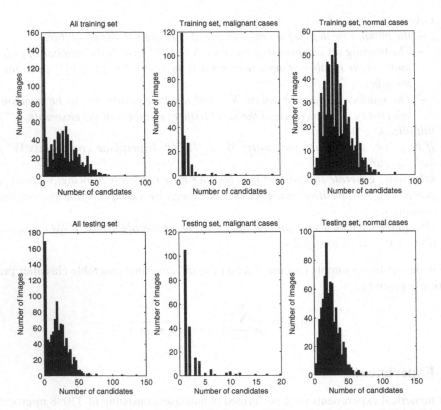

Fig. 1. Histograms for all the candidates, malignant candidates only, and for normal candidates. Notice that some of the outlier images in both the training and the testing set have an unusually large number of positive and negative candidates.

The number of positive candidates to be randomly chosen from each positive image is denoted as i. Therefore, the final number of positive candidates depends on the choice of i and the number of positive images. Since our training set contains 201 malignant images, when $i = 2$, this results in randomly choosing up to 402 positive candidates to be included in the training set. In other words,up to 2 candidates were chosen from each malignant image; some images may not have 2 positive clusters, in that case only one was picked. Our choice of $i = 1$ gave the best results. The number of classifiers in the ensemble k was empirically fixed to 101.

The idea behind this positive samples sampling scheme is to drive the ensemble classifier performance to be optimized to maximize the sensitivity per image instead of sensitivity per individual cluster. In other words, by sampling positive clusters uniformly across all the positive images, the classifier gets to learn a more heterogeneous concept of malignant clusters. By using all the positives candidates, the classifier may get biased by some of the rare images with an unusually large number of positive candidates (see Figure 1). These outlier images are not representative of the general population of positive images.

4.1 Comparison to a Standard SVM

We compared the accuracy of our algorithm against an efficient implementation of a SVM [6]. Since SVMs have a tuning parameter—the tradeoff between the accuracy and the regularization terms—we used cross-validation to select it based on the training set. Although most conventional methods for classifier design focus exclusively on maximizing accuracy at a cluster level, CAD applications are frequently evaluated in different terms. It is clinically important to also measure: (a) sensitivity while detecting images with malignant clusters; and (b) sensitivity while detecting patients with malignant clusters). Figures 2,3 and 4 show that our proposed method is considerable more robust and generalize better on the unseen data at all levels (per cluster, per image and per patient respectively).

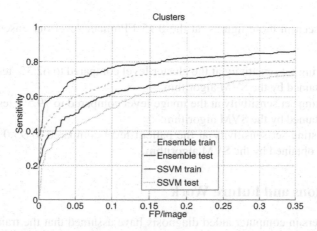

Fig. 2. Comparisons of a SVM and the proposed ensemble for cluster detection

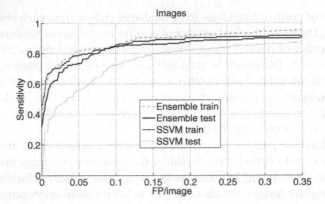

Fig. 3. Comparisons of a SVM and the proposed ensemble for correctly detecting at least one malignant cluster in an image (with a malignant cluster)

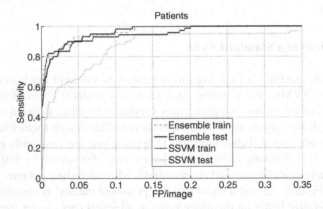

Fig. 4. Comparisons of a SVM and the proposed ensemble for correctly detecting at least one malignant cluster in a patient (with a malignant cluster)

As can be seen in these figures, at the 0.15 FP/image level our ensemble method obtained:

- 66.5% testing set sensitivity at the cluster level compared to 62.3% testing set sensitivity obtained by the SVM algorithm.
- 88.8% testing set sensitivity at the image level compared to 79.5% testing set sensitivity obtained by the SVM algorithm.
- 100.0% testing set sensitivity at the patient level compared to 95.0% testing set sensitivity obtained by the SVM algorithm.

5   Discussions and Future Work

Most researchers in computer aided diagnosis have assumed that the training data for learning classifiers satisfies some general assumptions like sample independence, and an identical distribution for all patients. Hence, many previously published papers in the mammography literature use general purpose algorithms to learn classifiers without acknowledging that their assumptions are commonly violated in CAD applications.

In this paper, we highlighted several characteristics of the data that make the use of standard algorithms inappropriate in digital mammography, *e.g.* samples from the same patient are strongly correlated. Further, all training samples are not drawn from the same (identical) distribution, *e.g.* the distribution of samples drawn from a very dense breast is clearly different from the samples drawn from a fatty breast. The results of this article show that explicitly accounting for these factors can improve the sensitivity and decrease the number of false positives per case, leading to a real clinical benefit. This improvement is particularly significant on an independent test set, especially in terms of per-image and per-patient sensitivity.

Nevertheless, even further gains in accuracy may be achievable by improving the statistical models for the data that are employed while learning these classifiers. Although our current model ignores this, in future work we intend to explicitly account for the fact that the correlation between samples is a function of the spatial distance between them. We are also investigating models that account for the fact that samples from the same patient are also correlated though they may be from different images.

References

1. Fu, J., Lee, S., Wong, S., Yeh, J., Wang, A., Wu, H.: Image segmentation, feature selection and pattern classification for mammographic microcalcifications. Comput Med Imaging Graph **9** (2005) 419–429
2. Pappadopolous, A., Fotiadis, D., Likas, A.: Characterization of clustered microcalcifications in digitized mammograms using neural networks and support vector machines. Artificial Intelligence in Medicine **34** (2005) 141–150
3. Wei, L., Yang, Y., Nishikawa, R., Jiang, Y.: A study of several machine learning methods for classification of malignant and benign microcalcifications. IEEE Transactions on Medical Imaging **24** (2005) 371–380
4. Brieman, L.: Bagging predictors. Machine Learning (1996)
5. Tipping, M.E.: Sparse Bayesian learning and the relevance vector machine. Journal of Machine Learning Research **1** (2001) 211–244
6. Lee, Y.J., Mangasarian, O.L.: SSVM: A smooth support vector machine. Computational Optimization and Applications **20** (2001) 5–22 Data Mining Institute, University of Wisconsin, Technical Report 99-03. ftp://ftp.cs.wisc.edu/pub/dmi/tech-reports/99-03.ps.

Computer-Aided Detection of Breast Cancer Using an Ultra High-Resolution Liquid Crystal Display: Reading Session Analysis

Yoshifumi Kuroki[1,*], Shigeru Nawano[1], Hidefumi Kobatake[2], Nachiko Uchiyama[4], Kazuo Shimura[3], and Kouji Matano[3]

[1] Natonal Cancer Center Hospital East, Chiba, Japan
[2] Tokyo University of Agriculture and Technology, Tokyo, Japan
[3] Fuji Photo Film Co., Ltd., Japan
[4] Research Center for Cancer Prevention and Screening

Abstract. We performed a reading session to examine the validity of computer-aided detection for mammograms using a 3-megapixel liquid crystal display (LCD). Digital mammograms of 225 patients (ROLAD M-IV and FCR9000, 100 µ/pixel), were divided into 3 data sets (each set consisting of 75 patients, including 30 with pathologically proven breast cancer) for this reading session. Fifteen physicians interpreted these three data set using 3 different imaging modalities; hard copy, LCD without computer-aided detection (CAD), and LCD with CAD. Then they categorized the images into 4 ranks according to the confidential levels of cancer. Sensitivity and specificity were calculated individually for each of the 3 different modalities, and then ROC analysis was performed. The sensitivity, specificity, and Az values showed no significant differences between LCD with out CAD and hard copy. Also, no significant differences were found between LCD with CAD and the other modalities for these 3 values. The results of this study indicate that it is reasonable to use a 3-megapixel LCD for interpretation of digital mammograms instead of conventional hard copy. Nevertheless, because the usefulness of the CAD system has not been fully ascertained, further studies are required.

1 Background

The morbidity and mortality rate of breast cancer in Japan are showing a tendency to increase. Since early detection of breast cancer is essential to decrease deaths from this disease, the importance of screening for breast cancer by mammography (MMG) is currently emphasized. Therefore, MMG will be introduced for breast cancer screening and the frequency of reading mammograms will increase rapidly as a result. However, it is feared that the number of interpreters specializing in diagnosis of mammograms will not be adequate to cope with such a rapid increase in demand. On the other hand, it has been reported that the false-negative rate of MMG for breast cancer screening is above the acceptable range. Since the quality of image interpretation largely depends on the training, experience, and diligence of the interpreter performing the task, it is important to develop an image reading system that can cope with such a rapid increase in the frequency of reading mammograms, while ensuring the high quality of interpretation.

---

* Corresponding author. E-mail address is ykuroki@east.ncc.go.jp

Susan M. Astley et al. (Eds.): IWDM 2006, LNCS 4046, pp. 92–96, 2006.
© Springer-Verlag Berlin Heidelberg 2006

Computer-aided detection (CAD) is one of the methods that can be used to solve this problem. Computer technology has made rapid advances in recent years, and CAD has been reported to be useful for cancer screening by chest CT. Application of CAD to MMG has been performed clinically since the U.S. Food and Drug Administration approved the first commercial CAD system in 1998. Digitization of information is essential for the use of CAD, and 2 methods are available for this purpose, which are 1) the digitization of conventional radiographic films and 2) direct use of digital data obtained by digital radiography, including computed radiography (CR). The diagnostic accuracy of MMG performed with CR (CR-MMG) is adequate in the case of hard copy. However, to use a system employing CAD more efficiently, it is obvious that a liquid crystal display (LCD) should be employed instead of the hard copy. However, it is necessary that the accuracy of image interpretation using LCD should be equal to that of using hard copy. In the present study, we performed a large-scale reading session to compare the diagnostic accuracy between LCD and hard copy in order to investigate the usefulness of a CR-MMG CAD system.

2 Materials and Methods

At the National Cancer Center Hospital East, CR-MMG was performed in 1,300 patients over 1 year from 1998 to 1999 using LORAD M-IV () and FCR9000 (Fuji Photo Film, Tokyo, Japan). The sampling size was 0.1 mm. From these 1,300 patients, 90 patients with pathologically confirmed breast cancers (≤20 mm) and 135 patients without breast cancer based on pathological examination or follow-up were selected. These 90 breast cancer patients and 135 patients without breast cancer (225 patients in total) were divided into 3 data sets, each of which comprised 75 patients including 30 with breast cancer. During the process of obtaining patients for the data sets, patients for whom it was excessively difficult to make a diagnosis and patients whose images were not obtained in adequate body positions were excluded by consensus between 3 radiologists who were experienced in reading mammograms, so that the difficulty of diagnosis was equalized among the data sets. Patients with bilateral breast cancer and a history of prior treatment for breast cancer were also excluded.

The LCD used for this reading session was an SL-IC300G (Fuji Photo Film, Tokyo, Japan). This was a so-called 3-megapixel LCD with a matrix of 2,048 × 1,536 pixels. The pixel size was 0.207 mm, the brightness was 500 cd/m², the contrast ratio was 600:1, and the gray scale resolution was 766. When reading the images, increasing the magnification and changing the window level/window width were possible. As the hard copy for this reading session, laser prints from a DryPix7000 (Fuji Photo Film, Tokyo, Japan) and DI-AL films (Fuji Photo Film, Tokyo, Japan) were used. We employed 12 bit D/A conversion, 0.05 mm writing, and 3.6 Dmax. For the characteristic curve of CR, pure T-gradation and pattern enhancement processing for mammography (PEM) were combined.

The CAD software used for this reading session was developed jointly by Tokyo University of Agriculture and Technology, Fuji Photo Film Co., Ltd., and us. Image data were transmitted directly from the FCR9000 to a computer for CAD. Candidate regions of tumor masses and microcalcifications were calculated separately using different programs. These regions were indicated with arrows and rectangles for masses and microcalcifications, respectively, on the LCD display. Approximately 2 minutes was required for assessment of 4 images from 1 patient. The performance of CAD with data sets used for this reading session was as follows; true positive rate of 91.5% (83% for masses and 100% for microcalcifications), and false positive of 2.8/case (1.4/case for masses and microcalcifications).

A total of 4 images obtained from each patient were used for this reading session. These were bilateral mediolateral oblique and craniocaudal views. The 3 data sets, each of which contained 75 patients including breast cancer patients, were assigned at random to 1 of 3 modalities: hard copy, LCD without CAD, and LCD with CAD. Images were diagnosed by 15 interpreteres qualified for MMG assessment who did not know the results. Before the image reading session, they received training in use of CAD for approximately 30 min with images of 10 patients who were not included in any of the data sets used for this session. In addition, they were given an explanation of the estimated number of breast cancer patients included in each data set and the performance of CAD. Each interpreter interpreted 900 films obtained from the 225 subjects with no duplications.

During image reading, the site of a suspected lesion was marked on the test paper, and the confidential level of cancer was expressed using the following 4 ranks; confidential level (0) "no cancer (no mark)," confidential level (1) "possible cancer," confidential level (2) "probable cancer," and confidential level (3) "definite cancer." Based on these confidential levels, ROC analysis was performed using ROCkit as software. Confidential levels (0) and (1) were considered negative, while confidential levels (2) and (3) were regarded as positive when performing the calculation of sensitivity and specificity. The imaging findings suggestive of breast cancer were classified as a mass lesions pattern, a microcalcifications pattern, and a mass lesions plus microcalcifications pattern. Then the mass lesions pattern was further classified as a typical mass lesions pattern and a FAD or architectural distortion (AD) pattern. Sensitivity of image interpretation was compared between LCD with CAD or without CAD.

3 Results

In the whole subjects, the sensitivity value was 0.64 for hard copy, 0.64 for LCD, and 0.59 for CAD. The specificity value was 0.95 for hard copy, 0.96 for LCD, and 0.97 for CAD. The Az value was 0.89 for hard copy, 0.90 for LCD, and 0.91 for CAD. There were no significant differences in the sensitivity, specificity, or Az values among the modalities used.

Overall results of three modalities

Modality	Az value	Sensitivity	Specificity
Hard copy	0.89	0.64	0.95
LCD without CAD	0.90	0.64	0.96
LCD with CAD	0.91	0.59	0.97

Breast cancer was detected in 174 images. A mass lesions pattern was noted in 136 images, while a microcalcifications pattern and a mass lesions plus microcalcifications pattern (CALC) were seen in the other 38 images. A mass lesions pattern was classified as typical mass lesions pattern (MASS) and a FAD or AD pattern (FAD/AD) noted in 75 images and 61 images, respectively. The table shows the relationship of each detection patterns by CAD and the sensitivity of each modality.

Correlation of sensitivity and modalities in MASS

Modality	CAD positive	CAD negative
LCD without CAD	0.95	0.40
LCD with CAD	0.93	0.30

Correlation of sensitivity and modalities in FAD/AD

Modality	CAD positive	CAD negative
LCD without CAD	0.65	0.42
LCD with CAD	0.72	0.29

Correlation of sensitivity and modalities in CAL

Modality	CAD positive	CAD negative
LCD without CAD	0.90	1.00
LCD with CAD	0.93	0.60

When we paid our attention to cases that CAD could point out lesions accurately (CAD positive), regardless of employment of CAD, sensitivity had no statistic difference about MASS, FAD/AD, neither of CALC. On the other hand, in cases of CAD could not point out lesions accurately (CAD negative), when CAD was employed, we understood that sensitivity was low statistically about FAD/AD, though there was no difference about MASS. Also when CAD failed to indicate microcalcifications, interpreters tend to overlook it.

4 Discussion

Introduction of CAD is considered essential for coping with an increase in the number of subjects undergoing MMG for breast cancer screening in the future and for ensuring the quality of mammogram interpretation. There is little doubt that Interpretation with CAD by using LCD is the most appropriate combination for efficient application of CAD.

As a prerequisite for image reading by LCD, it was necessary to confirm that the diagnostic accuracy of LCD was at least as high as that obtained with conventional hard copy. In the present study, the 3-megapixel LCD was clearly inferior to hard copy with regard to resolution and gray scale resolution, but there were no significant differences of Az value, sensitivity, or specificity between the two modalities. This was presumably because LCD images could be change imaging parameters such as window level/width and magnified ratio appropriately and enhanced by image processing techniques including PEM for the diagnosis of microcalcifications. Since CAD is excellent for detection of microcalcifications, a combination of CAD and LCD with image processing techniques and magnification may be very useful for the diagnosis of microcalcifications. For the diagnosis of mass lesions, it appears that the interpreters could make up for the disadvantage of lower gray scale resolution by adjusting the window level/width of LCD. Since the density of mammary glands varies in each patient, it is more appropriate to perform image reading while adjusting the window level/width according to the density of the mammary glands in each patient than with fixed settings as in hard copy. Owing to these characteristics of LCD, its diagnostic accuracy was presumably as high as that of hard copy despite the disadvantages of lower resolution and gray scale resolution.

In the present study, the Az value and specificity of CAD tended to be higher than those of LCD and hard copy, but no statistically significant differences were noted among the three modalities. When detection by CAD and its sensitivity were investigated in detail, there were no significant differences of sensitivity between the modalities in relation to the detection of typical mass lesions and microcalcifications for which diagnosis was relatively easy. On the other hand, in the FAD or AD group in which diagnosis was difficult, there were no significant differences of sensitivity between the modalities when candidate lesions could be indicated by CAD, while the sensitivity of CAD was significantly lower than that of LCD when candidate lesions could not be indicated by CAD. These results suggest that the interpreters tended to place too much confidence in the results of CAD when diagnosis was relatively difficult. CAD should not be regarded as a second interpreter, but should be used to prevent overlook. However, in the present study, the interpreters presumably used CAD as another interpreter and depended on its results when they had difficulty in making a diagnosis, in result CAD was not used appropriately. Prior to using CAD, interpreters should be given a full explanation of its performance and appropriate use and should be trained so that they can use it appropriately. It is conceivable that the inappropriate use of CAD was one of the causes of failure to statistically confirm its usefulness in the present reading session. Further studies will be necessary to define the value of CAD, including training methods for its appropriate use.

5 Conclusion

It was confirmed statistically by the present study that the diagnostic accuracy of 3-megapixel LCD was as high as that of interpreting conventional hard copy. The usefulness of CAD was not confirmed statistically, presumably because of insufficient training of the interpreters. It is therefore necessary to conduct further studies on the value of CAD, including training methods for appropriate using CAD.

References

1. Timothy W. Freer, Michael J. Ulissey, Screening Mammography with Computer-aided Detection: Prospective Study of 12,860 Patients in a Community Breast Center, Radiology 2001; 220:781-786
2. Mark A. Helvie, Lubomir Hadjiiski, Heang-Ping Chan, et.al, Sensitivity of Noncommercial Computer-aided Detection System for Mammographic Breast Cancer Detection: Pilot Clinical Trial, Radiology 2004; 231:208-214
3. S.M.Astley, F.J.Gilbert, Computer-aided detection in mammography, Clinical Radiology 2004; 59:390-399

Mammography Reading with Computer-Aided Detection (CAD): Performance of Different Readers

Susan M. Astley[1], Stephen W. Duffy[2], Caroline R.M. Boggis[3], Mary Wilson[3],
Nicky B. Barr[3], Ursula M. Beetles[3], Miriam A. Griffiths[3], Anil Jain[3], Jill Johnson[3],
Rita M. Roberts[3], Heather Deans[4], Karen Duncan[4], Geeta Iyengar[4],
Olorunsola Agbaje[2], Pamela M. Griffiths[1], Magnus A. McGee[5],
Maureen G.C. Gillan[6], and Fiona J. Gilbert[6]

[1] Department of Imaging Science & Biomedical Engineering, University of Manchester,
Manchester, UK
{Astley, Griffiths, sue.astley}@manchester.ac.uk
[2] Department of Epidemiology, Mathematics & Statistics, Wolfson Institute of
Preventive Medicine, London, UK
{Duffy, stephen.duffy}@cancer.org.uk,
{Agbaje, Olorunsola.Agbaje}@cancer.org.uk
[3] Nightingale Centre, Withington Hospital, Manchester,UK
{Boggis, Wilson, Barr, Beetles, Griffiths, Jain, Johnson,
Roberts, caroline.boggis}@dsl.pipex.com
[4] NE Scotland Breast Screening Centre, Aberdeen UK
{Deans, Duncan, Iyengar, heather.deans}@nhs.net
[5] Department of Public Health & General Practice, Christchurch School of Medicine, NZ
{McGee, magnus.mcgee}@chmeds.ac.nz
[6] Department of Radiology, University of Aberdeen, UK
{Gilbert, Gillan, f.j.gilbert}@abdn.ac.uk

Abstract. Computer-aided detection (CAD) systems place prompts in digital images to attract readers' attention to potential malignancies. A reader must then decide whether or not prompted regions correspond to genuine abnormalities and has the option of disregarding falsely prompted regions. In this paper we investigate different readers' performance with CAD in the context of breast screening. In a retrospective study, eight consultant radiologists each read over 1000 screening mammograms comprising normal cases, screen detected cancer cases and cases that were detected as cancers subsequently. We present their results in terms of cancer detection and recall rates, and relate this to their previous experience of film reading. Our results show that the detection of cancers did not differ significantly between readers, although more experienced film readers were less likely to recommend that normal cases should be recalled.

1 Introduction

Computer-aided detection (CAD) systems can be used to prompt abnormalities that might otherwise be overlooked by a film reader [1]. In order to achieve sufficient sensitivity to genuine abnormalities, CAD algorithms also prompt normal regions

Susan M. Astley et al. (Eds.): IWDM 2006, LNCS 4046, pp. 97–104, 2006.

which have some abnormal features [2]. It is the responsibility of the reader using the CAD system to decide whether prompted regions are actually abnormal, or whether the prompts should be disregarded.

Readers in the UK Breast Screening Programme are closely monitored and subject to a number of regulations to ensure good performance; readers must read more than 5,000 screening mammograms per year, participate in clinical meetings and assessment clinics, and have their performance evaluated on a set of difficult mammograms. Despite this, there is still variation in performance between readers. Some of this may be due to experience; the most experienced readers in the breast screening programme have read many tens of thousands of films, whilst newly eligible readers will have read a much smaller number.

Computer-aided detection has been suggested as a way of improving the performance of readers, but different readers may respond in different ways to CAD prompts [3]. In this paper we use data from a study comparing double reading to single reading with CAD to investigate whether there were significant differences in performance with CAD between the eight consultant radiologists who took part.

2 Methods

In the CAD Evaluation Trial (CADET) [4], 10,096 mammograms, originally double read in 1996, were re-read in 2003 by a single reader using an ImageChecker M1000 CM System (R2 Technology, Inc. Sunnyvale, CA) with software version 5.0, a CheckMate Ultra Display Unit with PeerView and Variable Sized Markers [5]. The case-mix was a cohort from the UK National Health Service Breast Screening Programme (NHSBSP) enriched by 50% by the random removal of normal cases. The cases were randomised in such a way that readers did not re-read in 2003 any cases that they had previously read in 1996.

The eight radiologist readers in the CADET study had between 2 and 15 years experience when the films were single read with CAD, and those who also participated in double reading in 1996 had between 1 and 8 years experience at that time. Other readers also participated in the double reading process, and overall the levels of experience of the readers in 1996 and 2003 were approximately similar.

The eight radiologists were based at two screening centres, each of which had different protocols for recalling cases. When single reading with CAD, these protocols were followed as closely as possible. In one of the screening centres (Aberdeen) a case was recalled when double reading if either reader recommended it. When single reading with CAD, a case was recalled if the single reader recommended it. In the second centre (Manchester) the recall process in double reading involved each of the readers scoring the case, and depending on the maximum score cases were either returned to normal screening, discussed with another reader or recalled. When single reading with CAD, cases were also scored and treated in a similar way. All readers in the CADET study underwent a two month training period in the use of CAD prior to commencing reading [6].

In this analysis we review the cancer detection rates for each reader (single reading the 1996 films with CAD) for those cases which had cancer detected by double reading in 1996, and those for which cancer was detected subsequently as interval cancers, at the next screen in 1999 or up to three years later. We also examine the recall rate for the cases that were normal (confirmed by two subsequent normal screens), and investigate whether differences are due to experience or to the different recall protocols at the two screening centres.

3 Results

Table 1 shows the breakdown of cases read with the aid of CAD by each of the eight consultant radiologists in CADET. The cancer cases labelled 'evaluation screen' are those detected in 1996 during the original double reading. It should be noted that those cancer cases labelled 'subsequent' were not detected in the 1996 films by the original double reading, nor were these films reviewed to determine whether they contained any visible signs of early cancer. The cancer detection rates for the cancer cases and recall rates for the normal cases are shown in table 2.

Table 1. Number of cases read using CAD by each of the eight radiologist readers in the CADET study. The cancer cases are split into those identified at the original double reading in 1996 (evaluation screen) and those detected as interval cancers or subsequently.

Reader		1	2	3	4	5	6	7	8
Cancer cases read with CAD	Evaluation screen	3	11	5	16	9	11	11	19
	Subsequent	29	22	40	52	16	32	24	15
Normal Cases		1210	1108	1202	1188	1253	1289	1301	1230

Cancers detected at the evaluation screen (the original double reading in 1996) were definitely visible in the images. It can be seen from table 2 that the proportion of these evaluation screen cancers amongst the cancer cases read with CAD varies from reader to reader. For example, less than 10% of those read by reader 1 were detected at the original double screening, whereas more than 55% of those read by reader 8 fell into this category.

The detection rates of cancers did not differ significantly between readers (p=0.8), although the number of cancer cases is relatively small. The recall rates of normal cases did, however, differ significantly among readers (p<0.001), with readers 6 and 7 having particularly high recall rates.

Table 2. Number (%) of cancer cases detected by each of the eight radiologist readers in the CADET study, and number (%) of normal cases recalled by each reader

Reader		1	2	3	4	5	6	7	8
Cancer cases detected with CAD	Evaluation screen	1 (33)	10 (91)	5 (100)	14 (88)	9 (100)	10 (91)	10 (91)	17 (89)
	Subsequent	6 (21)	3 (14)	8 (20)	11 (21)	2 (13)	10 (31)	7 (29)	3 (20)
Recalled normals		71 (6)	58 (5)	84 (7)	85 (7)	52 (4)	156 (12)	153 (12)	84 (7)

In 1996, only readers 1, 2, 3, 5 and 6 took part in double reading the CADET cases, and a number of other readers were also involved. During the double reading process the recall decision was made either as a result of both readers' judgements, or on the basis of a single reader's judgement, depending on the screening centre, so it is not possible to directly compare cancer detection rates and recall rates for individual readers with and without CAD. We do, however, have data showing the outcomes for cases in the CADET study that were double read in 1996 (table 3). Two of the readers (5 and 6) had particularly good sensitivity when double reading in 1996, although their recall rate for normal cases was similar to that of the other readers.

Table 3. CADET cases double read in 1996 by five radiologists who subsequently read with CAD. Note that all recall decisions were taken jointly with another radiologist.

Reader	Number of normal mammograms read in 1996	Number of normal cases recalled (%)	Number of cancer mammograms read in 1996	Number of cancer cases recalled (%)
1	2477	129 (5)	90	26 (29)
2	2253	131 (6)	81	12 (15)
3	1266	81 (6)	57	15 (26)
5	4849	276 (6)	135	59 (44)
6	2049	114 (6)	54	30 (56)

In figure 1, the recall rate for single reading with CAD is shown by years of screening experience for cancers that had been originally detected by double reading in 1996. Figure 2 shows recall rate for cases in which cancer was diagnosed subsequently. Logistic regression relating the probability of identification for recall to years of experience showed no significant effect, either for the 1996 screen detected cancers (p=0.9), subsequent cancers (p=0.9) or all cancers combined (p=0.5).

Figure 3 shows the recall rate by years of experience for the normal cases. There was a significant negative relationship between years of experience and proportion of normal subjects recalled (p=0.01). This is further illustrated in Table 4 where we split the readers by less than and more than ten years' experience. Those with 10 or more years of experience were less likely to recall normal subjects (OR = 0.83, 95% CI 0.71-0.92).

Table 5 shows recall rates by the single reader with CAD for normal cases, 1996 screen-detected cancers and subsequently diagnosed cancers. Manchester had significantly higher rates of recall both for normal women screened (p<0.001) and for all cancers combined (p=0.002). There was no significant difference between the two centres for 1996 cancers only, or for subsequent cancers only, although this may be due to low statistical power with relatively small numbers.

When centre and experience were assessed mutually adjusted in a multiple logistic regression analysis, these results remained unaltered: for normal cases there were significantly higher recall rates in Manchester and significantly lower recall rates for readers with more experience; for all cancers combined there were significantly

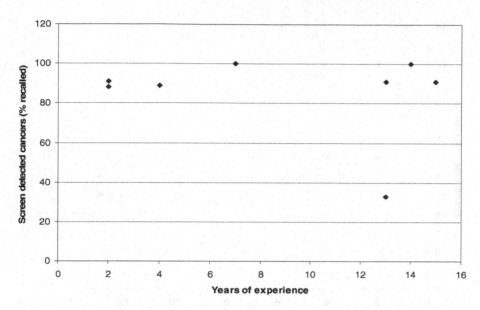

Fig. 1. The percentage of cancers screen found by double reading in 1996 that were detected by single reading with CAD, plotted against the number of years of previous breast screening experience for each reader

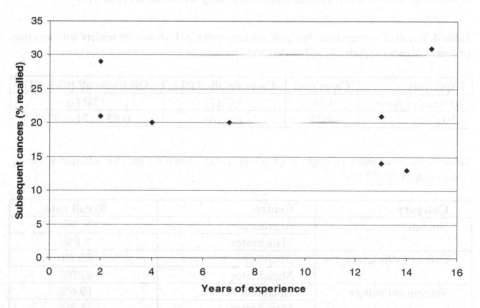

Fig. 2. The percentage of cancers found subsequently that were detected by single reading with CAD, plotted against the number of years of previous breast screening experience for each reader

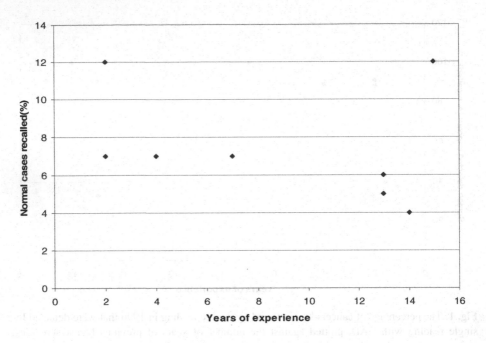

Fig. 3. The percentage of normal cases that were recalled by single reading with CAD, plotted against the number of years of previous breast screening experience for each reader

Table 4. Recall of normal cases by single reading with CAD, shown for readers with less than 10 years screening experience, and readers with 10 years or more screening experience

Experience	Cases read	Cases recalled (%)	OR for recall (95% CI)
10 years or more	4860	337 (7)	1.00 (-)
<10 years	4921	406 (8)	0.83 (0.71-0.97)

Table 5. Recall of cases by single reading with CAD, shown for the two different screening centres in the CADET trial

Category	Centre	Recall rate
Normal	Aberdeen	6.3%
	Manchester	8.8%
Cancer 1996 screen	Aberdeen	85.7%
	Manchester	92.0%
Subsequent cancer	Aberdeen	19.6%
	Manchester	25.3%
All cancers	Aberdeen	32.6%
	Manchester	49.6%

higher recall rates in Manchester, and no significant effects of experience; and no significant effects of centre or experience were observed within the 1996 cancers and within the subsequent cancers.

4 Discussion

CADET was a retrospective trial undertaken at two UK breast screening centres, comparing double reading and single reading with CAD. Although the dataset was relatively large (10,096 cases), it contained only a small proportion of cancer cases since the trial was intended to provide information about the performance of readers using CAD in a screening setting, where the vast majority of cases are normal. Consequently, the number of cancer cases read with the aid of CAD by each individual reader was small and we were not able to demonstrate a significant difference in sensitivity between the readers. Furthermore, there were two different categories of cancer cases: cases in which there were visible signs of cancer detected at the original 1996 screen by double reading, and cases in which cancer was identified at a later stage, some of which had visible signs of abnormality in the 1996 films, and some of which didn't. The proportions of these two categories allocated to the individual readers varied. It is possible that, with the small numbers of cancer cases allocated to different readers, differences in numbers and types of visible cancers could affect the results. In order to asses this, the cancer cases allocated to each reader would have to be reviewed to determine whether they were comparable in terms of visibility.

Previously published studies have shown either no increase in recall rate, or only a slight increase, with the use of CAD [1,7,8]. It is apparent that two of the radiologists in CADET had much higher recall rates of normal cases than the others, recalling 12% of normal cases. This level is greater than would be acceptable in clinical practice; even given the 50% enrichment of the CADET case-mix we would expect recall rates to be in the range 7-10%. There are a number of possible reasons for this. Firstly, CADET had a retrospective design, so the readers were aware that there were not the same constraints on them as there would be in routine reading, namely that women recommended for recall would not actually be subject to unnecessary further investigation should their mammograms turn out to be normal. There may have been a tendency for some readers to attempt to detect the very early cancers that were missed in the original double reading at the expense of the recall rate for normal cases. It is worth noting that both the readers who had high recall rates also had high cancer detection rates for the early cancers.

In 1996, when the cases were double read without CAD, all the readers who participated had broadly similar recall rates, albeit in conjunction with a second reader. Furthermore, when the cases were re-read all eight readers were participating in a national screening programme with stringent quality control procedures; when reading without the aid of CAD they were thus operating within normal limits. One possible reason for the significant variation in recall rates when reading with CAD is a difference in the ability or willingness of readers to dismiss prompts marking abnormal regions of the mammograms. This may resolve with further experience, but as yet there is insufficient data to determine how performance with a CAD system changes over time.

The results show that readers with greater experience of breast screening recalled significantly fewer normal cases when single reading with CAD than did less experienced readers. This could be due to more experienced readers having greater confidence in rejecting CAD markers placed in normal regions. Further analysis showed that this effect was not due to the difference in reading protocols between the two screening centres.

The results showed a significant difference in recall rates between the two screening centres, with higher recall rates for both normal and cancer cases in the centre that employed a form of arbitration to decide whether to recall equivocal cases. Some of this effect may be attributed to differences in the case mix between the two centres, but nevertheless it merits further investigation: it may be that in order to achieve sensitivities comparable to double reading, a single reader using CAD must refer a proportion of cases for arbitration by a second reader.

References

1. Burhenne, LW, Wood S, D'Orsi CJ, Feig SA, Kopans DB, O'Shaughnessy KF, et al. Potential contribution of computer-aided detection to the sensitivity of screening mammography. *Radiology* 2000; 215(2):554-62
2. Ciatto S, Ambrogetti D, Bonardi R et al Comparison of two commercial systems for computer aided detection (CAD) as an aid to interpreting screening mammograms. Radiol Med (Torino) 2004; 107 (5-6) : 480-488
3. Balleyguier C, Kinkel K et al Computer-aided detection (CAD) in mammography: does it help the junior or senior radiologist? Eur J Radiol 2005 54(1): 90-6
4. Gilbert FJ, Astley SM, McGee MA, Gillan MGC, Boggis CRM, Griffiths PM and Duffy SW. Comparison of double reading and single reading with CAD in the UK NHS Breast Screening Program: Computer Aided Detection Evaluation Trial. (CADET). *Radiology* (In press)
5. http://www.r2tech.com/mammography/home/index.php accessed 10.02.06
6. Astley S, Quarterman C, Al Nuami Y et al. Computer-aided detection in screening mammography: the impact of training on reader performance. In: IWDM 2004, Ed E. Pisano, 2005:231-236
7. Freer TW, Ulissey MJ. Screening mammography with computer-aided detection: prospective study of 12,860 patients in a community breast center. Radiology 2001; 220:781-786
8. Gur D, Sumkin JH, Rockette HE, et al. Changes in breast cancer detection and mammography recall rates after the introduction of a computer-aided detection system. J Natl Cancer Inst 2004; 96:185-190.

The Impact of Integration of Computer-Aided Detection and Human Observers

Nachiko Uchiyama[1], Noriyuki Moriyama[1], Takayuki Yamada[2], and Noriaki Ohuchi[3]

[1] Department of Cancer Screening, Research Center for Cancer Prevention and Screening, National Cancer Center 5-1-1, Tsukiji, Chuo-Ku, Tokyo, Japan, 104-0045
nuchiyam@ncc.go.jp
[2] Department of Radiology, Tohoku University 1-1, Seiryomachi, Aoba-Ku, Sendai, Miyagi, Japan, 980-8574
[3] Department of Surgical Oncology, Tohoku University 1-1, Seiryomachi, Aoba-Ku, Sendai, Miyagi, Japan, 980-8574

Abstract. We evaluated the impact of integration of CAD (Computer-Aided Detection) system and human observers in digital mammography. We com-pared the diagnostic efficacy of non-informed observers and informed observers regarding the CAD system's ability (average FP (false positive) per four images and sensitivity of microcalcifications and mass) to detect cancer. With the informed-group, we previously informed them of the accuracy of CAD. In each group, observers recorded the diagnosis before utilizing the CAD system and after utilizing the CAD system according to BI-RADs category and to six additional categories associated with diagnostic confidence. Regarding diagnostic accuracy, with the informed group, sensitivity and NPV were improved without an increase in FP. On the other hand, the diagnostic accuracy of human observers was in-fluenced by prior notification of CAD's accuracy and by CAD's performance in cancer detection itself.

1 Introduction

Recently, the performance of CAD has been improved and CAD is being used clinically in digital mammography[1-5]. In this paper, we evaluate the impact with respect to diagnostic accuracy of integrating CAD and human observers in a clinical environment, specifically that of digital mammography.

2 Methods

We utilized an indirect FFDM (full field digital mammography) system: Computed Radiography (CR) system (FCR 5000MA Plus: FUJIFILM, Japan) with 50 microns and non-commercial CAD developed by FUJIFILM, Japan. The CR images were diagnosed utilizing soft-copy reading system. The monitors were LCD (Liquid Crystal Display) with 5M pixels (EIZO NANAO CORPORATION, Japan). The clinical cases in this study were randomly selected from screening mammograms. The total number of cases was 50 including 23 malignant cases (five cases with masses and microcalcifications, five cases with masses, eight cases with microcalcifications, and five cases with FAD

Susan M. Astley et al. (Eds.): IWDM 2006, LNCS 4046, pp. 105–110, 2006.

(focal asymmetric density) or distortion) and 27 benign cases. The number of observers was ten. Three observers were radiologists and seven observers were breast surgeons. All of them were experienced at reading mammograms and passed the examination of reading mammograms in accordance with the committee in charge of the quality control manual for mammography screening in Japan. Their sensitivities and specificities were all over 85.0%. There were two randomly selected groups of observers: non-informed observers and informed observers with regard to the CAD system's accuracy. Before this study, we instructed observers in ten cases utilizing other cases including malignancies and normal cases in which CAD pointed out the lesion. The informed-observers were previously informed of the ability of the CAD system with regard to detection rate in microcalcifications and masses and the number of FP per four images. The non-informed observers were not given information regarding accuracy of CAD which was a follows: the average FP marker rate was 1.6 markers per normal 4-view case, sensitivity in calcification was 100.0% and sensitivity in mass was 71.1%. Observers recorded the diagnosis and the schema before utilizing CAD and after utilizing CAD according to BI-RADs category and to six categories associated with diagnostic confidence of malignancy (definitely malignant: 6, probably malignant: 5, maybe malignant: 4, maybe not malignant: 3, probably not malignant: 2, and definitely not malignant: 1). Categories 1 to 3 were evaluated as benign and 4-6 were evaluated as malignant. Diagnostic accuracy was evaluated with respect to sensitivity, specificity, NPV (negative predictive value), PPV (positive predictive value), and ROC analysis utilizing ROCKIT software (Version 0.9.1 BETA).

3 Results

1) Sensitivity, Specificity, PPV, and NPV (Table 1-2.)

Table 1. Sensitivity, Specificity, PPV, and NPV with the Non-Informed Group

a) Pre-CAD

	Sensitivity	Specificity	PPV	NPV
Observer1	0.739	0.974	0.895	0.967
Observer2	0.609	1.000	1.000	0.952
Observer3	0.782	0.974	0.900	0.972
Observer4	0.696	0.987	0.941	0.962
Observer5	0.783	1.000	1.000	0.973
Average	0.722	0.985	0.947	0.965

b) Post-CAD

	Sensitivity	Specificity	PPV	NPV
Observer1	0.739	0.974	0.895	0.967
Observer2	0.609	1.000	1.000	0.952
Observer3	0.782	0.974	0.900	0.972
Observer4	0.696	0.987	0.941	0.962
Observer5	0.783	1.000	1.000	0.973
Average	0.722	0.985	0.947	0.965

Table 2. Sensitivity, Specificity, PPV, and NPV with the Informed Group

a) Pre-CAD

	Sensitivity	Specificity	PPV	NPV
Observer1	**0.522**	1.000	1.000	**0.941**
Observer2	0.739	0.987	0.944	0.947
Observer3	0.739	0.961	0.850	0.967
Observer4	0.565	0.987	0.929	0.946
Observer5	0.739	0.948	0.810	0.966
Average	**0.661**	0.977	0.907	**0.953**

b) Post-CAD

	Sensitivity	Specificity	PPV	NPV
Observer1	**0.565**	1.000	1.000	**0.947**
Observer2	0.739	0.987	0.944	0.947
Observer3	0.739	0.961	0.850	0.967
Observer4	0.565	0.987	0.929	0.946
Observer5	0.739	0.948	0.810	0.966
Average	**0.669**	0.977	0.907	**0.955**

With the non-informed group, averaged data of sensitivity, specificity, PPV, and NPV in pre-CAD were 0.722, 0.985, 0.947, and 0.965. With the informed group, averaged data of sensitivity, specificity, PPV, and NPV were 0.661, 0.977, 0.907, and 0.953. There was no statistically significant difference between two groups with regard to each parameter by unpaired-t test (P=0.326, P=0380, P=0.352, P=0.115>0.05).

With the non-informed group, averaged data of sensitivity, specificity, PPV, and NPV did not show any changes with or without CAD. On the other hand, with the informed group, averaged data of sensitivity and NPV were improved compared to those in pre-CAD because one observer could detect malignant microcalcifications utilizing CAD. However, there was no significant difference between the data in pre-CAD and in post-CAD by paired-t test (P=0.897>>0.05 and P =0.873>>0.05).

2) ROC Analysis (Table3.)

The A(z) value showed that with the non-informed group, two observers in post-CAD showed better performances compared to those in pre-CAD, two observers showed worse performances in post-CAD, and one observer showed no difference. In average, there was no significant statistical difference between pre-CAD and post-CAD (P=0.382 > >0.05). On the other hand, with the informed group, four of five observers showed better performances in post-CAD. One observer showed no difference. Averaged data showed higher performances utilizing CAD, however, there was no significant difference between pre-CAD and post-CAD P=0.116>0.05).

Table 3. A(z) values by ROC Analysis with the Non-Informed Observers in Pre-CAD and Post-CAD

a) Non-Informed Group

	Pre CAD		Post CAD
Observer 1	0.889	>	0.888
Observer 2	0.930	<	0.950
Observer 3	0.881	=	0.881
Observer 4	0.835	>	0.830
Observer5	0.836	<	0.844
Average	0.874	<	0.879

Calculated by Paired-t Test
P=0.382>>0.05

b) Informed Group

	Pre CAD		Post CAD
Observer1	0.891	<	0.918
Observer2	0.949	=	0.949
Observer3	0.935	<	0.940
Observer4	0.955	<	0.957
Observer5	0.923	<	0.945
Average	0.931	<	0.942

Calculated by Paired-t Test
P=0.116 >0.05

3) Changes regarding diagnostic efficacy in pre-CAD and post-CAD (Table4.)

With the non-informed group, categorical changes were inconsistent both in benign cases and malignant cases. In particular, two observers under-diagnosed malignant cases. One case presented malignant microcalcifications where CAD pointed out the lesion and another was a malignant case with distortion in which CAD did not point out the lesion. With the informed group, no observers under-diagnosed malignant cases whether or not the CAD system pointed out the lesion. One observer over-diagnosed benign cases while four observers' diagnostic accuracy in malignant cases was improved. In addition, diagnostic efficacy regarding the cases with masses and microcalcifcations was improved in four cases and two in four cases were diagnosed as malignant. On the other hand, in two cases with distortion, the diagnostic efficacy was improved, though none was not diagnosed as malignant.

4 Discussion

We conducted this study in connection with a query and a hypothesis. Human observers could not depend 100% on CAD system unless the system had 100% reliability in cancer detection. Many papers have reported the usefulness of CAD systems[1)-5)] without mentioning this important point.

Table 4. Changes regarding Diagnostic Efficacy in Pre-CAD and Post-CAD

a) Non-Informed Group

	Benign			Malignant		
	Up /	No Change /	Down	Up /	No Change/	Down
Observer1	1 /	76 /	0	*1 /	22 /	0
				(microcalc)		
Observer2	0 /	74 /	3	0 /	23 /	0
Observer3	0 /	76 /	1	0 /	22 /	*1
						(microcalc)
Observer4	1 /	76 /	0	0 /	23 /	0
Observer5	0 /	76 /	0	*1 /	21 /	**1
				(FAD)		(distortion)

b) Informed Group

	Benign			Malignant		
	Up /	No Change /	Down	Up /	No Change/	Down
Observer1	0 /	77 /	0	*3 /	20 /	0
				(mass+nicrocalc:2, distortion:1)		
Observer2	0 /	77 /	0	0 /	23 /	0
Observer3	3 /	74 /	0	*1 /	22 /	0
				(distortion)		
Observer4	0 /	77 /	0	*1 /	22 /	0
				(mass+microcalc)		
Observer5	0 /	77 /	0	*1 /	22 /	0
				(mass+microcalc)		

*: CAD system detected
**: CAD system not detected

The present ability of CAD in mammography is limited. In cases with micro-calcifications, the CAD system can surpass human observers' diagnostic ability with accuracies approaching nearly 100%. On the other hand, in cases with masses, FAD, and distortion, the CAD system can not surpass experienced readers' ability. So it would be not useful to improve diagnostic accuracy in human observers even if they had experienced many cases over a long period. Rather than that, under current conditions, we should inform how good or bad the CAD system is and prioritize human observers' skill at diagnosis to revise CAD system's weak points. The study showed positive results that proved our hypothesis.

In accordance with the results of this study, diagnostic accuracy can differ with or without information about CAD system's ability. With the informed group that acknowledged the CAD system's performance from both strong aspects such as microcalcifications and weak aspects such as masses, distortion, and FAD, total diagnostic accuracy was improved. In particular, in cases with microcalcifications where the CAD system has 100% sensitivity and a relatively lower FP marker rate in this study, human observers can improve their diagnostic accuracy without an increase in FPs. On the other hand, with the non-informed group, some observers were confused by CAD's detection and as a result, their diagnostic accuracy deteriorated. Despite chances of ruling out malignant cases in accordance with CAD, they nevertheless diagnosed accurately by themselves without utilizing CAD.

In conclusion, human observers should be notified about the accuracy of the CAD system in cancer detection before they utilize it in order to improve the synergy between the CAD system and the human observers. Such a step will positively influence observers regarding the reliability of CAD system.

In addition, it might be effective to install test images to evaluate the human observers' and the CAD system's ability in cancer detection before utilizing the CAD system. This could help the users understand what particular aspects of the CAD system could assist them or in what ways they might have to compensate for the CAD system.

Acknowledgement

This study was supported by cancer research grant of Japanese ministry of health, labor and welfare, FUJIFILM, Japan and FUJIFILM Medical Japan (T. Komaki, K. Matano).

References

1. P. Taylor, R. Given-Wilson, H. Potts et al.: Assessing the Impact of CAD Compared to Double Reading by Radiologists. IWDM2004.
2. P. Skaane, A Kshirsagar, S Staplenton: False Positive CAD Marks on FFDM Acquired Normal Screening Mammograms. IWDM 2004.
3. S. M. Astley, C. R. M. Boggis, S. Walker et al.: An Evaluation of a Commercial Prompting System in a Busy Screening Centre. IWDM 2002, 471-475.
4. S. M. Astley, C. R. M. Boggis, V. F. Hillier: Should We Use Humans or Machine to Pre-Screen Mammograms? IWDM 2002, 476-480.
5. M. Yip, R. A. Jong, M. J. Yaffe: the Efficacy of a Digital Mammographic Computer-aided Detection System. IWDM2004.

Improving Access to Mammography in Rural Areas

Elizabeth A. Krupinski

Department of Radiology University of Arizona Tucson, AZ 85724
Krupinski@radiology.arizona.edu

Abstract. Many rural areas do not have reliable or adequate access to breast cancer evaluation facilities and care. With the advent of digital mammo-graphy it is possible to send high quality mammographic images across teleradiology/-telemedicine networks for interpretation at certified mammo-graphy centers. We have a statewide telemedicine network upon which telemammography is conducted with a number of very rural locations. Strict turn-around times for interpretation are guaranteed in contractual agree-ments. We are also testing the use of ultra-rapid pathology clinics for women with positive mammograms and real-time consultation with oncologists to reduce the time it takes for rural women to receive care.

1 Background

Breast cancer is the most common cancer of women in the United States. It is the second leading cause of cancer deaths. The National Cancer Institute predicted that 213,000 new breast cancer cases would be diagnosed in 2005, with 41,000 estimated deaths. [1] Breast cancer is typically detected during screening that, for the majority of women, relies on mammography and clinical breast exams. It is estimated that over 48 million mammograms are performed every year and the number is increasing. Less than one million (2-5%) require a subsequent biopsy. [2] However, the majority of biopsies (65% to 80%), result in benign diagnoses with malignancy being found in only 1 in 10 women who undergo breast biopsy. [3] In rural, medically underserved areas, mammo-graphy rates are lower for a variety of reasons, including lack of dedicated screening facilities and/or personnel, poor compliance and large distances between patients and clinics (making it difficult to return for follow-up care). Telemammography has been found to alleviate significantly this problem in many rural areas.

The entire breast cancer detection process from mammography to clinical consulta-tion with the oncologist is usually about 28 days. Once an abnormal mammogram is diagnosed, a diagnostic biopsy performed at the mammography center or by a surgeon typically follows. The tissue is then processed and read by a pathologist who generates a report and sends it back to the surgeon. If the diagnosis is malignant, the patient schedules a meeting with the medical oncologist for consultation and a treatment plan. The timeframe is even longer for women in rural areas who typically need to travel to an urban hospital for many of these procedures. Whether urban or rural, however, the long wait time between initial diagnosis, pathology results and

Susan M. Astley et al. (Eds.): IWDM 2006, LNCS 4046, pp. 111–117, 2006.
© Springer-Verlag Berlin Heidelberg 2006

possibly oncology consultation can be extremely stressful for the patient. Tele-medicine and digital radiology and pathology are ways to reduce those waiting times and the time it takes for a woman with breast cancer to receive definitive care. We describe here some of the ways that we have developed to help improve breast care for women in both rural and urban areas by reducing the waiting times for various steps in the breast care timeline.

2 Methods

Our telemedicine program (Arizona Telemedicine Program, ATP) has a scalable T-1/ATM (asynchronous transfer mode) broadband telecommunications system that connects over 150 sites using real-time and store-and-forward applications. The network is used for a variety of telemedicine related activities including clinical, educational and administrative. We began providing teleconsultations in May of 1997. Teleradiology represents the most common use of the network, with over 100,000 cases transmitted and interpreted in 2005. In 2005 seven rural sites used the telemammography service, sending over 3,500 cases to the hub for interpretation. Contracts with the sites for telemammography specify a turn-around time (from receipt to generation and trans-mission of a report back to the site) of no more than 30 minutes. We have tracked turn-around times to verify compliance with the agreements.

Pilot studies were carried out to study the feasibility of establishing ultra-rapid breast clinics. The first study surveyed patients at the university breast clinic to determine if and how much women would be willing to pay for faster pathology results if the needed a biopsy. A 13-question survey (available in both English and Spanish) was distributed to all patients signing in for an exam who agreed to participate (and signed a consent form) over a 2-month period. All questions were Likert-scale responses and non-parametric tests were used to statistically analyze the results.

In a separate investigation we studied digital scanning of pathology specimen slides to insure rapid processing and transmission for interpretation could accom-plished. Sixteen benign and 14 malignant surgical breast biopsy cases from an existing database were selected by a referee pathologist and scanned digitally. We used the DMetrix virtual slide processor that samples images at 0.47 microns/pixel to scan a series of breast specimen images for interpretation on a color computer display monitor compared to the original slide images (traditional light microscopy). Diagnostic accuracy and reading times were recorded. Readers (4 board certified pathologists) classified each image as benign, equivocal or malignant and rated image quality as excellent, good, fair or poor.

The final pilot study tested the teleoncology component. Patients requiring a core biopsy were approached sequentially for participation at the breast center. The study was explained to them and if they agreed to participate they entered the Ultra-Clinic arm of the study. To date, eight patients have participated. Following biopsy, tissue was processed by Vacuum Histoprocess and ultra-rapid fixation, converted to a digital image by the DMetrix scanner, and sent via the telemedicine network to be read via telepathology. The patient then went to the telemedicine suite to receive the results. The teleoncologist presented all results and all questions were answered. The time course of the entire process was recorded. Control data for the pilot study was obtained from a cohort of patients using patient charts that also recorded the times for each of the events studied.

3 Results

For the teleradiology component (an established service) we found over 90% compliance with the 30-minute turn-around time required in the service contracts at all sites. Discrepancies occurred for the most part due to transmission difficulties, not prolonged times once the images arrived at the interpretation workstation.

The willingness to pay for pathology services study had 312 responses. If diagnosed with cancer, 92% of the respondents in this study reported they would seek an expert second opinion. The data were unevenly distributed (χ^2 = 51.14, df = 4, p < .001) with 33% of the participants reporting a willingness to travel over 50 miles and 47% willing to travel between 11 and 50 miles (see Figure 1).

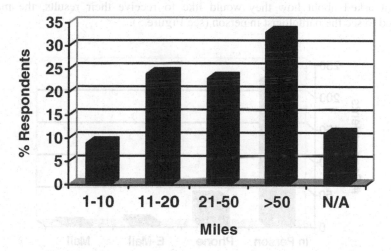

Fig. 1. Percentage of respondents corresponding to the number of miles they would drive to obtain a second opinion

When asked if they would pay a co-payment for a second opinion if their insurance covered the benefit, 97% of those surveyed responded affirmatively. Thirty-five percent of respondents reported they would pay more than $50 for such a service. The distribution of values suggested that significantly more of the individuals surveyed would be willing to pay $25 or more than those willing to pay less than $25 ($\chi^2$ = 139.52, df = 5, p < .0001) (see Figure 2).

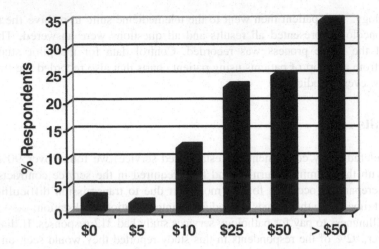

Fig. 2. Percentage of respondents corresponding to the amount of co-payment they would be willing to expend for a second opinion

When asked about how they would like to receive their results, the majority preferred to see the pathologist in person (see Figure 3).

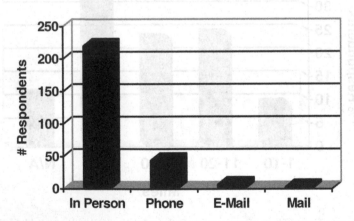

Fig. 3. Respondent preferences regarding mode of communication with pathologists

The diagnostic accuracy study comparing virtual (see Figure 4) versus traditional viewing of pathology specimens showed that performance with the digital slides viewed on a computer display are equivalent to viewing traditional slides (kappa greater than 0.90 for all readers). Out the 120 total diagnoses rendered (4 pathologists x 30 cases) there were only 3 incorrect diagnoses with the virtual slides, each by a different pathologist. The most experienced pathologist had no errors. Two pathologists read the same case as benign when it was malignant and another called a benign case malignant. In the light microscopy condition, all three of these cases were called equivocal so they were very difficult cases to begin with. In terms of image quality, 56.6% of the virtual images were rated excellent, 39.2% good, 4.2% fair and 0% poor. The viewing times however were significantly longer (> 1 minute per slide versus < 30 sec on average per slide for virtual versus traditional), although these are likely to decrease as better user interfaces are developed.

Fig. 4. Typical virtual pathology slide of breast core biopsy samples

For the ultra-rapid clinic pilot study, the elapsed time (from mammogram to definitive oncology care) data were analyzed comparing the control (patients receiving traditional care) and pilot groups (ultra-rapid) using the non-parametric Mann-Whitney U Test. Although the results did not reach statistical significance because of the very

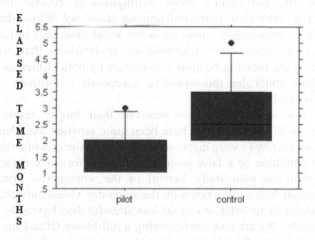

Fig. 5. Box plots of elapsed time from mammography to definitive oncology care

small sample size (Z = -1.804, p = 0.0713), there was a clear trend towards the pilot group having a shorter elapsed time to definitive oncology care. Figure 5 shows box plots of the two data sets. The median elapsed time for the pilot group was 2 months and for the control group was 2.5 months. The "whiskers" on the bar graph show the variability in the data, with 3 months being the longest elapsed time for the pilot group and 5 months being the longest for the control group.

4 Discussion

We have an established telemammography program that is serving a number of rural sites, providing diagnostic results within 30 minutes of receipt of the case. This allows women at the rural sites to receive follow-up care they may need on the same day or at least to schedule follow-up care on the same day. Without telemammography services, these women would either have no mammography services or the effort involved in getting to the clinic, getting results and coming back for more care would be too difficult. Many of these rural women simply do not get breast care without telemammography. There are a number of other teleradiology programs in the US and world and many include telemammography. We have not seen any data however on the business model that we use – requiring turn-around times within a specified period of time. It is our belief that by requiring reports back within a specified time of image acquisition, we are improving the care of rural patients.

The willingness-to-pay survey results show that women do want pathology results faster than they currently do and, at least for the urban women in our sample, are willing to pay for it and travel short distances for it. We still need to determine if rural women would respond in the same manner. Not surprisingly, the majority of women prefer to hear the news about their biopsy reports in-person with the pathologist. Receiving a phone call, letter or e-mail is generally not acceptable. In this survey we did not inquire about willingness to receive the news via videoconferencing. Although videoconferencing does not allow the patient to actually be with the pathologist, it does allow for a real-time, face-to-face encounter with the clinician. Most other telemedicine applications that use real-time videoconferencing are found to be quite satisfactory by both clinicians and patients and we have little doubt that this would be acceptable for women receiving the results of their breast biopsies.

So far, the few women who have received their biopsy results via video-conferencing in the Ultra-Clinic study have been quite satisfied with their results. So far 3 of the 8 patients (38%) were diagnosed with breast cancer while the other 5 had either a benign condition or a false positive result. No formal satisfaction surveys were distributed in the pilot study, but all of the women (no matter what the diagnosis) expressed high satisfaction with the same-day videoconferencing process. All noted that although stressful, it was far less stressful than having to wait days or weeks for the results. We are now implementing a full-blown Ultra-Clinic program at the breast center for same-day biopsy results and oncology consultations. [4] The goal is to have results within 3-4 hours rather than days or weeks.

References

1. National Cancer Institute. (2005). Breast Cancer Facts and Figures. http://www.cancer.gov/cancertopics/types/breast
2. Imaginis – The Breast Health Resource. (2005). Breast Biopsy: Indications and methods. http://imaginis.com/breasthealth/biopsy/#introduction
3. Susan G. Komen Breast Cancer Foundation. (2005). About Breast Cancer: Diagnosis and Types of Biopsies. http://www.komen.org/
4. http://www.uphkino.org/ultraclinics.htm

Dual Modality Surgical Guidance for Non-palpable Breast Lesions

Patricia Goodale Judy, Priya Raghunathan, and Mark B. Williams

University of Virginia, Radiology Research, 409 Lane Road,
Charlottesville, VA 22903
pgoodale@virginia.edu

Abstract. Currently, the majority of lumpectomy and excisional biopsy procedures are performed using the wire localization (WL) technique; however, this technique suffers from several drawbacks including inaccuracy in placement of the wire, possible displacement of the wire prior to surgery, and ambiguity of the lesion's location along the wire. We propose dual modality surgical guidance (DMSG) as a means to overcome many of the problems associated with WL. The approach uses a dual modality (digital mammography and breast scintigraphy) breast imaging system developed in our lab to place a small radioactive marker (a radiomarker), directly into the lesion. Here we present the results of measurements of the localization and injection accuracy of our system. The localization accuracy, evaluated by determining the difference between the known and measured inter-well separations, were within 0.76 mm (standard deviation of 0.46 mm) of the true distances for x-ray imaging and within 0.66 mm (standard deviation of 0.43) for gamma imaging. Our maximum error in injection accuracy in any of the three Cartesian coordinates was 1.8 mm. On average, the errors were 0.6, 0.4, and 0.9 mm for x, y, and z respectively. The results of these phantom tests provide encouragement that our upright digital mammography unit can accurately a) locate a lesion in three dimensions, b) inject a radiomarker into the lesion, and c) assess the offset between the lesion and radiomarker centers.

1 Introduction

Major clinical trials have shown that for patients with Stage II breast cancer, the survival rate of women receiving breast conservation therapy (lumpectomy/ radiation) is similar to that of women undergoing mastectomy [1]. Furthermore, no increased risk of second malignancies has been demonstrated in patients who select breast conservation therapy as opposed to mastectomy [2]. Thus, there has been a shift away from mastectomy and towards breast conserving procedures. Concurrently, recent advances in mammography have significantly improved the detection of early stage breast cancers, presenting surgeons with the increasingly difficult tasks of lesion localization and complete lesion excision.

Currently, the majority of lumpectomy and excisional biopsy procedures are performed using the wire localization (WL) technique. In WL, a guide wire is placed through the lesion on the day of surgery. Along with the mammographic images, the

Susan M. Astley et al. (Eds.): IWDM 2006, LNCS 4046, pp. 118–124, 2006.

surgeon uses the wire, which extends through the skin, to locate the tissue to be excised. Although this is the current standard of practice, the WL technique suffers from several drawbacks including, 1) ambiguity in the location of the lesion along the wire, 2) the possibility that the wire can get displaced prior to surgery, and 3) the fact that the entry point of the wire and its orientation within the breast cannot be relied upon as an optimum entry point and path for incision and dissection. One consequence of uncertain intraoperative lesion localization is the increased likelihood of positive margins, potentially necessitating a second surgery. Efforts to avoid this can result in the removal of needlessly large masses of breast tissue to reduce the risk of residual malignancy. Also, since WL must be performed on the day of surgery due to risk of displacement of the protruding wire, surgical procedures requiring it cannot be scheduled early in the surgical schedule. These consequences result in increased cost, morbidity and trauma for the patient, and increased logistical problems for the surgeons and radiologists involved, and have motivated the search for alternative, more accurate methods for intraoperative localization of nonpalpable breast lesions.

One possible solution to the problems associated with WL is to provide the surgeon with intraoperative guidance by means of a small radioactive marker, placed directly into the lesion. During surgery a hand-held gamma probe is used by the surgeon to locate and excise the marked lesion. Such an approach has been tested by researchers at the H. Lee Moffit Cancer Center at the University of South Florida (using implanted radiotherapy (^{125}I) seeds as radiomarkers) and investigators at the European Institute of Technology in Italy (using ^{99m}Tc-labeled macroaggregated albumin), and has shown promising results [3-6](De Cicco et al., 2002; Gennari et al., 2000; Gray et al., 2001). Our approach, known as dual modality surgical guidance (DMSG), uses an upright dual modality (digital mammography and breast scintigraphy) breast imaging system developed in our lab. A photo of the system is shown in figure 1. In this approach, the x-ray component of the dual modality breast scanner is used to identify the 3-dimensional location of the lesion within the breast. A 3-axis translation system, mounted on the mammography unit, is then used to accurately inject a small amount of a radiolabeled substrate (radiomarker) into the center of the lesion. The gamma imaging component is then used to verify the position of the radiomarker relative to the lesion as seen on the x-ray images.

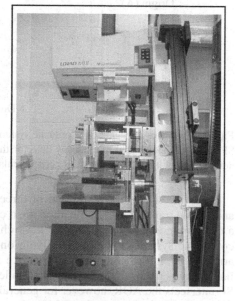

Here we present the results of measurements of the localization and injection accuracy of our system.

Fig. 1. Photo of the dual modality scanner modified to perform radiomarking

2 Methods

2.1 System Description

The scanner is based on a modified Lorad M-III upright mammography unit. The cassette holder and grid have been replaced with a CCD-based digital x-ray detector built under NIH funding [7]. A small field of view (10 cm x 10 cm) gamma camera is mounted on the gantry arm below the x-ray tube, and is positioned along the arm using a stepper-motor driven translation stage. The gantry arm is driven by a servo motor by way of a worm gear. Thus positioning of the x-ray tube, x-ray detector, and gamma camera are accomplished via computer control. The breast support, compression paddle, and 3-axis injection stage are mounted to the main mammography unit support frame by way of a stainless steel rod, but are independent of the rotational motion of the gantry arm itself. For accurate radiomarking, the scanner must first identify the location of the lesion within the breast, and then must move the needle tip precisely to that location.

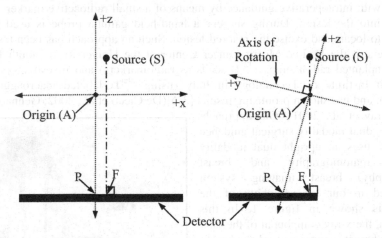

Fig. 2. Diagram of the common coordinate system defined by the x-ray system. The line segment SF is the surface normal to the x-ray detector that intersects the x-ray focal spot. The z-axis is defined so that it intersects the AOR perpendicularly at the point on the AOR nearest to SF.

Since the scanner is comprised of three separate subsystems (x-ray, gamma ray, and needle translation), each with its own coordinate system, it is necessary to define a common coordinate system. We have chosen to define the origin of this common coordinate system to be the point lying on the axis of rotation (AOR) of the gantry arm that is closest to the detector surface normal intersecting the source focal spot, line segment SF in figure 2. Note that under ideal gantry alignment, the line segment SF intersects the AOR, however for generality our localization equations do not make that assumption. The y-axis is defined to be the gantry arm rotation axis, with the positive y direction pointing away from the patient. The x-axis is defined to be along the line perpendicular to the AOR and to the line SF when the gantry arm is in its central ($\theta = 0$) position. Positive x points towards the patient's right. The z-axis is perpendicular to the AOR, but not necessarily parallel to SF, since in general the AOR may not be perpendicular to the detector surface normal. Positive z points towards the source.

2.2 Localization Studies

We have made preliminary measurements of the scanner's ability to localize objects in space using both x-ray and gamma ray imaging. The phantom consists of a thin-walled acrylic box with a 9 x 9 square array of holes in the bottom surface, each separated by 1 cm in both dimensions. A series of acrylic standoffs of various heights (0.5, 1.5, 2.5, 3.5, and 4.5 cm) can be attached to the inside of the bottom surface. A hole approximately 1 mm in diameter and 1 mm deep is drilled on the top surface of

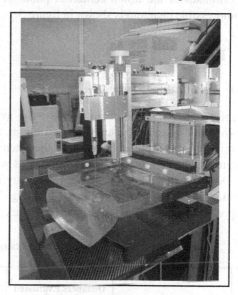

the standoffs to form wells to hold a few drops of a radioactive and radio-opaque solution. A mounting rod is attached to one end of the phantom, located on its symmetry axis, permitting the phantom to be mounted approximately on the rotation axis of the gantry arm of the scanner. Well-defined well positions within the phantom mean that the Euclidian distance (defined as the square root of the sum of the squares of the x, y, and z positions) between any two wells is precisely known. Since the absolute positions in space of the wells are not precisely known, we have evaluated the localization accuracy of the system in terms of its ability to measure the distance between pairs of wells. A stronger test of absolute localization accuracy is presented below in the needle positioning accuracy studies. For the

Fig. 3. Photo of the needle positioning system mounted on the gantry. The x-ray detector, angled for a stereotactic view, can be seen beneath the breast support.

localization tests, each well of the phantom was filled with approximately 50 µCi of a solution of ^{99m}Tc and Gd-DTPA, allowing the wells to be seen by both detectors. X-ray and gamma ray images were obtained at gantry arm angles of $\theta = \pm 15, 25, 30, 45$ and 60°. Well coordinates were calculated using stereo pairs of images (e.g. $\theta = \pm 30°$) and compared to the known locations [8].

2.3 Needle Positioning Accuracy Studies

Preliminary measurements have also been made of the scanner's ability to accurately position a needle at a precise point in space. A compressible, tissue equivalent breast phantom containing randomly distributed simulated lesions (Fluke Biomedical, Cleveland, OH) was positioned on the scanner and stereo images were obtained at gantry arm angles of $\theta = \pm$ 15, 25, 35 and 45°. The coordinates of several of the simulated lesions inside the phantom were determined using stereo pairs of x-ray images. For each lesion, the needle was then translated to the x and y positions given by the lesion coordinates. With the needle mounted to the z-stage, the needle was manually lowered to the z position of the lesion center. To confirm that the final location of the needle tip was coincident with the center location of the lesion, stereo views were again obtained of the phantom and the 3-D coordinates of the needle tip were determined. To test consistency, and to evaluate possible deflection of the lesion during needle insertion, these images were also used to re-calculate the 3-D coordinates of the lesion center. A photo of the needle positioning system and the compressible phantom is shown in figure 3.

3   Results

3.1 Localization Studies

Table 1 shows, for both modalities, the average absolute difference between the known and measured inter-well separations for stereotactic angles of $\pm$ 25 degrees. Similar results were obtained for other stereotactic angles between $\pm$ 10 and $\pm$ 60 degrees. The measured Euclidian distances were within 0.76 mm (standard deviation of 0.46 mm) of the true distances for x-ray imaging and within 0.66 mm (standard deviation of 0.43) for gamma ray imaging. The maximum Euclidian distance error reported by the two modalities was 1.63 mm.

Table 1. Error in the localization data obtained from x-ray and gamma ray imaging

	Number of Distances Evaluated	Average Error (mm)	Standard Deviation (mm)
X-Ray Imaging	15	0.76	0.46
Gamma Ray Imaging	6	0.66	0.43

3.2 Needle Positioning Accuracy Studies

Table 2 shows the errors between the measured lesion centers and the placement of the needle tip. For stereo angle pairs of $\theta = \pm$ 25 degrees the maximum error in any of the coordinates was 1.8 mm. On average, the errors were 0.6, 0.4, and 0.9 mm for x, y, and z respectively. The Euclidian errors were 1.0, 1.8, and 1.3 mm for lesions 1, 2, and 3 respectively. Similar results were obtained using stereotactic angles of $\pm$15, $\pm$35, and $\pm$45 degrees.

Table 2. Error between lesion center and needle tip placement

Lesion #	Stereo Angles	Error: Lesion Center-Needle Tip			Euclidian Error (mm)
		x (mm)	y (mm)	z (mm)	
1	± 25°	-0.4	-0.8	-0.4	1.0
2	± 25°	0.3	0.1	-1.8	1.8
3	± 25°	1.2	-0.2	0.4	1.3

4 Discussion

Accurate intraoperative guidance is necessary for reliable surgical biopsy and lumpectomy of nonpalpable breast lesions. The use of a radiomarker could potentially overcome some of the limitations of wire localization in this regard. A prototype integrated system for the x-ray-guided injection of the radiomarker and measurement of its location has been built. Preliminary evaluations of the system's ability to localize the lesion and to position the needle accordingly are encouraging, but further improvements can be made. Although the error between the lesion center and the needle tip is currently larger than our goal of ≤ 1 mm for two of the three measurements (maximum error = 1.8 mm), improved performance is likely to be obtained by fine tuning the orientation of the translation stages so that their translation directions are more precisely parallel to the x, y, and z axes of the common reference frame established by the x-ray imaging system. Also, the effects of operator variability in the identification of the locations in the stereotactic images of the lesion and needle tip must be further evaluated, as does possible flexing of the relatively small bore (20 gauge) needle. These improvements will be made prior to the beginning of clinical evaluation, scheduled for the fall of 2006.

Acknowledgements

We would like to thank Stan Majewski and the Detector and Imaging Group at the Thomas Jefferson National Accelerator Facility for building the gamma camera used in this project.

This project is supported in part by The Susan G. Komen Foundation (grant #IMG0402326) and the National Institutes of Heath (grant # P30 CA44579).

References

1. van Dongen,J.A., Voogd,A.C., Fentiman,I.S., Legrand,C., Sylvester,R.J., Tong,D., van der,S.E., Helle,P.A., van Zijl,K., and Bartelink,H. (2000). Long-term results of a randomized trial comparing breast-conserving therapy with mastectomy: European Organization for Research and Treatment of Cancer 10801 trial. Journal of the National Cancer Institute 92, 1143-1150.

2. Obedian,E., Fischer,D.B., and Haffty,B.G. (2000). Second malignancies after treatment of early-stage breast cancer: lumpectomy and radiation therapy versus mastectomy. Journal of Clinical Oncology *18*, 2406-2412.
3. Cox,C., Furman,B., Stowell,N., Ebert,M., Clark,J., Dupont,E., Shons,A., Berman,C., Beauchamp,J., Gardner,M., Hersch,M., Venugopal,P., Szabunio,M., Cressman,J., Diaz,N., Vrcel,V., and Fairclough,R. (2003). Radioactive Seed Localization Breast Biopsy and Lumpectomy Can Specimen Radiographs Be Eliminated? Annals of Surgical Oncology 10, 1039-1047
4. De Cicco,C., Pizzamiglio,M., Trifiro,G., Luini,A., Ferrari,M., Prisco,G., Galimberti,V., Cassano,E., Viale,G., Intra,M., Veronesi,P., and Paganelli,G. (2002). Radioguided occult lesion localisation (ROLL) and surgical biopsy in breast cancer. Technical aspects. Quarterly Journal of Nuclear Medicine 46, 145-151
5. Gennari,R., Galimberti,V., De Cicco,C., Zurrida,S., Zerwes,F., Pigatto,F., Luini,A., Paganelli,G., and Veronesi,U. (2000). Use of technetium-99m-labeled colloid albumin for preoperative and intraoperative localization of nonpalpable breast lesions. Journal of the American College of Surgeons *190*, 692-698
6. Gray,R.J., Salud,C., Nguyen,K., Dauway,E., Friedland,J., Berman,C., Peltz,E., Whitehead,G., and Cox,C.E. (2001). Randomized prospective evaluation of a novel technique for biopsy or lumpectomy of nonpalpable breast lesions: radioactive seed versus wire localization. Annals of Surgical Oncology *8*, 711-715
7. Williams MB, Simoni PU, Smilowitz L, Stanton M, Phillips WC, and Stewart A. Analysis of the Detective Quantum Efficiency of a Developmental Detector for Digital Mammography. Medical Physics 1999; 26(11):2273-2285
8. More, M.J., Narayanan, D., Goodale, P.J., Majewski, S., Welch, B., Wojcik, R., Williams, M.B., "X-ray stereotactic lesion localization in conjunction with dedicated scintima-mmography", *IEEE Transactions on Nuclear Science*, vol. 50, issue 5, part 2, pp. 1636-1642, Oct. 2003

Mammography Reading with Computer-Aided Detection (CAD): Single View *vs* Two Views

Olorunsola F. Agbaje[1], Susan M. Astley[2], Maureen G.C. Gillan[3],
Caroline R.M. Boggis[4], Mary Wilson[4], Nicky B. Barr[4], Ursula M. Beetles[4],
Miriam A. Griffiths[4], Anil Jain[4], Jill Johnson[4], Rita M. Roberts[4], Heather Deans[5],
Karen Duncan[5], Geeta Iyengar[5], Pamela M. Griffiths[2], Magnus A. McGee[6],
Stephen W. Duffy[1], and Fiona J. Gilbert[3]

[1] Department of Epidemiology, Mathematics & Statistics, Wolfson Institute of
Preventive Medicine, London, UK
[2] Department of Imaging Science & Biomedical Engineering, University of Manchester,
Manchester, UK
[3] Department of Radiology, University of Aberdeen, UK
[4] Nightingale Centre, Withington Hospital, Manchester, UK
[5] NE Scotland Breast Screening Centre, Aberdeen UK
[6] Department of Public Health & General Practice, Christchurch School of Medicine, NZ

Abstract. Two-view mammography is known to be more effective than one-view in increasing breast cancer detection and reducing recall rates. In addition, there is evidence that computer aided detection (CAD) systems are able to prompt malignant abnormalities that have been overlooked by a human reader. Using data from the UK NHS Breast Screening Programme (NHSBSP) we compared double reading with single reading using a CAD system, to assess the relationship between CAD and number of views in terms of the sensitivity of the screening regime to cancer detection and the recall rate of normal cases. CAD appeared to contribute to an increased cancer detection rate with single-view mammography without significantly increasing the recall rate. For two-view mammography, there was no significant change in sensitivity using CAD but a significantly higher recall rate. However, single-view mammography was used in incident rounds in which previous mammograms were available whereas two-view mammography was used in the prevalent round where no previous mammograms were available.

1 Introduction

It is known that two-view mammography has substantially superior sensitivity to single-view in screening and symptomatic examinations [1][2]. It is also known that computer aided detection (CAD) systems can prompt malignant abnormalities overlooked by a human reader [3][4]. In the UK National Breast Screening Programme, the policy of two-view mammography at first screen followed by single-view thereafter has recently been replaced by a policy of two-view mammography at every round. In this paper, we use data from a study comparing the original double reading with single reading using a CAD system, in which prevalent round mammograms were two-view and incident round mammograms were single-view, to

Susan M. Astley et al. (Eds.): IWDM 2006, LNCS 4046, pp. 125–130, 2006.

assess the relationship of the single reader using CAD and number of views in terms of the sensitivity of the screening regime to cancer detection rate and the recall rate of normal subjects.

2 Methods

In CADET [5], 10,096 mammograms, originally double read in 1996, and with the cancer casemix enriched by 50%, were reread by a single human reader assisted by the R2 ImageChecker CAD system with software version 5.0. Of the 10,096 mammograms 315 had cancers diagnosed at the original mammogram or up to six years later. We had data on number of views for all 315 of the cancers and for 9733 of the 9781 normal cases (99.5%). We retrieved prompt data on 309 cancers (98%). Reading conditions from 1996 were replicated in that incident round mammograms were hung with the previous examination undertaken three years earlier.

3 Statistical Analysis

We first compared two reading regimes for single-view with two-view mammograms separately, using the McNemar's test. Further analysis was by logistic regression estimating the effects of number of views, tumour size, breast density, and node status on the odds of being recalled by the original double reading and by the single reader with CAD. This yielded odds ratio estimates of the relative risk of being recalled, and the deviance chi-squared tests for the significance of the association of the factors with the chance of being recalled. In addition, for the single reader with CAD, we also estimated the association with when the tumour was diagnosed.

4 Results

Table 1 shows the detection rates of all cancers diagnosed at or after the original 1996 screen by number of views for the original double reading and for the single reading with CAD.

Table 1. Detection rate of cancers and recall rate of normal subjects by use of CAD and number of views

Outcome	Single View		Two view	
	CAD	No CAD	CAD	No CAD
Detection rate	95/241(39%)	73/241(30%)	31/74(42%)	30/74(41%)
Recall rate	420/6879(6%)	315/6879(5%)	319/2854(11%)	241/2854(8%)

For single-view there is a very significant difference in sensitivity (p=0.0003), with single reading using CAD being more sensitive than the previous double reading. However, it also confers a significant increase in recall of normal cases (p<0.0001). For two-view there is no significant difference in sensitivity (p=0.9), but again a significant increase in recall of normal cases with CAD (p<0.0001). There were no significant differences between single-view sensitivity and two-view sensitivity either with or without CAD. With CAD, two-view had significantly higher recall rates of normal cases than single-view (p<0.0001). Similarly, without CAD, the recall rates were significantly higher for two-view mammography (p<0.0001). It should be noted, however, that the results are confounded by incident/prevalent screen status. Due to the screening policy in place in 1996, the two-view cases were mostly prevalent screen and the single-view mostly incident screen where the previous round mammograms were hung for comparison.

Table 2 shows the CAD prompts (of the true tumour region as determined by retrospective review of all imaging and clinical/pathological information).

Table 2. CAD prompts in the tumour region by number of views and tumour feature on mammogram

| Feature | Single view | | | Two view | | |
	Prompted	Not Prompted	Prompted in MLO only	Prompted in CC only	Prompted in both views	Not Prompted
Mass	60 (54M)	108	6 (4M)	6 (5M)	11 (10M)	19
Microcalc	38 (29C)	36	3 (3C)	1 (0C)	9 (8M)	12

The figures in parentheses give the number actually prompted as that type of lesion. With single view mammography, 60 out of 168 masses were prompted, 54 with a mass prompt, six with a microcalcification prompt. With single view, 51% of microcalcifications and 36% of masses were prompted. This difference in prompt rates was significant (p=0.04). For two-view mammography, 57% of micro-calcifications and 55% of masses were prompted (no significant difference). In those with two view mammography, there was no significant difference between CC and MLO with respect to the likelihood of a prompt.

Table 3 shows the effects of number of views, tumour size, breast density and node status on the odds of recall by the original double reading. The only significant

Table 3. Univariate and multivariate logistic regression results for effects of number of views, tumour size node status and density on recall of cancers by double reading

| Factors | Category | Univariate | | Multivariate | |
		OR	95% CI	OR	95% CI
View	Double	1	-	1	-
	Single	0.63	(0.37, 1.08)	1.09	(0.48, 2.48)
Tumour size	1-9	1	-	1	-
	10-14	1.69	(0.80, 3.59)	2.91	(1.00, 8.46)
	15-20	2.12	(1.05, 4.25)	3.35	(1.18, 9.52)
	20+	0.70	(0.29, 1.69)	0.84	(0.25, 2.86)
Breast density	(per 1%)	1.01	(1.00, 1.02)	1.02	(1.00, 1.03)
Node status	Positive	1	-	1	-
	Negative	0.47	(0.24, 0.93)	0.54	(0.24, 1.21)
	Others	0.88	(0.40, 1.93)	1.56	(0.56, 4.39)

effects, whether in the univariate analysis or in the multivariate analysis with factors adjusted for each other, were those of tumour size and breast density. For tumour size, the chances of recall increase with size, except for the largest category, greater than 50mm, for which there were only 7 cases. In the adjusted analysis, the effect of the density was borderline significant (p=0.06), but the result suggested a 2% increase in density.

Table 4 shows the corresponding results for effects on recall by the single reader with CAD, with the addition of when the tumour was diagnosed. The only significant effects, both univariate and multivariate were the density and when the tumour was diagnosed. Recall was much more likely for tumours diagnosed at the original 1996 screen, reflecting the higher rate of agreement between double reading and single reading with CAD. There was a 2% adjusted increase in the odds of recall per 1% increase in density.

Table 4. Univariate and multivariate logistic regression results for effects of number of views, tumour Size, node status, density, and including when the tumour was diagnosed (outcome) on recall of cancers with single reading with CAD

		Univariate		Multivariate	
Factors	Category	OR	95% CI	OR	95% CI
View	Double	1	-	1	-
	Single	0.90	(0.53, 1.53)	1.29	(0.49, 3.39)
Tumour size	1-9	1	-	1	-
	10-14	1.03	(0.50, 2.13)	0.57	(0.17, 1.91)
	15-20	1.74	(0.90, 3.38)	1.52	(0.51, 4.51)
	20+	0.80	(0.36, 1.76)	0.61	(0.17, 2.16)
Breast density	(per 1%)	1.01	(1.00, 1.02)	1.02	(1.00, 1.04)
Node status	Positive	1	-	1	-
	Negative	0.57	(0.30, 1.07)	1.20	(0.47, 3.09)
	Others	0.82	(0.39, 1.74)	1.14	(0.33, 3.89)
Outcome	Cancer at 1996 screen	1	-	1	-
	Cancer at subsequent screens	0.03	(0.01, 0.07)	0.03	(0.01, 0.09)
	Intervals cancer	0.04	(0.02, 0.11)	0.04	(0.01, 0.14)

5 Discussion

The above suggests that with single-view mammography, CAD contributes to an increased cancer detection rate. The fact that this was achieved without a substantial increase in recall of normal cases is probably due to the fact that the single view mammograms pertained to incident screens and therefore, for these, there were previous mammograms available for comparison. This is due to the policy of the UK Breast Screening Programme in 1996. At that time, prevalent screens used two-view mammography and incident screens single-view. Thus, if the original 1996 mammography was single-view, this would imply that there would be pre-1996 mammography for comparison. If it was two-view, then the 1996 screen would have been a prevalent screen with no prior mammograms. The large increase in recall rate with CAD for two-view mammography is therefore similarly likely to be due to prevalent round examinations with no previous mammograms available.

There was no clear benefit of CAD observed for two-view mammography in terms of cancer detection, although this finding must be regarded as suggestive, since there was a relatively small number of two-view mammograms available for this study, and because of the confounding with incident/prevalent screen status. There was, however, a higher recall rate of normal subjects with CAD amongst the two-view subjects. Interestingly, the higher CAD prompt rate of tumours with two-view mammography applied mainly to masses. Prompts of calcifications were equally common for one-view and two-view mammography.

When considered in terms of factors influencing recall by the original 1996 double readers and the single reader with CAD separately, some interesting results emerged. With reading regimes (double and single with CAD) number of views did not affect cancer detection rates. For the original double reading, significant associations with recall of cancer cases were observed only for higher density and larger tumour size, except for the largest category, > 50 mm.

It is of interest that there was a greater likelihood of recall by either regime with increased breast density. Breast cancers occur more frequently in dense breasts, and there is probably greater uncertainty in reading dense mammograms. Human reader awareness of both of these facts probably contributes to the higher recall rates in dense breasts.

Cancers previously recalled by double reading were much more likely to be recalled by the single reader with CAD. This is consistent with our finding of very high agreement rates between the two reading regimes [5].

The major implication of this work is the clear increase in recalled cancers with CAD when there are prior mammograms for comparison. When prior mammograms are available, there is also a lesser human cost in terms of recalled normal subjects. The R2 system prompts a large proportion of mammograms and this can lead to increased false positive screens as can be seen from our results for two-view mammography (i.e. prevalence screen). This tendency is much mitigated if there are prior mammograms.

It is likely that future CAD system will aim at improving specificity, and more accurate prompting of masses, bringing the sensitivity in line with that for microcalcifications.

Acknowledgement

We thank all the staff of the Aberdeen and Manchester breast screening centres.

References

1. Wald NJ, Murphy P, Major P, Parkes,C, Townsend J, Frost C. UKCCCR multicentre randomised controlled trial of one and two view mammography in breast cancer screening. *BMJ* 2005; 311:1189-1193.
2. Blanks RG, Bennett RL, Patnick J, Cush S, Davison C, Moss SM. The effect of changing from one to two views at incident (subsequent) screens in the NHS breast screening programme in England: impact on cancer detection and recall rates. *Clinical Radiology* 2005; 60:674-680

3. Burhenne, LW, Wood S, D'Orsi CJ, Feig SA, Kopans DB, O'Shaughnessy KF, et al. Potential contribution of computer-aided detection to the sensitivity of screening mammography. *Radiology* 2000; 215(2):554-62.
4. Freer TW, Ulissey MJ. Screening mammography with computer-aided detection: prospective study of 12,860 patients in a community breast center. *Radiology* 2001; 220(3):781-6.
5. Gilbert FJ, Astley SM, McGee MA, Gillan MGC, Boggis CRM, Griffiths PM and Duffy SW. Comparison of double reading and single reading with CAD in the UK NHS Breast Screening Program: Computer Aided Detection Evaluation Trial. (CADET). *Radiology* (In press)

Automated Breast Tissue Measurement of Women at Increased Risk of Breast Cancer

Patel H.G.[1], Astley S.M.[1], Hufton A.P.[2], Harvie M.[3], Hagan K.[1], Marchant T.E.[2], Hillier V.[1], Howell A.[4], Warren R.[5], and Boggis C.R.M.[6]

[1] University of Manchester, Imaging Science and Biomedical Engineering
Stopford Building, Oxford Road, Manchester M13 9PT
Sue.Astley@Manchester.ac.uk
[2] North Western Medical Physics,
Christie Hospital, Wilmslow Road, Manchester M20 4BX
alan.hufton@physics.cr.man.ac.uk
[3] Room 8, 1st Floor, Home 4, Withington Hospital, Nell Lane, Manchester, M20 2LR
michelle.harvie@smtr.nhs.uk
[4] CRUK Department of Medical Oncology,
Christie Hospital, Wilmslow Road, Manchester, M20 4BX
Anthony.Howell@christie-tr.nwest.nhs.uk
[5] Addenbrooke's Hospital Cambridge
akd15@radiol.cam.ac.uk
[6] South Manchester University Hospitals Trust
caroline.boggis@manchester.ac.uk

Abstract. We have analysed data from a subgroup of thirty-nine women who had previously gained more than 10kg in adult life, and who were amongst those recruited from a family history clinic to a study examining the effects of diet and exercise on breast cancer risk. At entry to the study and after 12 months they underwent a series of investigations, including mammography during which markers were attached to the compression plate to allow accurate measurement of breast thickness. A calibrated stepwedge was placed adjacent to the breast to enable quantitative analysis. The proportions of glandular and fatty tissue were calculated at each pixel from the stepwedge and thickness data and from these, the percentage gland in the breast was computed, both by area and by volume. Statistical analysis showed that the volume of glandular tissue was not related to breast size. Over the 12 month period, the majority of the women lost weight, while some gained weight. It was found that weight change was correlated with change in the volume of fat in the breasts, with those women who lost the largest amount of weight showing the greatest reduction in volume. There was little change in volume of glandular tissue for any of the women. Percentage gland is often used as an indication of risk of developing breast cancer. These results suggest that measures of percentage of gland (e.g. Boyd groups) may be dominated by excess breast fat in overweight women.

1 Introduction

Increased breast density has been associated with an elevated risk of breast cancer by a number of researchers, most notably Wolfe [1] and Boyd [2]. This is of particular

Susan M. Astley et al. (Eds.): IWDM 2006, LNCS 4046, pp. 131–136, 2006.
© Springer-Verlag Berlin Heidelberg 2006

interest because whilst there are many different risk factors for breast cancer which cannot be altered (e.g. age, parity and family history), breast density can be modified by a variety of methods including diet, exercise and drugs.

Measurement of breast density is generally carried out by radiologists, either by categorising the parenchymal patterns into one of the groups proposed by Wolfe [1], or by estimating the percentage of dense tissue in the breast [2,3,4]. However, these forms of assessment are subjective and do not accurately reflect the three dimensional nature of the breast and its component tissues. The X-ray mammogram is a two-dimensional projection of a three-dimensional structure, with the brightness at any given point in the image depending on the thickness of glandular and other dense tissue projected onto that point. The arrangement of glandular tissue within the breast depends on the way in which the breast is compressed, so measures of the area occupied by dense tissue will vary depending on compression. Furthermore, the overall brightness of the image depends on the imaging parameters, which in turn vary depending on factors such as the degree of compression used, the positioning of the woman and the composition of the breast. The impact of these factors on radiologists' estimates of glandular density has not been quantified. There may also be ambiguity in locating the breast border over which percentage area is estimated. For example, in the medio-lateral view, the pectoral muscle is often excluded from the analysis, although in some mammograms, the glandular tissue may overlap this region. Finally, some approaches to measuring breast density rely on delineation of the breast border and glandular region, and hence calculation of the percentage of the *area* of the breast occupied by gland, whereas others attempt to take into account the relative densities of different regions and treat the density as a *volume*.

In recent years, semiautomated and automated methods have been developed to measure more accurately the proportion of dense tissue in the breast by means of analysis of X-ray mammograms. The most simple methods are designed to facilitate thresholding of images [5]; however, these suffer from many of the limitations described above. Apart from these there are three principal approaches: firstly, a method based on the physical parameters of the imaging process developed in Oxford [6]; secondly a technique using a step wedge to calibrate grey levels developed in Toronto [7] and thirdly another step-wedge based method developed in Manchester [8,9]. The advantage of these approaches is that they enable calculation not only of the percentage of dense tissue, but also of the volumes of dense and fatty tissue in the breast.

In this paper we describe the application of the automated method developed in Manchester to a group of women participating in a study examining the effects of diet and exercise on the risk of developing breast cancer, and present our results relating measures of gland and fat to weight change.

2 The Lifestyle Study

The lifestyle study [10] aims to evaluate the effect of diet and exercise on women at increased risk of developing breast cancer. Premenopausal women in the age range 35-45 were recruited to the study. All had a family history of breast cancer, and had gained at least 10kg of weight since the age of 18. Half the participants were offered specific dietary advice and encouraged to adhere to an exercise regime. All were assessed at baseline, and followed up at 12 and 24 months with a view to determining whether diet and exercise (and any resulting weight loss) have altered their risk of developing breast cancer. A variety of methods was used to assess these women, but the work described in this paper focuses on the relationship of weight change to change in breast density.

3 Method

Two methods of measuring the quantity of dense breast tissue were used in this study: an automated technique developed in Manchester [9] and expert radiologists' estimation of percentage gland. In the automated technique, a calibrated stepwedge is placed alongside the breast during mammography, and markers on the compression plate enable accurate measurement of compressed breast thickness, allowing for tilt of the compression plate. Data from the stepwedge and images was then used to measure total breast volume and glandular volume, and hence the percentage of dense breast tissue (by volume) and the volume of fat. Two radiologists experienced in estimating percentage gland also assessed every film by viewing digitised images on a computer screen. The films were re-randomised and the assessment repeated to enable calculation of intra observer variability.

At entry into the study (0 months), some of the women were not eligible for mammography with the stepwedge and compression markers, as they had recently undergone routine mammography. Some women also withdrew from the study during the twelve month period. The availability of images for automated assessment is summarised in table 1.

Table 1. Availability of data for automated measurement of breast density

	With stepwedge	Without stepwedge	Total
0 Months	160	116	276
12 Months	224	16	240
Total	384	132	516

4 Results

Some women in the group which had intervention (exercise and dietary advice) did lose weight, but for others, either no change or an increase in weight was measured at the end of the twelve month period. There was a similar pattern in the control group. For this reason, the data were analysed in terms of weight change rather than comparing control and intervention groups. The weight change data are represented in figure 1, and the results are summarised in figure 2.

Both radiologists were very consistent in estimating percentage gland, with intra class correlation coefficients of 0.936 and 0.964. The correlation between the two readers was 0.836, with a 4.1% difference between the means. The difference between the readers increased systematically with density.

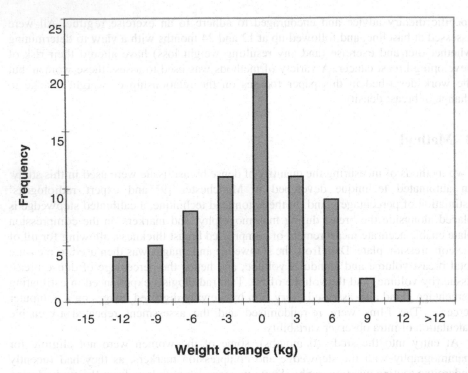

Fig. 1. Histogram of change in weight in kg of women in the study over a 12 month period

The most consistent radiologist's estimate was compared with the percentage gland calculated from the automated technique. Here the correlation coefficient was 0.806, but the difference between the means was much larger (17.8%). The automated method had the lower mean, and once more this was a difference that systematically increased with increasing density.

The breast volume measured using the automated technique was compared with the woman's weight to determine whether weight and breast volume were related. There was found to be a significant relationship with a correlation of 0.799 (p<0.001) at entry, and a similar result at 12 months, with heavier women having larger breast volumes. There was no significant relationship between weight and glandular tissue volume.

There was a significant correlation between change in weight and change in breast volume, with breast volume increasing in women who gained weight and decreasing in women who lost weight. The correlation coefficient was 0.787 (p<0.001). No statistically significant relationship was found between change in glandular volume and change in weight over the 12 month period. The correlation coefficient was -0.294 (p=0.091).

Figure 2 illustrates the changes in the parameters measured (breast volume, glandular volume and percentage gland) in women with weight loss greater than 5kg over the twelve month period, in those with weight loss less than 5kg and in those women who put on weight. It shows that there was little change in either glandular

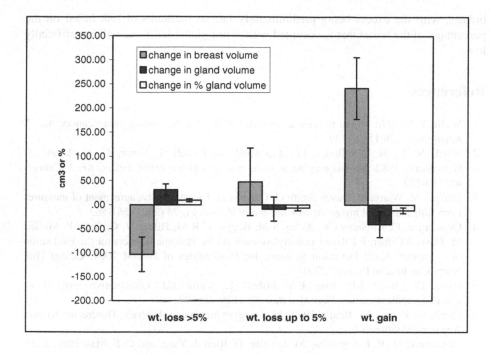

Fig. 2. Change in breast volume, glandular volume and percentage gland (by volume)

volume or percentage gland with weight change, and that these measures are dominated by the significant change in breast volume.

5 Discussion

In this study, an automated measure of breast density was used to investigate the effect of weight loss on a population at increased risk of developing breast cancer. The method was compared with an expert radiologist's assessments of percentage gland. It was found that the measures were correlated, but the mean percentage gland calculated automatically was nearly 18% lower than that estimated by the radiologist. This could in part be due to the method used to calculate percentage gland in the region where the breast is no longer in contact with the compression plate (near the edge of the breast). In the version of software used for this study, a rectangular profile was assumed; this error has subsequently been corrected, and an elliptical model has been incorporated in the method [9]. The results of the study show a significant decrease in breast volume with weight loss (and increase with weight gain). This is much larger than any measured change in glandular volume and dominates measures of change in percentage gland which are calculated from both breast volume and glandular volume. Previously, authors have noted that women with high body mass indices are less likely to have high-risk mammographic patterns [11]. Our results support this in that they suggest that women who are overweight tend to have larger breasts, with the excess being predominantly fat, so measures of risk based on the percentage of the breast that is occupied with dense glandular tissue will be artificially low.

References

1. Wolfe, J. N. 1976. Breast patterns as an index of risk for developing breast cancer. *Am. J. Roentgenol.* 126:1130-1139
2. Boyd, N. F., B. O'Sullivan, J.E. Campbell, E. Fishell, I. Simor, G. Cook and T. Germanson. 1982. Mammographic signs as risk factors for breast cancer. *Br. J. Cancer.* 45: 185-193.
3. Jeffreys M, Warren R, Davey Smith G, Gunnell D. Breast density: agreement of measures from film and digital image. *British Journal of Radiology.* 76 (2003) 561-563
4. Quarterman C, Al-Nuaimi Y, Astley S M, Boggis C R M, Hillier V, Griffiths P, McGee M, Duffy S,Gilbert F J Breast Density Assessment by Multiple Readers for the Evaluation of Computer Aided Detection Systems. In: Proceedings of IWDM 2004, Chapel Hill, North Carolina, ed Pisano E. 2004
5. Byng JW, Boyd NF, Jong RA, Fishell E, Yaffe MJ. Quantitative analysis of mammographic densities. *Phys Med Biol* 39: 1629-38. 1994
6. Highnam, R. and M. Brady. 1999. *Mammographic Image Analysis.* Dordrecht: Kluwer Academic Publishers.
7. Pawluczyk, O., B. J. Augustine, M. J. Yaffe, D. Rico, J. Yang, and G. E. Mawdsley. 2003. A volumetric method for estimation of breast density on digitized screen-film mammograms. *Med. Phys.* 30:352-364.
8. Smith J, Astley S, Graham J, Hufton A. The calibration of grey levels in mammograms *In* K Doi, ML Giger, R M Nishikawa, R A Schmidt (Eds.) *Digital Mammography* Elsevier 1996
9. Hufton A, Astley SM, Marchant T and Patel H. A method for the quantification of dense breast tissue from digitised mammograms. In: Proceedings of IWDM 2004, Chapel Hill, North Carolina, ed Pisano E. 2004
10. Harvie M, Mercer TH, Humphries G, Hopwood P, Adams J, Evans G, Sumner H, Astley S, Hayes L, Cooley J, Ashcroft L and Howell A (2002) The effects of weight loss and exercise on biomarkers of breast cancer risk – rationale and study design. In S Gandalai (Ed.), Recent research developments in nutrition: Volume 5. Kerala, India, Research Signpost, pp. 91-110.
11. Sala E, Warren R, McCann J, Duffy S, Luben R, Day N (1999) High risk mammographic parenchymal patterns and anthropometric measures: a case control study. *British Journal of Cancer* 81 (7) 1257-1261

Mammography Tomosynthesis System for High Performance 3D Imaging

Jeffrey W. Eberhard[1], Douglas Albagli[1], Andrea Schmitz[1], Bernhard E.H. Claus[1], Paul Carson[2], Mitchell Goodsitt[2], Heang-Ping Chan[2], Marilyn Roubidoux[2], Jerry A. Thomas[3], and Jacqueline Osland[3]

[1] GE Global Research, Niskayuna, NY
eberhard@research.ge.com
[2] University of Michigan, Ann Arbor, Michigan
[3] Via Christi Regional Medical Center, Wichita, Kansas

Abstract. Tomosynthesis provides a major advance in image quality compared to conventional projection mammography by effectively eliminating the effects of superimposed tissue on anatomical structures of interest. Early tomosynthesis systems focused primarily on feasibility assessment by providing 3-dimensional images to determine performance advantages. However, tomosynthesis image quality depends strongly on three key parameters: 1) detector performance at low dose, 2) angular range and number of projections acquired in the tomosynthesis scan, and 3) reconstruction algorithm processing characteristics used to create slice images from the measured projections. In this work, a new GE mammography tomosynthesis research system was developed that incorporates key improvements in each of these three areas compared to an early feasibility prototype system in use at Massachusetts General Hospital from 2000 to 2004. The performance gains that can be achieved by these enhancements are characterized, and clinical images acquired with the system at the University of Michigan Cancer and Geriatrics Center are presented. The advanced research system also provides the ability to acquire mechanically co-registered x-ray tomosynthesis and ultrasound images of the breast, and initial dual modality images are also presented.

1 Method

An x-ray tomosynthesis/ultrasound dual modality prototype system suitable for clinical evaluation has been developed to assess the potential to further improve breast cancer diagnosis. The tomosynthesis system is based on the Senographe DS image chain (GE Healthcare, Milwaukee, WI). Key x-ray subsystems include the x-ray source (tube and generator), the detector, the patient positioner, and the reconstruction and review hardware. The tube and generator from the Senographe DS digital mammography system have been modified to provide 50% higher current on the Rh target. This allows shorter x-ray exposure times and minimizes the possibility of patient motion during the tomosynthesis exam.

Susan M. Astley et al. (Eds.): IWDM 2006, LNCS 4046, pp. 137–143, 2006.
© Springer-Verlag Berlin Heidelberg 2006

The detector is a high performance, next generation a-Si/CsI flat panel design that achieves significant improvement in DQE at typical tomosynthesis dose levels [1]. It consists of a matrix of 1920 x 2304 pixel elements at a pitch of 100um. In order to enable low dose imaging, the noise floor of the detector was significantly reduced by altering the ratio of the electronic noise (EN) to the conversion factor (CF, signal per incident x-ray). This ratio describes the electronic noise of the detector in units of x-rays and governs how the DQE falls off with decreasing exposure (Figure 1). While 12-24 x-rays of noise may be acceptable for current 2D screening applications, 3-6 x-rays of noise are required for tomo applications, which may be acquired at 10 to 20 times lower dose per projection than a standard mammogram. By optimizing the scintillator and optical transport properties of the flat panel and adding a storage capacitor at each pixel, this electronic noise reduction was achieved while expanding the overall dynamic range of the detector.

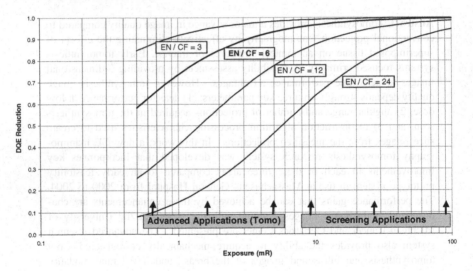

Fig. 1. DQE reduction factor vs. exposure as a function of electronic noise ratio (EN/CF) [1]

A specialized patient positioner was designed to provide a more flexible acquisition geometry with provision for dual modality XR/US imaging. During the tomosynthesis acquisition, the tube traverses an arc above the patient, with the point of rotation at the level of the breast support. The compressed breast remains stationary above the non-rotating detector surface during the examination. The system acquires 21 projection images over a wide angular range of 60 degrees in under 8 sec in order to minimize patient motion during the exam. Larger angular range provides greater depth resolution and more projections reduce the level of streak artifacts in the images. The prototype system installed at the University of Michigan is shown in Fig. 2.

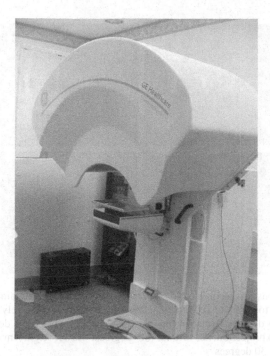

Fig. 2. Photograph of the prototype tomosynthesis system installed at the University of Michigan Cancer and Geriatric Center

Images from the research system are reconstructed using a generalized filtered backprojection (GFBP) reconstruction algorithm [2], consisting of a 2D filtering operation on the projections, followed by an order-statistics based backprojection step (OSBP). The slice images are typically reconstructed on a 100um x 100um grid (full detector resolution) with a slice spacing of 500um. The 2D filtering is effective in enhancing contrast of structures and managing statistical image noise (quantum and electronic), while the OSBP step is useful in managing out-of-plane artifacts. This flexible algorithm is non-iterative (i.e., fast) and flexible.

2 Results

Results of the analysis of reconstructed image quality using a wire phantom are illustrated in Figure 3. In particular, the figure shows vertical cross-sections through volumetric reconstructions of various wires, where the image gray scales are normalized such that the brightest point and the background in all images are at the same gray-scale. GFBP exhibits higher contrast and reduced artifacts as compared to simple backprojection. Also, the beneficial effects of larger angular range (leading to improved depth-resolution) and larger number of projections (leading to reduced artifact contrast) are demonstrated.

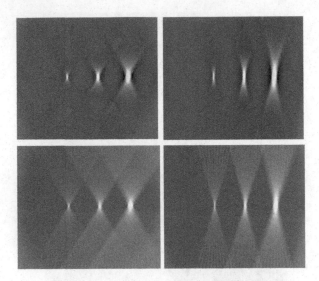

Fig. 3. Cross-sections of reconstructions of the wire phantom containing 4 wires, with diameters (from left to right) of 0.05, 0.79, 1.59, and 2.38mm respectively. Upper left image: GFBJ, 21 views, 60 degrees. Upper right image: GFBP, 11 views, 30 degrees. Lower left image: Simple Backprojection, 21 views, 60 degrees. Lower right image: Simple Backprojection, 11 views, 30 degrees.

Profiles through the wires are shown in Figure 4. Note that the horizontal resolution is essentially independent of number of projections and scanning angle, but that vertical resolution improves as scanning angular range is increased.

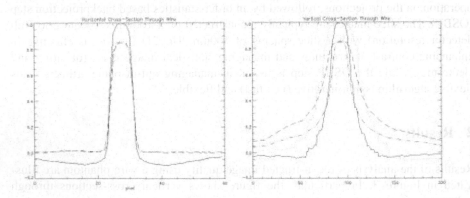

Fig. 4. a) Horizontal cross-section through reconstructed wire (left), and b) vertical cross-section through reconstructed wire (right); the x-axis is in 0.1mm (= 1 pixel) units. Solid: GFBP, 21 views, 60 degrees. Dotted: GFBP, 11 views, 30 degrees. Dash-dotted: Simple Backprojection, 21 views, 60 degrees. Dashed: Simple Backprojection 11 views, 30 degrees.

The research system is used routinely for research imaging of patients. Tomosynthesis images are reconstructed from 21 low-dose projection images acquired over an angular range of 60 degrees in less than 8 sec. Reconstruction of patient images is done with both the GFBJ [2] and the SART algorithm [3].

Projection images acquired with the system are presented in Figure 5. The first, middle and last images acquired in the projection sequence are presented to the technologist during the exam as an initial quality check. The technologist checks for correct positioning, patient motion, and generally appropriate exposure parameters.

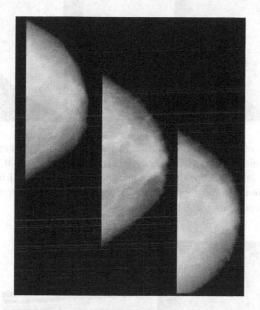

Fig. 5. Projection images acquired with the tomosynthesis research system at tube positions of a) –30 degrees, b) 0 degrees, and c) 30 degrees. Total dose in a tomo scan ranges from 150% to 200% of the dose in a standard mammographic view, so the dose in a single tomo projection is approximately 7 – 10% of that in a standard mammographic view.

A comparison of a conventional projection mammography image to two tomographic slices is shown in Figure 6. Note the soft tissue detail visible in the tomo slices and the enhanced visibility of the lateral vein in one tomographic slice, compared to the mammogram where only the thickest, central part is seen. The blood vessel present in the first tomographic slice has disappeared in the adjacent slice, 3 mm away.

A comparison of conventional mammography to an ultrasonic scan is shown in Figure 7. The ultrasound is a sagittal view at the location of the top arrow in the mammogram. Note the boundary between the anechoic and echogenic regions indicated by the arrow in the ultrasonic image.

Finally, a comparison of a conventional mammogram with the co-registered ultrasonic image is shown in Figure 8. Both tomosynthesis and ultrasonic images for all the slices through the breast are, of course, available from the physically co-registered acquisitions.

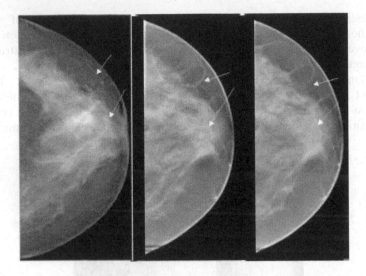

Fig. 6. Comparison of conventional digital mammogram with tomographic slices.   A. Mammogram in Cranio Caudal (CC) view. B. Tomographic slice at 25 mm deep.   C. Tomographic slice at 28 mm deep. Note the disappearance of much of the 3.8 mm diameter vessel (upper arrow) in this tomographic slice (C), separated by 3 mm from (B). Note also the changing soft tissue detail throughout the two slices.

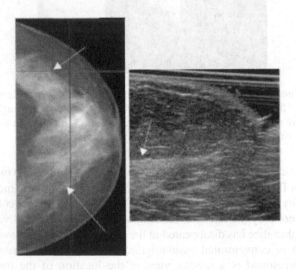

Fig. 7. Comparison of conventional mammogram to co-registered ultrasonic image. A. Mammogram in Cranio Caudal (CC) view. The bottom arrow denotes a glandular tissue boundary and the superficial vessel seen more clearly in the tomogram in Fig. 6.   B. Ultrasonic image in sagittal slices normally acquired for CC views (twice the scale of the mammogram).

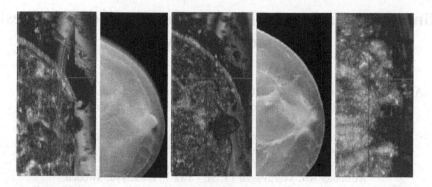

Fig. 8. Comparison of ultrasound images with tomographic slices in normal volunteer. A. Reconstructed axial ultrasound image (C scan). B. Tomographic slice showing subcutaneous vessel near the bottom of the image. C. Axial ultrasound slice 15 mm from the skin, D. Corresponding tomographic slice. E. Axial Ultrasound 25 mm deep, corresponding to tomographic image in Fig. 8B.

3 Discussion

A dual modality, x-ray tomosynthesis/ultrasound imaging prototype system has been designed, built, and tested, and characterized. Significant performance enhancements have been realized by incorporating a new, high performance aSi flat panel detector optimized for low dose acquisitions, a large tomosynthesis acquisition angular range with a substantially increased number of projections compared to previous systems, and a fast, flexible reconstruction algorithm with artifact management incorporated directly into the reconstruction process. The system is in clinical evaluation at the University of Michigan Cancer and Geriatric Center in Ann Arbor and at Via Christi Regional Medical Center in Wichita, Kansas.

This work was supported in part by Grant No. 5RO1 CA091713 from the National Cancer Institute and by Grant No. MDA9050210012 from the U.S. Office of Naval Research, through subcontract 65092 from the Henry M. Jackson Foundation for the Advancement of Military Medicine.

References

1. D. Albagli, S. Han, A. Couture, H. Hudspeth, C. Collazo, "Performance of an optimized amorphous silicon cesium-iodide based large filed-of-view detector for mammography", Proc **SPIE 5745**, 1078-1086 (2005)

2. B.E.H. Claus, J.W. Eberhard, J.A. Thomas, C.E. Galbo, W.P. Pakenas, S.L. Muller, "Preference Study of Reconstructed Image Quality in Mammographic Tomosynthesis", in H.-O. Peitgen (ed.), Digital Mammography IWDM 2002, Proceedings of the 6th Intl. Workshop on Digital Mammography, June 22-25, 2002, Bremen, Germany, Springer 2003.

3. Y. Zhang, H. Chan, B. Sahiner, J. Wei, M. M. Goodsitt, L. M. Hadjiiski, J. Ge, C. Zhou. "Tomosynthesis reconstruction with simultaneous algebraic reconstruction technique (SART) on breast phantom data", Proc SPIE, Medical Imaging 2006.

Clinical Evaluation of a Photon-Counting Tomosynthesis Mammography System

Andrew D.A. Maidment[1], Christer Ullberg[2], Tom Francke[2], Lars Lindqvist[2], Skiff Sokolov[2], Karin Lindman[2], Leif Adelow[2], and Per Sunden[3]

[1] University of Pennsylvania, Department of Radiology,
3400 Spruce Street, Philadelphia, PA USA 19104
andrew.maidment@uphs.upenn.edu
[2] XCounter AB, Svärdvägen 11, SE - 182 33 Danderyd, Sweden
{christer.ullberg, tom.francke, lars.lindqvist, skiff.sokolov, karin.lindman, leif.adelow}@xcounter.se
[3] Danderyds Sjukhus, Mammography Department,
AB 182 88 Stockholm, Sweden
per.sunden@ds.se

Abstract. Digital breast tomosynthesis promises solutions to many of the problems currently associated with projection mammography, including elimination of artifactual densities from the superposition of normal tissues and increasing the conspicuity of true lesions that would otherwise be masked by superimposed normal tissue. We have investigated the performance of a novel tomosynthesis system in a clinical setup. The novel system uses 48 photon counting, orientation sensitive, linear detectors which are precisely aligned with the focal spot of the x-ray source. The x-ray source and the digital detectors are scanned in a continuous motion across the patient; each linear detector collecting an image at a distinct angle. The results from an assessment of image quality and the initial clinical trial of this device are presented. Initial results provide anecdotal evidence supporting the superiority of tomosynthesis over projection mammography.

1 Background

There are a number of problems currently associated with projection mammography, including decreased conspicuity of true lesions that are masked by superimposed normal tissue and artifactual densities from the superposition of normal tissues [1]. Tomosynthesis is a promising solution to overcome these problems [2-5]. However, tomosynthesis systems based on area flat-panel detectors themselves suffer from a number of fundamental limitations. First, the requirement of sequential image acquisition limits the number of images acquired; acquiring an insufficient number of images results in image artifacts [6, 7]. Second, electronic noise, ghosting and lag found in each of the source projection images are added in the reconstruction process, resulting in excessive noise in the reconstructed images. Third, the long readout time of current flat panel detector technology results in image blurring, both from patient motion, and from the continuous scanning motion used in some systems.

Susan M. Astley et al. (Eds.): IWDM 2006, LNCS 4046, pp. 144–151, 2006.
© Springer-Verlag Berlin Heidelberg 2006

2 Imaging System

A novel tomosynthesis system has been developed [6-10]. The system uses 48 photon-counting, orientation sensitive, linear detectors which are precisely aligned with the focal spot of the x-ray source. The x-ray source and the digital detectors are scanned in a continuous motion across the patient; each linear detector collecting an image at a distinct angle.

The 48 simultaneously collected images are of very high image quality due to several special characteristics of this detector technology. First, the detectors are insensitive to scattered radiation; the detector geometry ensures that only primary photons emanating from the focal spot of the x-ray source will elicit a response from the detector. Second, the detector does not contribute any electronic noise; the strong gaseous amplification of each photon interaction allows a simple threshold to exclude electronic noise from being counted and included in the final image. Third, the image pixels are very small (60 μm) avoiding motion blurring from long scanning times of each sub-image. Finally, the detector technology does not have any residual image, ghosting or blooming artifacts.

Data appropriate for tomosynthesis is acquired over a region 24x30 cm^2 within 15 seconds. The resulting 48 projection images are then reconstructed using filtered back-projection to produce a volumetric data set of tomographic images. The images are presented on a dedicated primary review workstation for interpretation.

The imaging system is typically operated with a tube potential of between 30 and 40 kVp with a W-target anode and Al filtration. The mean glandular dose for a tomosynthesis image is typically less than or equal to a normal film/screen mammogram. The system is shown in Figure 1.

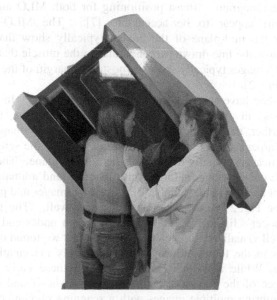

Fig. 1. The imaging system is shown. The system is capable of both projection mammography and tomosynthesis. The system is wider than conventional systems to accommodate the scanning detector and x-ray source.

3 Clinical Trial

Method: An initial clinical study of this novel tomosynthesis system has recently been completed. Enrolment was limited to 20 patients. The study was conducted with IRB oversight. All patients provided informed consent. Patient recruitment was limited to women having clinical and/or mammographic findings; specifically, they either had to be recalled after an abnormal screening mammogram or be referred by a physician after suspicious physical findings.

For each patient, analog film images were first taken at Danderyd Sjukhus (Danderyd, Sweden). Later the same day, digital tomosynthesis images were taken of the same breast by the same radiologic nurse. The digital tomosynthesis images were then reviewed by a trained radiologist.

Dosimetry: Twenty patients were enrolled in the clinical trial. The film-screen radiographs were acquired at either 30 or 31 kVp, with an average entrance skin air kerma (ESAK) of 6.68±4.83 mGy, and average glandular dose (AGD) of 1.46±0.73 mGy. By comparison, the tomosynthesis images were acquired at 30-35 kVp and 140-180 mA, resulting in an average ESAK of 4.98±0.61 mGy, and an AGD of 1.42±0.16 mGy.

Clinical Evaluation: Our initial goal was to seek anecdotal proof that the tomography system provided clinically acceptable breast images. Criteria included breast positioning, resolution of high-contrast structures such as calcifications and clips, and conspicuity of larger low-contrast objects such masses and cysts.

A preliminary analysis indicates that the image quality achieved to date is clinically acceptable. Figure 1 demonstrates the system being used for a medial-lateral oblique (MLO) mammogram. Breast positioning for both MLO and cranio-caudal (CC) mammograms appear to be acceptable [7]. The MLO images, when reconstructed near the mid-plane of the breast, typically show that the pectoralis muscle extends below the line drawn perpendicular to the muscle that passes through the nipple. The CC images typically show the posterior margin of the glandular tissue (for example, see Fig. 2).

The images to date have shown very high spatial resolution. In general, we see more calcifications in the tomosynthesis images than in the screen-film mammograms. Further, the calcifications in the tomosynthesis images are generally better resolved (sharper margins and higher contrast) than in the screen-film images. We find that calcifications rapidly disappear when out-of-plane. These observations are consistent with our previous findings with phantoms and animals, and are likely due to the choice of angular range, number of projection images and pixel size.[6]

The images (see Fig. 2) depict the breast anatomy well. The glandular tissue, adipose tissue, Cooper's ligaments, blood vessels, lymph nodes and other structures of the breast are well visualized. In the 20 women studied we found one cancer which was quite obvious in the tomosynthesis image, and only marginally visible in the screen-film image. While anecdotal, we believe that these early images provide convincing evidence of the superiority of both tomosynthesis and our approach of simultaneously acquiring multiple images with a scanning photon-counting detector. We believe that the system is capable of producing images with clinically acceptable

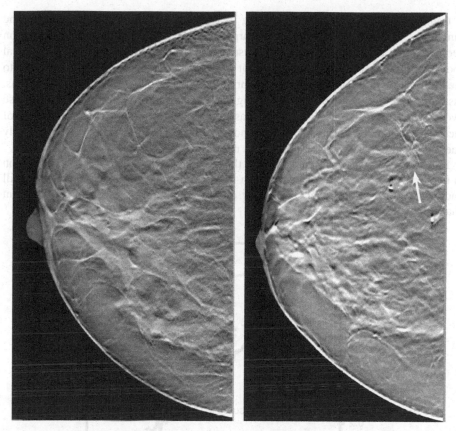

Fig. 2. Reconstructions from 2 patients. The patient on the left has numerous calcifications that are clearly seen. The patient on the right has a spiculated mass, which on biopsy was identified as a ductal carcinoma.

quality, and having adequate tissue penetration and breast positioning. Admittedly, these results are preliminary and lack statistical significance.

4 Assessment of Image Quality

Image quality has been assessed by multiple methods, including the assessment of the modulation transfer function (MTF) and the noise power spectrum (NPS).

MTF: The MTF in the scanning and strip (i.e., parallel to the linear detector strips) directions have been measured. The MTF was measured using a slanted edge method [11]. The edge was measured in an image reconstructed with simple back-projection, in the plane of the edge. Figure 3 shows the measured MTF in the scanning direction. These data are shown compared to theoretical calculations. The theoretical MTF can be decomposed into 2 main sources of blurring. The first is related to scanning unsharpness. The detector is read out each time the detector array is translated 60 μm. Thus, the scanning unsharpness can be represented by a sinc function. The second source of unsharpness is related to the image acquisition geometry; the collimator is at a fixed distance above the breast and the x-ray focal spot is of known size and shape. Thus, it is possible to calculate the blurring due to the collimator width and geometric unsharpness as the product of two sinc functions, assuming that the focal spot has a rectangular intensity profile. The product of these two sources of unsharpness is specified as the "Total" in Figure 3. The similarity of the measured and experimental data is noteworthy. The discrepancy seen is likely due to deviation from the assumption of a rectangular focal spot.

Figure 4 shows the measured MTF in the scan and strip directions. The resolution in the strip direction is lower than that in the scan direction. This degradation is still under investigation; however, it is likely due to simultaneous triggering of adjacent channels in the detector.

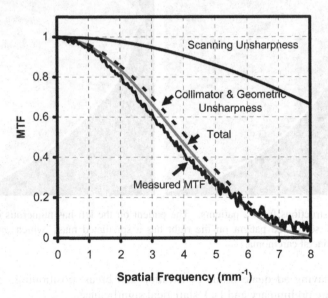

Fig. 3. System MTF of tomographic images in the scanning direction. Both measured and theoretical data are presented. The theoretical unsharpness is divided into two terms: scanning unsharpness, and collimator and geometric unsharpness. Their product is labeled "Total". The theoretical total MTF is quite similar to the measured MTF.

NPS: Images to calculate the NPS were acquired at 35 kVp with a W-target x-ray tube and 0.5 mm Al filtration. A uniform block of PMMA 40 mm thick was imaged. From these projection images, 128 planes with 0.3 mm separation were reconstructed using both simple backprojection and filtered backprojection. Using these data, a volume of interest (VOI) 38×60×200 mm (128×1024×3328 pixels) was selected with the largest dimension parallel to the chest wall. The VOI size and orientation were chosen to minimize the heel effect. A VOI 200 mm long is acceptable due to the scanning geometry. The VOI was then divided into 128×128×128 voxel cubes

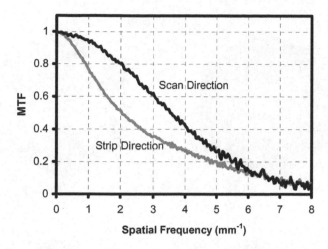

Fig. 4. MTF of tomographic images in the scan and strip directions. The MTF in the strip direction is reduced com-pared to the scan direction due to simultaneous trig-gering of adjacent channels.

overlapping by 64 pixels in both the x and y directions. A 3D spectral estimate was calculated for each cube, and these estimates were averaged to calculate the NPS.

The NPS are shown in Fig. 5 for the case of simple (a, c) and filtered (b, d) back-projection, presented logarithmically. The same grayscale is used for the simple and filtered spectra. The axes are labeled with the spatial orientation corresponding to the spatial frequencies shown, where X denotes the direction along the chestwall, Y denotes the orthogonal direction from the chestwall to the nipple, and Z is the direction perpendicular to the detector. The origin is located at the center of the cube.

There are many notable features in the NPS. As shown previously, the NPS of the projection images produced with the system are essentially white [7]. Restated, there is little correlation in the images. This can be seen in Fig. 1a and c, where the NPS can roughly be segmented into areas of white noise (the uniform light gray regions) and no noise (the uniform dark gray regions). This segmentation allows us to define the null space [12] of the imaging system as the latter region. An examination of the null space clearly demonstrates one of the benefits of photon-counting detectors in tomosynthesis, as there is virtually no noise in the regions of space not supported by the angular sampling. The complement to the null space clearly demonstrates which spatial frequencies are supported in the reconstruction.

Comparing Figs. 1a and c to Figs. 1b and d, the effect of the filter is made clear. In the example shown, the filter that was used suppressed high spatial-frequencies in the X-direction. This is consistent with the two large dark bands running vertically in the Z-direction on the lateral sides of the X-Z face (Fig 1b and d). Very low spatial frequencies in the X-direction are also suppressed, as can be seen by the dark vertical band that divides the X-Z face and X-Y face (Fig. 1b).

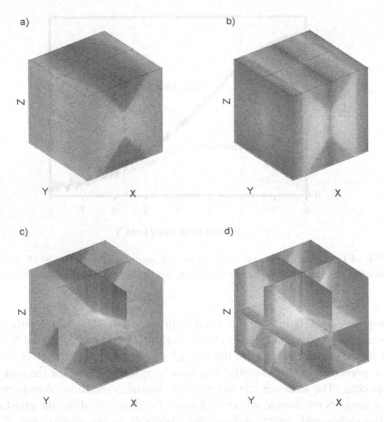

Fig. 5. The logarithm of the NPS is shown in 3D for the case of simple (a, c) and filtered (b, d) back-projection. The axes are labeled with the spatial orientation corresponding to the spatial frequencies shown (X, the direction along the chestwall; Y, the orthogonal direction from the chestwall to the nipple; Z, the direction perpendicular to the detector).

5 Discussion

A novel tomographic imaging system has been developed. The detector technology is the first to have been developed specifically for tomosynthesis imaging. As such, it offers numerous technical advantages over tomosynthesis with flat panel detectors. The first clinical trial of the system is complete. Initial clinical results demonstrate outstanding image quality and diagnostic value. To date, these results are anecdotal. A retrospective reader trial is planned to determine more quantitative measures.

The clinical trial was performed at a dose comparable to screen-film mammography. It is important to realize that the dose in a digital image is somewhat arbitrary, as the system is linear and has very wide dynamic range. However, there are two relevant questions: (1) is the resultant image x-ray quantum noise limited to high spatial-frequency; and (2) are the images of clinical quality. We believe that the NPS analysis establishes the former. We further believe that the outstanding image quality of the clinical images to date provide anecdotal proof of the latter. Thus, it is notable that the tomosynthesis images were acquired at a lower dose than the screen-film mammograms, yet appear to have comparable or superior image quality.

Acknowledgments

This work is funded in part by NIH grant PO1 CA85484-01.

References

[1] Ma L, Fishell E, Wright B, et al. Case-control study of factors associated with failure to detect breast cancer by mammography. Journal of the National Cancer Institute 1992;84(10):781-5.

[2] Dobbins JT, 3rd, Godfrey DJ. Digital x-ray tomosynthesis: current state of the art and clinical potential. Physics in Medicine & Biology 2003;48(19):R65-106.

[3] Niklason LT, Christian BT, Niklason LE, et al. Digital tomosynthesis in breast imaging. Radiology 1997;205(2):399-406.

[4] Rafferty EA. Tomosynthesis: New Weapon in Breast Cancer Fight. Decisions in Imaging Economics 2004;17(4).

[5] Wu T, Moore RH, Rafferty EA, et al. Breast tomosynthesis: Methods and applications. In: Karellas A, editor. RSNA Categorical Course in Diagnostic Radiology Physics: Advances in Breast Imaging - Physics, Technology, and Clinical Applications; 2004. p. 149-163.

[6] Maidment ADA, Albert M, Thunberg S, et al. Evaluation of a Photon-Counting Breast Tomosynthesis Imaging System. In: Flynn MJ, editor. SPIE Medical Imaging 2005; p. 572-82.

[7] Maidment ADA, Adelow L, Blom O, et al. Evaluation of a Photon-Counting Breast Tomosynthesis Imaging System. In: Flynn MJ, editor. Physics of Medical Imaging, Proc. SPIE 6142; 2006.

[8] Thunberg S, et al. Evaluation of a Photon Counting Mammography System. In: SPIE Medical Imaging 2002 p. 202-208.

[9] Thunberg S, Maidment ADA, et al. Dose reduction in Mammography with Photon Counting Imaging. In: SPIE Medical Imaging 2004; p. 457-465.

[10] Thunberg S, Maidment ADA, et al. Tomosynthesis with a Multi-line Photon Counting Camera. In: Pisano E, editor. 7th International Workshop on Digital Mammography; 2004; p. 459-465.

[11] Kao Y-H, Maidment ADA, Albert M, et al. Assessment of a software tool for measurement of the modulation transfer function. In: Flynn MJ, editor. Medical Imaging 2005: Physics of Medical Imaging; p. 1199-1208.

[12] Myers KJ, Barrett HH. Foundations of Image Science. New York, NY: John Wiley & Sons; 2004.

Three-Dimensional Digital Breast Tomosynthesis in the Early Diagnosis and Detection of Breast Cancer

Mari Varjonen

Tampere University of Technology, PL 692, 33101 Tampere, Finland
mari.johanna@sci.fi
Planmed Oy, Asentajankatu 6, 00880 Helsinki, Finland
mari.varjonen@planmed.com

Abstract. This paper presents doctoral thesis of three-dimensional digital breast tomosynthesis in the early diagnosis and detection of breast cancer. The purpose is to prove that digital breast tomosynthesis has the potential to provide clinically important information, which cannot be obtained with conventional breast imaging methods. Three-dimensional digital breast tomosynthesis seeks to (1) determine whether a mammographic finding is the result of a 'real' lesion or the superimposition of normal parenchyma structures, (2) detect subtle changes in breast tissue, which might otherwise be missed, and (3) to reduce the number of biopsies performed as well as verify the correct biopsy target if the procedure is needed. This study presents digital breast tomosynthesis in diagnostic mammography by comparing digital breast tomosynthesis with screen-film and digital mammograms clinical performance, evaluates Tuned Aperture Computed Tomography capability as a 3D breast reconstruction algorithm in the limited angle tomosynthesis system, and demonstrates technical performance of a real-time amorphous-selenium flat-panel detector in full field digital breast tomosynthesis. The results indicate that breast tomosynthesis has the potential to significantly advance diagnostic mammography. Tomosynthesis of the breast will increase specificity. Study also suggests that tomosynthesis might facilitate the detection of cancers at an earlier stage and a smaller size than is possible in two-dimensional mammography [1].

1 Introduction

Two-dimensional (2D) mammography plays a most important role in all aspects of breast cancer detection, diagnosis and treatment. Although it is well known that 2D mammography has limitations and it is not capable of detecting all breast cancers, there is no question that mammography is an important imaging technique for detecting and diagnosing breast cancer. Challenges of 2D mammography are structured noise, which is created by the overlap of normal dense tissue structures within the breast. This may obscure the findings causing lesions to be missed (reduction of diagnostic sensitivity). Breast tissue may also simulate the presence of a cancer that does not actually exist. This causes a loss of diagnostic specificity. Currently 2D mammography is the only x-ray imaging modality accepted for breast cancer screening, but for years researchers have tried to find improved technologies and new methods to

Susan M. Astley et al. (Eds.): IWDM 2006, LNCS 4046, pp. 152–159, 2006.

supplement 2D mammography and provide better sensitivity and specificity. Digital breast tomosynthesis (DBT) is a method that was first described many years ago, but could not be easily applied until the development of fast read-out digital detectors. The goal of breast tomosynthesis is to make available a method for screening and diagnostic mammography, which provides higher sensitivity and specificity than routine mammography [1], [2], [3].

1.1 Digital Breast Tomosynthesis

The ability to produce tomographic sections through the body with x-rays to eliminate structured noise was developed decades ago. In the late 1970's, linear and poly-cycloidal tomography was used to evaluate many organ systems. During exposures that lasted several seconds, the x-ray tube was moved in one direction while the film receptor was moved in the opposite direction. Only structures in the plane of interest stayed perfectly aligned and in sharp detail during the exposure, while structures that were out the plane on interest were blurred by the motion. Only the structures at the fulcrum of movement stayed registered. To see another plane, the fulcrum of the motion was shifted, and another exposure was made. Commonly used to evaluate other organ systems, such as kidney and chest, this technique was not feasible for breast evaluation. Breast tomosynthesis acquires multiple images as the x-ray source moves through an arc above the stationary compressed breast and digital imaging detector. As the acquisition begins, the beam moves through a series of positions in different degrees. Once the projections of the breast are obtained during a tomosynthesis sequency, they must be reconstructed into a data set and displayed in a manner suitable for review by a radiologist [2], [4], [5].

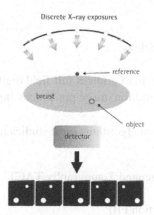

Fig. 1. Principle of breast tomosynthesis imaging

With stereotactic tubehead movement, the digital mammography system acquires a number of projection images with different angles, shown in figure 1. The total arc varies between 30° to 60°. The number of projection images varies from 7 to 25 exposures. The patient is seated during the tomosynthesis study since the complete set of exposures must be accomplished with the breast held in compression while the patient remains motionless. The time of complete acquisition varies from 8 to 90 seconds. After each exposure, the tube moves to the next position and stops to acquire the next image [1].

The projection images obtained during a tomosynthesis sequence must be reconstructed. As the x-ray source moves along an arc above the breast, algorithms allow reconstruction of arbitrary planes in the breast from limited-angle series of projections. Almost every research group has their own specific way to perform a tomosynthesis study. Many important parameters for breast tomosynthesis have an effect on quality of three-dimensional (3D) data, and are currently under evaluation among many research groups:

- Number of projection images
- Total dose of the tomosynthesis study
- Slice 'thickness'
- Number of slices
- Type of detector technology
- Type of detector motion
- Radiation source
- Quality of x-ray beam
- X-ray tube
- Acquisition time
- Detector calibration
- Reconstruction time
- 3D data visualization
- 3D workstation
- Compression force
- Reconstruction algorithms
- Post-processing
- Algorithm development of gridless full field digital mammography
- Angle dependent projection image pre-processing [1].

The following reconstruction algorithms have studies in breast tomosynthesis:

- Shift-and-add SAA
- Tuned Aperture Computed Tomography TACT
- Back Projection BP
- Filtered Back Projection FBP
- Iterative Matrix Inversion Tomosynthesis MITS
- Maximum-Likelihood Algorithm ML
- Algebraic Reconstruction Technique ART
- Gaussian Frequency Blending GFB.

2 Materials and Methods

2.1 Study Objectives

There were five main objectives in the study design [1]:

1. Investigate digital breast tomosynthesis in diagnostic mammography by comparing digital breast tomosynthesis images and screen-film or digital mammograms clinical performance. Study digital breast tomosynthesis as an improved clinical method having greater possibility to:
   - Distinguish possible malignant from benign
   - Analyze lesion margins
   - Interpret confidently the finding as a summation.
2. Evaluate Tuned Aperture Computed Tomography (TACT®) capability as 3D breast reconstruction algorithm in the limited angle tomosynthesis system.
3. Demonstrate technical and clinical performance of a real-time amorphous-selenium (a-Se) flat-panel detector (FPD) in full field digital breast tomosynthesis.
4. Feasibility study combining diagnostic breast tomosynthesis and ultrasound imaging of the breast with clinical information in diagnostic mammography.
5. Evaluate digital spot image quality (= tomosynthesis projection images) against screen-film and diagnostic mammography.

This paper concentrates on the first objective; investigate digital breast tomosynthesis in diagnostic mammography by comparing digital breast tomosynthesis images and screen-film or digital mammograms clinical performance and study digital breast tomosynthesis as an improved clinical method.

2.2 Clinical Patients

The patient data included in this thesis is comprised of 250 patients. 150 patients were enrolled in Finland and 100 were enrolled in the USA. Screen-film and digital mammograms included right and left mediolateral oblique (MLO) and craniocaudal (CC) views. Diagnostic mammography (also called work-up) included lateromedial (LM) and coned-down magnification views [1].

2.2.1 Helsinki University Central Hospital (HUCH) Mammography Department, Helsinki, Finland

Diagnostic digital breast tomosynthesis examinations were performed on 150 asymptomatic women. The key investigation, which was digital breast tomosynthesis in diagnostic mammography, consisted of 60 asymptomatic-women. The potential value of digital breast tomosynthesis was investigated by testing its ability to resolve ambiguities possible lesions in the screening examination. The women were selected for the study based on the fact that it was not possible to exclude the presence of breast cancer based on their screening mammography exams. Some abnormal findings seen on the images were architectural distortion, stellate look-a-like lesions, parenchymal asymmetry and density changes. Some lesions included micro-calcifications, which were either clusters or diffusely distributed. The morphology of the micro-calcifications was casting, granular, punctate, or miscellaneous. Adjunctive diagnostic methods were core biopsy, fine needle aspiration biopsy (FNAB) or vacuum assisted biopsy. Cytological and histological results for benign findings were: fibrocystic change, tumor phylloides, cysts, fibroadenomas, fibrosis, adenosis, atypical ductal hyperplasia (ADH), ductal cancer in situ (DCIS) and lobular cancer in situ (LCIS). Results for malignant findings were ductal and lobular cancers, both grades 1 and 2 were found. The pathological anatomy diagnosis (PAD) from the surgery specimens varied in the following ways: ductal, lobular, mucinosum, tubulobular, multifocal tubular, invasive micropapillare cancers, fibroadenomas, adenosis, DCIS, LCIS, radial scars, tumor phylloides, and papillomas. The grade of malignant tumor varied between 1 and 3[1], [4], [6], [7].

2.2.2 Jane Brattain Breast Center, Park Nicollet Clinic, Minneapolis, USA

The total number of women participating in the study were 100 (ages 45 to 80). All patients were recalled because additional information was needed to better determine treatment planning or because it was not possible to exclude the presence of breast cancer after screening mammography. A total of 43 invasive cancers and 3 ductal in situ carcinomas (DCIS) were detected and diagnosed. The 54 benign cases included lobular carcinoma in situ (LCIS), atypical ductal hyperplasia (ADH), fibrocystic change, fibroadenoma, cyst, scar, intracystic papilloma, hemangioma, benign microcalcifications, and summation of breast tissue [8].

2.3 Evaluation of Clinical Data

Clinical image quality was evaluated independently by three experienced radiologists using the Likert scale or specific breast tomosynthesis evaluation form. The statistical method which was used was *t* test.

2.4 Digital Breast Tomosynthesis Systems

A small field of view digital breast tomosynthesis system, Diamond-Delta 32 TACT (Instrumentarium Imaging, now part of GE Healthcare) and the prototype of full field

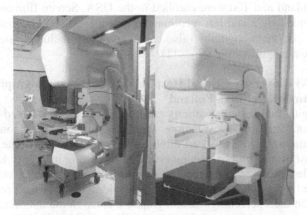

Fig. 2. On the left side Diamond Delta 32 for diagnostic breast tomosynthesis system. This system incorporates a CCD small-area detector with 48 μm pixel size, and is using TACT 3D technology. On the right side the prototype of tomosynthesis FFDM system (Diamond DX) based on *a*-Se technology with 85 μm pixel size.

digital breast tomosynthesis system, Diamond DX (Instrumentarium Imaging, now part of GE Healthcare) were the two tomosynthesis systems used mainly for the research of this thesis (figure 2.).

3 Results

3.1 *t* Test

The result of the *t* test shown in table 1 indicates that the clinical image quality is better in breast tomosynthesis slices than in SFM and DFM. The results indicate that breast tomosynthesis has the potential to significantly advance diagnostic mammography.

3.2 Specificity Analysis

The comparison of digital breast tomosynthesis slice images versus screening FFDM images and tomosynthesis volume model versus screening FFDM images were evaluated by three experienced radiologists. Results are presented in two tables. Table 2 summarizes the benefits of benign cases and table 3 explains the benefits of malignant cases. Digital breast tomosynthesis was found to be an improved method by providing greater opportunity to distinguish possible malignant from benign, analyze lesion margins and interpret confidently the finding as a summation.

Table 1. *t* test results [4], [6], [7]

(N=180)	*t* value	Std. Error	*t* test; (*P* < 0.001)
tomosynthesis slice images versus screen-film mammography (SFM) images	1.23	0.15	accept
tomosynthesis slice images versus diagnostic film mammography (DFM) images	0.82	0.15	accept

Table 2. Digital breast tomosynthesis (DBT) an improved clinical method studying the following benign cases [8]

Indication for digital breast tomosynthesis (DBT) clinical benefit	Number of cases where DBT was better (N=53)	Diagnostic benefit of tomosynthesis by increasing specificity
Probably benign lesion; analyze the lesion margins	20	38% (20/53 cases)
Summation of the breast tissue	14	26% (14/53 cases)
Number of unnecessary biopsies	36	68% (36/53 cases)
Analyze the finding; abnormality is present or not	40	75% (40/53 cases)
Reduce number of follow-up exams	30	57% (30/53 cases)

Table 3. Digital breast tomosynthesis (DBT) an improved clinical method studying the following malignant cases [8]

Indication for digital breast tomosynthesis (DBT) clinical benefit	Number of cases where DBT was better (N=47)	Diagnostic benefit of tomosynthesis by increasing specificity
Analyze tumor margins	30	64% (30/47 cases)
Multifocality, multicentricity	10	21% (10/47 cases)
Detection of small non-palpable breast cancers	3	6% (3/47 cases)

4 Discussions and Conclusion

Breast tomosynthesis shows promise of better breast cancer detection and diagnosis, even though there are many challenges in technology and clinical performance that lie ahead. Breast tomosynthesis needs clinical acceptance in order to play a successful role in breast cancer detection, diagnosis and treatment. In order to gain clinical acceptance a number of trials must be conducted which provide conclusive evidence that breast tomosynthesis screening is associated with a significant reduction in breast cancer mortality. Screening and diagnostic breast tomosynthesis trials have achieved good results with an acceptable increase in specificity and sensitivity for detecting and diagnosing challenging breast cancer cases. The goal of breast tomosynthesis is the detection of a high percentage of early stage breast cancers while maintaining an acceptable recall rate, biopsy rate and biopsy yield [1].

The first measure is sensitivity, which assesses the ability of radiologists to detect breast cancer on mammography, should be better than 85%. Follow-up on all cases, both positive and negative ones, is necessary to determine sensitivity accurately. Although the primary role of the radiologist is to detect early breast cancers, it is also important to have an acceptable recall rate. In mammography, the term 'false-positive' can be used to refer to two situations: recall for evaluation when cancer is not present or a biopsy recommendation for which benign disease is found. The number of false-positives should be as low as possible, without significantly reducing the breast cancer detection rate. Ideally the recall-rate should be less than 10%. Less than 1% of screening cases should lead to biopsy, and of those cases, the positive biopsy yield should be greater than 25% [9], [10].

Acknowledgements

My greatest gratitude and thanks goes to Dr Daniel Kopans, Dr Martin Yaffe, Dr Martti Pamilo, Dr Peter Dean, Dr Michael Nelson, Dr Leena Raulisto, and the personnel at the Helsinki University Central Hospital Mammography Department, Helsinki, Finland and the Jane Brattain Breast Center Park Nicollet Clinic, Minneapolis, USA. I would also like to acknowledge Dr Samuli Siltanen, Martti Kalke (MSc) and Timo Ihamäki (MSc).

References

1. Varjonen M. Three-dimensional (3D) digital breast tomosynthesis (DBT) in the early diagnosis and detection of breast cancer. Doctoral thesis. Tampere University of Technology publications 594, 2006.
2. Kopans DB. Digital mammography: Principles, equipment, technique and clinical results. Breast Imaging: RSNA Categorial course in Diagnostic Radiology 2005;77-82
3. Rafferty EA, Georgian-Smith D, Kopans DB, McCarthy KA, Hall DA, Moore R, Wu T. Comparison of full-field digital tomosynthesis with two view conventional film screen mammography in the prediction of lesion malignancy (abstr.). Radiology 2002;225(P):268.
4. Lehtimäki M, Pamilo M, Raulisto L, Roiha M, Kalke M, Siltanen S, and Ihamäki T. Diagnostic clinical benefits of digital spot and digital 3D mammography following analysis of screening findings. SPIE Proc 2003;5029:698-706.
5. Rafferty EA. Breast tomosynthesis. Advances in Digital Radiography: RSNA Categorical Course in Diagnostic Radiology Physics 2003;219-226.
6. Lehtimäki M, Pamilo M. Clinical aspects of diagnostic 3-dimensional mammography. Seminars in Breast Disease 2004;6:72-77.
7. Varjonen M, Pamilo M, Raulisto L. Clinical benefits of combined three-dimensional digital breast tomosynthesis and ultrasound imaging. SPIE Proc 2005;5745:562-571.
8. Lehtimäki M, Nelson M, Lechner M, Elvecrog E. Improved method for diagnosis in clinical mammography with breast tomosynthesis. Internatiol Workshop on Digital Mammography (IWDM) 2004.
9. D'Orsi CJ, Bassett LW, Berg WA, Feig SA, Jackson VP, Kopans DB, et al. Breast imaging reporting and data system. American College of Radiology 2003.
10. Farria DM, Monsees B. Screening mammography practise essentials. Radiol Clin N Am 2004;42:831-843.

Lesion Visibility in Low Dose Tomosynthesis

Andrew P. Smith, Loren Niklason, Baorui Ren, Tao Wu,
Chris Ruth, and Zhenxue Jing

Hologic Inc, 35 Crosby Drive,
Bedford, MA 02420 USA
asmith@hologic.com

Abstract. Visibility of lesions in mammography are significantly reduced by the presence of anatomical, or structure, noise. Breast tomosynthesis offers the possibility of reducing this noise. We have compared the detection of low contrast and microcalcification objects with tomosynthesis imaging as a function of dose to full field digital mammography (FFDM) performed at a standard screening dose. The measurements were performed with a variety of phantoms and complex backgrounds. The complex backgrounds greatly reduced object visibility using FFDM; much less so for the tomosynthesis images. In summary, visibility of low contrast objects using tomosynthesis was superior to visibility of these objects in FFDM, even when the tomosynthesis imaging was performed at 1/4 or less of a FFDM dose. Tomosynthesis also showed superior visibility to FFDM for 160-180 micron microcalcifications at 1/2 the FFDM dose.

1 Background

The sensitivity of conventional two-dimensional mammography can be limited by the presence of structures in the breast, which obscure detection of pathologies of interest[1]. Three dimensional imaging techniques reduce tissue overlap and improve visibility of low contrast details. Tomosynthesis is a method of performing high resolution limited angle tomography, at mammographic dose levels. Because the intrinsic contrast of tomosynthesis slices is very high, through the reduction of tissue overlap, it is of interest to estimate what tomosynthesis dose levels might provide equivalent detection efficiency compared to FFDM.

2 Method

Object visibility was measured using phantoms. Three types of phantoms were used. Two were contrast detail phantoms: the CDMAM phantom[2] and RMI-180 mammography contrast detail phantom[3]. The CDMAM phantom has gold discs with diameters from 0.06 to 2 mm and thickness 0.03 to 2 microns. The RMI-180 phantom has holes in acrylic with diameters from approximately 0.3 to 7 mm and depths from 0.06 to 1 mm. A third phantom contained calcifications grouped into sizes 160, 180 and 250 microns.

Susan M. Astley et al. (Eds.): IWDM 2006, LNCS 4046, pp. 160–166, 2006.
© Springer-Verlag Berlin Heidelberg 2006

These phantoms were imaged on top of complex backgrounds of varying types. The backgrounds were cadaverous 4.5 cm thick breast tissue and a piece of 2.5 cm thick beef.

The phantom/background combinations were imaged with a FFDM system at conventional U.S. screening dose (~1.7 mGy for 4.2 cm standard breast), and with a tomosynthesis system at a variety of doses (1.45, 0.73, 0.36, and 0.18 mGy for 4.2 cm standard breast).

Tomosynthesis acquisitions on a prototype system were performed, the raw data reconstructed, and the reconstructed slice at the appropriate height for the phantom objects was identified. Four experienced readers viewed all the images. For the microcalcification targets, the number of visible specks at each microcalcification size was totaled for each image and used as a scoring metric. For the contrast detail phantom, contrast detail curves were generated for the FFDM and the tomosynthesis images at the different doses.

2.1 Acquisition Method

The FFDM images were acquired on a standard digital mammography system (Selenia, Hologic, Inc.). The tomosynthesis images were acquired using a digital tomosynthesis prototype[4], which is a Selenia FFDM system modified to accommodate tomosynthesis acquisitions. This system acquired 11 views over a 15-degree scan. The phantoms were imaged twice at each dose level, moving the phantom relative to the background between exposures to avoid biasing the results by inadvertent arrangements between the objects and the obscuring background structures.

2.2 Reconstructions

The data acquired using the tomosynthesis systems were reconstructed using a filtered back projection algorithm. The images were reconstructed in a matrix with pixel spacing of 100 microns and a slice separation of 1 mm.

2.3 Reading and Scoring

Four experienced readers evaluated the images in a darkened room using a softcopy workstation with dual 3 MP flat panel monitors. Readers were free to magnify and window/level, and to spend as much time as desired on every image. In the case of the tomosynthesis images, only one slice was scored- the in-focus slice where the objects were visible with the greatest sharpness.

Contrast detail phantoms were scored using the following criteria. For each disc diameter, the score was the thinnest visible disc, not allowing skipping over larger sized invisible discs. No other corrections were made to these scores. With the CD-MAM phantom, only the central disc in each square was evaluated. The contrast detail results were averaged over the four observers and over the two sets of acquisitions for each phantom and background combination.

The microcalcification scoring proceeded differently. The phantom consisted of groups of microcalcifications of differing sizes. The number of microcalcifications in each size group was known from the phantom manufacturer, and from imaging the phantom in the absence of structured background, when they could all be seen. For each size group, the reader would count the number of visible microcalcifications.

3 Results

The phantom results are shown as a function of FFDM and tomosynthesis (tomo) dose. FFDM was imaged at only one dose, approximately 1.7 mGy for 4.2 standard breast, referred to a FFDM 1x dose. The tomo dose levels will be referred to as 1x, ½ x, ¼ x, 1/8 x, and correspond to the dose levels of 1.45, 0.73, 0.36, and 0.18 mGy for 4.2 cm standard breast.

3.1 Contrast-Detail Phantoms

Contrast detail curves at each tomosynthesis dose level and for the FFDM images were averaged over the four observers.   Without exception, the contrast detail performance of the tomosynthesis images at 1.45 mGy greatly exceeded the FFDM performance at similar 1.7 mGy dose. As the tomo dose was decreased, image noise predictably increased, but object visibility remained high relative to FFDM, due to the reduction of structure noise.

One example set of images is seen in Figure 1. The tomosynthesis image at 1/8x dose is grainy, but still has superior disc visibility to the FFDM image at 1x dose.

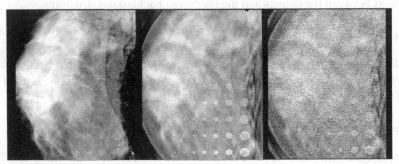

FFDM 1x dose   Tomo 1x dose   Tomo 1/8x dose

Fig. 1. RMI-180 contrast detail phantom with cadaverous breast tissue complex background imaged with both FFDM and tomosynthesis

Figs. 2-4 shows the contrast detail performance for two different complex backgrounds and the two different phantoms. The area of the cadaverous breast was too small to cover the CD-MAM phantom so that imaging combination was not performed. These results are averaged over the four observers and over the two relative positionings of the phantom and the background.

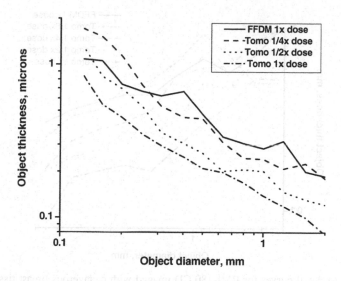

Fig. 2. Contrast detail curves for CD-MAM imaged with meat complex background

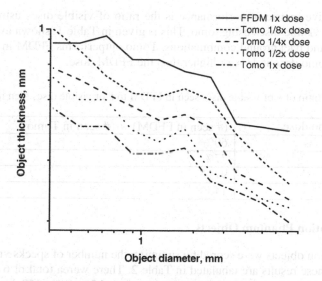

Fig. 3. Contrast detail curves for RMI-180 CD imaged with meat complex background

The CD-MAM phantom showed roughly equivalent contrast detail performance between FFDM at 1x dose and tomo at ¼ x dose. The RMI-180 phantom showed similar performance for tomo at ¼ -1/8x dose compared to FFDM. The slightly superior relative tomo performance with the RMI phantom compared to the CD-MAM phantom might be a reflection of the larger axial extent of the RMI phantom, and hence the greater blurring of the out-of-plane background texture.

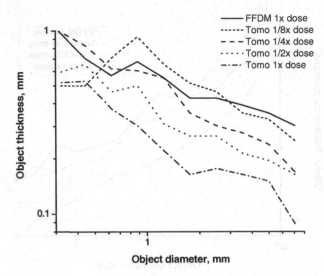

Fig. 4. Contrast detail curves for RMI-180 CD imaged with cadaverous breast tissue complex background

An alternative metric of performance is the ratio of visible discs using FFDM to the number of visible discs using tomo. This is given in Table 1, shown averaged over all phantoms and background combinations. Tomo outperforms FFDM in disc visibility when the tomo dose is 1/4x or higher than the FFDM dose.

Table 1. Ratio of # of visible discs seen in FFDM to # of visible discs seen in Tomo

Tomo dose	(# seen in FFDM) ÷ (# seen in Tomo)
1 x	60%
½ x	77%
¼ x	97%
$^1/_8$ x	146%

3.2 Calcification Phantom Objects

The calcification objects were scored by summing the number of specks visible at each object size. These results are tabulated in Table 2. There werea total of 6 calcification objects of size 160 microns, 18 of size 180 microns, and 20 of size 250 microns.

Table 2. Number of calcifications seen with FFDM and tomo at varying doses

Calcium object size, microns	FFDM score	Tomo score @ 1x dose	Tomo score @ ½ x dose	Tomo score @ ¼x dose	Tomo score @ $^1/_8$x dose
160	2.5	4	2.5	0	0
180	13.5	15	15	12	5
250	20	20	20	20	19.5

All the 250-micron calcium objects in a complex background could be seen both with FFDM and with tomosynthesis at all dose levels. The tomosynthesis images at 1/2x dose had similar detection performance to the FFDM images at the standard dose level for the 160 and 180 micron sizes.

3.3 Clinical Microcalcification Results

Clinical trials are being conducted whereby patients are imaged with both FFDM and the tomosynthesis prototype, at matched doses. The clinical protocol was approved by the hospital's Institutional Review Board and informed patient consent is obtained. Although the tomo acquisition is performed at only the 1x dose, we are able to simulate acquisitions at lower doses by reconstructing the data with a subset of the acquisition projections. We have studied this for two microcalcification cases performing reconstructions at 1x, ½x, and 1/3x the standard dose, and compared the results to the FFDM image at 1x dose.

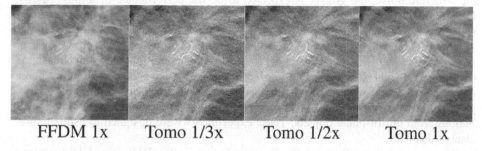

FFDM 1x   Tomo 1/3x   Tomo 1/2x   Tomo 1x

Fig. 5. Image of microcalcifications using FFDM at 1x dose, and tomo at 1/3, 1/2, and 1x doses

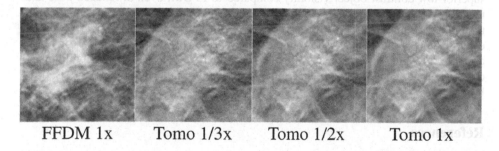

FFDM 1x   Tomo 1/3x   Tomo 1/2x   Tomo 1x

Fig. 6. Image of microcalcifications using FFDM at 1× dose, and tomo at 1/3, 1/2, and 1x doses

The linear microcalcifications in Fig 5 have a width of about 200-300 microns, and the individual microcalcifications seen in Fig 6 also have a size of about 200-300 microns. For both of these patients, the contrast and overall visibility of these micro-calcifications was superior with tomo at reduced dose compared to the FFDM at standard dose. In other patients, especially where there was little tissue structure noise, there was no advantage in tomo relative to FFDM.

4 Discussion

These studies suggest that tomosynthesis can provide similar low contrast detection performance at reduced dose relative to conventional two-dimensional digital mammography. In general, the FFDM visibility of low contrast objects in the contrast detail phantom was severely degraded by the addition of structure noise. Readers of FFDM could only visualize 60% of the discs visible on tomo images at matching doses. FFDM scoring matched tomo scoring when tomo was approximately 1/4x the FFDM dose. Calcification objects were less affected by structure noise of the complex backgrounds, however tomosynthesis still offered a detection advantage at a similar dose to FFDM.

These experiments do not perfectly simulate the imaging task in a real breast, as the objects for detection were at a different plane from the structure noise. They were separated by 5-10 mm. In a real breast, the lesions are interspersed amongst the breast parenchyma. Clearly, the further away the plane of the objects is from the source of the structure noise, the greater is expected to be the performance of tomosynthesis. Despite this experimental limitation, the results are still relevant for a number of reasons. A typical breast is perhaps 5 cm thick, so if the lesion is randomly located in this volume it will likely be separated in depth from the majority of breast tissue by 1 or more cm, and thus this experiment approximates this condition. The other reason is that tomosynthesis is not expected to offer any imaging advantage to FFDM when a object is embedded within a homogeneous region of breast tissue with similar radiographic density. Tomosynthesis is designed to improve imaging by removing contributions from out-of-plane objects. These experiments were designed to estimate precisely this effect.

Quantum noise is often not the limiting factor in the detection of low contrast objects in mammography. We have demonstrated that tomosynthesis images offer superior low contrast object visibility compared to FFDM, even at reduced dose and therefore higher quantum noise. Microcalcification visibility was also superior, although less dramatically than for larger masses. Preliminary patient images of microcalcifications, for example, show improved contrast with tomo at similar or lower dose to FFDM in some, but not all, cases. Clinical validations of these preliminary conclusions are underway, to determine a clinically adequate tomosynthesis dose level.

References

1. Breast Imaging 2nd edition. DB Kopans. Lippincott-Raven. 1998.
2. Artinis Contrast-Detail Phantom CDMAM 3.4 www.artinis.com
3. RMI-180 Contrast-Detail Phantom Gammex RMI www.gammex.com
4. Smith AP, Ren B, Ruth C, DeFreitas K, Shaw I, Jing Z, Stein JA. Initial Experience with Selenia Full Field Digital Breast Tomosynthesis. In: Proceedings of IWDM 2004, Durham North Carolina, Ed. Etta Pisano

Generalized Filtered Back-Projection Reconstruction in Breast Tomosynthesis

Bernhard E.H. Claus[1], Jeffrey W. Eberhard[1], Andrea Schmitz[1], Paul Carson[2], Mitchell Goodsitt[2], and Heang-Ping Chan[2]

[1] GE Global Research, One Research Circle, Niskayuna, NY
claus@research.ge.com
[2] University of Michigan, Ann Arbor, Michigan

Abstract. Tomosynthesis reconstruction that produces high-quality images is a difficult problem, due mainly to the highly incomplete data. In this work we present a motivation for the generalized filtered backprojection (GFBP) approach to tomosynthesis reconstruction. This approach is fast (since non-iterative), flexible, and results in reconstructions with an image quality that is similar or superior to reconstructions that are mathematically optimal. Results based on synthetic data and patient data are presented.

1 Tomosynthesis Reconstruction – Background

Tomosynthesis focuses on one of the most important problems in mammography, namely superimposed normal tissue being interpreted as suspicious or hiding a lesion. The goal of advanced tomosynthesis reconstruction approaches is to overcome the following problems:

1. Reduced contrast of structures (the contrast of a structure in a projection image is a function of its attenuation and its thickness – ideally, however, only the attenuation should be reflected in the reconstructed gray scale values, while the thickness is reflected in the spatial distribution of the data);
2. Artifacts and so-called "structured noise" (due to out-of-plane structures);
3. Image noise ("statistical noise" - quantum and detector noise).

Until recently, simple backprojection (BP), which is also referred to as "shift-and-add" reconstruction, has been considered the standard reconstruction approach in tomosynthesis. However, it addresses only the image noise problem. Improvements due to other, more advanced reconstruction approaches are generally limited, and may have significant drawbacks. For example, the high-pass filtering in a filtered back-projection (FBP) type approach [1,2] (although differently motivated) addresses the contrast enhancement requirement. However, it also increases the contrast of artifacts, and creates potentially "noisy" reconstructions, unless the filter is suitably optimized. Artifact management is addressed in order-statistics based backprojection (OSBP) approaches [3,4], but these techniques do not result in any contrast enhancement. Other advanced reconstruction approaches (e.g., ML-maximum likelihood [5,6], algebraic reconstruction technique (ART) [7], matrix inversion tomosynthesis (MITS)

Susan M. Astley et al. (Eds.): IWDM 2006, LNCS 4046, pp. 167–174, 2006.

[8]) are more involved, and a straightforward interpretation and evaluation of their effects on image quality and their effectiveness in addressing the problems above, becomes difficult. These approaches generally aim at maximizing the agreement (in some mathematical sense) of the reconstructed 3D volume with the acquired projection data.

The number of alternative reconstruction algorithm families, and the different choices within each family make a fair comparison of algorithms difficult. In one comparison study [1], ML was found to represent a good compromise in image quality (when compared to BP and FBP), while another comparison study [2] found generalized filtered backprojection (GFBP) superior, followed by ART (compared against OSBP and FBP). Some other comparisons [4,5] found tomosynthesis image quality superior to standard projection images, with varying results for the comparison among reconstruction algorithms. However, the scope of all of these studies has been too limited to even hint at a definitive answer as to what reconstruction algorithm may be "best", although they help illustrate some of the desirable properties of a "good" reconstruction algorithm. An additional problem in the comparison of reconstruction algorithms is that, unlike in CT reconstruction where complete or nearly complete data exist, in tomosynthesis the data are highly incomplete, and consequently most mathematical optimality criteria (which are used in many reconstruction algorithms) may not be appropriate as a measure for image quality.

2 Superior Reconstructions That Are "Non-optimal"

As an example of a mathematically optimal reconstruction we consider the so-called "minimum-norm solution", which is achieved (theoretically) by several different reconstruction algorithms (e.g., MITS and additive ART). Although generated in a different manner, this solution can be represented as a simple backprojection of "suitably modified" projection images; this is obvious from the fact that the basis functions that span the vector space containing the minimum-norm solution is spanned by the intersection of individual rays with the imaged volume.

From this basic observation it follows that the minimum-norm solution, although optimal in a mathematical sense, is not very effective in managing the artifact problem (since the backprojection operator, by its very definition, creates "streaks"). Furthermore, the minimum-norm solution can be seen to have a high-pass filtering characteristic, but only in the scanning direction of the x-ray tube. That is, it enhances the contrast, but favors one orientation over another. Both properties are illustrated in Figure 1, which shows reconstructions (BP, ART, GFBP) from simulated projections of identical wires of 1cm length and 1mm diameter, in two different orientations. The images are normalized such that the brightest point and the background assume the same gray level in all images. Note the out-of-plane artifacts from the wires, as well as the different in-plane appearance of the two wires, for the ART reconstruction (center column).

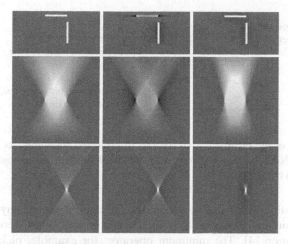

Fig. 1. Reconstructions of a phantom containing 1cm long wires with 1mm diameter. 1st row: in-plane reconstruction; 2nd and 3rd row: vertical slices through the reconstructed dataset, through each of the wires. Left column: BP; center column: ART; right column: GFBP. The images are based on simulated data: 21 projections, acquired over 60 degrees total angular range.

These observations suggest that the minimum-norm solution can be approximated by a filtered-backprojection type reconstruction that is similar to the standard FBP approach; specifically, a 1D high-pass filter followed by simple backprojection. However, due to the mentioned drawbacks, a strong argument exists for a reconstruction approach with improved image quality (as compared to the minimum-norm solution), as described in the following section.

3 Generalized Filtered Backprojection (GFBP)

The proposed GFBP reconstruction approach consists of the following two steps: (1) 2D high-pass filtering of projections, optimized as a compromise between balanced contrast enhancement and noise management, and (2) backprojection with artifact management.

The 2D high-pass filter is designed as a "scale-enhancing" filter. The projection image is decomposed into different scales (corresponding to different size structures), and each scale is enhanced with a factor that is given by the ratio of the overall thickness of the compressed breast to the size of the structure, therefore boosting the contrast of a structure to its "optimal" level. This enhancement factor is based on an isotropic shape assumption, and designed to reverse the relative loss of contrast for small structures, which is illustrated in Figure 2. For fine scales, this factor is modified to reduce image noise in the reconstruction. In this approach, a certain "scale" of the image is generated as the difference of the image convolved with (unit-integral) Gaussian kernels of different width. Note that the contrast enhancement in this approach is independent of orientation of the imaged structure, as illustrated in Figure 1 (top right).

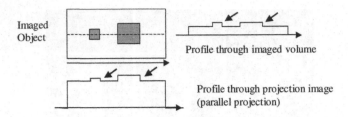

Fig. 2. Illustration of the relative loss of contrast in projected structures, for structures of the same attenuation. Note the reduced contrast of the small structure as compared to the bigger structure (indicated by the arrows).

Initial work with OSBP for artifact management did not include any image filtering and only the minimum or maximum of the backprojected values were chosen at any given voxel location [4]. The minimum operator, for example, picks at any given location the darkest backprojected grayscale value, therefore essentially eliminating bright out-of-plane artifacts due to high-contrast calcifications. Only where *all* backprojected images have a high grayscale value (thus indicating "calcification present") will a bright structure appear in the reconstruction. In a more general scenario, the average value of all but the N_{min} smallest and N_{max} largest values is taken [3]. Since the high-pass filter will enhance the contrast of (small) structures, and also create some "overshoot", a small number of largest *and* smallest values need to be disregarded for efficient artifact management. Some effects of this artifact management strategy are illustrated in Figure 1, as well as in Figure 4 (below).

4 Results

The GFBP reconstruction was performed on datasets acquired with a tomosynthesis prototype (see [9] for details), acquiring 21 projections aver a total tomographic angle of 60 degrees. Each acquisition is performed in less than 8 seconds. The scale-enhancing filter for this angular range was chosen to be non-isotropic: The high-pass filtering is two-dimensional, but with a general preference for the scanning direction (see also discussion below). In Figure 3 we show three different tomosynthesis slices of a patient dataset, separated by approximately 8mm.

In Figure 4 we show an artifact comparison for 11 vs. 21 projections, and we illustrate the additional benefit of the artifact management in the backprojection. The imaged object was a spherical, relatively high-contrast marker. The 11 view reconstruction is based on a subset of 21 projections, spanning the same angular range. All the images are normalized such that in each reconstruction the marker itself, as well as the background, were at the same respective gray scale levels.

It is clear that the increased number of projections alone already reduces the relative impact of the artifacts. The added benefit of the artifact management is also obvious. Note that the 11 projection reconstruction uses a subset of the images, and corresponds therefore to an acquisition with about 50% of the dose of the 21 projection dataset (with the corresponding relative increase in quantum noise).

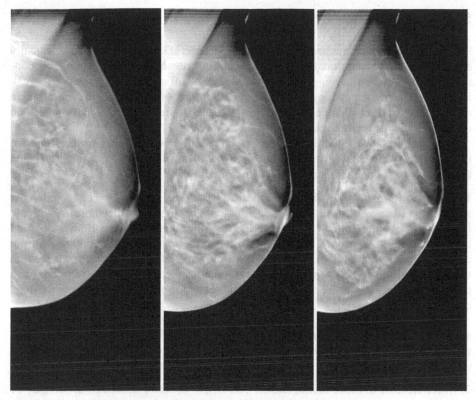

Fig. 3. Slices through a reconstructed patient dataset, about 8.0 mm apart. Note the varying anatomical characteristics as a function of depth.

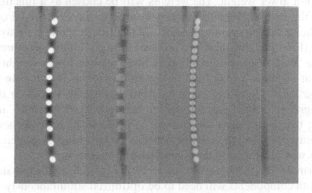

Fig. 4. Reconstructions comparing out-of-plane artifacts due to a spherical marker. From left to right: GFBP, 11, views, no artifact management; GFBP, 11, views, with artifact management, GFBP, 21 views, no artifact management; GFBP, 21 views, with artifact management. The images were normalized such that the respective gray values for the background and the marker itself were the same in all datasets.

5 Further Improvements

As discussed above, mathematical optimality criteria alone do not automatically ensure a superior image quality: the corresponding reconstructions may exhibit non-isotropic high-pass filtering characteristics, and insufficient management of streak artifacts. Instead of pursuing a suitable modification of the optimality criterion (a complicated and challenging task), our present strategy is to focus solely on optimizing reconstruction image quality.

Modifications to the outlined GFBP reconstruction method that further improve image quality (potentially moving further away from theoretical "optimality") and that are easy to implement include the following options.

1) Optimization of the filter functions. A purely isotropic (i.e., rotationally symmetric) filter works best for small tomographic angles, while more anisotropic filters will be more suitable for larger tomographic angles (in the limit we would expect the filter to approach the 1D ramp-filter in the scanning direction known from computer tomography (CT)). The filter functions may also be varying from view to view. The fine-scale (or high-frequency) enhancement should be chosen as a compromise between noise management and enhancement of fine structures (e.g., calcifications).

An additional criterion in the filter optimization may be the out-of-plane spread of structures, where the edge-enhancing properties of the filter can be tuned such that enhanced (interior) contrast of structures and (exterior) overshoot enable a canceling effect, thereby improving the depth-resolution in the reconstruction.

2) More flexible artifact management. The OSBP operator described above may be replaced, for example, with a weighted backprojection operator. Here the simple averaging of backprojected values (as performed in a simple backprojection reconstruction) is replaced by a weighted averaging, where low and high gray scale values are given a lower weight. The weights will be chosen as a function of the gray scale values in the image. The effect is very similar to the OSBP-type operator: If all projections indicate "calcification present", then all corresponding gray scale values have a similar (low) weight, therefore reconstructing a bright structure. If only few images indicate "calcification present", then their relative lower weights will tend to suppress the out-of-plane artifact due to the calcification. By choosing the weights and the (maybe locally varying) mapping from gray scale values to the associated weights, the degree of artifact suppression can be tuned to an "optimal" image quality. Note, however, that with increasing number of projection images generally the total image quality improves, and the relative benefit due to artifact management strategies decreases. This was illustrated in the comparison in Figure 4.

Note furthermore that, due to the interaction between artifact management and filter design, both components will need to be optimized simultaneously.

3) Using additional image information. The previous arguments for filter design and artifact management were established with the interior of the imaged breast in mind. The artifact management will also be efficient, for example, in managing out-of-plane artifacts due to the skinline. However, with an easily accomplished prior segmentation of the breast in the projection images, there is now an even simpler tool for managing this type of effects: The segmentation can be used to label pixels in the projections as "air" or "tissue", and any location in the reconstruction where a single backprojected image indicates "air", the reconstruction is set to zero (= attenuation of air).

One can observe that the filter also artificially enhances the skinline contrast (since the argument used for the design of the scale-enhancing filter does not fully apply near the skinline). Therefore, in combination with the skinline segmentation, one may choose to apply a thickness compensation (see, e.g., [10]) to the projection images, i.e., adjusting the low-frequency content of the image (within the breast) to counteract the reduced tissue thickness near the skinline. Typically this compensation sets the local dc value in the images near the skinline to a value corresponding to about 100% fatty tissue (of the full compressed thickness), without changing the fine-scale image content. Now setting the "air" pixels in the projection images to this same gray scale value, the artificial enhancement of the skinline can be avoided.

6 Summary

By optimizing the GFBP reconstruction algorithm outlined in this paper, one will obtain an image quality that is optimal for the class of "direct", i.e., non-iterative reconstruction algorithms. This class of algorithms requires significantly less computational power (or time) than iterative algorithms (e.g., ART, ML). Furthermore, the potential image quality benefits of the iterative methods (which generally optimize some mathematical criterion) have yet to clearly materialize. As laid out above, mathematical optimality alone is by no means a guarantee for good image quality, unless measured with the appropriate (and yet to be developed?) criterion. Indeed, in [1] the author states that "...the BP algorithm provided best SDNR [signal difference to noise ratio] for low-contrast masses,...; the FBP algorithm provided the highest edge-sharpness for microcalcifications; the information of both were well restored with balanced quality by the ML algorithm,...".

Obviously, although based on a mathematical optimality criterion, ML only achieved the best *compromise* in image quality between the algorithms considered, but didn't show outstanding results in a single one of the considered image quality criteria. On the other hand, both BP and FBP are part of the GFBP family of algorithms, both exhibiting relatively poor image quality. By using "optimized" GFBP, clearly a compromise with similar, if not superior image quality than ML can be reached, at a significantly lower computational cost. A similar conclusion can be drawn, e.g., when comparing reconstruction image quality in GFBP against ART or other iterative reconstruction approaches.

References

1. T. Wu, R. Moore, E. Rafferty, D. Kopans: "A comparison of reconstruction algorithms for breast tomosynthesis", Med Phys. 31 (9), 2636-2647, 2004.
2. B.E.H. Claus, J.W. Eberhard, J.A. Thomas, C.E. Galbo, W.P. Pakenas, S.L. Muller: Preference Study of Reconstructed Image Quality in Mammographic Tomosynthesis, in H.-O. Peitgen (ed.), Digital Mammography IWDM 2002, Proceedings of the 6th IWDM, June 2002, Bremen, Germany, Springer 2003.

3. B.E.H. Claus, J.W. Eberhard: "A New Method for 3D Reconstruction in Digital Tomosynthesis", Proc. SPIE Vol. 4684, Medical Imaging 2002.
4. S. Suryanarayanan, A. Karellas, S. Vedantham, S.P. Baker, S.J. Glick, C.J. D'Orsi, R.L. Webber: "Evaluation of Linear and Nonlinear Tomosynthetic Reconstruction Methods in Digital Mammography", Acad. Radiol. 8:219-224, 2000.
5. S. Suryanarayanan, A. Karellas, S. Vedantham, S.J. Glick, C.J. D'Orsi, S.P. Baker, R.L. Webber: "Comparison of Tomosynthesis Methods Used in Digital Mammography", Acad. Radiol. 7: 1085-1097, 2000.
6. T. Wu, A. Stewart, M. Stanton, W. Phillips, T. McCauley, D.B. Kopans, R.H. Moore, J.W. Eberhard, B. Opsahl-Ong, L. Niklason, M.B. Williams: "Tomographic mammography using a limited number of low-dose cone-beam projection images", Med. Phys. 30 (3), 365-380, 2003.
7. B. Wang, K. Barner, D. Lee: "Algebraic Tomosynthesis Reconstruction", Proc. SPIE Vol. 5370, p. 711-718, Medical Imaging 2004.
8. J.T. Dobbins, D.J. Godfrey: "Digital x-ray tomosynthesis: current state of the art and clinical potential", Phys Med Biol. 48:R65-R106, 2003.
9. J.W. Eberhard, D. Albagli, A. Schmitz, B.E.H. Claus, P. Carson, M. Goodsitt, H.-P. Chan, M. Roubidoux, J.A. Thomas, J. Osland, "Mammography Tomosynthesis System for High-Performance 3D Imaging", Proceedings of Intl. Workshop on Digital Mammography, IWDM2006, June 18-21 2006, Manchester, UK.
10. J. W. Byng, J. P. Critten, and M. J. Yaffe, "Thickness-equalization processing for mammographic images," Radiology 203, 564–568 (1997).

Adaptation of Image Quality Using Various Filter Setups in the Filtered Backprojection Approach for Digital Breast Tomosynthesis

Jasmina Orman, Thomas Mertelmeier, and Wolfgang Haerer

Siemens AG, Medical Solutions, 91050 Erlangen, Germany
{jasmina.orman, thomas.mertelmeier,
wolfgang.haerer}@siemens.com

Abstract. The main limitations of conventional projection mammography consist in tissue overlap and missing depth information. These deficiencies are intended to be reduced by the new technique of digital breast tomosynthesis. From a set of radiographic projections, acquired at different view angles in a linear tomosynthesis research system setup, 3-D slices of the scanned breast region are reconstructed. As the method of choice for the reconstruction we use filtered backprojection. By applying different filters with task-adapted parameters this method allows to control the image quality regarding noise, spatial resolution and artifacts. In order to investigate the basic effects of the various settings in the filtering step the method is first applied to simulated data. The impact of the selected filter functions is then demonstrated with clinical data.

1 Introduction

To overcome the limitations of tissue overlap and missing depth information in conventional (digital) mammography, the application of 3-D imaging methods to the breast seems appropriate. Digital breast tomosynthesis benefited by the progress in several key technologies such as flat detectors, reconstruction and post-processing algorithms, has become an interesting research topic within the last few years. Initial investigations on this technique have been promising and provide the opportunity to overcome drawbacks of conventional mammography by acquiring several views of the breast from different angles and reconstructing a 3-D data set. Separating lesions from overlapping dense fibroglandular tissue, tomosynthesis is expected to improve both detectability and characterization, while the applied dose can be kept comparable to mammography.

In Ref. [1] Grant described 1972 a type of geometric tomography he called tomosynthesis, which uses a conventional X-ray source and a digital detector to produce a virtually unlimited number of tomographic images at arbitrary depth in the patient. To date successful reconstruction and post-processing algorithms have included filtered backprojection, traditional shift-and-add reconstruction coupled with matrix inversion or constrained iterative restoration deblurring methods, and algebraic iterative reconstruction procedures [2-6]. The challenge for reconstruction algorithms consists in optimizing the image quality from the limited, incomplete sampling of the object.

Susan M. Astley et al. (Eds.): IWDM 2006, LNCS 4046, pp. 175–182, 2006.
© Springer-Verlag Berlin Heidelberg 2006

In this paper, we present results of the filtered backprojection with various filtering setups, carried out for a prototype breast tomosynthesis system. In section 2 we describe the optimized filtered backprojection method and the corresponding filter design. The achieved image quality of the reconstruction results for simulated and clinical data is presented in section 3.

2   Filtered Backprojection for Linear Tomosynthesis

The acquisition system we employ is based on the Siemens full-field digital mammography x-ray generator modified for linear tomosynthesis. The X-ray tube moves over an arc of up to $\pm 25°$ relative to the pivoting point. During a single X-ray scan, multiple X-ray pulses are generated synchronized with the detector read/integrate cycle and X-ray tube motion.

The reconstruction approach described here is based on filtered backprojection [3]. It allows a systematic filter design, an optimized image quality specific to the application and strategies for reducing artifacts caused by inherent incomplete sampling. It can also easily be implemented. Due to its pipelined structure pre- and postprocessing steps can be taken into account as well.

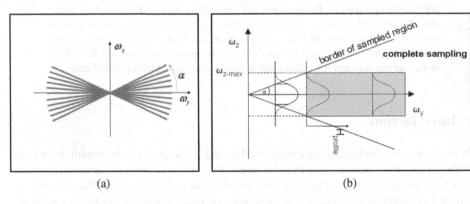

(a)   (b)

Fig. 1. (a) Moving the X-ray tube over an arc from angle $-\alpha$ to α the Fourier space data are acquired in a double wedge domain. (b) The introduction of a slice profile filter function $H_{profile}$ (ω_z) ensures a constant depth resolution over a wide range of spatial frequencies.

The tube motion on an arc over the stationary detector is a linear sampling path in y-orientation with varying magnification and can be treated in parallel beam approximation. This approximation is acceptable for the filter design since the associated inaccuracies are small compared to the effects induced by the incomplete tomosynthetic sampling. The backprojection step for the filtered data is performed with the appropriate high accuracy by using projection matrices for each view, which are determined from the angular information provided by the system [7].

The filtering operations are derived in 3-D Fourier space and can be performed herein. Advantageously, they may be transformed into 2-D projection frequency space by a simple coordinate transformation. The Fourier-Slice theorem states that, in Fourier space, to each projection of the object a plane perpendicular to its beam direction corresponds. Collecting the projections during one tomosynthesis scan will thus not fill the entire Fourier space but only a double wedge region as shown in Fig. 1a.

We assume that the system modulation transfer function (MTF) can be split into a filter function and a projection-backprojection part [8]: $H(\omega) = H_{filter}(\omega) \cdot H_P(\omega)$.

Then, an appropriate filter function in Fourier space for linear sampling in y orientation can be chosen as

$$H_{filter}(\omega_y, \omega_z) = H_{spectrum}(\omega_y) \cdot H_{profile}(\omega_z) \cdot H_{inverse}(\omega_y, \omega_z) \tag{1}$$

where $H_{inverse}$ inverts the modulation transfer function H_P of the projection–backprojection process in the double wedge frequency region and is proportional to a ramp-type filter. With realistic noisy data, the ramp filter is known for emphasizing noise. In order to suppress high frequencies and thereby noise an appropriate spectral filter $H_{spectrum}$ may be employed. We choose a von Hann ('Hanning') window with adjustable parameter A (A>0) for this purpose.

After inversion and even after applying a spectral filter in ω_y, the ω_z-border of the sampled region in Fourier space (cf. Fig 1b) still consists of a sharp step-function in ω_z. This discontinuity will create a corresponding ringing in the spatial domain, increasing the out-of-plane artifacts already present from the incomplete sampling. Therefore, a slice profile function can suppress these artifacts [3] controlling the spatial slice thickness. This behavior can be achieved with the third filter part $H_{profile}(\omega_z)$, which we call 'slice profile function' or 'slice thickness filter':

$$H_{profile}(\omega_z) = \begin{cases} 0.5\left(1 + \cos\left(\dfrac{\pi\omega_z}{B}\right)\right) & \text{for } |\omega_z| < B \quad \text{and} \quad |\omega_z| < \tan(\alpha)||\omega_y| \\ 0 & \text{elsewhere.} \end{cases} \tag{2}$$

The parameter B (B>0) controls the cutoff-frequency in ω_z and thus, via inverse Fourier transformation of $H_{profile}$, also the width of the slice profile function in object space. The incomplete sampling generally prevents from obtaining a constant slice thickness and thus generates out-of-plane artifacts. Fig. 1b illustrates how these can be largely reduced for spatial frequencies ω_y above a certain limit. If the cutoff on the z-frequency scale is inside the sampling region, a slice thickness is well defined here. For small y-frequencies, i.e. for $\omega_y < \omega_{z\text{-max}}/\tan(\alpha)$, however, the slice thickness increases with decreasing y-frequencies. Thus in tomosynthesis, the slice thickness cannot be held constant, with its effective value depending on the frequency content of the object.

The ramp-type behavior of the inverse MTF filtering, in case of incompletely sampled data, leads to suppression of low frequencies, which might be visible in clinical data as intensity drop towards the breast center. Motivated by this issue, we designed a new filter, labeled as 'frequency selective contrast enhancement filter' (FSCE), with two adjustable filter parameters C and D:

$$H_{FSCE}(\omega_y) = \begin{cases} C + (1-C) \cdot 0.5\left(1 - \cos\left(\dfrac{\pi\omega_y}{D}\right)\right) & \text{for } |\omega_y| < D \\ 1 & \text{elsewhere.} \end{cases} \tag{3}$$

A closer look at the filter definition reveals that the filter splits into two parts: the constant component C and the remaining second addend. The constant transmits all frequencies and thus determines the level of blending with the unfiltered projections. The second term is designed for replacing the inverse MTF filtering. In order to retain a low noise level, the spectral filtering $H_{spectrum}$ should be combined.

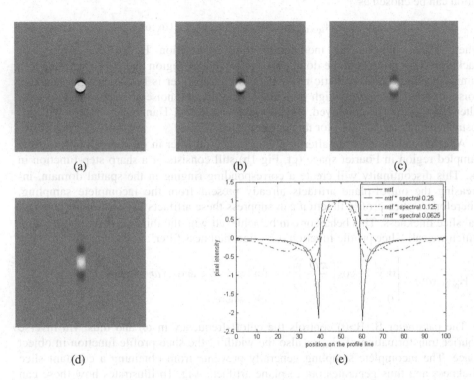

(a)   (b)   (c)

(d)   (e)

Fig. 2. Slice through the center of the ball of 2 mm diameter for MTF inversion filtering only (a) and for MTF and spectral filtering with different cutoff parameters: (b) MTF * spectral [A=0.25ω_N], (c) MTF * spectral [A=0.125ω_N], (d) MTF * spectral [A=0.0625ω_N]. The scan direction is vertical (y). (e) Profiles through the different reconstructions of the ball in scan direction. The unit of the horizontal axis is the reconstruction voxel size (0.1 mm). ω_N is the Nyquist frequency of the projections.

3   Results and Discussion

3.1   Filter Evaluation on Phantom Data

The influence of the various filters on the image quality is first studied on simulated data. This ensures 3-D slices to be free from artifacts caused by noise, object movement or possibly inexact geometry computation and enables quantitative evaluation.

Fig. 2 shows the impact of the spectral filter on the visual acuity of the reconstructed object. The simulation phantom, in this example, consists of a high-contrast ball with 2 mm diameter. With the decreasing filter parameter A of the Hanning window the ball looses sharpness in scan direction. At the same time the artifact amplitude coming from the incomplete MTF inversion (ramp-type) is reduced as well, which can be seen from the profile through the ball (Fig. 2e).

The effect of the slice thickness filter is demonstrated in Fig. 3. Slices reconstructed solely with MTF inverse filtering (Fig. 3a) exhibit very strong long-range out-of plane artifacts. In case of objects aligned in scan direction, as in our example, the out-of-plane artifacts even interfere with each other and may give the false impression of an existing object in neighboring slices. Employing, additionally to the MTF inversion filter, the slice thickness filter, with an appropriate value for the parameter B, the reconstructed object will be more uniformly spread out over the slice as a consequence of defining an appropriate slice sensitivity profile. The out-of-plane artifacts are visibly reduced (Fig. 3c) and thus also their mutual interference on the neighboring slices.

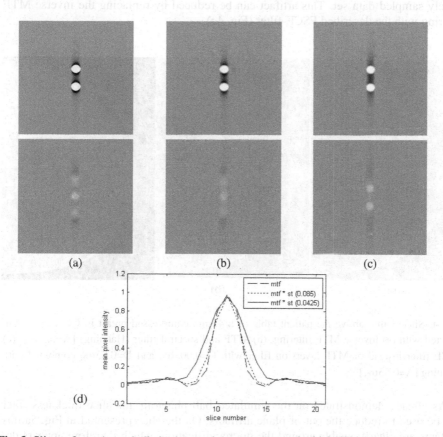

Fig. 3. Slices of two 1 mm balls in the xy-plane reconstructed with MTF inversion filter solely (a) and in combination with the slice thickness filter with parameter $B = 0.085\omega_N$ (b) and $B = 0.0425\omega_N$ (c). The first row presents the central slices through the balls' center and the second row shows slices at a distance of 3 mm. (d) Mean intensity z-profile plot of the upper ball through 21 slices.

3.2 Application to Clinical Data

In this section we present results obtained with clinical data. All tomosynthesis data sets were acquired over an angular range of ±25° with 25 or 49 projections. The total dose was approximately the same as for the corresponding screen/film mammogram.

The slices presented in Fig. 4 nicely demonstrate the impact of different reconstruction parameters on the image quality. This 45 mm compressed left breast received a tomosynthesis scan in cranio-caudal (CC) position. The slice is located 3 mm above the patient table. In the backprojection method with only MTF inverse filtering the image noise is emphasized (Fig. 4a). Applying in addition the spectral filter will lead to noise suppression (Fig. 4b). The effect of noise reduction depends on the filter parameter A. Decreasing A and thus the cutoff frequency, leads to more noise suppression, but also to lower visual acuity. The intensity decrease towards the breast middle is visible in both cases and is caused by the ramp-type filtering of the incompletely sampled data set. This artifact can be reduced by replacing the inverse MTF filtering with the described FSCE-filter (Fig. 4c).

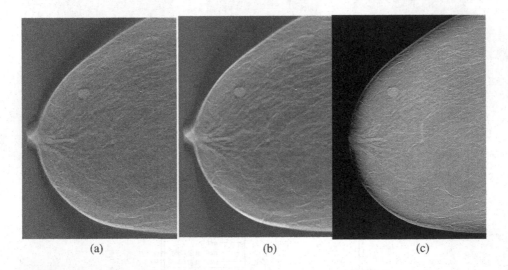

(a)   (b)   (c)

Fig. 4. Slice 3 mm above the patient table of a 45mm compressed breast in CC view reconstructed with (a) inverse MTF filtering, (b) MTF and spectral filter (Hanning) $[A=0.5\omega_N]$, (c) FSCE-filter instead of MTF inversion filter with $C=0.003\omega_N$ and $D=0.85\omega_N$ combined with Hanning $[A=0.55\omega_N]$

As already demonstrated on the simulated ball phantom, the slice thickness filter can be used to reduce the out-of-plane artifacts. On the slice presented in Fig. 5a this artifacts are clearly visible around the microcalification, which therefore appears deformed. Applying the slice thickness filter will reduce this artifacts leading to a better definition of the microcalcification (Fig. 5b). The risk to overlook existing microcalcifiation may be reduced. Since the slice thickness filter smoothes the image, the parameter A of the combined spectral filter has to be adjusted.

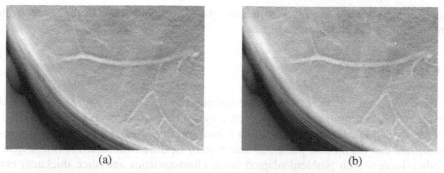

(a)   (b)

Fig. 5. Reconstruction of a slice 47 mm above the patient table of a 60 mm compressed breast in MLO view with (a) MTF inversion filter and spectral filter with A = $0.5\omega_N$, (b) MTF inversion filter with spectral filter [A = $1.5\omega_N$] and slice thickness filter [B = $0.07\omega_N$]

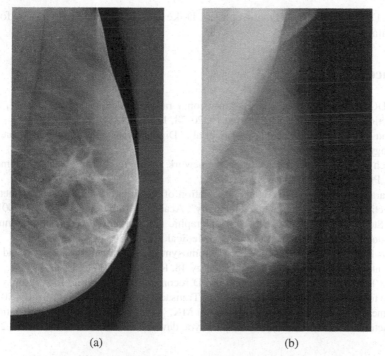

(a)   (b)

Fig. 6. Reconstructed 'mammogram' (a) by applying the slice thickness filter forming a 'total volume slice' and (b) the digitized analog mammogram (Duke University Medical Center)

The application of the slice thickness filter for generating a certain slice thickness can be considered as an alternative to the averaging over several consecutive slices to form thicker slabs. Reconstructing one single slice, we call it 'total volume slice', with the thickness of the total compressed breast and using the slice thickness filter, it is even possible to retrieve a mammogram of the scanned breast. Figure 6a shows a 'total volume slice' of a 6 cm compressed breast in comparison to the screen/film mammogram of the same breast (Fig. 6b).

4 Conclusion

We have demonstrated the effects of the various filter processes with simulated and with clinical data acquired with a research tomosynthesis system. Whereas the simulations provide basic insight into the filter operations, the clinical tomosynthesis scans demonstrate that the method presented here is very flexible with regard to image quality. Slice images with problem-adapted noise characteristics and slice thickness can be obtained, even 'mammograms' can be reconstructed as thick slabs.

Acknowledgement

We thank Dr. Jay Baker and Dr. Joseph Lo, Duke University Medical Center, for the clinical data.

References

1. Grant DG, "Tomosynthesis: a three-dimensional radiographic imaging technique", IEEE Transactions on Biomedical Engineering 19, 20-28, 1972
2. Niklason LT, Christian BT, Niklason LE, et al., "Digital tomosynthesis in breast imaging", Radiology 205, 399-406, 1997.
3. Lauritsch G, Haerer WH, "A theoretical framework for filtered backprojection in tomosynthesis", Proc. SPIE 3338, 1127-1137, 1998
4. Suryanarayanan S, Karellas A, et al., "Evaluation of linear and nonlinear tomosynthetic reconstruction methods in digital mammography", Academic Radiology 8, 219-224, 2001.
5. Wu T, Stewart A, Stanton M, et al., "Tomographic mammography using a limited number of low-dose cone-beam projection images", Medical Physics 30, 365-380, 2003.
6. Dobbins III JT, Godfrey DJ. "Digital x-ray tomosynthesis: current state of the art and clinical potential", Physics in Medicine and Biology 48, R65-R106, 2003.
7. Wiesent K, Barth K, et al. W, "Enhanced 3-D reconstruction algorithm for C-arm systems suitable for interventional procedures", IEEE Transactions MI, vol. 19(5), 391-403, 2000
8. Mertelmeier T., Orman J., Haerer W, Dudam MK, "Optimizing filtered backprojection reconstruction for a breast tomosynthesis prototype device", Proc.SPIE 6142, 131-142, 2006

Optimization of Contrast-Enhanced Digital Breast Tomosynthesis

Ann-Katherine Carton, Jingjing Li, Sara Chen, Emily Conant,
and Andrew D.A. Maidment

University of Pennsylvania, Department of Radiology,
3400 Spruce Street, Philadelphia, PA, USA, 19104
{ann-katherine.carton, sara.chen, emily.conant,
andrew.maidment}@uphs.upenn.edu

Abstract. Digital breast tomosynthesis (DBT) is a tomographic technique in which individual slices through the breast are reconstructed from x-ray projection images acquired over a limited angular range. In contrast-enhanced DBT (CE-DBT) functional information is observed by administration of an radiographic contrast agent. The uptake of iodine in the breast is very small and causes changes in x-ray transmission that are smaller than 5%. This presents significant technical challenges if quantitative assessment of contrast agent concentration in tissue is desired. We modeled CE-DBT acquisition by simulating x-ray spectra from 40 to 49 kV. Comparison of attenuation data of our simulated and measured spectra were found to agree well. We investigated the effect of patient motion and scatter on iodine uptake. These parameters were evaluated by means of experiments and theoretical modeling.

1 Background

Digital breast tomosynthesis (DBT) is a tomographic technique for imaging the breast morphology at a dose comparable to digital mammography. However, as breast tumor growth and metastasis are accompanied by neoangiogenesis, a functional tomographic imaging technique is desired. Contrast-enhanced digital breast tomosynthesis (CE-DBT) [1] would potentially integrate the benefits of both CE digital mammography [2, 3] and DBT [4-7]; thus, providing both functional information and improved breast cancer morphology by minimizing the superimposition of nonadjacent breast tissues that occurs with projection mammograms. Temporal analysis of contrast enhancement may further help to distinguish benign and malignant lesions.

The uptake of iodine in the breast is very small and thus causes only small changes in x-ray transmission; typically less than 5%. This presents significant technical challenges if quantitative assessment of contrast agent uptake is desired [1]. Technical factors that significantly influence quantitative analysis of CE-DBT exams are exposure reproducibility, linearity of the detector as a function of position, temporal response of the detector, scatter and patient motion. In this paper, we will discuss scatter, and patient motion.

Susan M. Astley et al. (Eds.): IWDM 2006, LNCS 4046, pp. 183–189, 2006.
© Springer-Verlag Berlin Heidelberg 2006

2 Methods

We have used a modified GE 2000D under IRB approval to gain initial experience in CE-DBT. In the experiments described, we have used temporal subtraction. High energy images are acquired before and after administration of an iodinated contrast agent. Logarithmic subtraction of these images is then performed. The signal intensities (SI) of the resulting images are proportionally to the uptake of iodine.

2.1 Spectrum

To model the acquisition process, x-ray spectra in the range of 40 to 49 kV were simulated by extrapolating Boone's model [8]. We validated our simulations using a least-squares comparison (χ^2 values) between attenuation data from our simulated spectra and attenuation data measured with the GE Senographe 2000D. We used high-purity Al filters to determine the attenuation curves. Minimum χ^2 values were found by adjusting the kV ($kV_{equivalent}$) and adding or subtracting Al ($Al_{equivalent}$) to the simulated spectra. We also compared the half value layers (HVL) and quarter value layers (QVL) of the simulations and the measurements. In this paper, we compare simulated and measured attenuation data from a Mo-target with 1 mm Al filtration, and a Rh-target with 0.27 mm Cu filtration.

2.2 Scatter

We performed CE-DBT without a grid. Scatter, S, was estimated by extrapolation of signal intensity measurements under Pb-disks with diameters of 3.9 to 23 mm to a disk of zero diameter. Scatter fractions (SF) were then calculated as the fraction of S to the SI value in the open field at the same position, which consist of S and primary radiation, P. These measurements were repeated as a function of position in 50% glandular-50% adipose breast equivalent phantoms (CIRS, Norfolk, VA), and various breast equivalent thickness. The phantoms were positioned so as to mimic the MLO breast position, including higher order scatter from the chest. A 49 kV spectrum with a 0.27 mm Cu filter was applied.

As part of our clinical CE-DBT trial, we have measured SF in the MLO projection images of 6 patients. Pb-disks 12 mm in diameter were positioned on top of the compression plate while the breast was compressed and a series of projection images was acquired over a 50° arc (as measured at the fulcrum, 20 cm above the breast support). SF were then calculated from the SI measured in the shadows of the Pb-disks, giving S, and the SI was also measured at the same position in the previously acquired pre-contrast projection images, thus giving $P + S$. The SF in the clinical data were compared with the SF calculated from the 12 mm Pb-disks in the phantom images. The same mammography unit and spectrum were used as in the phantom measurements.

We modeled the effect of scatter on the quantification of the iodine concentration for various breast thicknesses. We simulated a Senographe 2000D tube operated at 49 kV with a Rh target and 0.27 mm Cu filtration. Our simulation includes the attenuation of the Be-window, Cu-filter, compression plate, air, ICRU-44 breast tissue, and the CsI detector material. We used the SF measured near the center of the breast equivalent phantoms. We calculated the contrast as a function of iodine uptake for the various breast thicknesses and then calculated the error in the iodine concentration estimate due to the scatter.

2.3 Patient Motion

In temporal subtraction, pre- and post-contrast images are subtracted. Any breast motion between series will result in artifacts and an erroneous estimate of the iodine uptake will be calculated. In our clinical trial, the total acquisition time could exceed 10 minutes, depending on the experimental protocol. Thus, breast motion is inevitable.

We developed a measure to demonstrate the effect of breast motion on the estimated iodine uptake. In 12 patient images, we selected ROIs where the breast thickness was constant. The relative SI variations, corrected for scatter by using measured SF, were calculated between pixel positions that are Δx apart from each other. We varied Δx from 1 to 128 pixels (0.1 - 12.8 mm). These measurements were calculated for displacements in the horizontal and vertical direction. The relative SI variations were related to corresponding iodine concentrations using our simulation. These simulations considered a Senographe 2000D x-ray tube operated at 49 kV with a Rh-target and 0.27 mm Cu filtration. The simulation includes the attenuation of the Be-window, Cu-filter, compression plate, air, ICRU-44 breast tissue, and the CsI detector material.

3 Results

3.1 Spectrum

A comparison of the simulated and measured attenuation data are presented in Tables 1 and 2. The measured attenuation data in Table 1 are from a GE Senographe 2000D operated with a Rh-target and 0.27 mm Cu filtration. The tube has a 0.69 mm Be window, and a 2 mm compression plate was in the x-ray beam. The measured attenuation data in Table 2 are from a GE DMR. The Mo-target x-ray source was used with 1 mm Al filtration. The x-ray tube window was composed of 0.69 mm thick Be and a 2 mm compression plate was again in place.

Table 1. Comparison of the measured and simulated attenuation data for a Rh-target tube filtered with 0.27 mm Cu

nominal kV	$kV_{equivalent}$	$Al_{equivalent}$	Measured		Simulated		χ^2
			HVL	QVL	HVL	QVL	
34	33.5	0.0	1.711	3.532	1.713	3.579	0.00009
40	39.4	0.0	2.232	4.750	2.238	4.738	0.00012
46	45.5	0.0	2.779	5.978	2.787	5.978	0.00005
49	48.4	0.0	3.060	6.619	3.063	6.578	0.00006

Table 2. Comparison of the measured and simulated attenuation data for a Mo-target tube filtered with 1 mm Al

nominal kV	$kV_{equivalent}$	$Al_{equivalent}$	Measured		Simulated		χ^2
			HVL	QVL	HVL	QVL	
22	21.1	0.075	0.388	1.285	0.385	1.286	0.00007
28	28.0	0.100	0.538	1.844	0.540	1.841	0.00005
34	35.0	0.050	0.607	2.050	0.609	2.197	0.00009
40	39.4	0.100	0.654	2.420	0.649	2.442	0.00070
46	45.4	0.150	0.698	2.734	0.686	2.736	0.00071
49	49.0	0.175	0.739	2.907	0.703	2.911	0.00422

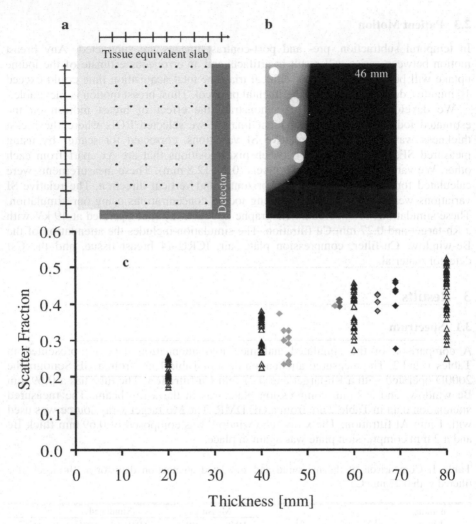

Fig. 1. *(a)* Geometry of the scatter measurements; 50% glandular, 50% adipose breast equivalent phantoms were used. The black dots indicate the positions where SF were measured. The distance between the ticks on the horizontal and vertical rulers is 2 cm. *(b)* Image of 12 mm diameter Pb-disks exposed on top of a breast in the MLO position. Breast thickness is shown in the upper right corner. *(c)* SF as a function of breast thickness in 0° projection images of 50% glandular-50% adipose breast equivalent phantoms (open triangles) and six clinical breast images (solid diamonds).

Shown are kV$_{equivalent}$ and Al$_{equivalent}$ of the simulated spectra for a nominal kV that results in the smallest χ^2. The measured and simulated estimates of the HVL and QVL are also presented. The simulated values are those that minimize the χ^2. The results in both tables demonstrate that the extrapolation of the Boone's spectral models agree well with our measurements.

3.2 Scatter

Figure 1a and b show the geometry used for the scatter measurements in the breast tissue-equivalent phantoms and in the patient data. Using the method of extrapolating the SF to zero disk diameter in breast equivalent phantoms demonstrates that scatter fraction increases with thickness, as expected. We measured SF = 0.29 for a 20 mm phantom, 0.43 for a 40 mm phantom, 0.52 for a 60 mm phantom, and 0.57 for a 80 mm phantom as measured near the center of the phantom.

Figure 1c illustrates SF derived from the shadows under 12 mm Pb-disks as a function of breast thickness. The SF correspond to the various positions in the field of view as indicated in Fig 1a and b. This analysis shows that the SF in real mammograms are similar to the SF measured in breast-equivalent phantoms for corresponding thicknesses.

Figure 2 shows the extent to which the iodine concentration will be underestimated if a correction for scatter is not applied. The amount by which the iodine concentration will be underestimated is dependent upon the breast thickness. Consider, for example, the situation were the breast has an actual iodine concentration of 2 mg/cm^2. Failure to correct for scatter will result in an error in the estimated iodine concentration of 29% for a 20 mm thick compressed breast and 50% for a 80 mm thick compressed breast. Note that even if images are produced with a grid, the iodine concentration is still underestimated. This has relevance for those attempting to perform contrast-enhanced digital mammography.

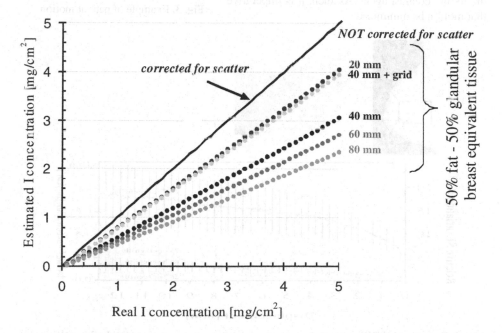

Fig. 2. Iodine concentration will be underestimated if not corrected for scatter. The simulation used a Rh target, 49 kV and 0.27 mm Cu filter. No grid was used if not specified.

3.3 Patient Motion

Figure 3 shows a clinical example of patient motion. The image was produced by subtracting a post-contrast reconstructed image of the breast from a pre-contrast reconstructed image. Two lead BBs are shown attached to the skin near the nipple. The arrows indicate patient motion. In our clinical trial, we consistently noted the greatest motion in the dependent (lower) portion of the breast.

We have attempted to estimate the magnitude of motion artifacts by simulating breast motion. Figure 4 illustrates the influ- ence of displacements simulating patient motion on the relative SI variation and equiv- alent iodine concentration. The data were calculated from images of 12 women. As an example, 25% of the 6 mm displacements have on average a 1% relative SI variation; this corresponds with a 0.5 mg/cm^2 iodine uptake. However, it is relevant to note that a displacement of as little as one pixel can result in more than a 5% change in signal intensity, which can potentially exceed the anticipated signal from the iodine contrast agent. As such, it is imperative that motion be minimized.

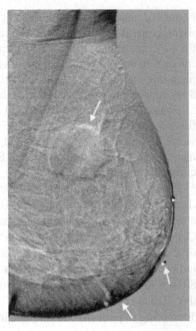

Fig. 3. Example of patient motion

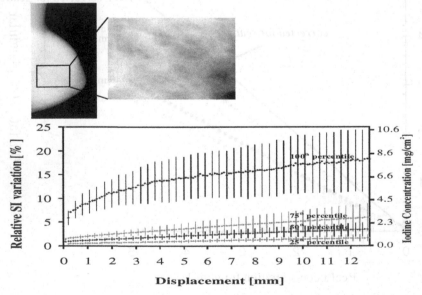

Fig. 4. Example of a ROI extracted from a projection mammogram acquired with a Rh-target x-ray tube at 49 kV with 0.27 mm Cu filtration (left). Relative SI variation between pixel displacements and the corresponding equivalent iodine concentration from 12 projection images are shown (below). The error bars represent standard deviations.

4 Conclusion

CE-DBT offers the potential to visualize the vascular characteristics of breast lesions as an adjunct to mammography. Based upon our initial clinical experience, and the work reported here, it is clear that the quantization of the iodine uptake for CE-DBT is complex. For the design of a CE-DBT system, attention should be paid to scatter and patient motion. At the current time, we are working on the reduction of patient motion and we are evaluating alternative subtraction methods using dual energy CE-DBT. We expect that these may minimize patient motion artifacts.

Acknowledgements

This work was funded in part by NIH grant PO1 CA85484 and a Philips Medical Systems/RSNA Research Seed Grant.

References

[1] Carton A-K, Li J, Albert M, et al. Quantification for contrast-enhanced digital breast tomosynthesis. In: Flynn MJ, Hsieh J, editors. Medical Imaging 2006: Physics of Medical Imaging; p. 111-121.

[2] Jong RA, Yaffe MJ, Skarpathiotakis M, et al. Contrast-enhanced digital mammography: Initial clinical experience. Radiology 2003;228:842-850.

[3] Skarpathiotakis M, Yaffe MJ, Bloomquist AK, et al. Development of contrast digital mammography. Medical Physics 2002;29(10):2419-26.

[4] Maidment ADA, Adelow L, Blom O, et al. Evaluation of a Photon-Counting Breast Tomosynthesis Imaging System. In: Flynn MJ, editor. Physics of Medical Imaging, Proc. SPIE 6142; 2006.

[5] Wu T, Moore RH, Rafferty EA, et al. Breast tomosynthesis: Methods and applications. In: Karellas A, editor. RSNA Categorical Course in Diagnostic Radiology Physics: Advances in Breast Imaging - Physics, Technology, and Clinical Applications; 2004. p. 149-163.

[6] Dobbins JT, 3rd, Godfrey DJ. Digital x-ray tomosynthesis: current state of the art and clinical potential. Physics in Medicine & Biology 2003;48(19):R65-106.

[7] Niklason LT, Christian BT, Niklason LE, et al. Digital tomosynthesis in breast imaging. Radiology 1997;205(2):399-406.

[8] Boone JM, Fewell TR, Jennings RJ. Molybdenum, rhodium, and tungsten anode spectral models using interpolating polynomials with application to mammography. Medical Physics 1997;24(12):1863-74.

Development of an Analytic Breast Phantom for Quantitative Comparison of Reconstruction Algorithms for Digital Breast Tomosynthesis

I. Reiser, E.Y. Sidky, R.M. Nishikawa, and X. Pan

Department of Radiology, The University of Chicago,
Chicago, IL 60637, USA

Abstract. We are developing an analytic breast phantom that allows for quantitative comparison of reconstruction algorithms for digital breast tomosynthesis. The phantom consists of simple shapes and aims at capturing the main features of the breast. Projection data can be computed analytically. We present volumes reconstructed from the phantom data using the filtered backprojection, expectation maximization and total variation algorithms. Our results indicate that the TV algorithm achieves highest contrast for mass lesions and best in-depth resolution.

1 Introduction

Digital Breast Tomosynthesis (DBT) is an emerging modality for breast imaging [1, 2]. Currently, several manufacturers have produced prototype units [1, 3, 4] using different imaging geometries and reconstruction algorithms, such as filtered back projection (FBP) [4, 3], iterative transmission expectation maximization (TEM) [1, 5], and matrix inversion tomography [6].

Researchers and manufacturers have presented clinical images produced by their systems, allowing only for qualitative image comparison. However, no quantitative comparison of imaging systems or reconstruction algorithms exist. Wu and coworkers [2] have compared image-quality parameters in volume images of the ACR phantom, reconstructed with the TEM, FBP and simple backprojection algorithms. The purpose of this current work is to develop a breast phantom that is composed of simple shapes, to allow researchers to easily compute analytic projection data for quantitative algorithm evaluation. A similar phantom, the well-known Shepp-Logan phantom, has been used in CT reconstruction work as a standard phantom simulating the human head.

While the Shepp-Logan phantom does not reflect every detail of a human head, it captures prominent features that can cause reconstruction artifacts, such as the highly attenuating scull. Projection data for such simple phantoms can be computed analytically, eliminating quantization errors.

The breast phantom that we are presenting in this work represents the breast as a truncated ellipsoid. It includes representations of a pectoralis muscle and fibroglandular tissue regions. In the current implementation, mass lesions are

Susan M. Astley et al. (Eds.): IWDM 2006, LNCS 4046, pp. 190–196, 2006.

also included in different tissue backgrounds. If necessary, other structures, such as microcalcifications, can also readily be incorporated into the phantom. We have used existing FBP and expectation-maximisation (EM) algorithms and a new total variation (TV) algorithm to reconstruct the breast volume from a sequence of projection data generated from this new breast phantom. Imaging geometry is similar to that of the first GE prototype unit [1].

2   Methods

The breast phantom, as shown in Fig. 1, is composed of several components. Each component is either an ellipsoidal object, or a volume bound by intersecting surfaces. Surfaces can be either planar, ellipsoidal, cylindrical, or conical. This set of surfaces allows one to construct a large number of shapes while enabling analytic computation of the path integrals. In our phantom, the overall shape of the breast was a truncated ellipsoid. The pectoralis muscle was represented by a rectangular slab. The ensemble of ductal structures was represented by a crescent shaped object, created from two intersecting ellipsoids. Three mass lesions were included in the breast phantom, located within the fatty tissue, embedded in dense fibroglandular tissue, and one mass lesion within the fatty tissue but with overlaying dense tissue.

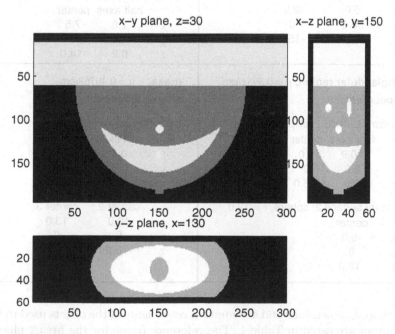

Fig. 1. Slices through the breast phantom along the three spatial directions. The difference in attenuation coefficient between the crescent-shaped fibroglandular tissue and the mass within that dense tissue is only 0.015 cm^{-1}. Axis units are mm.

Table 1. Dimensions and attenuation coefficients of the objects used to build the breast phantom. Length units are cm.

breast volume, $\mu = 0.245$/cm shape: truncated ellipsoid	nipple, $\mu = 0.245$/cm shape: truncated cylinder
boundary surface 1: ellipsoid 　　half axes center 　x　　12.0　　5.0 　y　　10.0　　0 　z　　5.0　　-15.0 boundary surface 2: plane $\hat{n} = \hat{z}$ z = -12.5 boundary surface 3: plane $\hat{n} = -\hat{z}$ z = -17.5 boundary surface 4: plane $\hat{n} = -\hat{x}$ x = 5.0	boundary surface 1: cylinder 　r = 0.5 　l = 12.5 　axis along $\hat{x}$ boundary surface 2: ellipsoid 　　half axes center 　x　　12.0　　5.0 　y　　10.0　　0 　z　　5.0　　-15.0
pectoralis muscle, $\mu = 0.3972$/cm shape: rectangular box	**dense tissue region,** $\mu = 0.3931$/cm shape: ellipsoid
side length　center 　x　　5.0　　　2.5 　y　　30.0　　　0 　z　　5.0　　　-15.0	boundary surface: ellipsoid 　　　half axes center 　x　　1.0　　7.5 　y　　1.0　　0 　z　　0.2　　-14.0
fibroglandular region, $\mu = 0.3931$/cm shape: crescent	**mass,** $\mu = 0.40768$/cm shape: ellipsoid
boundary surface 1: ellipsoid 　　half axes center 　x　　10.0　　5.0 　y　　8.0　　0 　z　　3.0　　-15.0 boundary surface 2: sphere, r = 12.0 　　　center 　x　　-5.0 　y　　0 　z　　-15.0	boundary surface: ellipsoid 　　half axes　center 1 　x　　0.5　　7.5 　y　　0.5　　0 　z　　0.3　　-16.0 　　　center 2　center 3 　x　　10.0　　13.0 　y　　0　　　0 　z　　-15.0　　-15.0

The shapes, dimensions and attenuation coefficients of the obects used to build the phantom are listed in Table 1. The reference frame for the breast phantom is such that the breast points towards the positive x-direction. The x-ray source motion is in the $y - z$-plane at $x = 0$. The coordinate origin is located at the source pivoting point.

3   Materials

Attenuation coefficients for breast tissues were taken from Johns and Yaffe [7] and from the online table of NIST x-ray data for 30 keV photons. We generated projection images from the new breast phantom at 11 projection views at equally spaced angular intervals, with the x-ray source covering an arc of 50 degrees. The source pivoting point was located 20cm above the detector surface. Source to detector distance was 66 cm. Pixel size in the projection data array was 1 mm.

We used FBP, EM and TV algorithms to reconstruct volume images from the data generated as described above. The FBP algorithm involved a simple ramp filter. The EM algorithm and TV algorithms are described in [8, 9].

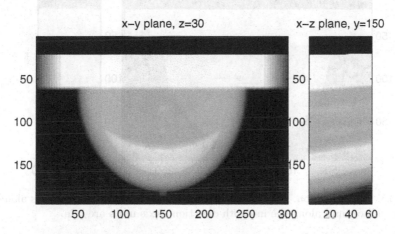

Fig. 2. FBP reconstruction. Slices through the reconstructed image volumes along the detector surface, and along the in-depth direction. Axis units are mm.

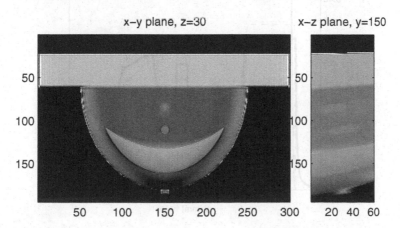

Fig. 3. EM-reconstruction. Slices through the reconstructed image volumes along the detector surface, and along the in-depth direction. Axis units are mm.

4   Results

Slices through the reconstructed volumes for the three algorithms investigated are shown in Figs. 2-4. The main features of the phantom are reproduced by all algorithms, namely the fatty and dense portions of the breast. The mass in the fatty region of the breast is conspicuous in all reconstructions. The mass in the fibroglandular region of the breast cannot be perceived in the FBP reconstruction. Resolution along the in-depth direction is lowest for FBP recon-

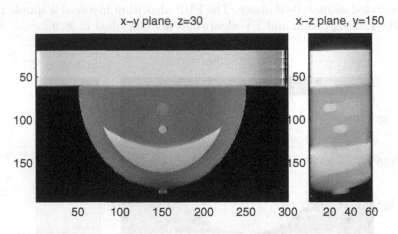

Fig. 4. TV reconstruction. Slices through the reconstructed image volumes along the detector surface, and along the in-depth direction. Axis units are mm.

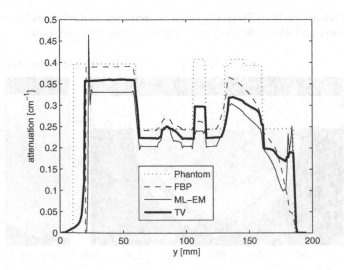

Fig. 5. Attenuation coefficients perpendicular to the source motion, at the center of the phantom, and in the in-depth direction

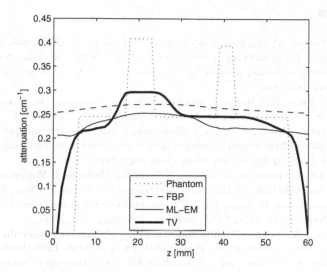

Fig. 6. Attenuation coefficients perpendicular to the source motion, at the center of the phantom, and in the in-depth direction

struction. EM produces spikes along the border. For quantitative comparison, profiles through the reconstructed volumes are shown in Fig. 5 perpendicular to the source motion, and in Fig. 6 along the in-depth direction. EM and TV reconstruction resolve the mass within dense tissue. Along the in-depth direction, TV reconstruction is the only algorithm that reproduces the overall shape of the breast. None of the algorithms maintain a constant attenuation from the edge of fibroglandular tissue out to the skin border.

5   Discussion and Conclusion

We have developed a new breast phantom that allows for quantitative comparison of reconstruction algorithm properties. The phantom and therefore the reconstructed image volumes are relatively simple, allowing to investigate algorithm properties in the absence of noise. The performance of the FBP algorithm will likely improve with an improved filter design. However the goal of this work was the development of the phantom, rather than algorithm development. Furthermore, results presented here are obtained with one imaging geometry. This phantom also allows to investigate how imaging geometry affects the reconstructed image volume. We hope that this phantom will prompt other researchers to quantitatively compare their algorithms. In the future, the breast phantom can be readily extended to include additional features, such as microcalcifications. In addition, physical factors, such as the spectrum of the x-ray beam, can be included.

References

1. T Wu, A Stewart, M Stanton, T McCauley, W Phillips, D B Kopans, R H Moore, J W Eberhard, B Opsahl-Ong, L Niklason, and M B Williams. Tomographic mammography using a limited number of low-dose cone-beam projection images. *Med. Phys.*, 30:365–380, 2003.
2. T Wu, R H Moore, E A Rafferty, and D B Kopans. A comparison of reconstruction algorithms for breast tomosynthesis. *Med. Phys.*, 31:2636–2647, 2004.
3. B Ren, C Ruth, J Stein, A Smith, I Shaw, and Z Jing. Design and performance of the prototype full field breast tomosynthesis system with selenium-based flat panel detector. In *Proc. SPIE*, volume 5745, page 550, 2005.
4. M Bissonnette, M Hansroul, E Masson, S Savard, S Cadieux, P Warmoes, D Gravel, J Agopyan, B Polischuk, W Haerer, T Mertelmeier, J Y Lo, Y Chen, J T Dobbins III, J L Jesneck, and S Singh. Digital tomosynthesis using an amorphous selenium flat panel detector. In *Proc. SPIE*, volume 5745, page 529, 2005.
5. K Lange and J A Fessler. Globally convergent algorithms for maximum a posteriori transmission tomography. *IEEE Trans. Med. Imag.*, 4:1430–1338, 1995.
6. D J Goodfrey, R J Warp, and J T Dobbins III. Optimization of matrix inversion tomosynthesis. In *Proc. SPIE*, volume 4320, pages 696–704, 2001.
7. P C Johns and M J Yaffe. X-ray characterisation of normal and neoplastic breast tissues. *Phys. Med. Biol.*, 32:675–695, 1987.
8. H H Barrett and K J Myers. *Foundations of Image Science*. Wiley Interscience, 2003.
9. EY Sidky, CM Kao, and X Pan. Accurate image reconstruction from few-views and limited-angle data in divergent-beam CT. *Journal of X-Ray Science and Technology*, 2006.

X-Ray Mammogram Registration:
A Novel Validation Method

John H. Hipwell, Christine Tanner, William R. Crum, and David J. Hawkes

Centre for Medical Image Computing,
Malet Place Engineering Building,
University College London, Gower Street,
London, WC1E 6BT
j.hipwell@ucl.ac.uk

Abstract. Establishing spatial correspondence between features visible in x-ray mammograms obtained at different times has great potential to aid assessment of change in the breast and facilitate its quantification. The literature contains numerous non-rigid registration algorithms developed for this purpose, but quantitative estimation of registration accuracy is limited. We describe a novel validation method which simulates plausible mammographic compressions of the breast using an MRI derived finite element model. Known 3D displacements are projected into 2D and test images simulated from these same compressed MR volumes. In this way we can generate convincing images with known 2D displacements with which to validate a registration algorithm. We illustrate this approach by computing the accuracy for a non-rigid registration algorithm applied to mammograms simulated from three patient MR datasets.

1 Introduction

In order to determine the presence or classification of breast cancer from x-ray mammograms, radiologists routinely compare images. This comparison may be made with mammograms obtained on a previous occasion, with alternate views of the same breast obtained during the same screening visit, or with the same view of the other breast as a means of determining any asymmetry that might be present. Clearly this comparison helps to confirm or refute the radiologist's appraisal of the disease and may enable an assessment of change and hence disease progression to be made.

While there have been several proposed methods for registering x-ray mammograms they are all generally flawed as they fail to take into account the complex 3D displacements of anatomy that contribute to the changes seen on the conventional x-ray projection of the compressed breast. In other words the applied transformations are diffeomorphic in the 2-dimensional plane, specifying a one to one correspondence between points in the registered images. In addition quantitative validation, when performed, is most commonly limited to the error associated with matching particular lesions identified by a clinician. This

Susan M. Astley et al. (Eds.): IWDM 2006, LNCS 4046, pp. 197–204, 2006.

approach is limited to the region of the lesion and dependent upon the visibility of the lesion in each view.

We propose a new method for evaluation of strategies for establishing this correspondence which uses 3D displacements obtained from computational bio-mechanical models of the breast. Our method simulates plausible mammographic compressions of the breast using an MRI derived finite element (FE) model. The resulting 3D displacements are then projected into 2D. X-ray mammograms are simulated from these same compressed MR volumes, generating convincing images with known 2D displacements with which to perform a registration validation. To illustrate this approach we compute the accuracy of non-rigid registrations of mammograms simulated from three patient MR datasets. The registration algorithm evaluated has previously proved accurate in 3D MR breast registrations [1].

We intend to use this method to aid development of new registration algorithms.

2   Methods

2.1   An MR Derived FE Model of Breast Compression

At the heart of our validation method is data describing the typical relative displacement of breast tissue caused by compression applied during routine x-ray mammography on separate occasions. This data was obtained using a FE model of the breast, constructed from segmented MR images and implemented using the FE software package ANSYS [2].

The FE models consisted of between 40,000 and 70,000 10-noded tetrahedral elements. Plate compressions were simulated by applying surface displacement boundary conditions, with displacements only specified in the direction perpendicular to the plates. This allows slippage along the plates to occur. Nodes adjacent to the pectoral muscle were constrained to have zero displacements as in [3]. All other nodes were allowed to move freely. Fatty, glandular and tumourous tissues were modelled as homogeneous, isotropic materials with linear elasticities of 1kPa and 1.5kPa, respectively, in accordance with tests extending the work reported in [4, 5]. Elasticity of tumorous tissue was varied between 3.6kPa and 10.8kPa to produce realistic variation in the data. In comparison to previous studies, our FE configuration was selected based on the accuracy of linear, non-linear and hyperelastic models to predict the location of internal breast structures after a 20% in-vivo compression for two volunteers [5]. This evaluation included models covering the wide range of reported elastic properties [6, 7] and variations to it [8, 9]. Linear models performed as well as non-linear models for these deformations. The three tissue types (fat, glandular and tumourous) were manually thresholded from the MR volume (after correction for inhomogeneities), and implausible regions resulting from this segmentation were removed in a subsequent manual processing step. A Poisson's ratio of 0.475 was chosen to allow for volume changes due to reduced blood volume as a result of the compression.

Cranio-caudal compressions for different patient visits were simulated by varying both the percentage compression, α, and the angle from the cranio-caudal axis (in the coronal plane) at which this compression is applied, β. Combinations of these two parameters produced N FE model deformations, $C_i(\alpha_i, \beta_i) : i = 1 \ldots N$, and these in turn generated multiple pairs of compression differences, $\{C_{pq}([\alpha_p, \beta_p],$ $[\alpha_q, \beta_q]) : \alpha_p \neq \alpha_q \text{ or } \beta_p \neq \beta_q\}$, for each patient, where each difference encapsulates the relative deformation of breast tissue that might occur between mammograms acquired on two separate occasions.

2.2   3D to 2D Projection

Using a perspective ray-casting algorithm both the MR volumes and their respective displacement fields can be projected into two dimensions as follows.

The 3D data set is placed at a particular location, t_{xyz}, and orientation, θ_{xyz}, in 3D space (for a given patient), relative to the virtual x-ray source position (the origin) and close to the 512×512 pixel, 0.5×0.5mm resolution simulated detector plane. The focal length of this virtual x-ray set was fixed at a mammographically realistic 660mm (*i.e.* parameters k_1 and k_2, the ratios of the x-ray pixel sizes to the focal length, equal 660), and for the purposes of these experiments the position of the x-ray normal from source to detector, (u_0, v_0), was placed at the centre of the detector plane ($u_0 = v_0 = 128mm$).

The equation of a ray, ψ, passing through the 3D data set from the x-ray source to a point, (u, v), on the 2D detector plane is obtained by solving:

$$P(k_1, k_2, u_0, v_0) \, T(t_{xyz}) \, R(\theta_{xyz}) \cdot \begin{pmatrix} x \\ y \\ z \\ 1 \end{pmatrix} = \lambda \begin{pmatrix} u \\ v \\ 1 \end{pmatrix}, \qquad (1)$$

where the perspective projection matrix $P(k_1, k_2, u_0, v_0)$, translation vector $T(t_{xyz})$, and rotation about x, y and z axes $R(\theta_{xyz})$, describe the pose and projection of the 3D data set relative to the detector. λ is an arbitrary perspective magnification factor.

The trajectory of ray, ψ, will cause it to traverse n_a axial, n_c coronal and n_s sagittal planes of voxels in the 3D data set, V. The highest sampling of the ray's profile is obtained by sampling V at planes, ρ, such that the greatest number of intersections with the ray is obtained, i.e.

$$\rho = \begin{cases} \text{axial if } n_a \geq n_c \text{ and } n_a \geq n_s \\ \text{coronal if } n_c > n_a \text{ and } n_c \geq n_s \\ \text{sagittal if } n_s > n_a \text{ and } n_s > n_c \end{cases}. \qquad (2)$$

The ray's profile is then given by

$$\begin{aligned} \psi(t_{xyz}, \theta_{xyz}, u, v) &= \{\psi(t_{xyz}, \theta_{xyz}, u, v, \iota) : \iota = 1 \ldots n_\rho\} \\ &= \{V(x_\iota, y_\iota, z_\iota) : \iota = 1 \ldots n_\rho\}, \end{aligned} \qquad (3)$$

where $V(x_\iota, y_\iota, z_\iota)$ is the intensity value from bi-linearly interpolating the neighbouring pixel values at the intersection of the ray with the ι'th ρ plane.

2.3   X-Ray Simulation from MR

Simulation of x-rays from MR enables us to generate realistic images with which to test a registration algorithm. In addition, because these digitally reconstructed radiographs (DRRs) are by definition in correspondence with the 3D MR and the 3D displacement field, we know the ground truth deformation between any given pair of DRRs generated in this way (figure 1).

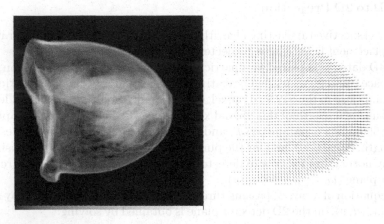

Fig. 1. Left: cranio-caudal x-ray mammogram simulated from an MR volume with compression, $C(50\%, 0°)$ for patient 'C'. Right: the relative mean displacement field between two compressions, $C_p(60\%,-5°)$ and $C_q(50\%, 5°)$, for this same patient.

In the DRR calculation described here we have ignored the contribution from fat because it is much more transparent to x-rays than either glandular tissue or tumour, but also because it contributes little to the texture of a mammogram and hence to the task of establishing correspondence between mammograms.

The manual segmentation described in section 2.1 was also used here to estimate the probability of glandular and tumourous tissue with MR intensity (I_{MR}), for the production of DRRs. A look-up table, L, was generated for this purpose from the ratio of the histograms of combined glandular and tumourous tissue intensities, H_G, and total intensity, H_T:

$$L(I_{MR}) = \frac{H_G(I_{MR})}{H_T(I_{MR})} . \tag{4}$$

Rays were cast through the MR volume, V, from each pixel location, (u, v), in the DRR as described in section 2.2. The look-up table was then used to convert the MR intensities to an estimated probability of glandular tissue or tumour, and these values were integrated to produce the DRR intensity $D_{RR}(u, v)$:

$$D_{RR}(u, v) = \cos(\phi) \sum_{\iota}^{n_\rho} L\left(\psi_{MR}(t_{xyz}, \theta_{xyz}, u, v, \iota)\right) , \tag{5}$$

where the term ϕ is the angle between the ray, ψ_{MR}, and the detector plane normal.

2.4 2D Displacement Fields

The 3D relative-displacement fields for a pair of compressions $C_p(\alpha_p, \beta_p)$ and $C_q(\alpha_q, \beta_q)$, are projected into 2 dimensions by treating the 3 displacement components as 3 images and creating ray profiles using the method described in 2.2. Corresponding points on the three component rays, $\delta_x(\iota), \delta_y(\iota), \delta_z(\iota)$, are then combined to create a ray profile of 3D displacements, $\psi_{\Delta_{pq}}$,

$$\psi_{\Delta_{pq}}(t_{xyz}, \theta_{xyz}, u, v) = \{\delta_x(\iota), \delta_y(\iota), \delta_z(\iota) : \iota = 1 \ldots n_\rho\} . \tag{6}$$

Each of these 3D vector displacements are then projected into 2D using the perspective projection matrix, M, where:

$$M = P(k_1, k_2, u_0, v_0)\, T(t_{xyz})\, R(\theta_{xyz}) \tag{7}$$

obtained by solving equation 1.

2.5 Registration Error Calculation

The output of a registration algorithm can be expressed as a list of "shipments" $m_{REG}(u, v, j)$ from pixel coordinates $(u, v) \in K_p$ in the source image to (continuous) pixel coordinates $(u', v') \in K_q$ in the target image. In general, for a conventional 2D registration, a single displacement (in the opposite direction: from target to source), is obtained at each pixel in the image (*i.e.* $j = 1$) and the mass associated with this displacement (or shipment) is equal to the pixel intensity in the source image. By considering the more general case of multiple shipments at each point in the image, we allow for subsequent registration developments which produce solutions closer to the true 3D movement of tissue in the mammogram.

For each experiment described below, we are establishing the transformation between two DRRs simulated from a pair of compressions, $C_p(\alpha_p, \beta_p)$ and $C_q(\alpha_q, \beta_q)$ (section 2.1). In the following we have dropped the t_{xyz}, θ_{xyz}, $[\alpha_p, \beta_p]$, $[\alpha_q, \beta_q]$ parameterisation for clarity. For each combination of C_p and C_q we know the corresponding 3D deformation and hence can calculate the 3D displacements, $\psi_{\Delta_{pq}}(u, v, \iota)$ and associated intensities, $\psi_{MR}(u, v, \iota)$, to transform the source volume into the target volume. By projecting these displacements and intensities into 2D, we obtain

$$m_{GT}(u, v, \iota) = \cos(\phi)L\left(\psi_{MR}(u, v, \iota)\right), \tag{8}$$

$$\delta_{GT}(u, v, \iota) = M(\psi_{\Delta_{pq}}(u, v, \iota)), \tag{9}$$

where M represents the projection from 3D to 2D obtained by solving equation 1. From equations 8 and 9 we can generate a ground truth registration for each pixel in the source DRR, which specifies a list of intensities, $m_{GT}(u, v, \iota)$, and their displacements, $\delta_{GT}(u, v, \iota)$, at each point, (u, v), in the image.

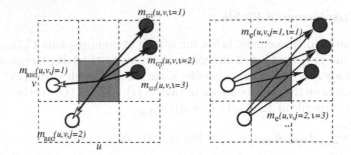

Fig. 2. The registration error at each pixel (u, v) is equal to the minimum work $\sum m_e(u, v, j, \iota) \, d_e(u, v, j, \iota)$ required to redistribute the computed registration "shipments" $m_{REG}(u, v, j)$ (open circles) to coincide with the ground truth shipments $m_{GT}(u, v, \iota)$ (closed circles)

As illustrated in figure 2, the registration error at each pixel is then defined as the minimum work, $e(u, v)$, required to reconcile the shipments computed by the registration algorithm, m_{REG}, with these ground truth shipments, m_{GT}:

$$e(u, v) = \sum_j \sum_\iota m_e(u, v, j, \iota) \, d_e(u, v, j, \iota)$$

$$: \quad m_e(u, v, j, \iota) \geq 0 , \tag{10}$$

where $d_e(u, v, j, \iota)$ is the corresponding Euclidean distance moved. To obtain the mean registration error for a pair of compressions $C_p(\alpha_p, \beta_p), C_q(\alpha_q, \beta_q)$ we simply sum over all the pixels in the source image and normalise by the total mass moved:

$$E_{pq} = \frac{\sum_{(u,v) \in K_p} e(u, v)}{\sum_{(u,v) \in K_p} \sum_j \sum_\iota m_e(u, v, j, \iota)} . \tag{11}$$

E_{pq} represents the mean registration error, for glandular tissue, in mm.

3   Results

To illustrate our validation methodology we have computed the registration error for a non-rigid registration algorithm [1] applied to a set of test images.

The test set of cranio-caudal image pairs was created for percentage compressions, $\alpha = \{50\%, 60\%, 70\%\}$ and orientations, $\beta = \{-10°, -5°, 0°, 5°, 10°\}$. Each combination of α and β produced 15 FE model deformations, $C(\alpha, \beta)$, and these in turn generated 210 pairs of compression differences, $(C_{pq}([\alpha_p, \beta_p], [\alpha_q, \beta_q]) : \alpha_p \neq \alpha_q$ or $\beta_p \neq \beta_q)$, for each patient.

Table 1 shows the mean errors for performing non-rigid registrations on these test images. This "fluid" registration algorithm registered the images to a mean accuracy of between 1.0 and 2.3mm, reducing the initial mean misregistrations which varied between 1.3 and 3.3mm.

Table 1. Registration errors for each of three patients and all compression combinations. The last column, $N_{F<N}$, gives the percentage of these 210 registrations for each patient for which the non-rigid registration gave an overall error less than that observed when no registration is performed.

Patient	No Reg'n Mean (Var)		Non-Rigid Reg'n Mean (Var.)		Success $N_{F<N}$
A	2.4	(1.0)	1.6	(0.5)	96%
B	1.3	(0.3)	1.0	(0.2)	89%
C	3.3	(2.1)	2.3	(1.1)	84%

The initial mean misregistration figures of 2.4, 1.3 and 3.3mm are low due to including percentage compressions which were the same for both target and source, (*i.e.* $\alpha_p = \alpha_q$), with only the angle at which this compression was applied varying, (β_p, β_q). The initial misregistration for this subset of test images varied from 0.3 to 4.6mm, whereas when the difference between the applied compressions was 20% (*i.e.* $\{\alpha_p, \alpha_q\} \in \{70\%, 50\%\}$: $\alpha_p \neq \alpha_q$) the range of initial misregistrations increased to 1.4 to 7.2mm.

Of the "failed" registrations in table 1 (registrations for which the non-rigid registration failed to decrease the overall misregistration), all correspond to compression pairs, C_{pq}, where the percentage compressions were the same for both target and source images ($\alpha_p = \alpha_q$), and only the angles, (β_p and β_q), at which the compressions were applied varied. The differences between these image pairs are caused by the different layers of breast tissue moving over one another. This is exactly the deformation that we know cannot be recovered by a two-dimensional diffeomorphic transformation. Such transformations imply a one-to-one correspondence between points in the source and target images. Clearly this is not the case for x-ray mammograms due to the perspective projection of the variably compressed 3D breast. For this reason new registration algorithms are required which produce non-diffeomorphic transformations that can capture the point-locus nature of the correspondence problem (*i.e.* "multiple registration shipments", $m_{REG}(u, v, j) : j > 1$). We are developing such an algorithm and will be able to use the same approach described here to validate the resulting program. It is necessary to develop such an evaluation strategy if we are to judge whether or not a particular algorithm is improving spatial correspondence.

4   Conclusion

This paper describes a novel validation technique for x-ray mammogram registration. Our approach uses real MR breast images from which realistic x-ray mammograms are simulated. By applying known compressions at a range of orientations we reproduce plausible deformations of the breast which might have occurred during mammography on separate occasions. Projections of these known deformations can then be used to compute the accuracy of a registration algorithm. It is our intention to use this validation technique to develop new registration algorithms which will be able to distinguish 3D movement of tissue between two x-ray mammograms from changes in the volume of (normal or abnormal) glandular tissue. In addition further assessment of the FE model accuracy for larger deformations will clarify the adequacy of the current model configuration.

Acknowledgments

We are grateful to the MARIBS study [10] and Guy's and St. Thomas' NHS Foundation Trust for providing the image data used in this study. This work was performed as part of the Medical Images and Signals IRC (EPSRC GR/N14248/01) and via UK Medical Research Council Grant No. D2025/31.

References

1. W.R. Crum *et. al.*, "Anisotropic Multiscale Fluid Registration: Evaluation in Magnetic Resonance Breast Imaging," *Phys. Med. Biol.*, vol. 50, 5153–5174, 2005.
2. ANSYS Inc., 2002.   275 Technology Drive, Canonsburg, PA 5317, USA. http://www.ansys.com.
3. P. Pathmanathan, D. Gavaghan, J. Whiteley, M. Brady, M. Nash, P. Nielsen, and V. Rajagopal. Predicting Tumour Location by Simulating Large Deformations of the Breast Using a 3D Finite Element Model and Nonlinear Elasticity. In *Medical Image Computing Computer-Assisted Intervention - MICCAI 2004, Pt 2, Proceedings*, volume 3217, pages 217–224, 2004.
4. C. Tanner, A. Degenhard, J. A. Schnabel, A. D. Castellano-Smith, C. Hayes, L. I. Sonoda, M. O. Leach, D. R. Hose, D. L. G. Hill, and D. J. Hawkes. Comparison of Biomechanical Breast Models: a Case Study. In *Medical Imaging 2002: Image Processing, Vol 1-3*, volume 4684, pages 1807–1818, 2002.
5. C. Tanner, J. A. Schnabel, M. O. Leach, D. R. Hose, D. L. G. Hill, and D. J. Hawkes. Factors Influencing the Accuracy of Biomechanical Breast Models. *Medical Phys.*, In Press.
6. T. A. Krouskop, T. M. Wheeler, F. Kallel, B. S. Garra, and T. Hall. Elastic Moduli of Breast and Prostate Tissues Under Compression. *Ultrasonic Imaging*, 20:260–274, 1998.
7. P. S. Wellman. *Tactile Imaging*. PhD thesis, Harvard University, 1999.
8. F. S. Azar, D. N. Metaxas, and M. D. Schnall. A Finite Model of the Breast for Predicting Mechanical Deformations during Biopsy Procedure. In *Proc. MMBIA'00*, pages 38–45, 2000.
9. A. Samani, J. Bishop, M. J. Yaffe, and D. B. Plewes. Biomechanical 3D Finite Element Modeling of the Human Breast Using MRI Data. *IEEE Trans. Med. Imag.*, 20(4):271–279, 2001.
10. J. Brown, D. Buckley, A. Coulthard, and A. K. Dixon. Magnetic Resonance Imaging Screening in Women at Genetic Risk of Breast Cancer: Imaging and Analysis Protocol for the UK Multicentre Study. *Magnetic Resonance Imaging*, 18:765–776, 2000.

A Probabilistic Approach for the Simultaneous Mammogram Registration and Abnormality Detection

Mohamed Hachama, Agnès Desolneux, and Frédéric Richard*

MAP5, University Paris 5,
45, rue des Saints Pères,
75006 Paris, France
{hachama, desolneux, richard}@math-info.univ-paris5.fr

Abstract. In this paper, we present a new method for simultaneously registering mammograms and detecting abnormalities. We assume that pixels can be divided into two classes: normal tissue and abnormalities (lesions). We define the registration constraints as a mixture of two distributions which describe statistically image gray-level variations for both pixel classes. The two distributions are weighted at each pixel by the probability of abnormality presence. Using the Maximum A Posteriori, we estimate the registration transformation and the probability map of abnormality presence at the same time. We illustrate the properties of our technique with some experiments and compare it with some classical methods.

1 Introduction

Mammograms are often interpreted by comparing left and right breast images or different mammograms of a same patient. Mammogram comparisons help radiologists to identify abnormalities and determine their clinical significance [1]. In the CAD context, image comparisons are not straightforward. The registration of images must be carried out to compensate for some normal differences that can cause high false-negative rates in abnormality detection schemes [2].

Several researchers have used the subtraction of registered images as a comparative means by which to detect abnormalities [3]. The obtained asymmetry image is then thresholded to extract suspicious regions. Thus, the success of the detection task depends on the preliminary registration process.

On the other hand, the registration problem is usually expressed as a minimization of an energy composed of a regularization term and a similarity term. Usually, similarity criteria rely on some assumptions about gray-level dependencies between images [4], which are not valid in the presence of abnormalities. The registration can be improved by including in the model some knowledge about these abnormalities, as it was done in [5, 6, 7] and for the optical flow estimation in [8].

---

* This work was supported by the grant "ACI Young Researchers 2003 (French Ministry of Research)" No. 9060.

In this paper, we present a mixture-based technique where pixels are classified into a normal tissue class and an abnormality class. The registration constraints are then defined as a mixture of two distributions describing gray-level character-istics of the two classes and which are weighted at each pixel by the probability of abnormality presence. The main feature of our model is the possibility to com-bine image registration and the detection of abnormalities, so as to take proper advantage of the dependence between the two processes.

The mixture-based technique and its mathematical formulation are presented in Section 2. In Section 3, we illustrate the method behavior on some examples and compare it with some classical techniques.

2   Method

Let I and J be two images defined on a discrete grid Ω_d associated to $\Omega = [0,1]^2$ and called respectively source image and target image. Image coordinates are matched using transformations ϕ which map Ω_d into itself. We assume that lesions may be present in the images. Let L be the lesion map which associates to each pixel of Ω_d its probability to belong to a lesion in I or J. Assuming that all variables are realizations of some random fields, Bayes rule can be expressed as:

$$p(\phi, L | I, J) = \frac{p(I, J | L, \phi) \, p(\phi) \, p(L)}{p(I, J)}.$$

For the sake of simplicity, we have assumed in the above formula that the de-formation ϕ and the lesion map L are independent (i.e. $p(\phi, L) = p(\phi)p(L)$). We can estimate the pair (ϕ, L) as the solution of the Maximum A Posteriori (MAP):

$$(\widetilde{\phi}, \widetilde{L}) = \arg\max_{(\phi, L)} \; p(I, J | \phi, L) \, p(\phi) \, p(L).$$

To ensure that the transformations remain smooth, we assume that they arise from the Gibbs distribution:

$$p(\phi) = \frac{1}{Cst} e^{-H_d(\phi)}, \tag{1}$$

where H_d is a discrete elasticity potential [9] (a continuous version is given by Equation (5)). We also assume that the lesion map arises from a Gibbs distribution:

$$p(L) = \frac{1}{Cst} e^{-R_d(L)}, \tag{2}$$

where R_d is a discrete energy of regularization. We use in this paper an energy restricting the amount of abnormal pixels in the images via a real parameter α_L:

$$R_d(L) = \alpha_L \sum_{x \in \Omega_d} L(x).$$

More specific terms should be defined to describe the spatial configurations of each type of lesion. We will investigate the use of such energies in the future.

In order to define the likelihood $p(I, J|\phi, L)$, we assume that, given the transformation ϕ, the probability of the pair of images (I, J) depends only on the registered images $I_\phi = I \circ \phi$ and J, and that pixels are independent. Hence, we can write

$$p(I, J|\phi, L) = \prod_x p(I_\phi(x), J(x)|L(x)).$$

The probability of the pair $(I_\phi(x), J(x))$ depends on the class of the pixel x. Each class is characterized by a probability distribution, denoted by p_N for the normal tissue and p_L for the lesion. Thus, the probability distribution $p(I_\phi(x), J(x)|L(x))$ can be defined as a mixture of the two class distributions

$$p(I_\phi(x), J(x)|L(x)) = (1 - L(x))p_N(I_\phi(x), J(x)) + L(x)p_L(I_\phi(x), J(x)). \quad (3)$$

The normal tissue class. We assume that image differences generated by normal tissue have a discrete centered Gaussian distribution with variance σ^2:

$$p_N(I_\phi(x), J(x)) = \frac{1}{Cst} \exp(-\frac{|I_\phi(x) - J(x)|^2}{2\sigma^2}),$$

The lesion class. For the sake of simplicity, we assume that a lesion is present in the target image J. We simply characterize the lesion as a region which is brighter in the target image than it is in the source image. Hence, we get the following distribution

$$p_L(I_\phi(x), J(x)) = \begin{cases} 0 & \text{if } I_\phi(x) > J(x) \\ Cst & \text{otherwise,} \end{cases}$$

Numerical resolution

Up to now, we have formulated a Bayesian registration model in a discrete setting. We now transform the discrete model into a continuous model so as to be able to use variational resolution techniques. First, using the negative-log function, we rewrite the MAP estimate as an energy minimization problem. Then, we define a continuous version of the obtained energy by interpolating all functions by the finite element method and replacing sums on the pixel grid Ω_d by integrals on Ω. Thus, we have to minimize the energy:

$$E(\phi, L) = H(\phi) + R(L) - \int_\Omega \log(p(I_\phi(x), J(x))) \, dx, \quad (4)$$

where the probability distribution $p(I_\phi(x), J(x))$ is the obtained continuous version of the mixture distribution given by Equation (3). $H(\phi)$ is the elasticity potential defined as

$$\sum_{i,j=1,2} \int_\Omega [\lambda \frac{\partial u_i(x)}{\partial x_i} \frac{\partial u_j(x)}{\partial x_j} + \mu(\frac{\partial u_i(x)}{\partial x_j} + \frac{\partial u_j(x)}{\partial x_i})^2] dx, \quad (5)$$

where $u = \phi - id$, and λ and μ are the Lame elasticity constants.

The term $R(L)$ is the following energy:

$$R(L) = \alpha_L \int_\Omega L(x) \, dx.$$

As in [10, 6], we use a gradient descent algorithm on the energy E and finite elements to approximate solutions of the minimization problem.

3　Results

3.1　Experiment 1: Comparison Results

We illustrate the characteristics of this mixture-based technique by comparing its performance with two other registration techniques. The first one is the minimization the Sum of Square Differences (SSD). The second one is a registration technique proposed in [6], which is related to M-estimation in robust Statistics. We apply the algorithms to the pair of bilateral mammograms (21, 22) of the MIAS database [11], for which the target image contains an asymmetric density (bright circular region at the bottom of Image 1(b). Registrations obtained with the SSD and the M-estimation techniques tend to incorrectly match the lesion with the bright tissue in the source image and thus reduce image differences due to the lesion (Images 1(d),1(e)). This is corrected by the mixture-based technique where images are correctly registered while differences due to the lesion are preserved (Image 1(f)).

In order to test the detection performance of the mixture-based technique, we compare a lesion binary image obtained by thresholding the lesion map $\tilde{L}$, to the ones obtained with the SSD and the M-estimation methods by thresholding the images of differences. Figures 1(g)-(i) show the binary lesion images obtained with the three techniques for the same amount of abnormal pixels. We can notice that the mixture-based method reduces the number of false-positives.

For evaluating and comparing the three algorithms without the influence of a threshold value, we have presented on Figure 2 the FROC curves obtained with the three methods. The FROC curve plots the sensitivity (fraction of detected true positives, calculated by using the expert segmented image) as a function of the number of false positives. For the mixture-based technique, we have presented the FROC curve obtained with $\alpha_L = 0.1$. When using different values of the weight α_L, we have obtained similar FROC curves.

As observed on Figure 2, the FROC curve associated to the mixture-based method is the highest. So, the detection by the mixture-based technique is more sensitive. For instance, for 10000 false positive pixels (2% of image pixels), the detection rate grows from 0.632 for the SSD and 0.627 for the M-estimation based method, to 0.947 for the mixture based method.

3.2　Experiment 2: The Prior Lesion Term

In this experiment, we study the influence of the weight associated to the regularization term $R_L(L) = \alpha_L \int_\Omega L(x)$ of the lesion map L. We use the pair

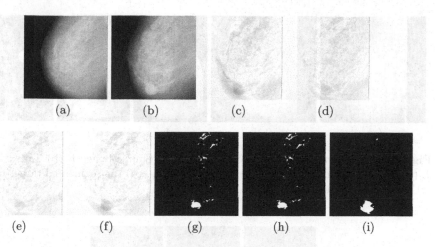

Fig. 1. Registration of bilateral mammograms. (a) Source image I, (b) Target image J, (c) The difference between the images before registration. The difference between the images after the registration using (d) the SSD method, (e) the M-estimation method, (f) the mixture-based method. Detection results containing 4180 pixels obtained with (g) the SSD method, (h) the M-estimation based method, (i) the mixture-based method.

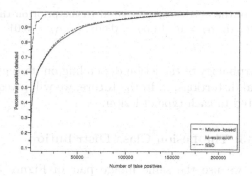

Fig. 2. FROC curves for the three detection methods

(117 − 118) of the MIAS database (Images 3(a) and 3(b)) ; the images are segmented and the registration is initialized using a geometric approach based on the matching of the contours [2].

We have applied the mixture-based technique to the pair of images (3(c), 3(d)), using the lesion class distribution described in Section 2, for different values of the weight α_L. Results are presented in Figure 4.

As shown on Figure 4, we can use the weight α_L to limit the quantity of lesion pixels present in the image. High values of this weight restricts the amount of lesion pixels. However, the lesion map contains isolated pixels which, clearly, do not belong to any lesion. The use of the sum of the lesion map as the prior potential does not take this into account. More sophisticated terms should take

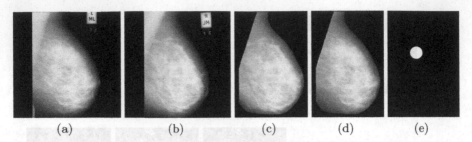

(a)   (b)   (c)   (d)   (e)

Fig. 3. Registration of bilateral mammograms. (a) Source image I, (b) Target image J, (c) the segmented and pre-registered source image, (d) the segmented target image, (e) the expert-segmented image.

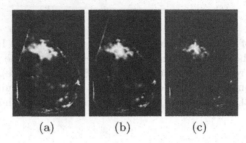

(a)   (b)   (c)

Fig. 4. The influence of the weight α_L associated to the prior on the lesion map. The lesion map obtained for (a) $\alpha_L = 0$, (b) $\alpha_L = 0.001$, (c) $\alpha_L = 0.01$.

into account the morphology of the lesion depending on its type: masses, calcifications, architectural distortions, ... In the future, we will investigate the design of prior terms adapted to each type of lesion.

3.3   Experiment 3: The Lesion Class Distribution

In this experiment, we use the same image pair of Figure 3. We apply the mixture-based method with different lesion class distributions.

First example. If we have no information about the photometric characteristics of the lesion, we should use an uniform distribution:

$$p_L(I_\phi(x), J(x)) = \frac{1}{Cst}.$$

Second example. As explained in Section 2, one can also suppose that a lesion is just a region in one image that is more bright that its correspondent in the second image. If we assume that the lesion is present in the target image, we get:

$$p_L(I_\phi(x), J(x)) = \begin{cases} 0 & \text{if } I_\phi(x) > J(x) \\ Cst & \text{otherwise,} \end{cases}$$

Third example. If we have more precise information about the gray-level values of lesion pixels, we can use a probability distribution of the form:

$$p_\text{L}(I_\phi(x), J(x)) = \begin{cases} 0 & \text{if } I_\phi(x) > J(x) \\ \frac{1}{Cst}\ \exp(-\frac{(J(x)-m)^2}{2\sigma^2}), & \text{otherwise,} \end{cases}$$

where m is the mean value of the lesion brightness and σ its standard deviation. In this experiment, m and σ are determined using the images and the expert-segmented lesion image ($m = 215$ and $\sigma = 5$). More generally, one can use a full database to estimate these parameters. Detection results (lesion maps) obtained with these three terms are shown on Figure 5.

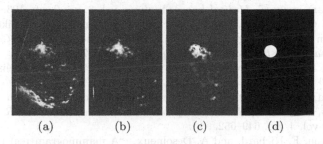

(a)   (b)   (c)   (d)

Fig. 5. Detection results with different lesion class distributions. Lesion map obtained with: (a) the first model, (b) the second model, (c) the third model. (d) Expert-segmented lesion.

As shown on Figure 5(a), when using an uniform model (which corresponds to the case when the lesion can be present either in the target image or in the source one), the algorithm tends to consider all asymmetric regions as lesions. The detection results are improved by using more information. If we suppose that the lesion is present in the target image, we can use the second distribution which produces better results. In practice, this is the case for the detection of the apparition, or change, of a lesion in a temporal sequence. In the third case, we have more precise information about the gray-level values of lesion pixels in the form of a Gaussian distribution with a known mean value and standard-deviation. With the third distribution, we get the best detection results: false positive are reduced and the lesion map is concentrated on the real lesion. In practice, one can estimate the parameters of the Gaussian distribution from a database.

4   Conclusion

We have presented a method for simultaneously registering mammograms and detecting abnormalities. Thanks to a combined approach, the mixture-based method improves the mammogram registration and reduces the false-positives rate for the lesion detection. In the future, we will focus on the design of lesion models for different types of lesions, and the estimation of the distribution parameters for both lesion and normal tissue classes. Furthermore, we will test the mixture-based method on a mammogram database.

References

1. L. Tabar and P. Dean, *Teaching atlas of mammography*, Thieme Inc., Stuttgart, 1985.
2. C. Graffigne F. Richard, "An image matching problem for the registration of temporel or bilateral mammogram pairs," *Proc. of the 5th International Workshop on Digital Mammography (toronto, Canada)*, june 2000.
3. M.Y. Sallam and K. Bowyer, "Registration and difference analysis of corresponding mammogram images," *Medical Image Analysis*, vol. 3, no. 2, pp. 103–118, 1999.
4. A. Roche, G. Malandain, and N. Ayache, "Unifying Maximum Likelihood Approaches in Medical Image Registration," *International Journal of Computer Vision of Imaging Systems and Technology*, vol. 11, pp. 71–80, 2000.
5. D. Hasler, L. Sbaiz, S. Susstrunk, and M. Vetterli, "Outlier modeling in image matching," *IEEE Trans. on Patt. Anal. and Match. Intell.*, pp. 301–315, 2003.
6. F. Richard, "A new approach for the registration of images with inconsistent differences," in *Proc. of the Int. Conf. on Pattern Recognition, ICPR*, Cambridge, UK, 2004, vol. 4, pp. 649–652.
7. M. Hachama, F. Richard, and A. Desolneux, "A mammogram registration technique dealing with outliers," in *IEEE International Symposium on Biomedical Imaging ISBI'06, Arlington, Virginia, USA*, April 2006.
8. A. Jepson and M.J. Black, "Mixture models for optical flow computation," in *IEEE Conf. on Computer Vision and Pattern Recognition*, 1993, pp. 760–761.
9. F. Richard, "A comparative study of markovian and variational image-matching techniques in application to mammograms," *Pattern Recognition Letters*, vol. 26, no. 12, pp. 1819–1829, 2005.
10. F. Richard and L. Cohen, "Non-rigid image registration with free boundary constraintes: application to mammography," *Journal of Computer Vision and Image Understanding*, vol. 89(2), pp. 166–196, 2003.
11. J. Suckling, J. Parker, and D. Dance, "The MIAS digital mammogram database," *In Proc. of the 2nd Int. Workshop on Digital Mammography, England*, july 1994.

Mammographic Registration: Proposal and Evaluation of a New Approach*

Robert Martí[1], David Raba[1], Arnau Oliver[1], and Reyer Zwiggelaar[2]

[1] Computer Vision and Robotics Group, University of Girona
Av. Lluís Santaló 17071, Spain
{marly, draba, aoliver}@eia.udg.es
http://eia.udg.es/~marly
[2] Department of Computer Science, University of Wales,
Aberystwyth Ceredigion, SY23 3DB, Wales, UK
rrz@aber.ac.uk

Abstract. The detection of architectural distortions and abnormal structures in mammographic images can be based on the analysis of bilateral and temporal cases. This paper presents a novel method for mammographic image registration inspired by existing robust point matching approaches. This novel method is compared with other registration approaches proposed in the literature using both quantitative and qualitative evaluation based on similarity metrics and ROC analysis (ground truth provided by an expert radiologist). Initial evaluation is based on mammographic data of 64 women with malignant masses which indicates the accuracy and robustness of our method.

1 Background

Image registration has been widely used in medical applications for quite a while now, and the analysis of mammographic images is not an exception. An added difficulty of trying to register mammographic images is their projective nature. Nevertheless, different approaches have been adopted to obtain an alignment and minimise effects due to acquisition factors such as patient movement, breast compression and other image related factors (film exposure and energy). Most of the published approaches (including the early works of Sallam and Bowyer [1] and Karssemeijer and te Brake [2]) use breast boundary information as it is relatively easy to extract and provides important information about the breast deformation. Another group of approaches can be classified as being intensity based, where the deformation is recovered maximising a measure of similarity between images. The use of an intensity measure to recover global transformations has been reported to obtain robust results [3], but can not account for severe local distortions and additional steps are needed. In addition to the breast boundary, information about the deformation of internal regions is also necessary in order to obtain a robust registration. This has been used by different authors [4,5,1].

---

* Research partiallly supported by the *Juan de la Cierva* Programme and research grant no. TIN2005-08792-C03-01

Susan M. Astley et al. (Eds.): IWDM 2006, LNCS 4046, pp. 213–220, 2006.

Although non-linear registration (warping methods) of mammographic images has been regarded by some authors as non-appropriate [3], it is our belief, which is corroborated by other authors [5], that non-linear transformation can also be successfully used. However, special care has to be taken in choosing the transformation function and its parameters (in particular, regularisation factors which ensure smoothness and continuity). It is true that a naive implementation can lead to non-realistic transformations.

The method presented here is an evolution of our initial proposal [4], focusing now on providing a robust framework for establishing point correspondence between mammograms. The novelty of this paper is twofold. Firstly, we introduce and adapt different concepts of robust point matching approaches to the proposed registration approach. Secondly, an evaluation is presented comparing our method to other existing approaches in terms of similarity measures and ROC curves using a relatively large number of cases. Although initial results, this work shows that image registration can be successfully used to asses temporal changes in mammograms such as involution of breast tissue, the detection of masses or architectural distortions.

2 Method

The registration methodology presented here is based on robustly matching interest points in two mammographic images of the same view (either MLO or CC). The algorithm extracts interest points found in the boundary and the internal breast region, and applies a robust point matching approach obtaining a non-linear transformation. Registered images are used for detecting possible abnormalities in contralateral mammograms (comparing left and right breasts) by subtracting images and measuring local measures of similarity.

An initial pre-processing step segments the breast boundary and extracts interest points from the boundary and internal regions. A distinction between boundary and internal structures is made. Boundary information is used to restrict the detection area of internal structures and is also a good initial estimate of the breast deformation. In this paper, the breast boundary is obtained by simple thresholding and morphological opening operations. Subsequently, interest points are obtained from this boundary by computing their maximal local curvature. Interest points internal to the breast are also extracted using a criteria of local maximal curvature after a line detection algorithm is applied to the breast region. This pre-processing is similar to the one presented in [4].

2.1 Point Matching Algorithm

The idea behind the registration methodology of this paper is inspired by robust point correspondence methods proposed by various authors [6,7,8]. The common approach from the cited methods is the use of an iterative process in order to minimise correspondence errors. Those errors are related to a cost matrix (C_{ij}) which describes the cost of matching one point i in one image (row i) with a point j in the second image (column j). The elements of this matrix are obtained using different point error measures such as Euclidean distance, shape contexts [7], local intensity information, gradient, etc. Additionally, relaxation labelling or soft assign methods can be applied to the cost matrix in order to minimise ambiguous matchings as in [8]. Relaxation methods are not applied in this work but will be investigated in the future. The minimisation of the cost matrix yields potential point matches which are used for transforming one point set (p) in order to match the other (q). The transformed points p and q are used for building the cost matrix for the next iteration. The stopping criteria of the iterative process is usually stated in terms of a maximum number of iterations or if the number of matches does not change with respect the last iteration.

Cost matrix. The Euclidean distance between points has perhaps been the most common distance measure for point matching. This is the case of Closest Iterative Point based methods (ICP) [6]. Shape Contexts (SC), originally proposed by Belongie et al. [7] are rich shape descriptors based on building local point distribution histograms. Thus, at a point level p_i, SC provide information about point distribution relative to that point p_i. A cost of matching points in both images can be obtained by comparing those local histograms. Normalised Cross-Correlation (NCC) is a well known measure of similarity which has been used for many applications in computer vision. Perhaps one of the most common is template matching, obtaining the position of a known template in a larger image. NCC computed within a local grey-level neighbourhood will be used as our third distance measure. The main drawback of using local similarity measures is that shape and point relationships are under-represented. For this reason, NCC will be used in combination of the above measures to ensure topological point relationships. Given the set of costs C_{ij}, one-to-one matches are obtained minimising the total matrix cost $H(\pi) = \sum_i C(p_i, q_{\pi(i)})$, where $\pi(i)$ denotes all permutation. This minimisation (optimal assignment problem) is obtained using the Hungarian method, as in [7].

Transformation. Points are transformed using the matches found in the previous step. In the first iteration, an affine transformation is used in order to recover global misregistration. In subsequent iterations, the Thin-Plate Splines (TPS) is used to obtain a smooth transformation between matched points. For a set of d dimensional points x, the Thin-Plate approximation function is defined as a sum of d independent functionals J_m^d minimising a measure of bending energy (related to m order derivatives, $m = d = 2$ is used here).

$$J_m^d(u) = \sum_{k=1}^{d} J_m^d(u_k) \qquad (1)$$

The solution, $u(x)$, is obtained by solving a linear system of equations,

$$u(x) = \sum_{\nu=1}^{M} a_\nu \phi_{nu}(x) + \sum_{i=1}^{n} w_i U(|p_i - x|) \qquad (2)$$

where $\phi_{nu}(x)$ defines the TPS behaviour away from the control points, U are the thin plate basis functions and a_ν and w_i are the parameters of the transformation. The smoothness of the TPS transformation can be controlled by introducing a regularisation term (λ) in the transformation (see [9]) weakening the interpolation condition ($q_i = u(p_i)$).

$$J_\lambda(u) = \frac{1}{n} \sum_{i=1}^{n} |q_i - u(p_i)|^2 + \lambda J_m^d(u_k) \qquad (3)$$

For λ values close to zero, the transformation interpolates exactly for each control point (the original TPS transformation), while for larger values we obtain smoother approximating transformations. This regularisation is used in the iterative process, where larger λ values are used in the initial iterations decreasing its value depending on an error fitness measure.

Outliers. The Hungarian method obtains optimal matches for all points in the cost matrix. For some applications, and mammographic registration is one of them, a large number of outliers is expected in both images. In this sense, the original cost matrix is enlarged with a percentage of dummy points, points to which real points will be assigned if a better match is not found. The number of dummy matches depends on two parameters defined experimentally: the cost of matching to a dummy point (which should be small enough to allow dummy matches but at the same time large enough to obtain a significant number of real matches) and also the number of dummy points allowed (as a percentage of the total number of points). Experimentally, and although exact values are not particularly critical, we have experienced that a dummy point percentage of $30 - 40\%$ with a cost of 0.1 provide the best results. Moreover, not all matches are taken into account, only those with minimal cost compared to its neighbourhood are selected as final matches. This neighbourhood criteria is implemented as a graph proximity problem.

3   Results

3.1   Qualitative Results

Here we qualitatively show the results of the registration algorithm. The described point matching algorithm is applied in two different steps. Initially, breast boundary points alone are used as interest points for finding potential matches. Subsequently, a second matching process is started in order to obtain matches for the internal points. The matching in this second step is constrained by the transformation found in the boundary matching process. This constraint is applied to the cost matrix where matches for boundary points are enforced to remain constant. Fig. 1 shows the different steps of the registration.

Fig. 2 shows original images and registration results and the difference image using the proposed method (rpm) of the example matched in Fig. 1.

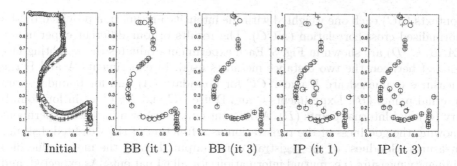

| Initial | BB (it 1) | BB (it 3) | IP (it 1) | IP (it 3) |

Fig. 1. Registration using breast boundary (BB) and internal points (IP) in different iterations. Crosses (circles) refer to control points from the reference (target) images.

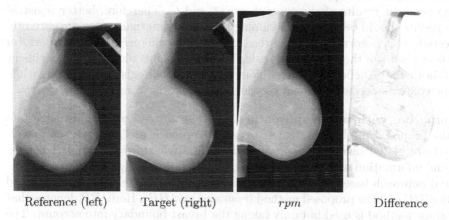

| Reference (left) | Target (right) | *rpm* | Difference |

Fig. 2. Example of registration results using the *rpm* approach

3.2   Quantitative Evaluation

A total of 128 mammographic images obtained from the DDSM mammographic database [10] are used as initial evaluation. These include 64 different patients with left and right MLO images where a malignant mass has been detected and annotated as ground truth. The difference image (after histogram matching) is computed from the registered images for each patient. In the ideal case of a perfect registration, this image is likely to highlight the suspicious region. The idea is that results from the difference image could be used for mass detection or at least to reduce the number of false positives in mass detection algorithms. An evaluation on the distance parameters of the proposed method is firstly given, and subsequently, a comparison with other approaches is performed.

Distance Function. As mentioned before, different distance measures can be used for computing the cost matrix. Various experiments have been carried out in order to assess the benefits of each distance measure and its relative importance. Distance measures evaluated are Euclidean distance (E) and shape contexts (SC) each one weighted with the intensity information provided by the normalised cross-correlation (NCC). The results of four different experiments (A, B, C, D) are shown in Fig. 3. Each experiment evaluates the weighting factor (α) between the two distance measures used. In experiments A and B the measures evaluated are E and NCC for boundary (A) and for boundary and internal points (B). Experiments C and D use SC and NCC again for boundary (C) and internal points (D). A different curve is shown for each experiment showing the goodness of the registration as a function of the weighted distance measures. Goodness of the registration is computed using the mean value of a similarity measure (i.e. mutual information) for all 64 patients. As expected, and corroborated by visual inspection of the registered images, the worst results are obtained using only breast boundary points (experiments A and C). For experiments using internal points $(B$ and $D)$, boundary matches are initially found using the best results of the experiments A and C. Therefore, better registration results should be obtained assuming that those internal points are correctly detected. This is corroborated by the experiments, where B and D outperform the best results of the experiments using boundary points alone. The experiment also shows that Euclidean distance alone provides good registration results while shape contexts needs additional grey level information to reach similar levels.

Comparing with other approaches. This section shows the initial results of the proposed method compared to other approaches. The approaches evaluated are global image registration using affine transformation maximising a mutual information measure $(miat)$, image registration using our previously presented approach based on point matching and thin-plate splines [4] $(linreg$ and $linregBB)$ and the proposed method $(rpm$ and $rpmBB)$. Here, BB denotes that the same method is used but only taking the breast boundary into account. The

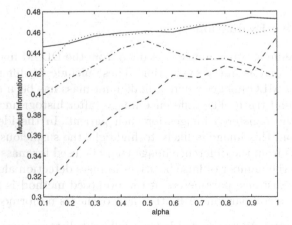

Fig. 3. Evaluation results of the relative importance of the distance measures in the final registration result: Experiments A (dashed), B (solid) and C (dot dashed) and D (dotted)

miat implementation is similar to one of the evaluated methods presented in [3]. Fig. 4a shows evaluation results in terms of box plots computed from similarity measures (mutual information) between the reference image (left breast) and the registered image (right breast) using the different approaches. From the plots, we can conclude that the proposed method obtains a similar accuracy to the *linreg* method with a slightly higher mean value and more robust and stable results (note the outlier in the *linreg* method). Results also show, as reported by various authors, that although using breast boundary information alone obtains good results, accuracy and robustness is increased when information from the internal breast structure is included. Additional evaluation results are shown in Fig. 4b, which shows ROC curves obtained from the difference image compared to the annotation ground truth provided by radiologists. The ROC curve is build by measuring the true positive and false positive fraction as a function of a threshold of the difference image compared to manual segmentations provided by a radiologist. In this case, although curves get close for the cases of *linreg*, *linregBB* and *rpm*, analysing the Area Under the Curve (*AUC*) value our proposal has a slightly worst results.

In summary, the proposed method obtains better results compared to the *miat* method which is in contrast with the results published in [3]. This will need further investigation but could be due to particular implementations or to pre-processing steps (i.e. pectoral muscle suppression). Compared to the *linreg* method, similar but more robust results are obtained. Both approaches share common methodologies which explains the similarity of the results. A comparison with other recently published approaches [5] can not be directly stated from this work but additional evaluation procedures will be proposed and included in the future work.

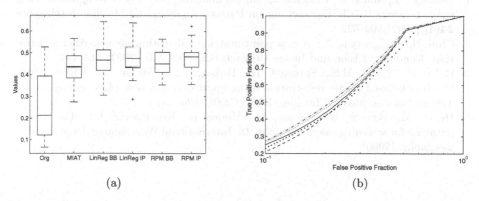

(a)   (b)

Fig. 4. (a) Box plots and (b) ROC curves for different registration methods: *miat* (bold dotted), *linregBB* (dotted), *linreg* (dash dotted), *rpmBB* (dashed) and *rpm* (solid). *AUC* values for each method are 0.714, 0.739, 0.747, 0.722 and 0.730, respectively.

4   Conclusions

A novel registration algorithm has been presented based on the application of robust point matching concepts. Quantitative and qualitative results have been presented that show the validity of our approach. Although initial results are presented, a comparison with other approaches has been provided, showing reduced error rates for the developed method. Future work will focus on extending the number of cases including temporal studies from our local database. Additional evaluation in terms of landmark error measures will be presented with the aim to obtain better comparison with other approaches.

References

1. Sallam, M., Bowyer, K.: Registration and difference analysis of corresponding mammogram images. Medical Image Analysis 3(2) (1999) 103–118
2. Karssemeijer, N., Brake, G.T.: Combining single view features and asymmetry for detection of mass lesions. In Karssemeijer, N., Thijssen, M., Hendriks, J., van Erning, L., eds.: 4th International Workshop on Digital Mammography, Kluwer Academic (1998) 95–102
3. van Engeland, S., Snoeren, P., Hendriks, J., Karssemeijer, N.: A comparison of methods for mammogram registration. IEEE Transactions on Medical Imaging 22(11) (2003) 1436–1444
4. Marti, R., Zwiggelaar, R., Rubin, C.: Automatic point correspondence and registration based on linear structures. International Journal of Pattern Recognition and Artificial Intelligence 16(3) (2002) 331–340
5. Marias, K., Behrenbruch, C.P., Parbhoo, S., Seifalian, A., Brady, M.: A registration framework for the comparison of mammogram sequences. IEEE Transactions on Medical Imaging 24(6) (2005) 782–790
6. Besl, P.J., McKay, N.D.: A method for registration of 3-D shapes. IEEE Transactions on Pattern Analysis and Machine Intelligence 14(2) (1992) 239–256
7. Belongie, S., Malik, J., Puzicha, J.: Shape matching and object recognition using shape contexts. IEEE Transactions on Pattern Analysis and Machine Intelligence 24(4) (2002) 509–522
8. Chui, H., Rangarajan, A.: A new point matching algorithm for non-rigid registration. Computer Vision and Image Understanding 89(2-3) (2003) 114–141
9. Rohr, K., Stiehl, H.S., Sprengel, R., Buzug, T.M., Weese, J., Kuhn, M.H.: Landmark-based elastic registration using approximating thin-plate splines. IEEE Transactions on Medical Imaging 20(6) (2001) 526–534
10. Heath, M., Bowyer, K., Kopans, D., Moore, R., Kegelmeyer, P.: The digital database for screening mammography. In: International Workshop on Digital Mammography. (2000)

Image Similarity and Asymmetry to Improve Computer-Aided Detection of Breast Cancer

Dave Tahmoush[1,2] and Hanan Samet[1]

[1] Computer Science Department, Center for Automation Research, Institute for Advanced Computer Science, University of Maryland, College Park, USA
tahmoush@cs.umd.edu, hjs@umiacs.umd.edu
[2] Applied Physics Laboratory, Johns Hopkins University, Laurel, Maryland, USA

Abstract. An improved image similarity method is introduced to recognize breast cancer, and it is incorporated into a computer-aided breast cancer detection system through Bayes Theorem. Radiologists can use the differences between the left and right breasts, or asymmetry, in mammograms to help detect certain malignant breast cancers. Image similarity is used to determine asymmetry using a contextual and then a spatial comparison. The mammograms are filtered to find the most contextually significant points, and then the resulting point set is analyzed for spatial similarity. We develop the analysis through a combination of modeling and supervised learning of model parameters. This process correctly classifies mammograms 84% of the time, and significantly improves the accuracy of a computer-aided breast cancer detection system by 71%.

1 Introduction

Breast cancer remains a leading cause of cancer deaths among women in many parts of the world. In the United States alone, over forty thousand women die of the disease each year [1]. Mammography is currently the most effective method for early detection of breast cancer [2]. For two-thirds of the women whose initial diagnosis of their mammogram is negative but who actually have breast cancer, the cancer is evident upon a second diagnosis of their mammogram [2]. Computer-aided detection (CAD) of mammograms could be used to avoid these missed diagnoses, and has been shown to increase the number of cancers detected by more than nineteen percent [3]. Measuring asymmetry, which consists of a comparison of the left and right breast images [4], is a technique that could be used to improve the accuracy of CAD. An automated prescreening system only classifies a mammogram as either normal or suspicious, while CAD picks out specific points as cancerous [5]. One of the most challenging problems with prescreening is the lack of sensitive algorithms for the detection of asymmetry [6]. This paper presents a simple and effective algorithm for the detection of asymmetry and extensions to improve upon it. We improve on our earlier results [7] and incorporate image similarity into a CAD system.

Mammograms are an excellent candidate for image similarity techniques to be effective because there are images of both the left and right breasts, which should be similar if there is no cancer present. Image similarity has been often utilized for

Susan M. Astley et al. (Eds.): IWDM 2006, LNCS 4046, pp. 221–228, 2006.
© Springer-Verlag Berlin Heidelberg 2006

content-based image retrieval (CBIR) from image databases [8, 9, 10, 11]. Both contextual and spatial comparisons are used [8]. Medical image databases have also used image similarity, from rule-based systems for chest radiographs [12] to anatomical structure matching for 3D MR images [13]. However, the focus is often on the non-cancerous structures, while it is the cancerous structures that are of principle interest here. In this paper we combine the image similarity concept of contextual then spatial comparison to the problem of detecting breast cancer in mammograms.

The majority of work on CAD analysis of mammograms has focused on determining the contextual similarity to cancer, finding abnormalities in a local area of a single image [14, 15]. This paper focuses on combining this with a spatial comparison in order to complete an image similarity measure. The majority of work has used methods ranging from filters to wavelets to learning techniques, but a detailed discussion of various imaging techniques is beyond the scope of this paper. Problems arise in using filter methods [14] because of the range of sizes and morphologies for breast cancer, as well as the difficulty in differentiating cancerous from non-cancerous structures. The size range problem has been addressed by using multi-scale models [15]. Similar issues affect wavelet methods, although their use has led to reported good results [16] with the size range issue being improved through the use of a wavelet pyramid [17]. Learning techniques have included support vector machines [18] and neural networks [16].

Detecting breast cancer is challenging because the cancerous structures have many features in common with normal breast tissue. This means that a high number of false positives or false negatives are possible. Asymmetry can be used to help reduce the number of false positives so that true positives are more obvious. Previous work utilizing asymmetry has used wavelets or structural clues to detect asymmetry with correct results as often as 77% of the time [4, 19]. Additional work has focused on bilateral or temporal subtraction, which is the attempt to subtract one breast image from the other [20, 21]. This approach is good because it does try to utilize the multiple images taken with the same machine by the same technician and analyzed using the same process in an effort to reduce the systematic differences that can be introduced. However, bilateral subtraction is hampered by the necessity of exact registration and natural asymmetry of the breasts. We introduce a measure of asymmetry that is more approximate in nature and seems more robust to the large amount of noise in the data, using learning to determine a highly constrained number of model parameters. Minimizing the number of parameters that are learned makes the model less subject to overfitting the noise in the data at the possible expense of accuracy.

Comparing multiple mammograms using learning techniques has been shown to be effective in CBIR [10, 22]. Our application lends itself well to supervised learning because the data set has already been screened for cancer and thus classified by expert radiologists. However, care must be taken since the expert classification is known not to be perfect [2].

We believe that developing ways to better utilize asymmetry is consistent with a philosophy of trying to use methods that can capture measures deemed important by doctors thereby building upon their knowledge base, instead of trying to supplant it. However, measuring asymmetry means comparing multiple images, and thus it is a more complicated process.

In order to more fully understand the effectiveness of incorporating asymmetry into CAD systems, we utilize Bayes Theorem as a simplified method for combining a global measurement of asymmetry with the local measure of the probability of having a cancer. Significant improvement is shown over the system without asymmetry.

The rest of this paper is organized as follows. Section 2 presents our method for measuring asymmetry between the mammogram images and incorporating the measure into a CAD system. Section 3 discusses the evaluation of the performance of the measure and compares the results with other work. Section 4 describes future work, while Section 5 discusses the conclusions that can be drawn from this work.

2   Asymmetry Measurement and CAD

Our work utilizes filtering followed by spatial analysis to determine an overall measure of similarity by combining the contextual similarity of the filtering with the spatial similarity of the analysis. This can be a useful measure for prescreening mammograms since only an overall determination is required. It can also be incorporated into CAD as we demonstrate using Beyesian statistics. A secondary goal of our work is to determine the importance of similarity or asymmetry in the computer analysis of mammograms.

Our analysis starts with filtering to find the contextually similar suspicious points that could be cancers in the mammograms. The filtering step is the same as we used in [7]. This yields a set of potential detection sites that can be analyzed for asymmetry. Although it may not be the optimal choice of either filtering or ranking, the spatial analysis that we used can be applied to any technique that can rank the suspiciousness of areas. The number of points returned by the filtering step is one of the variables that can be adjusted to optimize the analysis. Alternatively, we can also make use of a threshold on the suspiciousness value instead of taking the top few. However, we chose to take the top few in order to be insensitive to image processing choices that might bias the analysis.

The analysis for similarity or asymmetry that we used does a comparison of the values of the sets of suspicious points. Two separators are learned with a training set of images. A model for a separator in 3D is a plane with the parameter set mx, my, b. Parametric learning is used to determine the best parameters based on the training set. A separator breaks the set of suspicious points in both images into two groups, and the populations in the groups are compared between the images. This is based upon the assumption that the presence of cancer will distort the distribution of suspicious sites, and that the distribution will be very similar from left to right breasts when there is no cancer. This is similar to comparing histograms whose parameters are learned from a test set. We used learning techniques to determine the optimal structure and parameters for the separator from the data. For this application, the importance of correct classification of the cancerous cases is much more important than the non-cancerous cases. To reflect this, the associated weighting of the cancerous cases was varied, and we evaluate the performance of various weightings.

The two separators break the areas in 3-space into groups labelled L_1, L_2, L_3, R_1, R_2, R_3, and each has its associated occupancy of suspicious points. A measure of asymmetry D is then calculated as $D = \sum_j |L_j - R_j|$. A more flexible measure would consider each set of groups as a separate measure with its own threshold. In order to use this measure to classify each case as either cancerous or non-cancerous, a threshold needs to be applied. This threshold is another parameter that is learned.

To incorporate asymmetry into a CAD system, we made use of Bayes Theorem, $P(CancerSite|Asym) = \frac{P(Asym|CancerSite)P(CancerSite)}{P(Asym)}$. The sites where asymmetry is measured are thus given an increased probability of being cancerous, while sites where asymmetry is not measured are given a reduced probablity of being cancerous. Since the asymmetry measurement is currently done on an entire case, all of the sites in those cases are affected similarly. The effect can be seen in Figure 1. Using Bayes Theorem to incorporate asymmetry into CAD is shown to work well at low numbers of false positives per image, but the overall performance is still strongly dependent on the effectiveness of the CAD system. The true positive fraction of the asymmetry measurement is essential in order to prevent true positives from having their probabilities diminished, and the false positive fraction is important for improving the effectiveness of the CAD system. At high levels of false positives per image, the incorporation of asymmetry has minimal effect, but this is expected since using Bayes Theorem merely reduces the probability of the false positives and does not eliminate them.

3   Evaluation and Results

The groups of suspicious points in the left and right mediolateral oblique (MLO) mammogram views were compared to evaluate the asymmetry measure. The analysis was done with cases that were normal mammograms and mammograms with malignant spiculated lesions from the Digital Database for Screening Mammography [23]. Spiculated lesions are defined as breast cancers with central areas that are usually irregular and with ill-defined borders. Their sizes vary from a few millimeters to several centimeters in diameter and they are very difficult cancers to detect [17]. The training set had 39 non-cancerous cases and 37 cancerous cases, while the test set had 38 non-cancerous cases and 40 cancerous cases. The data is roughly spread across the density of the breasts and the subtlety of the cancer. The breast density and subtlety were specified by an expert radiologist. The subtlety of the cancer shows how difficult it is to determine that there is cancer. The training data set was used to determine optimal parameters for the

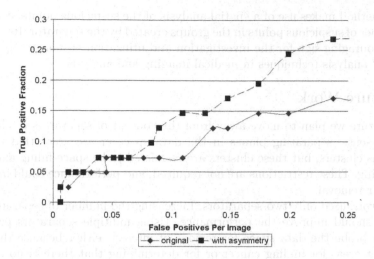

Fig. 1. Comparison of the CAD system before and after the addition of asymmetry. The improvement in performance is good at a small number of false positives per image.

separators used in the classification. These cases indicated that a difference in the groups of one or more suspicious points indicated cancer.

Our results are good on all cases of the test set, correctly classifying 84% on the test set. This shows that spatial distribution of suspicious points is changed by the presence of a cancer. However, it is much more important to correctly classify the cancerous cases, and by heavily weighting the importance of the cancerous cases, we correctly classify 97% of the cancerous cases but only 42% of the non-cancerous cases. Neither the subtlety nor the density of the cancer had an effect on the results. The comparison with a commercial system shows that the results are surprisingly good. Correct classification results of 96% of the cancerous cases and 33% of non-cancerous cases are possible using the R2 ImageChecker system [6]. Our method showed correct classification results on 97% of cancerous cases and 42% of the non-cancerous cases. This demonstrates the importance of asymmetry in pre-screening, since using only asymmetry achieves a better performance than a complete comercial system. The inclusion of additional factors other than asymmetry in the method should improve the results. However, the data sets used are different, as the R2 ImageChecker data contains all cancer types and our method has only the difficult to detect spiculated lesions. The R2 ImageChecker data set also had a much higher proportion of non-cancerous mammograms to cancerous cases.

The results on using Bayes Theorem to incorporate asymmetry into CAD were good, increasing the accuracy by up to 71% at a set level of false positives per image, as is shown in Figure 1. The improvement is most apparent at low levels of false positives. At higher levels of false positives, the effectiveness of the CAD technique dominate because the Bayes technique does not actually remove any false positives, it merely reduces their probability of being cancerous.

Our method makes use of a spatial analysis of the suspicious points, counting the number of suspicious points in the groups created by the separator. Its success is an encouraging sign for the investigation and utilization of more complicated non-local analysis techniques in medical imaging and analysis.

4   Future Work

In the future we plan to move away from the concept of separators to clusters. In some sense, separating planes in the data space create areas that can be defined as clusters, but these clusters are restricted to be space-filling and non-overlapping. These restrictions are not required, and performance could improve with their removal.

This work used only two separators. Increasing the number of separators, or clusters, should improve the performance. Using multiple separators provides a way to probe the data space for regions of interest, either because they are important areas for finding cancer or for determining that there is no cancer. The initial analysis has discovered a small region of interest for diagnosing a mammogram as non-cancerous.

This algorithm is not expected to work well on every case because there are to many types of breast cancer and breast characteristics. Tuning the algorithm to the characteristics of the breasts should improve the results. Additionally, letting the algorithm decide when it can do well and when it cannot should also improve performance.

One of the parameters that are learned is the optimal number of suspicious points to use in the analysis. Initial results are always at or near the top of the range that we used, varying from 28 to 31 points depending on the model and weightings. This was surprising because the cancer was usually in the top sixteen if not the top eight points. However, the suspicious points do tend to cluster around a cancer, so including more suspicious points may create a greater distortion of the underlying distribution than fewer points. The learning algorithm does not get the number of points directly, only the cluster differences, so the inclusion of more data should not result in overfitting.

A further improvement might be possible by first transforming the data before filtering, such as applying wavelet analysis to the images before simply thresholding or applying the filter. This has been successfully attempted previously [4] with good results. However, an optimal solution would first combine all of the various filtering and transform methods which create meaningful suspicious points, and then learn an effective analysis from them. This is similar to the effective combination of weak classifiers into a single strong classifier through ensemble learning methods like boosting, which has been successfully used before in tumor classification [24].

5   Conclusion

The overall results of using our techniques are good, our experiments yielded 84% accuracy suggesting that asymmetry is an important measure to incorporate into prescreening or CAD software. Incorporating the technique into CAD shows up to a 71% improvement in the accuracy at a set level of false positives. The technique can be tuned to be more effective at diagnosing cancerous cases, reaching 97% accuracy. We suggest several ways to improve on the methods that we used to measure asymmetry. One method is to convert a mammogram into a connected graph structure of suspicious points and utilize known graph comparison methods for the measure. Another is to use registration of suspicious points from one breast to the other and reduce the suspiciousness of points that have a similar counterpart. Alternatively, increasing the number of separators could improve the method.

Our work has demonstrated the potential of utilizing techniques like image comparisons and other non-local methods with medical imaging. We have shown that we can effectively measure doctor-defined quantities like asymmetry. We believe that in the future, the combination of capturing doctor-defined quantities like asymmetry and machine learning of parameters could be a powerful method for improving the quality of research in medical imaging, and this is one of the avenues of research that we intend to pursue.

Acknowledgements

The support of the National Science Foundation under Grants EIA-00-91474 and CCF-0515241, Microsoft Research, and the University of Maryland Graduate Research Board is gratefully acknowledged.

References

1. American Cancer Society. *Breast Cancer Facts and Figures 1999-2000*. American Cancer Society, Inc., Atlanta, GA, 1999.
2. J. Linda, W. Burhenne, S.A. Wood, C.J. D'Orsi, S.A. Feig, D.B. Kopans, K.F. O'Shaughnessy, E.A. Sickles, L. Tabar, C.J. Vyborny, and R.A. Castellino. Potential contribution of computer-aided detection to the sensitivity of screening mammography. *Radiology*, 215(554–562), 2000.
3. T.W. Freer and M.J. Ulissey. Screening mammography with computer- aided detection. *Radiology*, 220:781–786, 2001.
4. R.J. Ferrari, R.M. Rangayyan, J.E.L. Desautels, A.F. Frere. Analysis of asymmetry in mammograms via directional filtering with Gabor wavelets. *IEEE Trans. on Medical Imaging*, 20(9), 2001.
5. S. Astley, T. Mistry, C.R.M. Boggis, V. F. Hillier. Should we use humans or a machine to pre-screen mammograms? In *Proc. of the Sixth Int. Workshop on Digital Mammography*, pp 476–480, 2002.
6. S. Astley and F.J. Gilbert. Computer-aided detection in mammography. *Clinical Radiology*, 59:390–9, 2004.
7. D.A. Tahmoush and H. Samet. Using image similarity and asymmetry to detect breast cancer. In *Proc. SPIE Int. Soc. Opt. Eng.*, vol. 6144, 2006.
8. A. Soffer and H. Samet. Pictorial queries by image similarity. In *Proc. of the 13th Int. Conf. on Pattern Recognition*, vol. 3, pp 114–119, 1996.

9. V. Gudivada and V. Raghavan. Design and evaluation of algorithms for image retrieval by spatial similarity. *ACM Trans. on Inf. Sys.*, 13(2):115–144, 1995.

10. I. El-Naqa, Y. Yang, N.P. Galatsanos, R.M. Nishikawa, and M.N. Wernick. A similarity learning approach to content based image retrieval: application to digital mammography. *IEEE Trans. on Medical Imaging*, 23(10):1233–1244, 2004.

11. J. Goldberger, S. Gordon, and H. Greenspan. An efficient image similarity measure based on approximations of kl-divergence between two gaussian mixtures. In *Proc. of the Ninth IEEE Int. Conf. on Computer Vision*, pp 487–493, 2003.

12. H.A. Swett and P.L.Miller. Icon: a computer-based approach to differential diagnosis in radiology. *Radiology*, 163:555–558, 1987.

13. A. Guimond and G. Subsol. Automatic mri database exploration and applications. *Pattern Recognition and Artificial Intelligence*, 11(8):1345–1365, 1997.

14. M.D. Heath and K.W. Bowyer. Mass detection by relative image intensity. In *The Proc. of the 5th Int. Conf. on Digital Mammography*, Medical Physics Publishing, Madison, WI, 2000.

15. P. Sajda, C. Spense, and L. Parra. Capturing contextual dependencies in medical imagery using hierarchical multi-scale models. In *Proc. of the IEEE Int. Symp. on Biomedical Imaging*, pp 165–168, 2002.

16. B.L. Kalman, S.C. Kwasny, and W.R. Reinus. Diagnostic screening of digital mammograms using wavelets and neural networks to extract structure. Technical Report 98-20, Washington University, 1998.

17. S. Lui, C.F. Babbs, and E.J. Delp. Multiresolution detection of spiculated lesions in digital mammograms. *IEEE Trans. on Image Processing*, 6:874–884, 2001.

18. R. Campanini, A. Bazzani, A. Bevilacqua, D. Bollini, D. Dongiovanni, E. Iampieri, N. Lanconelli, A. Riccardi, M. Roffilli, and R. Tazzoli. A novel approach to mass detection in digital mammography based on support vector machines. In *Proc. of the 6th Int. Workshop on Digital Mammography*, 2002.

19. P. Miller and S. Astley. Detection of breast asymmetry using anatomical features. In *Proc. of the Int. Society for Optical Engineering Conf. on Biomedical Image Processing and Biomedical Visualization*, 1905:433-442, 1993.

20. M.A. Wirth and A. Jennings. A nonrigid-body approach to matching mammograms. In *Proc. of the IEEE Image Processing and its Applications*, pp 484–7, 1999.

21. F.F. Yin, M.L. Giger, K. Doi, C.E. Metz, C.J. Vyborny, and R.A. Schmidt. Computerized detection of masses in digital mammograms: analysis of bilateral subtraction images. *Medical Physics*, 18:955–63.

22. I. Gondra and D.R. Heisterkamp. Learning in region-based image retrieval with generalized support vector machines. In *Proc. of the Computer Vision and Pattern Recognition*, p 149, 2004.

23. M.D. Heath, K.W. Bowyer, D. Kopans et al. Current status of the digital database for screening mammography. *Digital Mammography*, Kluwer Academic Publishers, pp 457–60, 1998.

24. M. Dettling and P. Buhlmann. Boosting for tumor classification with gene expression data. *Bioinformatics*, 19(9)1061–1069, 2003.

Potential Usefulness of Multiple-Mammographic Views in Computer-Aided Diagnosis Scheme for Identifying Histological Classification of Clustered Microcalcification

Ryohei Nakayama[1], Ryoji Watanabe[2], Kiyoshi Namba[3], Koji Yamamoto[4],
Kan Takeda[1], Shigehiko Katsuragawa[5], and Kunio Doi[6]

[1] Department of Radiology, Mie University School of Medicine, 2-174 Edobashi,
Tsu,514-8507, Japan
{nakayama, takeda}@clin.medic.mie-u.ac.jp
[2] Hakuaikai Hospital, 1-28-25 Sasaoka, Fukuoka, 810-0034, Japan
watanabe@hakuaikai.or.jp
[3] Breastopia Namba Hospital, 2-112-1 Maruyama, Miyazaki, 800-0052, Japan
k-namba@breastopia.org
[4] Medical Informatics Section, Mie University School of Medicine, 2-174 Edobashi,
Tsu, 514-8507, Japan
yamamoto@clin.medic.mie-u.ac.jp
[5] Department of Health Sciences, Kumamoto University School of Medicine, 4-24-1,
Kuhonji, Kumamoto, 862-0976, Japan
katsur@hs.kumamoto-u.ac.jp
[6] Kurt Rossmann Laboratories for Radiologic Image Research, Department of Radiology,
The University of Chicago, 5841 South Maryland Avenue, Chicago, Illinois 60637
k-doi@uchicago.edu

Abstract. The purpose of this study was to investigate the usefulness of multiple-view mammograms in the computerized scheme for identifying histological classifications. Our database consisted of mediolateral oblique (MLO) and craniocaudal (CC) magnification mammograms obtained from 77 patients, which included 14 invasive carcinomas, 17 noninvasive carcinomas of comedo type, 17 noninvasive carcinomas of noncomedo type, 14 mastopathies, and 15 fibroadenomas. Five features on clustered microcalcifications were determined from each of MLO and CC images by taking into account image features that experienced radiologists commonly use to identify histological classifications. Modified Bayes discriminant function (MBDF) was employed for distinguishing between histological classifications. For the input of MBDF, we used five or ten features obtained from MLO and/or CC images. With ten features, the classification accuracies for each histological classification ranged from 70.6% to 93.3%. This result was higher than that obtained with only five features either from MLO or CC images.

1 Introduction

It is difficult to make correct clinical decisions for biopsy or follow-up on clustered microcalcifications on mammograms. Therefore, many investigators have developed various computer-aided diagnosis (CAD) schemes for assisting radiologists in their

Susan M. Astley et al. (Eds.): IWDM 2006, LNCS 4046, pp. 229–236, 2006.

assessment of clustered microcalcifications. Most of these CAD schemes are based on the analysis of single-view standard mammograms.

Routine mammographic projections are mediolateral oblique (MLO) projection and craniocaudal (CC) projection. MLO image is the single most useful mammographic projection for the breast.[1] CC image is generally used for complementing MLO image. Two views can permit an appreciation of three dimensional structures which may be helpful in distinguishing overlapping structures when single-view mammogram is read. In this study, therefore, we investigated the usefulness of multiple-view mammograms in the CAD scheme for identifying histological classification of clustered microcalcification.

2 Materials and Methods

2.1 Database

Our database consisted of MLO and CC magnification mammograms obtained from 77 patients at the Breastopia Namba Hospital, Miyazaki, Japan. It included 48 malignant clustered microcalcifications (14 invasive carcinomas, 17 noninvasive carcinomas of the comedo type, and 17 noninvasive carcinomas of the noncomedo type) and 29 benign clustered microcalcifications (14 mastopathies and 15 fibroadenomas). The histological classifications of all clustered microcalcifications were proved by stereotaxic core needle biopsy.

The magnification mammograms were acquired with a Kodak MinR-2000/MinR-2000 screen/film system. The magnification factor of magnification mammograms was 1.8. The mammographic x-ray system included an x-ray tube with a 0.1 mm focal spot and a molybdenum anode, 0.03-mm-thick molybdenum filter, and a 5:1 reciprocating grid. These mammograms were digitized to a 512x512 matrix size with a 0.0275 mm pixel size and a 12-bit gray scale by the use of an EPSON ES-8000 digitizer.

2.2 Methods

The methods for the segmentation of microcalcifications, the determination of cluster margin and the extraction of five features are the same as those used in our previous study[2]. Therefore, we briefly describe them here.

2.2.1 Segmentation of Microcalcifications and Definition of Cluster Margin

For segmentation of individual microcalcifications within a cluster on mammograms, we first enhanced the microcalcifications by the use of a novel filter bank[3]. A gray-level thresholding technique[4] was then applied to the enhanced image. In order to segment all microcalcifications in our database, we used a 600-pixel value as a threshold value empirically. By using such a fixed threshold value, however, 12 breast tissues were also segmented as the candidates for microcalcifications. In this paper, we employed a manual method to remove these candidates which were not identified as a microcalcification by an experienced radiologist.

In order to obtain the information about the shape of the distribution of clustered microcalcifications, the cluster margin was automatically determined by our CAD scheme. We first drew circles at the center of gravity of each microcalcification. The diameter of these circles was increased from 20 to 60 pixels until all circles within a cluster were connected. We then employed a binary morphologic closing operator[5] to smooth the edge of the region connecting the circles. This smoothed edge was finally determined as the cluster margin.

2.2.2 Extraction of Five Features

In our previous study[2], we selected five features to identify histological classification by taking into account the differences in image features between five histological classifications. We then showed that these features were statistically significant for identifying histological classifications of clustered microcalcifications. In this study, therefore, we used the same features. These features were: (1) the variation in size of microcalcifications within a cluster; (2) the variation in pixel values of microcalcifications within a cluster; (3) the irregularity measure in shape of microcalcifications within a cluster; (4) the extent of linear and branching distribution of microcalcifications; and (5) the distribution of microcalcifications in direction toward the nipple. These features were quantified based on the segmented microcalcifications and the cluster margin.

2.2.3 Identification of Histological Classification and Evaluation of Classification Performance

In our previous study[2], Bayes discriminant function (BDF)[6] was employed for identifying histological classification of clustered microcalcification. The relationship between the covariance matrix $_l\Sigma$ of each class l based on histological classifications, its i-th eigenvalue $_l\lambda_i$ $\left(_l\lambda_i \geq {}_l\lambda_{i+1}\right)$, and its i-th eigenvector $_l\Phi_i$ satisfy the following equation:

$$_l\Sigma = \sum_{i=1}^{n} {}_l\lambda_{il} \,{}_l\Phi_{il} \,{}_l\Phi_{i}^{t}, \tag{1}$$

when n is the number of dimensions of the feature vector. Therefore, BDF is defined as

$$g_0^l(x) = \sum_{i=1}^{n} \frac{\left(x - {}_l\mu, \,{}_l\Phi_i\right)^2}{{}_l\lambda_i} + \ln\prod_{i=1}^{n} {}_l\lambda_i. \tag{2}$$

Here, x and $_l\mu$ are the input feature vector and the mean vector of class l, respectively. In BDF, the estimation error of the eigenvectors becomes large when the number of training samples is not large enough compared with the number of dimensions of the feature vector.[7] Especially, the estimation error of higher-order eigenvectors is much larger than that of lower-order eigenvector.[7] The trained BDF would be influenced by this problem because our database was relatively small. In this study, therefore, we employed Modified Bayes discriminant function (MBDF)[8] which solves this problem to distinguish between the five different types of histological classifications. MBDF is given by

$$g^l(x) = \sum_{i=1}^{k} \frac{(x-_l\mu, _l\Phi_i)^2}{_l\lambda_i} + \sum_{i=k+1}^{n} \frac{(x-_l\mu, _l\Phi_i)^2}{_l\lambda_{k+1}} + \ln\left(\prod_{i=1}^{k} {}_l\lambda_i \prod_{i=k+1}^{n} {}_l\lambda_{k+1}\right), \quad (3)$$

where $k\,(1 \le k < n)$ is an integer. Here, the estimation error of higher-order eigenvectors is reduced by using $_l\lambda_{k+1}$ as an approximate value of $_l\lambda_i\,(i = k+2, \cdots, n)$. In the case of $k = n-1$, MBDF is equal to BDF. When k is about one-third of the number of dimensions of the feature vector, it is known to show the highest classification performance.[9] In this study, therefore, k was given as a one-third of the number of dimensions of the feature vector.

For the input of MBDF, we used five or ten features obtained from MLO and/or CC images. The output of MBDF provided five values indicating the likelihood of each class based on histological classifications. The class yielding the smallest output value was considered to be the result of the distinction among the five types of histological classifications. A leave-one-out (round-robin) testing method[10] was used for training and testing of MBDF. In this method, the training was carried out for all cases except one case in the database, and the one case not used for training was applied for testing with the trained MBDF. This procedure was repeated until every case in our database was used once.

3   Results and Discussion

3.1   Features Obtained from Two-Views Magnification Mammograms

Figure 1 shows the mean values and the standard deviations of each feature for the five different types of histological classifications in MLO and CC images. These features were normalized in each of MLO and CC image. The differences in five features between five histological classifications for MLO image appeared to be nearly similar to those for CC image. This trend of the features also corresponded to radiological findings[1,2] of microcalcifications in each of histological classifications.

Table 1 shows the results of tests for univariate equality of group means in features for each of MLO and CC images. In each of five features, the Wilk's lambda[11] and the F value[11] for MLO image and those for CC image were almost equal. This result indicates that there was no large difference between MLO and CC images in the contribution to identify histological classifications of clustered microcalcifications. In the variation in size and the irregularity measure in shape, the Wilk's lambdas were smaller than any other features, and the F values were larger than other features. Therefore, these features made a larger contribution to identifying five histological classifications of clustered microcalcifications. The p values[11] for all features reached the level of statistical significance. Therefore, ten features obtained from MLO and CC images were statistically significant for identifying histological classifications of clustered microcalcifications.

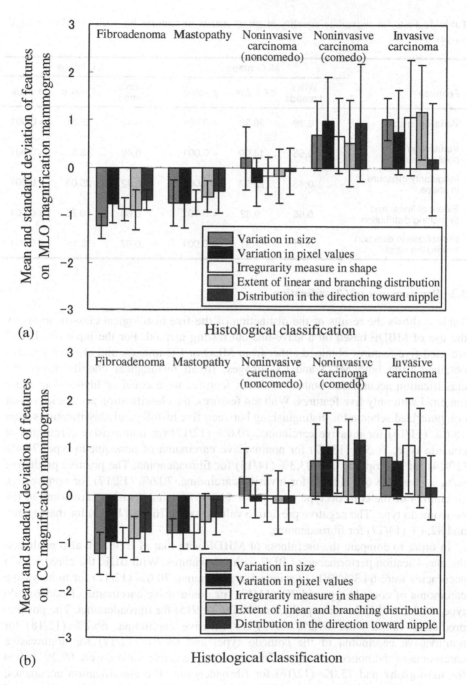

Fig. 1. Mean values and standard deviations of each feature for the five different types of histological classifications in MLO images and CC images

Table 1. Tests for univariate equality of group means in features for each of MLO and CC images

Features	MLO image			CC image		
	Wilk's Lambda	F value	p value	Wilk's Lambda	F value	p value
Variation in size	0.38	28.98	< 0.001	0.42	25.31	< 0.001
Variation in pixel values	0.56	14.09	< 0.001	0.49	18.82	< 0.001
Irregularity measure in shape	0.43	23.97	< 0.001	0.42	25.03	< 0.001
Extent of linear and branching distribution	0.66	9.32	< 0.001	0.63	10.72	< 0.001
Distribution in direction toward the nipple	0.71	7.31	< 0.001	0.67	9.15	< 0.001

3.2 Performance of Classification

Table 2 shows the results of the distinction of the five histological classifications by the use of MBDF based on a leave-one-out testing method. For the input of MBDF, we used five features obtained either from MLO or CC images, and also ten features obtained from both MLO and CC images. In all histological classifications, the classification accuracies obtained with ten features were equal or higher than those obtained with only five features. With ten features, the classification accuracies of our computerized scheme for distinguishing between five histological classifications were 78.6% (11/14) for invasive carcinoma, 70.6% (12/17) for noninvasive carcinoma of comedo type, 76.5% (13/17) for noninvasive carcinoma of noncomedo type, 71.4% (10/14) for mastopathy, and 93.3% (14/15) for fibroadenoma. The positive predictive values[12] were 78.6% (11/14) for invasive carcinoma, 70.6% (12/17) for noninvasive carcinoma of the comedo type, and 81.3% (13/16) for noninvasive carcinoma of the noncomedo type. The negative predictive values[12] were 76.9% (10/13) for mastopathy and 82.4% (14/17) for fibroadenoma.

In order to compare the usefulness of MBDF with that of BDF, we also evaluated the classification performance of BDF with ten features. With BDF, the classification accuracies were 64.3% (9/14) for invasive carcinoma, 70.6% (12/17) for noninvasive carcinoma of comedo type, 64.7% (11/17) for noninvasive carcinoma of noncomedo type, 64.3% (9/14) for mastopathy, and 80.0% (12/15) for fibroadenoma. The positive predictive values were 69.2% (9/13) for invasive carcinoma, 66.7% (12/18) for noninvasive carcinoma of the comedo type, and 64.7% (11/17) for noninvasive carcinoma of the noncomedo type. The negative predictive values were 69.2% (9/13) for mastopathy and 75.0% (12/16) for fibroadenoma. The classification accuracies, the positive predictive values and the negative predictive values were improved substantially by the use of MBDF.

Table 2. Comparisons of the computerized classification results obtained by Modified Bayes discriminant functions with five features and ten features

Pathological diagnosis	Computer output		
	With five features for MLO images	With five features for CC images	With ten features for MLO and CC images
Invasive carcinoma (14)	10 (71.4%)	9 (64.3%)	11 (78.6%)
Noninvasive carcinoma of the comedo type (17)	11 (64.7%)	12 (70.6%)	12 (70.6%)
Noninvasive carcinoma of the noncomedo type (17)	11 (64.7%)	13 (76.5%)	13 (76.5%)
Mastopathy (14)	10 (71.4%)	9 (64.3%)	10 (71.4%)
Fibroadenoma (15)	12 (80.0%)	13 (86.7%)	14 (93.3%)

4 Conclusion

We investigated the classification accuracies obtained with computerized analysis of single-view mammogram and those of multiple-views mammograms. The results indicated that the CAD scheme for multiple-view mammograms was more accurate in identifying histological classification of clustered microcalcification. This computerized scheme may be useful in assisting radiologists in their assessment of clustered microcalcifications.

References

1. D. B. Kopans: Breast imaging. 2nd edn. Lippincott-Raven publishers, New York (1997).
2. R. Nakayama, Y. Uchiyama, R. Watanabe, S. Katsuragawa, K. Namba, and K. Doi: Computer-aided diagnosis scheme for histological classification of clustered microcalcifications on magnification mammograms. Med. Phys. Vol.31 (2004) 789-799.
3. R. Nakayama, Y. Uchiyama: Development of new filter bank for detection of nodular patterns and line patterns in medical images. IEICE Trans. Inf. and Sys. J-87-D-II (2004) 176-185.
4. R. C. Gonzales and R. E. Woods: Digital Image Processing. Addison-Wesley, MA (1992).
5. J. Sera: Image Analysis and Mathematical Morphology. Academic Press, London (1982).
6. R. O. Duda, P. E. Hart, and D. G. Stork: Pattern Classification. 2nd edn. John Wiley & Sons, NY (2001).
7. F. Kimura, K. Takahashi, S. Tsuruoka, and Y. Miyake: On avoiding peaking phenomenon of the quadratic discriminant function. IEICE. J-69-D (1986) 1328-1334.
8. S. Tsuruoka, M. Kurita, T. HARADA, F. Kimura, and Y. Miyake: Handwriting 'KANJI' and 'HIRAGANA' character recognition using weighted direction index histogram method. IEICE. J70-D (1987) 1390-1397.

9. Tsuruoka, H. Morita, F. Kimura, and Y. Miyake: Handwritten character recognition adaptable to the writer. IEICE. J-70-D (1987) 1953-1960.

10. M. Aoyama, Q. Li, S. Katsuragawa, H. MacMahon, and K. Doi: Automated computerized scheme for distinction between benign and malignant solitary pulmonary nodules on chest images. Med. Phys. 29 (2002) 701-708.

11. R. A. Johnson and D. W. Wichern: Applied Multivariate Statistical Analysis. Prentice-Hall, Englewood Cliffs NJ (1992).

12. C. P. Langlotz: Fundamental measures of diagnostic examination performance - Usefulness for clinical decision making and research. Radiology 228 (2003) 3-9.

Exploitation of Correspondence Between CC and MLO Views in Computer Aided Mass Detection

Saskia van Engeland and Nico Karssemeijer

Radboud University Nijmegen Medical Centre
Department of Radiology
The Netherlands

Abstract. In this paper we investigate the effect of reclassification of CAD findings using correspondences in MLO and CC views, with the aim of reducing false positives and inconsistencies. We use a method to link regions identified as suspicious in both projections and add a two-view classifier to an existing CAD scheme. The input of this two-view classifier was a feature vector containing the likelihood of malignancy of the region, the likelihood of malignancy of the corresponding region in the other view, and a number of features that describe the resemblance between the both regions. Using FROC analysis we show that detection results improve when using two-view information.

1 Introduction

Most methods for computer aided detection of masses in mammograms are limited to analysis of single views. Radiologists, on the other hand, are trained to judge different views in combination. They make comparisons between patterns in the left and right breast, and compare features of suspect abnormalities projected in different views. In mammography it is common to make a medio lateral oblique (MLO) and a cranio caudal (CC) view of each breast. By processing these views independently, CAD systems often mark abnormalities only in one view, even if they appear rather similar visually. This is due to the fact that differences in features computed in the two views may cause a relatively large difference in the levels of suspiciousness assigned to the lesions by the CAD system. By using a fixed display threshold for the CAD markers the lesion may be rendered in one view while in the other it is not. Radiologists tend to complain when this occurs because they find this behavior of the CAD system inconsistent. Moreover, in recent studies it is reported that it is more likely that radiologists ignore CAD marks if they only mark a lesion in one view [1] [2].

In this paper we investigate if correspondence can be utilized to reduce false positives of a mass detection method. We expect that false positives in different projections will be less correlated than true positives. By reclassification of CAD findings using two-view information we aim at decreasing the suspiciousness of false positives while maintaining the strength of the true positives. Moreover, by combining information from two views the difference between the CAD output of true positive projections in two views will be reduced, which will improve consistency of the system.

Susan M. Astley et al. (Eds.): IWDM 2006, LNCS 4046, pp. 237–242, 2006.
© Springer-Verlag Berlin Heidelberg 2006

Figure 1 presents a schematic overview of the method, which is a cascaded system of three classifiers. The output of the first classifier $L_1(x, y)$ is a measure of suspiciousness at every location in the breast. The mass likelihood $L_2(i)$ is obtained after region segmentation at selected locations i with a high likelihood of malignancy. Finally, $L_3(i)$ is the output of the two-view detection method, in which correspondence between projections is used. Details of the single view stages of the algorithm may be found in [3] [4].

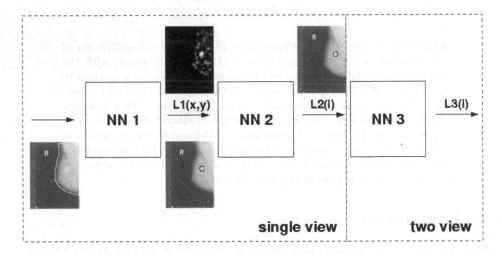

Fig. 1. Schematic overview of our CAD scheme

2 Finding Corresponding Regions

In our method we determine correspondence between potentially suspicious areas determined by a CAD scheme in MLO and CC views, using the nipple as a landmark. Many radiologists use distance to the nipple to correlate a lesion in MLO and CC views. It is generally believed that this distance remains fairly constant, although other methods are used as well, such as distance to the chest wall/pectoral, or distance of the nipple to a projection of the lesion on a line perpendicular to the chest wall/pectoral (cartesian straight line method). In an attempt to take the effect of compression into account, Kita *et al* [5] used a model-based method to find a curve in the MLO view which corresponds to the potential positions of a point in the CC view. Our choice for distance to the nipple, also referred to as the arc method, was based on experimental evidence and on the fact that it is easy to implement. Chang *et al* [6] provide experimental evidence that the arc method is at least as good as the cartesian straight line method. Further evidence is found in previous studies, where it was found that correlation between distances to the nipple determined in CC and MLO views is high [7], [8].

In the present study we use an automatically determined nipple location to define an annular search area in the other view. The nipple location was roughly estimated using a simple approach, in which we determined the point on the skin contour with the largest distance to the chest or the pectoral muscle (for the MLO views). The pectoral line was determined using a Hough transform based method [9]. The width of the annular search area search area was 48 mm. It was found that in 79 percent of the cases the distance to the nipple does not deviate more than 1.5 cm between both views.

To find corresponding regions, for all possible combinations of candidate regions a feature vector is determined. Features represent the difference in distance of the candidate regions to the nipple, gray scale correlation between both regions and the mass likelihood $L_2(i)$ of the regions. Next, Linear Discriminant Analysis (LDA) is used to compute a correspondence measure for every possible combination. For every region in the original view the region in the other view with the highest correspondence score is selected as the corresponding candidate region.

3 Two-View Classification

Application of the linking algorithm results for every region in a corresponding region in the other view with accompanying correspondence score. If no corresponding region is found, the correspondence measure is set to zero. Otherwise a two-view feature vector is computed for the region to be classified. Features included are the single view likelihood of suspiciousness of the region itself and of its corresponding projection in the other view, the correspondence score, and a number of features representing similarity of the two regions. To select the features for the two-view classifier a forward feature selection algorithm is used, using a LDA classifier and Receiver Operating Characteristic (ROC) analysis. To avoid that feature selection biased results we used cross validation. The final two-view classifier used was a 3-layer neural network with three hidden nodes, with the selected features as input. The net was trained with back-propagation.

Our two-view detection scheme was evaluated on a data set containing 412 abnormal cases, and 537 normal cases. All cases had four-view mammograms. The total number of images processed was 3796. The set of normal cases was roughly matched with respect to acquisition period to the set of abnormal cases. These normal cases did not include benign abnormalities, and were verified to be normal by an experienced radiologist. The set of abnormal cases was a random sample of screen-detected or interval cancers (90%) and of priors of cancer cases with a visible abnormality (10%).

The two-view classifier was tested using cross validation with 95 percent training and 5 percent testing. The performance was compared with the single-view detection results using FROC analysis and we present both an image and a case based evaluation. In the case based evaluation, a case is by definition regarded as a true positive (TP) case if in at least one of the two views the lesion is detected by our CAD scheme.

Both the output of the single-view and the two-view CAD scheme were standardized using only images from the normal cases. To this end, we computed for every region the number of normal regions per image with values lower than that of the current region. We refer to this as the *normality score*. In other words, this is the frequency of occurrence in normal mammograms of regions that are at least as suspicious as the region at hand.

Our method for finding correspondence between views was not able to link projections of cancers in two views correctly in all cases. To investigate to what extent this influenced results we prepared a data set which contained only normals and cases with correctly linked true positive regions. Also for this data set the performance of two-view and single-view detection was compared.

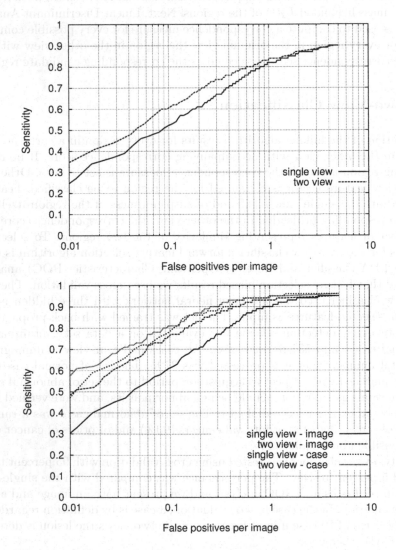

Fig. 2. Image based FROC evaluation of single- and two-view mass detection is shown in the upper graph. Results in the lower graph were obtained by excluding 18% of the abnormal cases in which no correct correspondence was obtained.

4   Results

Using forward feature selection we determined the optimal set of features for the two-view classifier. The first feature that was selected was the output of the single-view CAD scheme L_2, which is understandable as this represents an overall measure of suspiciousness based on local region features. The features that were selected next were all two-view features: the correspondence measure, a pixel based correlation measure, suspiciousness of the corresponding region, difference in distance to the nipple, and a histogram correlation measure.

The performance of the two-view classifier and of the single view CAD scheme is shown in figure 2. On the left the result of the image based evaluation is presented, and an improvement due to the use of correspondence can be observed. In the case based evaluation, however, we found no improvement. On the right in figure 2 we show results for the subset of cases where true positives in the two projections were correctly linked, and all the normal cases. This was 82% of the total number of abnormal cases. In 18% no correct link was found, where it is remarked that in 8% there was no possibility to link a true positive region because the lesion was visible only in one view.

5   Discussion

We found that by establishing correspondence between regions detected in two views detection performance can be improved, but that improvements thus far are only seen in image based evaluation. This is important though, as this means that results of the CAD system become more consistent: It happens less often that a lesion is only marked in one view. This may lead to increased confidence of radiologists in the system.

Only a the few studies have been published thus far on the use of MLO and CC information to improve detection results. Paquerault et al [8] developed a two-view matching method resulting in a correspondence score for each possible mass pair. By combining this score with their single view detection score in a fusion analysis, based on ranking of the scores in each case, their detection results improved significantly. Earlier, Good et al. [10] reported a preliminary attempt of matching computer-detected objects in two views by exhaustive pairing of the detected objects and feature classification.

The fact that case based results did not improve in our study is not entirely surprising. In case based results a lesion is counted as detected if it is marked in one view at least. The main effect of correlation on true positives is that the weaker findings get boosted if a strong correlation with the other view exists. This does not affect case sensitivity, as this is determined by the strongest finding. Another effect of two-view classification is that the suspiciousness of false positives is reduced when no correspondence is found. This effect appears to be small, and counterbalanced by a small fraction of true positives that become less suspicious because of the absence of a correct link with the other view. This was demonstrated by the fact that if incorrect links are removed also case based performance increases. From this we may conclude that it will be worthwhile to further improve the linking scheme.

References

1. R M Nishikawa, AEdwards R A Schmidt, J Papaioannou, and M N Linver. Can radiologists recognize that a computer has identified cancers that they have overlooked? *SPIE Medical Imaging*, 6146, 2006.
2. B Zheng, D Chough, P Ronald, C Cohen, C M Hakim, G Abrams, M A Ganott, L Wallace, R Shah, J H Sumkin, and D Gur. Actual versus intended use of CAD systems in the clinical environment. *SPIE Medical Imaging*, 6146, 2006.
3. N Karssemeijer and G M te Brake. Detection of stellate distortions in mammograms. *IEEE Trans Med Imag*, 15:611–619, 1996.
4. G M te Brake and N Karssemeijer. Segmentation of suspicious densities in digital mammograms. *Medical Physics*, 28:259–266, 2001.
5. Y. Kita, E. Tohno, R. Highnam, and M. Brady. A CAD system for the 3D location of lesions in mammograms. *Med Image Anal*, 6(3):267–73, 2002.
6. Y. H. Chang, W. F. Good, J. H. Sumkin, B. Zheng, and D. Gur. Computerized localization of breast lesions from two views. an experimental comparison of two methods. *Invest Radiol*, 34(9):585–588, 1999.
7. S van Engeland and N Karssemeijer. Matching breast lesions in multiple mammographic views. In W Niessen and M Viergever, editors, *Medical Image Computing and Computer-Assisted Intervention*, volume 2208, pages 1172–1173. Springer, LNCS, 2001.
8. S. Paquerault, N. Petrick, H. P. Chan, B. Sahiner, and M. A. Helvie. Improvement of computerized mass detection on mammograms: fusion of two-view information. *Med Phys*, 29(2):238–47, 2002.
9. N Karssemeijer. Automated classification of parenchymal patterns in mammograms. *Phys Med Biol*, 43:365–378, 1998.
10. W F Good, B Zheng, Y-H Chang, X H Wang, G Maitz, and D Gur. Multi-image cad employing features derived from ipsilateral mammographic views. *SPIE 1999 Image processing*, 3661:474–485, 1999.

Breast Composition Measurements Using Retrospective Standard Mammogram Form (SMF)

Ralph Highnam[1], Xia-Bo Pan[1], Ruth Warren[2], Mona Jeffreys[3],
George Davey Smith[4], and Michael Brady[5]

[1] Siemens Molecular Imaging Ltd, Oxford, UK
[2] Consultant Radiologist, Addenbrooke's Hospital, Cambridge, UK
[3] Senior Lecturer in Public Health, Massey University, Wellington, NZ
[4] Professor of Clinical Epidemiology, University of Bristol, UK
[5] Professor of Information Engineering, University of Oxford, UK
rphighnam@aol.com

Abstract. Standard Mammogram Form (SMF), is a standardized, quantitative representation of a breast x-ray that can be easily estimated. From SMF it is possible to compute the volume of non-fat tissue and measures of breast density, both of which are of significant interest in determining breast cancer risk. Previous theoretical analysis of SMF suggested that a complete and substantial set of calibration data (such as mAs and kVp) would be needed to generate realistic breast composition measures, which is problematical since there have been many interesting trials that have retrospectively collected images with no calibration data. In this paper, we show how implementations of SMF include self-compensation mechanisms, so that SMF can be applied retrospectively to data for which calibration parameters are not (or only partially) available. To illustrate our findings, the current implementation of SMF (version 2.2β) was run over 4,028 digitized film-screen mammograms taken from 6 sites during the years 1988-2002, both with and without using the known calibration data. Results show that the SMF implementation running with no calibration data generates results which display a strong relationship with those obtained using a complete set of calibration data. More importantly, they bear a close relationship to an expert's visual assessment of breast composition using established techniques.

1 Background

The Standard Mammogram Form (SMF) representation of an x-ray mammogram is a standardized, quantitative representation of the breast (Highnam & Brady 1999) from which the volume and percentage of non-fat tissue can straightforwardly and automatically be estimated. Both the volume and percentage of dense tissue appear to be of significance for determining breast cancer risk (Boyd et al 1998, Heine and Malhotra 2002, Hufton et al 2004, Pawluczyk et al 2003). Recent work on SMF has shown that the estimate of percentage of non-fat tissue (SMF%) correlates strongly with an expert's visual assessment of breast density (Jeffreys et al. 2006), and SMF-based estimates of both volume (SMF Volume) and density show a small but

Susan M. Astley et al. (Eds.): IWDM 2006, LNCS 4046, pp. 243–250, 2006.
© Springer-Verlag Berlin Heidelberg 2006

significant association with age as well as correlation with important known breast cancer risk measures such as body mass index (Jeffreys et al. 2003a).

We have previously reported (Highnam and Brady 1999) that implementations of SMF require a characterisation of the imaging system in the form of a set of calibration data, including parameters such as mAs, kVp and breast thickness. Furthermore, we presented a theoretical (Taylor's series) analysis that aimed to determine the errors in SMF values as a function of errors in the parameters, eg mAs. Unfortunately, and particularly when seeking to apply SMF to quantify films retrospectively, it is often the case that insufficient calibration data is available. In this paper, we present a new analysis of the implementations of SMF which show that they are in fact able to overcome both a lack of calibration data, and errors in the provided calibration data. The results contained in this paper are from SMF implementation 2.2β.

2 Calibration Parameter Compensation

The Taylor-series-based theoretical analysis of SMF by Highnam and Brady (1999) firmly conclude that both SMF% and SMF Volume are highly susceptible to errors in the calibration data. As a specific example, the analysis implied that a change in breast thickness of just 0.1cm changes SMF% by approximately 5%. However, documented evidence about errors in breast thickness readings from most mammography machines (Burch and Law 1995) and the lack of recorded breast thickness readings for many mammograms, led to an implementation of SMF which always estimates breast thickness directly from the image. The upshot is that, though apparently subtle, this implementation detail has a profound consequence: errors in the calibration data are used in the estimation of breast thickness, so the calibration data parameters are not independent, and, as a consequence, the Taylor's series analysis turns out to be massively overly pessimistic. Instead, we realise that the SMF process embodies a set of mutual constraints between parameter values, and these have the welcome property of automatically correcting for errors in the calibration data by the use of "ground truth" from the image. This constraint propagation process we call *Calibration Parameter Compensation (CPC)*.

Following the approach of Tromans (2006), we illustrate CPC by considering SMF as a transfer function from input pixel value to thickness of non-fat tissue (h_{int}). Now consider that from the image itself, via the breast thickness estimation method, we know that a certain pixel value maps to $h_{int}=0$. It does not matter what the calibration data is, that mapping will remain constant and the breast thickness will be adjusted to keep it so. In short, the breast thickness is adjusted to compensate for any and all calibration data errors by using image-derived ground truth.

As an example, refer to Figure 1. The thick black line shows the "true" transfer function, that is, using the correct values of 61mAs and H=5.0cm. It also shows the transfer functions for the case where the mAs is deliberately made erroneous by a large amount: continuous thin line 40mAs (squares) and 100mAs (triangles) but breast thickness estimation (CPC) is not used. Finally, we show as dotted lines the resulting transfer functions when CPC is used. The legend notes the breast thicknesses estimated. Clearly, with CPC the transfer function is evidently far better than without. Also, despite the entirely wrong mAs, the transfer function is almost identical to the true case. We note that the previous theoretical analysis (Highnam & Brady 1999) suggested that errors in mAs would translate the h_{int} values up or down, likewise with breast thickness H. Given that, it is perhaps no surprise that the transfer functions with CPC are almost identical no matter what the mAs is.

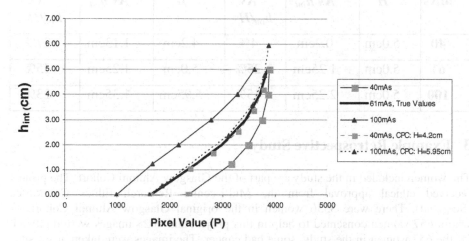

Fig. 1. SMF with wrong mAs: transfer function with and without CPC and with wrong mAs. The "true" values are 29kVp, Mo/Mo filter/target, H=5.0cm and 61mAs, see the black curve. The two continue curves are for wrong mAs (40, 100)) but with using the true H=5.0cm and the two dotted curves are for when CPC is used with those wrong mAs. Note the breast thicknesses estimated in the legend.

Consider next the quantitative values for our example pseudo-breast where "Av h_{int}" is taken to be the value corresponding to a pixel value of 2500 (note that this equates to a film density of 1.5, a reasonable average film density for many automatic exposure controls) and should be regarded as being closely related to volume of glandular tissue (SMF Volume) and that average divided by H as being closely related to breast density (SMF%), see Table 1.

Table 1 shows that with CPC, the changes in the average h_{int} are much smaller than without CPC, and that CPC shows a remarkable ability to compensate for errors especially in the pseudo-SMF% values. For example, using an incorrect mAs of 100 leads to an SMF% of 45%, without CPC, whereas with CPC the result is 23%, just 2% difference from the "real" value.

The experiments presented in this section, as well as a host others which assess errors in other calibration data, and which are being prepared for publication, strongly suggest that CPC is capable of correcting for some of the inevitable errors in the calibration data, so long as the ground truth is reliable. However, equally, if the calibration data that we estimate is at the extreme end to the actual values then although CPC can limit the errors passed through to the breast composition measures, they do still exist and can be substantial.

Table 1. Wrong mAs and Breast Composition: The mAs used is shown in the left column and then we have the breast thickness (H) and breast composition measures, Av h_{int} is closely related to SMF Volume and Av h_{int}/H is closely related to SMF%:

mAs	Without CPC			With CPC		
	H	Av h_{int}	Av h_{int}/H	H	Av h_{int}	Av h_{int}/H
40	5.0cm	0.2cm	4%	4.2cm	1.13cm	27%
61	5.0cm	1.25cm	25%	5.0cm	1.25cm	25%
100	5.0cm	2.25cm	45%	5.95cm	1.35cm	23%

3 Example Retrospective Study

The women included in the study are part of the Glasgow Alumni Cohort. The project received ethical approval from the Multi-centre Research Ethics Committee (Scotland). There were 3556 women in the original Glasgow Alumni Cohort, of whom 657 women consented to help in this project and 4028 images were digitized. Of the 657 women in the study, some had cancer. The images were taken at six sites throughout Scotland over a 15 year period (1988 to 2002). Included women were aged between 40 and 76 with the median age of 57.

Data inspection revealed several mismatches and errors in the data entry. Of the 4028 images, 3873 had mAs, 3983 had a valid kVp (between 25 and 32), and 3867 had both mAs and a valid kVp. 3515 of the images had a recorded breast thickness. No separate tuning of the SMF algorithm was required or performed for each site. We ran the SMF software over all the data using all the calibration data and not using any of it and compared the outputs.

When we ran without any calibration data, the SMF implementation defaults the data, in particular it assumes:

- A Mo/Mo, filter/target combination
- 28kVp tube voltage
- A typical film-screen combination
- An mAs estimated from the projected breast area.

3.1 Results

Table 2 shows the consistency of the breast composition measures with and without calibration data. The consistency of these results is estimated as the median difference between mammograms taken for the same woman on the same day, of the same view for left-right comparisons, and the same side for CC/MLO comparisons see Table 3. Importantly, overall, there are no significant differences in left/right or CC/MLO consistency, depending on whether SMF% or SMF volume are estimated using calibration data or without.

Table 2. Consistency with and without calibration data, median values

	With CD	Without CD
SMF Volume	64.5cm^3	57.1cm^3
SMF %	23.9%	26.7%
H$_{estimated}$	4.9cm	3.6cm
H$_{recorded}$ − H$_{estimated}$	0.0cm Signed 0.5cm Abs	1.1cm Signed 1.2cm Abs

Table 3. Median signed differences (inter-quartile range) in SMF results

	With CD	Without CD
Left-Right Difference		
SMF volume	1 cm^3 (-8 to 10)	1 cm^3 (-9 to 10)
SMF%	-0.1% (-2.6 to 2.3)	-0.1% (-3.4 to 2.7)
MLO-CC Difference		
SMF volume	5 cm^3 (-5 to 17)	4 cm^3 (-8 to 15)
SMF%	-0.6% (-3.7 to 2.3)	-1.2% (-4.9 to 2.1)

Finally, comparing the results of SMF% without calibration data versus a visual assessment using the six category (Boyd et al 1998) and Wolfe (1976) classifications revealed a similar correlation to when calibration data is used (Jeffreys et al 2006) , see Fig 2 and Fig3.

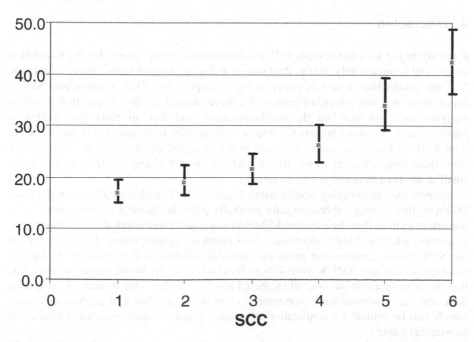

Fig. 2. SCC v SMF% when generated using no calibration data, the median values and inter-quartile ranges are shown

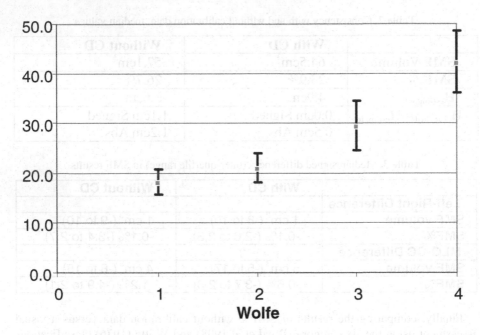

Fig. 3. SCC v SMF% when generated using no calibration data, the median values and inter-quartile ranges are shown

4 Discussion

It is easy to see how the current SMF implementation compensates for the translation errors, and is not entirely able to deal with non-linear changes in the transfer function. Yet, the results shown in this paper strongly suggest that SMF Volume and SMF% (even more so) are robust to errors. We have argued in this paper that previous analyses have not matched the implementation, and that, in particular, SMF% is robust because for most breasts the Breast Volume (the denominator) is much greater than SMF Volume (the numerator, and is not changed by the CPC process) so that even quite large changes in the Breast Volume do not change SMF% significantly; small dense breasts might not be so robust.

Despite the encouraging results using *GenerateSMF* without calibration data, we also note that having calibration data generally provides more accurate results. It is important to note that the estimated SMF Volume increases when the calibration data is known, whereas SMF% decreases. This cautions against using absolute levels of the SMF breast composition measures between databases. For example, if for one database we declare SMF% over 37% to be class 4 on the Wolfe scale, we may find that the next database has overall increased levels of SMF% due to lack of calibration data, and many women have (apparently) class 4 breasts. We will explore this issue, which will be critical for application to cross-population epidemiological studies, in subsequent papers.

On a related point, the database used in this work is from the UK where most mammograms were routinely performed (following national screening standards) at 28kVp with a Mo/Mo filter/target combination. Consequently, the defaults used in this work (namely 28kVp, Mo/Mo) are likely to be good estimates. Anecdotal evidence suggests that mammograms in the US and elsewhere have a higher degree of variability in technique and thus it may be that the current SMF implementation would be less good at compensating for errors over a large, US database for which almost nothing is known about the imaging of the mammograms. This is, of course, a very pessimistic assumption. Note also that newer systems have a wider variety of kVp and target/filter combinations, only some of which are set automatically. If these are not known, then again the defaults might not give satisfactory results. Of course, the defaults can easily be changed.

5 Conclusions

Retrospective use of SMF, and use of SMF without calibration data, are possible and yield quantitative results which strongly correlate with SCC. We propose that this is because *SMF implementations* automatically and effectively corrects for errors in the calibration data by using image-based ground truth when estimating breast thickness. We have proposed an analysis of this automatic *Calibration Parameter Compensation* using transfer functions.

Acknowledgments

The work of Pat Forrest in collecting data is greatly appreciated. The Centre for Public Health Research is supported by a Programme Grant from the Health Research Council of New Zealand. Dr Jeffreys (née Okasha) was previously employed at the University of Bristol, and she is grateful for financial support from Breast Cancer Campaign, Breast Cancer Research Trust and World Cancer Research Fund International. Part of this work was funded by the EU MammoGrid project. Finally, many thanks to Chris Tromans for useful discussions around SMF and for showing the benefits of the transfer function approach.

References

Boyd N., Lockwood G., Byng J., Tritchler D., Yaffe M (1998), "Mammographic densities and breast cancer risk", *Cancer Epidemiol Biomarkers Prev* 7:1133-1144.
Burch A, Law J, (1995), "A method for estimating compressed breast thickness during mammography", British J Radiology, 68:394-399, 1995.
Heine J, Malhotra P (2002). "Mammographic tissue, breast cancer risk, serial image analysis, and digital mammography. Part 1: Tissue and related risk factors", *Acad Radiol,* 2002; 9(3), 298-316.
Highnam R., Brady M. (1999), "Mammographic Image Analysis", Kluwer Academic Publishers.

Hufton A, Astley S, Marchant T, Patel H. (2004) "A method for the quantification of dense breast tissue from digitised mammograms". *Proceedings of the IWDM 2004* 2; in press.

Jeffreys M, Warren R, Gunnell D, McCarron P, Highnam R, Davey Smith G (2003a). "Body Mass Index in young adulthood and breast cancer risk (abstract)". Australasian Epidemiologist 2003;10(3):17.

Jeffreys M, Warren R, Highnam R & Davey Smith G (2006), "Initial experience of using an automated volumetric measure of breast density: the standard mammogram form (SMF)", British Journal of Radiology, 2006 (in press).

Pawluczyk O, Augustine BJ, Yaffe MJ, Rico D, Yang J, Mawdsley GE, (2003) "A volumetric method for estimation of breast density on digitized screen-film mammograms". *Med. Phys.* 2003;30(3):352-64.

Tromans C (2006), "Measuring breast density from x-ray mammograms", DPhil. Thesis to be submitted March 2006, University of Oxford.

Wolfe JN (1976). Breast patterns as an index of risk for developing breast cancer. Am J Roentgenol 1976;126(6):1130-1137.

A Scatter Model for Use in Measuring Volumetric Mammographic Breast Density

Christopher Tromans and Michael Brady

Wolfson Medical Vision Laboratory, Department of Engineering Science,
University of Oxford, Parks Road, Oxford, UK, OX1 3PJ
cet@robots.ox.ac.uk

Abstract. In order that accurate measurements of volumetric breast density may be made, a model of the scattered radiation present within an image is required: such a model is presented here. The model has the advantageous property of utilising a model of photon scattering, allowing cross sections to be calculated, and thus allowing scatter to be modelled for any object. An analysis is presented which uses the model to quantify the effect of varying small angle scattering properties of breast tissues; and the effect of the height within the breast at which tissues are present. Since the details of the anatomical structure of the breast under measurement are unknown, their precise effect on scatter cannot be calculated, but this model is used here to establish error bounds on the scatter estimate, which is a significant contribution to the error in breast density measurement.

1 Introduction

The study of the correlation between radiological features of the breast and the likelihood of the breast containing, or subsequently developing, a malignant lesion, is termed breast density. In particular, volumetric measurement techniques calculate the quantities of fibroglandular and adipose tissue present in the cone between a detector pixel, and the x-ray focal spot, using the x-ray attenuation coefficients of these tissues. Highnam and Brady [1] originally pioneered the h_{int} representation which utilises this technique to produce a normalised image of anatomical structure. Over recent years, a second generation of this model has been developed which harnesses the extra power made available by modern computers to remove several of the simplifying assumptions made in the original model. Features of the enhanced model include: a ray tracing architecture, removing the parallel beam approximation; consideration of self-filtration within the tube target to model spatial inhomogeneity of the x-ray beam; a theoretical scatter model removing the need for interpolation from empirical data; and a enhanced detector calibration procedure.

We present here an overview of the novel scatter model, and an analysis gleaned through use of the model of the effect on scatter of two properties of the breast.

Two scattering phenomena occur within the breast: coherent (Rayleigh) and incoherent (Compton). Coherent scattering is elastic and involves the energy of the x-ray photon being completely absorbed and subsequently re-emitted in a random direction

Susan M. Astley et al. (Eds.): IWDM 2006, LNCS 4046, pp. 251–258, 2006.

by an electron of a single atom. Incoherent scattering is inelastic, and occurs when a x-ray photon collides with one of the outer shell electrons of an atom. The outer shell electron is bound to the atom with very little energy, and essentially all of the energy lost by the x-ray photon in the collision is transferred as kinetic energy to the electron, which as a result is ejected from the atom. Energy and momentum are conserved in the collision, so the resulting energy and direction of the photon depends on the energy transferred to the electron. In the mammographic energy range, coherent scattering is dominant at low photon energies, whilst incoherent phenomena become steadily dominant as energy increase. High energy photons are present in increased numbers in the spectra employed in clinical use, and so the majority of scatter is incoherent.

The variation in electron density across a molecule resulting from the bonding between constituent atoms provides a significant contribution to the scattering characteristics of photons undergoing coherent phenomena. Variations in molecular bonding therefore manifest themselves within the scattering characteristics, particularly at small angles. Incoherent scatter, resulting from a different physical phenomena, does not exhibit such variation, and is largely independent of molecular bonding. Significant differences in small-angle ($3°$ to $10°$) coherent scattering patterns measured from thin excised breast tissue samples have been found. A study by Kidane et al [2] catalogued scattering signatures for 100 excised tissue samples for which histological analysis was available, and found the signature to be useful in differentiating healthy, benign and malignant breast tissue. They reported that shapes of the scatter signatures were "significantly different" between the various tissue types, and hence concluded that "if particular values of momentum transfer are monitored, a discriminating signal could be obtained". The effect of varying small angle scattering properties of the tissues within the breast, on the total scattered radiation present within a mammographic image, is therefore considered in this paper.

The second property under investigation is the effect of the vertical position of tissue structures within the breast in the plane perpendicular to the detector. The details of both properties investigated are unknown for a breast under examination, and so the analysis in this paper allows the limitations of the scatter model to be established, and thereby the accuracy of subsequent measurements.

2   Overview of the Scatter Model

The cross-section describing the coherent scatter incident on a Cartesian area element (an image pixel) is given in equation 1. For reasons of space we consider only coherent scatter, although a similar relation to that in equation 1 exists in the incoherent case, and the remaining algorithmic details are equally applicable.

$$\sigma_{coherent, pixel} = \int_{y_1}^{y_2} \int_{x_1}^{x_2} \frac{r_e^2}{2} \left(1 + \cos^2 \phi\right) F_m^2 \left(\frac{\sin \phi}{\lambda}\right) \frac{c}{r^3} dx dy \qquad (1)$$

The scatter model uses equation 1 to calculate the cross section describing the scatter originating from each infinitesimally small traversal of the primary beam, destined, subject to further interaction, for each of the image receptor pixels in the surrounding area. An attenuation coefficient is calculated for each cross section, and hence the scattered spectrum is found. The number of photons undergoing multiple scatterings is assumed negligible, and so the scattered spectrum is attenuated by the photoelectric absorption along the path between the scatter origination point and image receptor. The scatter component at each image pixel is calculated from the sum of incident scattered spectra, arising from the scattering points in the cone of tissue above.

2.1 Small Angle Scattering

The molecular form factor, F_m, encodes not only information about the various elements present in a material, but also the bonding and the structural arrangement of the molecules. Theoretical calculation of the form factor is possible if the electron density is known, which is likely in the atomic case, but rare for molecules since the correlation between the electrons of the various atoms must be considered. The molecular form factor may be approximated from the form factors of the constituent atoms using the independent atom model (IAM). This model assumes a gas for which no bonding between atoms exists. The form factors are calculated as a linear combination of the constituent element form factors, weighted using abundance by mass.

Form factors including consideration of bonding are generally gleaned from empirical studies. Unfortunately Kidane et al [2] do not include form factors in their paper. Poletti et al [3] include measurements for a range of phantom materials, as well as healthy adipose and fibroglandular tissue, but for no further histopathological cases. Figure 1 shows the variation with scattering angle of the scattering coefficient, for form factors approximated using the IAM, and those measured by Poletti et al.

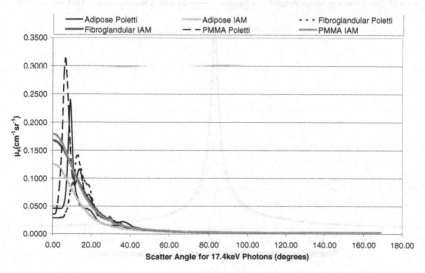

Fig. 1. Angular scatter attenuation coefficients for adipose and fibroglandular tissue

Inspection of figure 1 shows significant variation below 30° at the energy of the K_α edge of Molybdenum. These scatter profiles apply at a infinitesimal point, but it is the combined effect along the traversal path that is of interest.

2.2 Variation in Mammographic Scatter

The difference in angular scatter profile between the IAM and empirical form factors in figure 1 is of a similar, if not slightly greater, magnitude to that between the various histopathologically discriminated tissue samples presented by Kidane et al [2]. It is therefore assumed here, in the absence of other form factor data, that the resulting variation within a mammographic image will be similar to that arising from the variation seen here.

In order to investigate the effect on a mammographic image, a single primary ray was simulated, passing through a 60mm thick, 33% fibroglandular - 67% adipose, tissue phantom. Empirical and IAM approximated form factors, for both adipose and fibroglandular tissue were tested; as well as forming the phantom of both a homogenous mix of tissue, and a inhomogenous mix where the entirety of the fibroglandular tissue is concentrated at the centre. Figure 2 shows a graph of the results, where inspection reveals a minimal difference between the scatter "kernels". The median average difference in energy imparted to the detector across the spatial area considered, between the simulations using the empirical and IAM form factors is 6.6% and 7.1%, for the homogeneous and inhomogeneous cases respectively. Similarly, the average difference between the homogeneous and inhomogeneous cases is 5.1% and 1.2%, for the empirical and IAM form factors respectively.

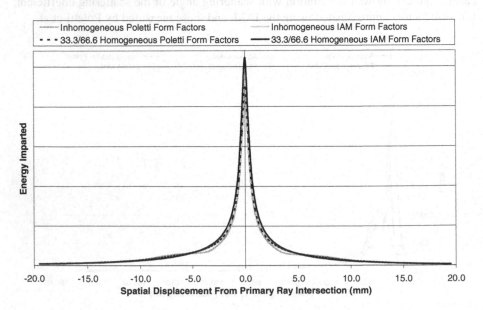

Fig. 2. The scatter profile arising from the complete traversal of a 60mm phantom

2.3 Experimental Validation of the Scatter Model

Experimental validation is performed through the comparison of simulated images calculated using the complete model of image acquisition, with those acquired using a GE Senographe 2000D in current clinical use. The model is configured to match the design of the 2000D, and the x-ray tube and image receptor are calibrated to match the specific machine according to the procedure described in [4]. Polymethyl methacrylate (PMMA) sheets of varying thickness are used as a phantom.

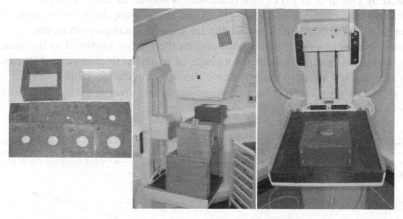

Fig. 3. The experimental setup: the apertures, phantom, and phantom side shielding (left), measurement of the primary beam (centre), measurement of scatter characteristics (right)

Although it is only the scatter component under consideration, the whole model is required since it is not possible to "decouple" this single component for measurement. A further complication arises from the impracticality of measuring the scatter "kernel" arising from the traversal of a single primary ray since a conventional x-ray tube is unable to deliver a sufficiently high exposure, mainly due to heat dissipation constraints, so that the resulting scattered energy is of a sufficient magnitude to adequately expose a mammographic image receptor. An indirect measurement technique, known as the beam stop method is therefore employed. A series of lead apertures of varying diameters are placed on top of the phantom, which itself sits on the breast table. The sides of the phantom are shielded using lead to prevent any radiation reaching the image receptor which has not passed through the aperture. The diameter of the aperture governs the volume of scattering material contributing to the energy incident upon the small group of detector pixels at the centre of the aperture shadow. The scattering characteristics of the material dictate the magnitude of the energy contributed by each infinitesimally small scattering point, and thus measuring the pixel intensities at the centre of the shadow provides an indirect measure of the characteristics, together with the attenuation between the scatter origination point and the image receptor. The median pixel intensity for a circle of pixels covering an area of approximately 1mm is used as the aforementioned measurement in order to provide a degree of robustness to noise. The primary component is measured through the use of a magnification tower which holds the phantom and the smallest diameter aperture as close to the tube window as possible (around 450mm above the breast table on the 2000D). The pixel intensity is measured in an identical fashion, through averaging across a 1mm diameter circular area in the centre of the aperture shadow. Due to the magnifying effect of the large distance between the scatter originator and the image receptor only photons scattered over a very limited range of angles will be present, and so the measurement will consist almost solely of the primary component.

Figure 1 shows a clear difference between the angular scatter characteristics calculated using the form factors approximated using the IAM, and those empirically measured by Poletti et al [3] (a difference that is similar to that seen in the breast tissues that are also included on the chart). Simulations using both sets of form factors are therefore investigated and compared to the experimental measurements.

Figure 4 illustrates the relationship between the energy imparted to the image receptor, and the aperture diameter for a range of phantom thicknesses. The exposure values are selected so as to use points on the detector transfer characteristics which are as similar as possible in order that the effect of any error arising in the calibration of this function is minimised.

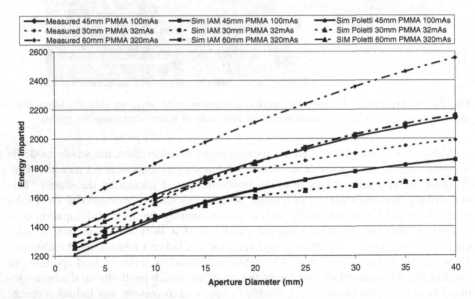

Fig. 4. The variation in energy imparted with aperture diameter for a range of phantom thicknesses, exposed at 28kVp, Mo-Mo

Table 1 presents the numerical results gleaned from the 45mm phantom. The '% Uncertainty' column holds the relative magnitude, expressed as a percentage of the energy experimentally measured, of twice the standard deviation of the pixel intensities within the 1mm circular area at the centre of the aperture shadow (that from which measurements are taken). This value thereby quantifies the stochastic noise present in the measurement, arising from such phenomena as quantum effects. The '% Error IAM' and '% Error Poletti' columns show the error, expressed as a percentage,

Table 1. The experimental and simulated results of the scatter model validation using a 45mm phantom, exposed at 28kVp, Mo-Mo, 100mAs

Aperture Diameter	% Uncertainty	% Error IAM	% Error Poletti	% Difference IAM-Poletti
Primary	2.18	11.90	14.95	3.46
2	1.77	9.73	12.76	3.35
5	1.87	9.49	11.86	2.62
10	1.74	9.65	10.45	0.89
15	1.37	9.52	9.92	0.45
20	1.66	10.22	10.54	0.36
25	1.51	10.75	10.85	0.12
30	1.89	11.74	11.74	0.00
35	1.67	12.51	12.46	-0.05
40	1.54	13.40	13.26	-0.16

between the experimental measurements on the 2000D, and the simulated results using the IAM approximated, and empirically measured form factors respectively. The '% Difference IAM-Poletti' column shows the difference, between the simulated results using the two sets of form factors, expressed as a percentage of the IAM result.

Inspection of Figure 4 and Table 1 suggests a good agreement between the simulated and measured imparted energies. The error in the primary beam measurement suggests inaccuracies elsewhere in the model, which inevitably have a consequential effect on the scatter results. The variation in error with aperture diameter remains approximately constant, particularly given the magnitude of the uncertainty due to noise. In order that the results may be seen excluding the effect of the error in the primary beam, Figure 5 includes a graph of the results for which the energy of the primary beam has been subtracted from all measurements.

Inspection of Figure 5 suggests a good degree of correspondence between the measured and simulated results, particularly at small aperture diameters. Small diameters include only the small angle scatter components, which are those that are most likely to pass through a anti-scatter device. It would appear that a slight advantage is gleaned for aperture diameters in this region from the use of the empirical form factors; however the advantage is almost negligible given the level of experimental uncertainty. The error in the primary component is likely to be due to the modelled tube spectra being softer than that in reality, resulting in a imparted energy that is too low (the total beam energy is calibrated). A lower beam quality will also have an effect at high aperture diameters where the distance over which scattered radiation is attenuated increases. In order to verify this hypothesis the primary beam was measured for constant exposure conditions, for 30 and 45mm phantoms. The ratio of the energy imparted through 45mm to that at 30mm in the experimental case is 0.319, compared to 0.307 in the simulation. Calculating the ratio removes the effect of the transfer characteristics of the image receptor, and so the magnitude of the error in attenuation is seen in the results. Whilst a number of factors are likely to contribute to this error, for example, material impurities, noise, and errors in the photoelectric absorption cross sections; an error in beam quality is likely to contribute a major component.

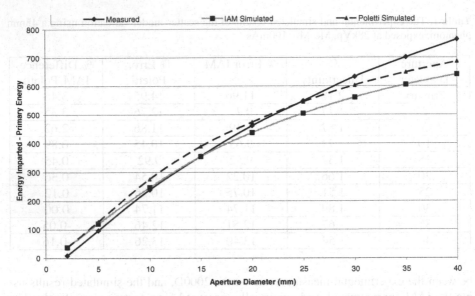

Fig. 5. The relationship between aperture diameter and the difference between energy imparted and the primary beam energy, using a 45mm phantom, exposed at 28kVp, Mo-Mo, 100mAs

3 Conclusion

The variation arising from both the vertical distribution in tissue heights, and the small angle scattering arising from molecular structure, has been seen to be so small as to have negligible effect. It can be concluded therefore that a breast model approximating scattering properties using the independent atom model, and assuming a homogenous mix of tissues, of proportions that vary spatial across the image, is sufficient for approximating scattered radiation when measuring breast density.

The minimal effect of small angle scattering presents a demanding challenge for those wishing to exploit such properties for use in in-vivo x-ray biopsy techniques. Were such techniques available they would be particular beneficial in quantifying stromal composition, a factor that has been suggested to be highly influential in determining the biological basis for the radiographic variations observed.

References

[1] R. Highnam and M. Brady, *Mammographic image analysis*. Dordrecht; London: Kluwer Academic, 1999.

[2] G. Kidane, R. D. Speller, G. J. Royle, and A. M. Hanby, "X-ray scatter signatures for normal and neoplastic breast tissues," *Phys Med Biol*, vol. 44, pp. 1791-802, 1999.

[3] M. E. Poletti, D. Goncalves, and I. Mazzaro, "X-ray scattering from human breast tissues and breast-equivalent materials," *Phys Med Biol*, vol. 47, pp. 47-63, 2002.

[4] C. Tromans, "DPhil Thesis: Measuring Breast Density from X-Ray Mammograms," in *Engineering Science*: Oxford University, to be submitted.

Using a Homogeneity Test as Weekly Quality Control on Digital Mammography Units

R.E. van Engen, M.M.J. Swinkels, L.J. Oostveen, T.D. Geertse, and R. Visser

Radboud University Nijmegen Medical Centre, National Expert and Training Centre for Breast Cancer Screening (577) P.O. box 9101, 6500 HB Nijmegen, The Netherlands
R.vanEngen@lrcb.umcn.nl

Abstract. In the Netherlands a number of (screening) trials with digital mammography equipment have been started since 1999. In this paper results from the weekly QC procedure are given. It seems that the homogeneity test as described in the addendum to the European protocol is able to detect detector problems and flat field calibration problems. However, visual inspection remains necessary. For the CR system in the trials the homogeneity test did not find many problems. Either the homogeneity test is not effective and other tests might be more appropriate or this CR system does not have relevant image quality variations and therefore might not require weekly quality control.

1 Introduction

In the Netherlands a number of (screening) trials with digital mammography have been started. The first trial began in 1999, in which digital mammography was tested in a clinical environment. For this purpose a GE Senographe 2000D was installed in the Radboud University Nijmegen Medical Centre. In 2002 the second trial started at a static screening site in Utrecht with a Lorad Selenia system. In this trial digital mammography was evaluated in a screening environment. In 2004 two more trials with mobile digital screening units were started. In these trials a Fuji FCR Profect and an Agfa DM 1000 system were installed in the screening units.

2 Methods and Materials

In the trials technical quality control is performed on all mammography units according to the European Guidelines for screening mammography [1]. Part of this quality control is a (weekly) evaluation of the stability of the mammography unit and homogeneity of the digital images [2].

For this weekly evaluation the radiographers image a homogeneous block of PMMA, covering the whole detector, under clinical conditions (fully automatic mode, compression paddle present). The resulting unprocessed image is sent to the physics section of the National Reference Centre in Nijmegen. The image is evaluated using a self-made software program, which is made available via internet (*www.euref.org*).

In this program an ROI is chosen (for our purpose: 0.5 cm by 0.5 cm) in the upper right corner of the image. This ROI is moved in steps of half ROI size over the whole image. For each ROI the average pixel value and standard deviation are determined and Signal-to-Noise Ratio (SNR) is calculated as pixel value over standard deviation.

Susan M. Astley et al. (Eds.): IWDM 2006, LNCS 4046, pp. 259–265, 2006.

The pixel value and SNR in each ROI are plotted in surface plots as function of position on the detector. Besides this the program checks for pixel values which deviate significantly (>30%) from the mean value in each ROI. These pixels are suspected to be uncorrected bad pixels. The images are also evaluated visually for artefacts smaller than the ROI size using a DICOM viewer with small window width. In this paper this whole procedure is referred to as a homogeneity test.

The homogeneity test is performed weekly. However, for the Lorad and Agfa systems the radiographers have to perform a flat field calibration weekly. In this calibration a number of images of a homogeneous PMMA block are made in order to determine the gain and offset for each detector element. For these systems the homogeneity test is performed twice a week, just before and right after the flat field calibration.

3 Results

3.1 Typical 'Normal' Output of the Homogeneity Test

For DR systems, the surface plot, in which pixel value is plotted as function of position on the detector, is expected to be flat due to the flat field calibration, which is performed. For CR systems however, pixel values are expected to decrease towards nipple and lateral sides due to the heel and geometric effects. For both DR and CR systems it is expected that SNR will decrease towards nipple and lateral sides due to the same effects. In figure 1 an example of the output of the homogeneity test software is given for a DR system.

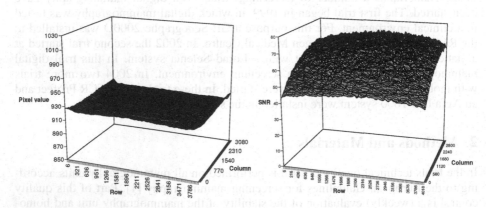

Fig. 1. Output of the homogeneity test on a DR system, a: pixel value plotted as function of psition on the detector, b: SNR plotted as function of position on the detector

3.2 Problems with Homogeneity

In the digital mammography trials a number of homogeneity problems have been observed. These problems can be divided into two subclasses:

1. Image receptor problems
2. Calibration procedure problems

Some examples of homogeneity problems are discussed in the paragraphs below. The homogeneity test did not find many problems with the CR system in the trials. Only some minor ghosting problems have been observed.

3.2.1 Image Receptor Problems

3.2.1.1 Sensitivity Change of the Image Receptor. In the long-term use of some DR systems and imaging plates of a CR system, it is observed that the sensitivity of the image receptor changes spatially. On the images this change in sensitivity presents itself as a ghost image, which increases over time. This can be explained as difference in ageing of the image receptor due to intensity differences of the incident X-rays. At chest wall side the sensitivity of the image receptor is higher because this part of the image receptor receives less radiation over a great number of exposures. Therefore on homogeneity images a faint breast-shaped structure is visible.

3.2.1.2 Lag. Several papers report the visibility of previously taken images in subsequent images [3] [4]. These images might be caused by either some residue of a previous image (lag) or by a change of sensitivity of the detector due to previous exposures. Both have been observed on homogeneity images. In most cases this effect is very small and was not visible on clinical images. However, at one site the manufacturer tried to speed up the readout of the detector a number of times because of complaints of limited patient throughput. As a result previously taken images were clearly visible both on homogeneity and clinical images. Up to four previous images could be identified on the homogeneity images, see figure 2. On the clinical images one previous image was clearly visible.

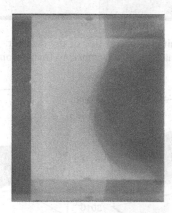

Fig. 2. Four previously taken images visible on a homogeneity image after speeding up the readout of the detector

3.2.1.3 Crystallization of the Detector Material. Crystallization of amorphous selenium occurs at relatively low temperatures and depends on the amount of stabilizers added to the selenium, temperature and other ambient conditions [5]. In both amorphous selenium detectors in the trials crystallization occurred two times (so the crystallization problem has been observed four times in total). Due to the position of readout electronics the detector temperature is expected to be highest at lateral sides, therefore crystallization was observed first at the far lateral sides of the detector and is seen to expand towards the middle of the detector in all four cases, see figure 3. However, it is known from other sites that crystallization might also start somewhere in the middle of the detector. Due to the spreading of signal in the selenium crystals the standard deviation of the signal will decrease leading to an artificial increase in SNR in the homogeneity test, see figure 4. Due to the irreversible nature of this problem, the detectors were replaced.

Crystallization can be detected with the homogeneity test when the area of crystallization is very small (under two millimeters length) and it can be seen very clearly that the problem increases over time, see figure 3 and 4. Using visual inspection only, it is very difficult to identify the crystallization problem at this early stage.

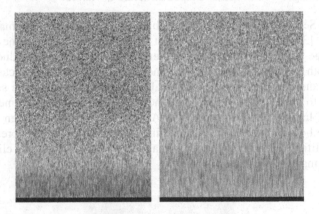

Fig. 3. Crystallization of selenium at lateral side of the detector. The size of the area shown is approximately 3 by 4 cm. a: Image from November, b: Image from January.

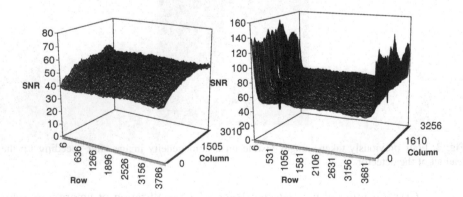

Fig. 4. On homogeneity graphs an increase in SNR can be observed in the area where crystallization has occurred, a: The area of crystallization is approximately two millimeter wide, b: The area of crystallization is over one centimeter wide

3.2.1.4   Defective Detector Element Calibration (Bad Pixel Calibration). On some DR systems the defective detector element (del) calibration is performed during service. Dels that become defective between two calibrations are detected by the homogeneity test. In all cases only a few bad pixels were found.

3.2.1.5   Blooming Artefact. According to a service engineer this artefact was caused by a detector element, which could not be read out. Due to the build up of charge at the position of the dead detector element, charge flowed to neighbouring dels causing a circle-like artefact on a homogeneity image. Due to the size of the artefact (a few pixels in diameter) this artefact proved very hard to detect with the software. However, this artefact is clearly seen by visual inspection. This is an example of a problem that is not observed with the automated homogeneity test, see figure 5.

Fig. 5. Blooming artifact on a homogeneity image

3.2.2 Calibration Procedure Problems

For two systems in the digital mammography trials the flat field procedure has to be performed weekly by the radiographers. It has been observed that a number of calibration procedure problems occurred. These problems can be divided in problems in the calibration procedure itself and calibration in the presence of a lag image.

3.2.2.1   Flat Field Calibration Problems. During calibration the radiographers have to image a homogeneous block of PMMA covering the whole detector multiple times. On three occasions it was noticed that the PMMA block did not always cover the detector area fully during calibration. As a consequence on all images after calibration an area with lower pixel values at lateral side was visible (see figure 6).

In one case the calibration procedure was aborted by the radiographers after imaging the block of PMMA only once. It was noticed that the flat field calibration was performed imperfectly in all subsequent images. The old calibration file was apparently already deleted and the new calibration file was either incorrect or flat fielding was not performed at all.

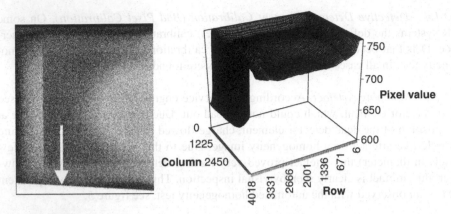

Fig. 6. During (part of the) flat fielding procedure the detector was not covered completely causing an area with deviating pixel values

3.2.2.2   Presence Lag Image During Calibration. Figure 7a shows the presence of lag in the detector on a homogeneity image just before calibration. The flat fielding masks the lag. Therefore on the homogeneity image made right after calibration the image appears homogeneous (Figure 7b). However, because the lag disappears over time, an inversion of the lag is visible on homogeneity images, which have been made some time after calibration (Figure 7c).

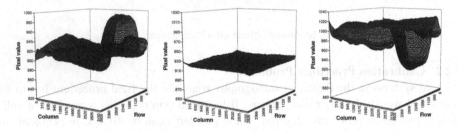

Fig. 7. a: A lag was present just before calibration. b: After flat fielding the lag is masked and the pixel value is equal over the whole image, c: Some time after the calibration the inversed lag from figure a. can be seen on the image.

In one case the PMMA did not cover the detector fully when the homogeneity image before calibration was made. In this case the resulting lag image was present during calibration and after calibration (and disappearance of the lag image) an inverted lag image was observed.

4   Discussion and Conclusions

The homogeneity test seems useful in determining problems at DR systems. However it is noticed that small artefacts are not detected and therefore visual inspection remains necessary.

Visual inspection however is time-consuming and knowledge about possibly occurring problems and their appearance on a homogeneity image is required. Therefore the homogeneity test needs to be improved in a future version of the European guidelines and a public database has to be set up with examples of known problems.

The homogeneity test did not find many problems with the CR system in the trials. Only some minor ghosting problems have been observed. However a weekly test for this ageing problem does not seems very useful. The fact that no major problems have been observed might have two causes:

1. The CR system in the trials does not have relevant image quality variations and weekly QC might be overtesting.
2. Readout problems might not be detected by the present homogeneity test (small effects might be obscured by the presence of the geometric and heel effect in the images) and other tests might be more relevant.

In our future work we might perform weekly QC with a phantom with diagonal lines to test the applicability for QC measurements on CR systems.

References

1. van Engen R, Young K, Bosmans H, Thijssen M: Addendum on digital mammography to chapter 3 of: European guidelines for Quality assurance in mammography screening, version 1.0, Euref (2002), www.euref.org
2. Oostveen LJ, van Engen RE, Visser R, Thijssen MAO: Technical quality control in digital mammography, in E. Pisano (ed.), proceedings IWDM 2004, Chapel Hill (2005)
3. Zhao B, Zhao W: Temporal performance of amorphous selenium mammography detectors, Medical Physics 32(1), 2005
4. Siewerdsen JH, Jaffray DA: Spatio-temporal response characteristics of an indirect-detection flat-panel imager, Medical Physics 26(8), 1999, 1624-1641.
5. Kasap SO, Rowlands JA: Review X-ray photoconductors and stabilized a-Se for direct conversion digital flat panel X-ray image-detectors, Journal of materials science: materials in electronics (11) 2000, 179-198.

Automated and Human Determination of Threshold Contrast for Digital Mammography Systems

Kenneth C. Young, James J.H. Cook, and Jennifer M. Oduko

National Coordinating Centre for the Physics of Mammography
Royal Surrey County Hospital, Guildford GU2 7XX, UK
ken.young@nhs.net

Abstract. European Guidelines for quality control in digital mammography specify minimum and achievable standards of image quality in terms of threshold contrast, based on readings of images of the CDMAM test object by human observers. However this is time-consuming and has large inter-observer error. To overcome these problems a software program (CDCOM) is available to automatically read CDMAM images and can be used to predict the threshold contrast for a typical observer. The results of threshold contrast determination by a panel of 3 human observers was compared in this study to predicted human readings for different types of digital mammography system to determine whether this provides a viable method of automated quality control and comparison with existing European Guidelines.

1 Background

European Guidelines for the quality control of mammography provide quality control procedures and minimum standards of performance for digital mammography [1]. The image quality standard is based on contrast-detail measurements using the CDMAM phantom (version 3.4, UMC St. Radboud, Nijmegen University, Netherlands) [2]. The minimum standards were chosen to ensure that digital systems are as good or better than current film screen systems [3]. Such contrast detail measurements rely on a large number of observer readings and suffer from significant inter-observer error, which undermines the reliability and confidence in the measurements. The use of human observers is also very time consuming. A possible solution to these problems is the use of the CDCOM program, which automatically reads CDMAM images [4,5,6,7]. It has been noted that the threshold contrasts determined using this program are lower than those found by human observers [4,5]. However recently the relationship between automatic and human observer scoring has been explored and a means of predicting typical human threshold contrast described [8]. This method is used here along with a panel of human observers to assess threshold contrasts for a variety of digital mammography systems and to compare these with the standards in European Guidelines.

2 Method

The CDMAM phantom was radiographed on each of the digital systems shown in Table 1. (One of the systems is identified only as Test CR as the manufacturer has

Susan M. Astley et al. (Eds.): IWDM 2006, LNCS 4046, pp. 266–272, 2006.
© Springer-Verlag Berlin Heidelberg 2006

suggested that the system may have been faulty and its performance not representative of normal operation.) The phantom was positioned with a 20 mm thickness of PMMA blocks above and below. This combination has a total attenuation approximately equivalent to 50 mm of PMMA. This has been shown to be equivalent to breasts of typical composition with a compressed thickness of 60 mm [9]. Expanded polystyrene spacers were added at the edges of the phantom to create a total thickness of 60 mm and a standard compression of 100N applied. This arrangement was imaged using the factors automatically selected by the X-ray set and shown in Table 1. Where possible the effect of dose on threshold contrasts was assessed using further sets of 8 CDMAM images obtained on each system by manually selecting mAs values that were approximate multiples of 2 higher or lower than selected using the AEC control. The tube voltage and target/filter combinations were kept the same. (It was not possible to adjust the dose for the Sectra system across a wide range.) The unprocessed CDMAM images were transferred to disk for subsequent analysis at our laboratory.

Table 1. Digital mammography systems tested

Imaging system (pixel size)	X-ray set	kV target filter
Fischer Senoscan	n/a	29kV W Al
Sectra Microdose	n/a	32kV W Al
Siemens Novation	n/a	28kV W Rh
GE Senographe DS	n/a	29kV Rh Rh
Fuji Profect (50 μm)	GE Senographe DMR+	26kV Mo Rh
Kodak Directview CR 850 (50μm)	GE Senographe DMR+	29kV Mo Rh
Test CR	GE Senographe DMR+	27kV Mo Rh

For each exposure the factors used when imaging the CDMAM phantom with the additional PMMA were recorded. The x-ray setting output, half-value layer (in mm of aluminium) and the distance from the focus to table top were measured allowing the entrance surface air kerma at the top of a 50mm thickness of PMMA to be calculated. The method described by Dance et al. was used to calculate the mean glandular dose (MGD) to typical breasts with a 60 mm compressed breast thickness and an attenuation equivalent to a 50 mm thickness of PMMA [9]. The average of these MGD values for each set of similar CDMAM images was then calculated. The maximum acceptable MGD in the European Guidelines is 3 mGy at this thickness.

The CDCOM outputs for the 8 CDMAM images were combined to determine the proportion of correctly identified discs for each detail diameter and thickness. A data smoothing algorithm was applied and a psychometric curve fitted for each detail diameter as described previously [8].

The threshold gold thickness was determined for each diameter as the point on the fitted curve with a probability of detection of 0.625. This probability is used because it lies midway between random guessing at 0.25 and complete accuracy at 1.0. These threshold gold thicknesses were converted to threshold contrast for a nominal 28 kV Mo/Mo combination as described in European Guidelines. A contrast detail curve was then fitted to improve the reproducibility of the measurements. Predicted threshold contrasts for a typical human observer were obtained by multiplying those determined automatically by factors of 1.50 and 1.82 for the 0.1 and 0.25 mm detail sizes, respectively. These factors were determined from the linear relationship found previously between human and automatic threshold contrasts [8]. The results focus on these two detail sizes as the threshold contrast requirements for the smallest details are the most difficult to meet and necessitate the highest doses.

The human readings were obtained by displaying the CDMAM images using a diagnostic quality 3 Mega Pixel DICOM calibrated display. The contrast and brightness of each image was adjusted to optimally display the details in the test object, before scoring. The observer could use as much electronic zoom as needed and background illumination was kept to a minimum. The manual for the CDMAM phantom explains how to apply a nearest neighbour correction to the scores for each reading of a CDMAM image. These rules were applied to each of the images read by a human observer. After applying these rules the smallest gold thickness for a correctly indicated disc was noted for each diameter. For each set of CDMAM images three observers each scored 4 images the average threshold gold thickness determined for each diameter. The average threshold contrast for each detail diameter for each set of images was fitted with a curve to improve the reproducibility.

The MGDs corresponding to the minimum and achievable threshold contrast limits for 0.1 and 0.25 mm detail sizes were determined for each system by fitting Eq. 1 to the automated and human threshold contrast data as a function of dose.

$$C = kD^{-n} \tag{1}$$

where C is the threshold contrast, D is the MGD for the equivalent breast and k and n are coefficients to be fitted. It is expected that n will have a value of approximately 0.5 due to quantum noise. The presence of other noise sources such as electronic and structure noise may modify this value. Equation 1 was fitted independently to the threshold contrast determined by the human and automated method. Where there were insufficient data points to determine n this was set to 0.5 and only k was fitted (i.e. Fischer and Sectra systems).

3 Results

The predicted and measured human threshold contrasts for 0.1 and 0.25 mm details are shown for different systems in Figs 1 to 5. (The human threshold contrasts were not completed at the time of writing for the GE Senographe DS system, and are therefore missing from Fig 5. In each case the threshold contrast declined as expected with increasing dose. The measured and predicted threshold contrasts generally agree within experimental error although the curves do not match perfectly. The errors in the predicted threshold contrasts were smaller at 0.25 mm than 0.1mm [8]. It is thought that this is caused by the absence of discs with sufficient gold thickness at the smallest detail sizes. It is likely that the reproducibility could be improved by a change in the test object design. The doses corresponding to the minimum acceptable and achievable threshold contrast in European Guidance are shown for these detail sizes in Tables 2 and 3.

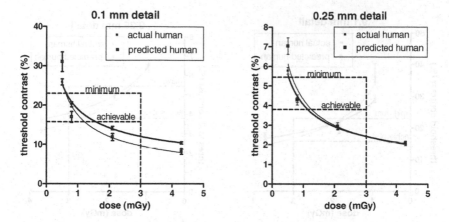

Fig. 1. Comparison of measured and predicted threshold contrasts at 0.1 and 0.25 mm details sizes against the minimum acceptable and achievable limits in the European Guidelines for a range of doses with a Siemens Novation. Error bars indicate 1 SE.

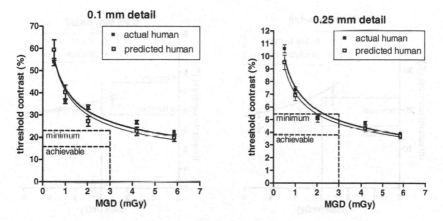

Fig. 2. Comparison of measured and predicted threshold contrasts at 0.1 and 0.25 mm details sizes against the minimum acceptable and achievable limits in the European Guidelines for a range of doses with the Test CR system. Error bars indicate 1 SE.

Table 2. MGD to equivalent 60mm thick breast required to reach the minimum threshold contrasts for 0.1mm and 0.25 mm detail sizes in the European Protocol. (Errors are 1 sem)

System	MGD (mGy) for 0.1 mm		MGD (mGy) for 0.25 mm	
	Human	Predicted	Human	Predicted
Fischer Seno.	0.55 ± 0.08	0.42 ± 0.06	0.48 ± 0.07	0.53 ± 0.08
Sectra MDM	0.60 ± 0.09	0.82 ± 0.12	0.67 ± 0.10	0.46 ± 0.07
Siemens Novation	0.63 ± 0.04	0.61 ± 0.17	0.52 ± 0.04	0.63 ± 0.13
GE DS		0.82 ± .07		0.83 ± .08
Fuji Profect CR	1.67 ± 0.12	1.78 ± 0.16	1.45 ± 0.02	1.35 ± 0.07
Kodak CR	3.46 ± 0.03	2.49 ± 0.13	1.49 ± 0.12	1.33 ± 0.12
Test CR	4.52 ± 0.35	4.17 ± 0.14	2.33 ± 0.07	2.12 ± 0.05

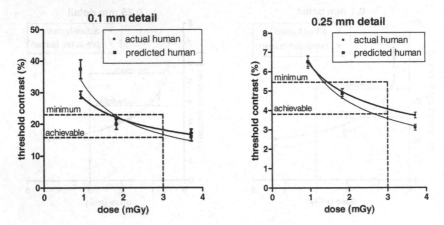

Fig. 3. Comparison of measured and predicted threshold contrasts at 0.1 and 0.25 mm details sizes against the minimum acceptable and achievable limits in the European Guidelines for a range of doses with the Fuji Profect CR system. Error bars indicate 1 SE.

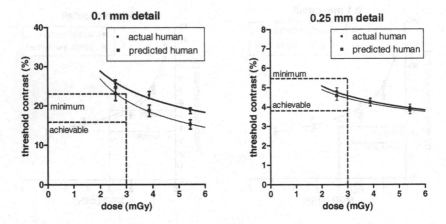

Fig. 4. Comparison of measured and predicted threshold contrasts at 0.1 and 0.25 mm details sizes against the minimum acceptable and achievable limits in the European Guidelines for a range of doses with the Kodak Directview CR system. Error bars indicate 1 SE.

Table 3. MGD to equivalent 60mm thick breast required to reach the achievable threshold contrasts for 0.1mm and 0.25 mm detail sizes in the European Protocol. (Errors are 1 sem)

System	MGD (mGy) for 0.1 mm		MGD (mGy) for 0.25 mm	
	Human	Predicted	Human	Predicted
Fischer Seno.	1.16 ± 0.17	0.90 ± 0.13	0.98 ± 0.15	1.09 ± 0.16
Sectra MDM	1.27 ± 0.19	1.74 ± 0.26	1.37 ± 0.21	0.95 ± 0.14
Siemens Novation	1.56 ± .03	1.21 ± .07	1.14 ± .05	1.27 ± .13
GE DS		1.57 ± .07		1.87 ± .07
Fuji Profect CR	4.26 ± 0.66	3.29 ± 0.44	3.52 ± 0.03	2.65 ± 0.03
Kodak CR	7.74 ± 0.71	5.56 ± 0.26	6.28 ± 0.25	5.60 ± 0.17
Test CR	11.5 ± 2.8	9.9 ± 1.1	5.96 ± .53	5.63 ± 0.26

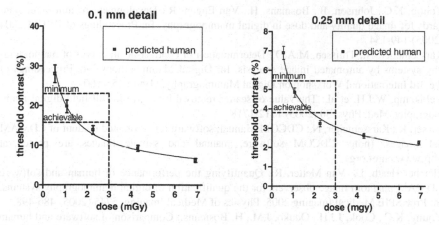

Fig. 5. Predicted threshold contrasts at 0.1 and 0.25 mm details sizes against the minimum acceptable and achievable limits in the European Guidelines for a range of doses with the GE Senographe DS system. Error bars indicate 1 SE.

4 Discussion

The use of predicted human threshold contrasts provided results for the digital systems across a range of doses that were generally within experimental error of those found using our panel of human observers. These data also demonstrated the large difference in performance between DR systems and CR systems. The two scanning systems, Fischer and Sectra, had as would be expected relatively low doses at the minimum and achievable levels. The two flat panel DR systems, Siemens Novation and GE Senographe DS, required similar or slightly higher doses. All four DR systems reached the achievable standard for image quality for a relatively low doses of about 1.5 mGy or less, well within the upper dose limit of 3 mGy set for this thickness in the European Guidelines. (It should be noted that, currently the Sectra MDM systems is limited to doses of about 0.7 to 1.0 mGy which are not sufficient to reach the achievable level.) Only one of the CR systems was able to meet the minimum standard within the dose limit, and this system did not meet the achievable limit within this dose constraint. Several manufacturers are introducing improved CR systems for digital mammography, which have not been reported on here, and these may meet the minimum standards. However, from the evidence currently available even the best CR systems seem to need much higher doses for the same image quality as the DR systems studied here.

References

1. Van Engen R., Young K.C., Bosmans H. and Thijssen M.: The European protocol for the quality control of the physical and technical aspects of mammography screening. Part B: Digital mammography. In: European Guidelines for Breast Cancer Screening, 4th Edition. Luxembourg: European Commission, 2006 (In press and available in draft online at www.euref.org)
2. Bijkerk, K.R., Thijssen, M.A.O., Arnoldussen, Th.J.M..: Modification of the CDMAM contrast-detail phantom for image quality of Full Field Digital Mammography systems. In: M. Yaffe (ed.): Proceedings of IWDM 2000. Medical Physics Publishing, Madison, WI, Toronto, (2000) 633-640

3. Young, K.C., Johnson, B., Bosmans, H., Van Engen, R.: Development of minimum standards for image quality and dose in digital mammography. In: Proceedings of IWDM 2004 (2005) 149-154

4. Karssemeijer, N., Thijssen, M.A.O.: Determination of contrast-detail curves of mammography systems by automated image analysis. In: Digital Mammography '96. Proceedings of the 3rd International Workshop on Digital Mammography. (1996) 155-160

5. Veldkamp, W.J.H. et al.: The value of scatter removal by a grid in full field digital mammography. Med. Phys. 30 (2003) 1712-1718

6. Visser, R., Karssemeijer, N.: CDCOM Manual: software for automated readout of CDMAM 3.4 images. (note: CDCOM software, manual and sample images are posted at http:www.euref.org)

7. Fletcher-Heath, L., Van Metter, R.: Quantifying the performance of human and software CDMAM phantom image observers for the qualification of digital mammography systems. In: Proc SPIE Medical Imaging 2005: Physics of Medical Imaging, 5745 (2005) 486-498

8. Young, K.C., Cook, J.J.H., Oduko, J.M., H. Bosmans.: Comparison of software and human observers in reading images of the CDMAM test object to assess digital mammography systems. In: Flynn MJ, Hsieh J (eds): Proceedings of SPIE Medical Imaging 2006, 614206 (2006) 1-13.

9. Dance, D.R., Skinner, C.L., Young, K.C., Beckett, J.R., C.J. Kotre.: Additional factors for the estimation of mean glandular breast dose using the UK mammography dosimetry protocol. Phys. Med. Biol. 45 (2000) 3225-3240

Beam Optimization for Digital Mammography – II

Mark B. Williams[1], Priya Raghunathan[1], Anthony Seibert[2], Alex Kwan[2],
Joseph Lo[3], Ehsan Samei[3], Laurie Fajardo[4], Andrew D.A. Maidment[5],
Martin Yaffe[6], and Aili Bloomquist[6]

[1] University of Virginia
[2] University of California-Davis
[3] Duke University
[4] University of Iowa
[5] University of Pennsylvania
[6] University of Toronto

Abstract. Optimization of acquisition technique factors (target, filter, and kVp) in digital mammography is required for maximization of the image SNR, while minimizing patient dose. The goal of this study is to compare, for each of the major commercially available FFDM systems, the effect of various technique factors on image SNR and radiation dose for a range of breast thickness and tissue types. This phantom study follows the approach of an earlier investigation [1], and includes measurements on recent versions of two of the FFDM systems discussed in that paper, as well as on three FFDM systems not available at that time. The five commercial FFDM systems tested are located at five different university test sites and include all FFDM systems that are currently FDA approved. Performance was assessed using 9 different phantom types (three compressed thicknesses, and three tissue composition types) using all available x-ray target and filter combinations. The figure of merit (FOM) used to compare technique factors is the ratio of the square of the image SNR to the mean glandular dose (MGD). This FOM has been used previously by others in mammographic beam optimization studies [2],[3]. For selected examples, data are presented describing the change in SNR, MGD, and FOM with changing kVp, as well as with changing target and/or filter type. For all nine breast types the target/filter/kVp combination resulting in the highest FOM value is presented. Our results suggest that in general, technique combinations resulting in higher energy beams resulted in higher FOM values, for nearly all breast types.

1 Introduction

The criteria for optimization of tube voltage and external filtration in full field digital mammography (FFDM) differ from those used in screen-film mammography. This is in part because the separation of the processes of acquisition and display in the former permits the contrast of individual structures to be adjusted when the image is viewed. Thus, rather than maximization of contrast within the constraint of acceptable film darkening and patient dose, beam optimization in digital mammography requires maximization of the image SNR, constrained by acceptable patient dose [4]. In recent

Susan M. Astley et al. (Eds.): IWDM 2006, LNCS 4046, pp. 273–280, 2006.
© Springer-Verlag Berlin Heidelberg 2006

years, four FFDM systems have gained FDA approval, with others soon to follow. Most of those systems are equipped with mechanisms for automatic selection of at least some technique factors including mAs and in some cases kVp, filtration, and target material. In some units, different acquisition modes are available in which different look-up-tables are utilized to emphasize either subject contrast (with lower kVp and higher mAs) or low dose (with higher kVp and lower mAs). It is the goal of this study to examine, for three simulated breast compositions, and three simulated breast thicknesses, the effect on the image SNR and the mean glandular dose (MGD) of varying kVp, and target and filter type.

2 Methods

Five different FFDM systems, the GE Healthcare Senographe 2000D, the Siemens Mammomat Novation, the Lorad Selenia, the Fischer/Hologic Senoscan, and Fuji's mammographic storage phosphor system, were used to image a common set of phantoms made of blocks of breast equivalent material (CIRS, Inc., Norfolk, VA). Nine different phantoms were assembled and imaged, simulating breasts of three different thicknesses (3 cm, 5 cm, and 7 cm), and three different attenuation equivalent adipose/fibroglandular mass ratios (30/70, 50/50, and 70/30). Two 5 mm thick blocks were placed on the top and bottom of each stack, to simulate skin (Fig. 1). The skin blocks were 100% adipose equivalent material.

In each phantom stack assembled, the centrally located block in the stack (the signal block) contained two stepwedges, one each of calcification equivalent and mass equivalent material. The mass equivalent stepwedge has the same x-ray attenuation as 100% glandular equivalent material, and the microcalcification equivalent step wedge is composed of calcium carbonate (Fig. 2). The thickness of all signal blocks is 2 cm.

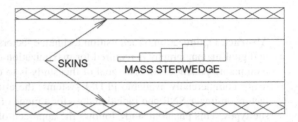

Fig. 1. Side view of a 5 cm phantom with a 2 cm signal block at the center, two 1 cm blank blocks and two 0.5 cm skins on the surface

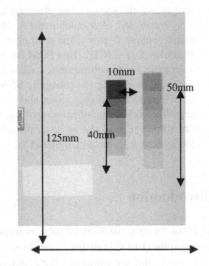

Fig. 2. Image of the phantom showing calcification (left) and mass equivalent step wedges.

Images were obtained in manual mode with the phantoms positioned at the chest wall edge of the receptor, centered left to right. Exposure time was selected to give approximately the same average pixel value in the phantom background area for each phantom/technique combination. For each combination, two images were obtained with identical exposure times for the purpose of image subtraction, taking care not to move the

Table 1. FFDM Units tested

System	Target	Filter	kV Range
Siemens	Mo, W	Mo,	23 – 35
Selenia	Mo	Mo,	23 – 39
Fischer	W	Al	28 – 37
GE	Mo, Rh	Mo,	24 – 32
Fuji	Mo	Rh	24 – 34

phantom between the two exposures. At each site, entrance exposures (mR/mAs) and half value layers (HVLs) were measured for each target/filter/kVp combination used. Table 1 lists the target and filter combinations and range of kVps used for each FFDM system tested in the study. Signal was defined as the difference between the average pixel values in a region of interest (ROI) centered on an individual step, and an equal sized ROI located immediately adjacent to the step, but containing only background.

To quantify the image noise, the two images of a given phantom, obtained at a common technique, were subtracted. Image subtraction was performed to remove fixed pattern noise associated with phantom defects, detector nonuniformity, and heel effect. Noise in a single image was defined as the standard deviation of the pixel values in an ROI within the difference image, divided by the square root of two.

The MGD for each phantom was calculated using its known thickness, composition and the measured HVL and mR/mAs values from each FFDM system. For Mo/Mo and Mo/Rh spectra, the parameterized dose tables of Sobol and Wu were utilized to obtain the glandular dose per unit exposure [6]. For the W/Al spectra, normalized (to entrance exposure) MGD values were obtained from the data of Stanton et al. [7]. Their data were extrapolated to 3 cm breast thickness, and interpolation between their published HVL curves was used to obtain correction factors for the particular glandular volume fractions (0.22, 0.40, and 0.61, corresponding to glandular mass fractions of 0.30, 0.50, and 0.70, respectively) used in our study. For the W/Rh spectra, the calculations of Boone were utilized, interpolating between his published HVL and adipose/ fibroglandular composition values [5]. All FOM values were obtained by dividing the square of the SNR by the MGD expressed in units of 10^{-5} Gy (1 mRad).

3 Results

For a given phantom/target/filter combination, the form of the dependence of the signal on kVp was the same for all the steps of each stepwedge; only the magnitudes of the signals differed. Therefore, the results presented in this paper will use only the 0.3 mm thick microcalcification step for calculation of the signal. The plots of Figures 3 and 4 show examples of the dependence of SNR and dose per exposure, respectively, on changing kVp. In these examples, the FFDM systems are the Loard Selenia and Senography 2000D, respectively and the phantoms had 0.50 mass fraction. In Figure 3, the calculated SNR has been normalized by the average pixel value in the background region of the phantom image since the average pixel values were not exactly the same for all kVps tested.

The acquisition parameters chosen by the GE Senographe 2000D using its intrinsic Automatic Optimization of Parameters (AOP) system were recorded for every phantom thickness and composition combination. Automatically selected acquisition parameter values for other units equipped with such systems are currently in the process of being obtained.

Table 2 lists the target, filter and kVp that resulted in the maximum value of FOM for each breast type and system.

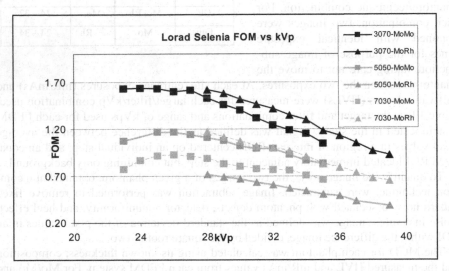

Fig. 3. Lorad Selenia : Square of SNR normalized by the average ADU value in the background, 50/50 composition

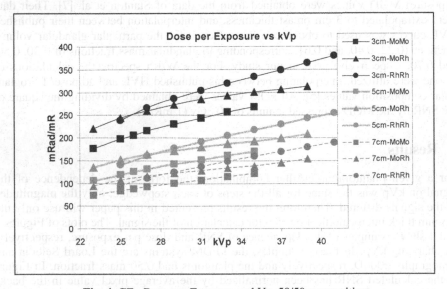

Fig. 4. GE : Dose per Exposure vs kVp, 50/50 composition

Table 2. Acquisition parameters resulting in maximum FOM. Table entries are in the form Target / Filter / kVp.

		30/70	50/50	70/30
GE	3cm	Mo / Mo / 25	Mo / Mo / 29	Mo / Mo / 29
	5cm	Rh / Rh / 27	Rh / Rh / 29	Rh / Rh/ 29
	7cm	Rh / Rh / 29	Rh / Rh / 29	Rh / Rh / 29
Lorad	3cm	Mo / Mo / 24	Mo / Rh / 28	Mo / Rh / 28
	5cm	Mo / Mo / 24	Mo / Mo / 25	Mo / Rh / 28
	7cm	Mo / Rh / 28	Mo / Rh / 28	Mo / Rh / 28
Siemens	3cm	W / Rh / 26	W / Rh / 29	W / Rh / 26
	5cm	W / Rh / 26	W / Rh / 26	W / Rh / 29
	7cm	W / Rh / 29	W / Rh / 29	W / Rh /29
Fuji	3cm	Mo / Mo / 24	Mo / Mo / 24	Mo / Rh / 30
	5cm	Mo / Mo / 24	Mo / Mo / 24	Mo / Rh / 30
	7cm	Mo / Rh / 30	Mo / Rh / 30	Mo / Rh / 31
Fischer	3cm	W / Al / 27	W / Al / 27	W / Al / 27
	5cm	W / Al / 29	W / Al / 30	W / Al / 30
	7cm	W / Al / 41	W / Al / 41	W / Al / 42

4 Discussion and Conclusions

The shape of the FOM vs. kVp curves for a given target/filter/phantom combination was found to be independent of step thickness, and was similar for mass and calcification equivalent signals. Figures 5-9 suggest that, for 5 cm breast thickness, for 50/50 as well as 70/30 compositions, the hardest beams result in higher FOM values in all systems tested. Furthermore, for 5 cm breast thickness and molybdenum target

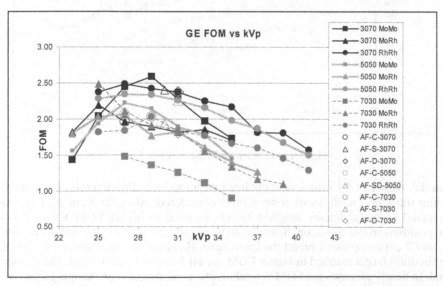

Fig. 5. GE : FOM vs. kVp, 5cm (AF : Autofilter, C : Contrast mode, S : Standard mode, D : Dose mode)

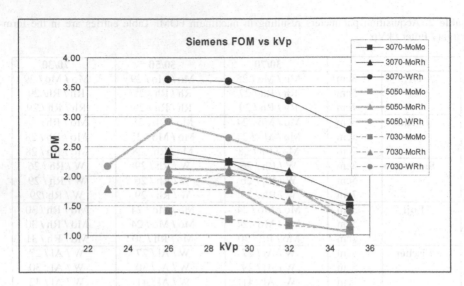

Fig. 6. Siemens : FOM vs. kVp, 5 cm

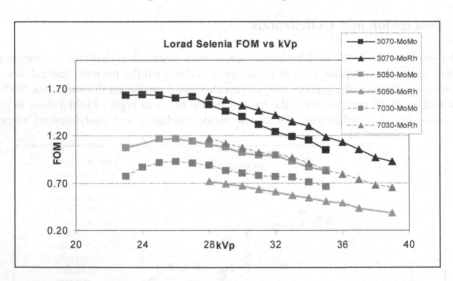

Fig. 7. Lorad Selenia : FOM vs. kVp, 5 cm

material, higher FOM values were obtained with rhodium filtration relative to molybdenum filtration for all breast compositions considered. Also, for 5 cm thick breasts,
compared to molybdenum, tungsten targets resulted in higher FOM values for all
compositions in the Novation. Space limitations prevent us from presenting data for 3
cm and 7 cm compressed breast thickness here. However, for the Senographe 2000D,
the rhodium target resulted in higher FOM for all 5 cm and 7cm breasts. On the other
hand, in nearly all cases the FOM is a relatively weak function of changing kVp, with
few well-defined maxima.

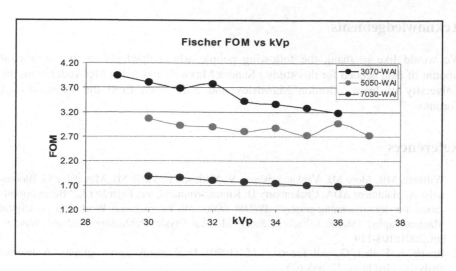

Fig. 8. Fischer : FOM vs. kVp, 5 cm

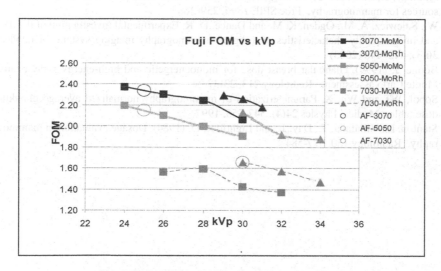

Fig. 9. Fuji : FOM vs. kVp, 5 cm (AF : AutoFilter)

These data suggest that the choice of target material and external filtration is more significant in determination of the overall FOM of a DM system than is choice of tube voltage. Figures 5 and 9 show the target/filter/kVp combination chosen by the Automatic Optimization of Parameters (AOP) and Autofilter systems of the GE Senographe 2000D and the mammography units used in testing the Fuji storage phosphor system. The selected techniques are indicated by the single, open symbols. As the figure shows, the technique factors selected by the AOP system are in most cases quite close to those that produced the highest FOM values in our study. A complete description of automated parameter selection performance across all manufacturers will be presented at the meeting.

Acknowledgements

We would like to thank the following people who helped obtain the significant amount of data needed for this study : Sandra Maxwell and Allen McGruder from the University of Iowa., Gordon Mawdsley and Sam Shen from the University of Toronto.

References

1. Williams MB, More MJ, Venkatakrishnan V, Niklason L, Yaffe MJ, Mawdsley G, Bloomquist A, Maidment ADA, Chakraborty D, Kimme-Smith C, and Fajardo LL. "Beam optimization for digital mammography". IWDM 2000: 5th International Workshop on Digital Mammography. (Martin J. Yaffe, Editor). Medical Physics Publishing. Madison, Wisconsin, 2001; 108-119
2. Boone, J., Shaber, G., and Tecotzky, M. (1990). Dual energy mammography: A detector analysis. Med.Phys. *17*, 665-675
3. Jennings, R.L., Quinn, P.W., Gagne, R.M., and Fewell, T.R. (1993). Evaluation of x-ray sources for mammography. Proc SPIE *1896*, 259-268
4. W., Sajewicz, A. M., Ogden, K. M. and Dance, D. R. Experimental investigation of the dose and image quality characteristics of a digital mammography imaging system. Med. Phys. **30**(3), 442–448 (2003)
5. Boone, J. (1999). Glandular breast dose for monoenergetic and high-energy x-ray beams: Monte Carlo assessment. Radiology 213, 23-37
6. Sobol, WT and Wu, X. Parameterization of mammography normalized average glandular dose tables. Medical Physics 24(4), 547-555. 1997
7. Stanton, L., Villafana, T., Day, J., and Lightfoot, D. (1984). Dosage evaluation in mammography. Radiology 150, 577-584

Image Qualities of Phase-Contrast Mammography

Chika Honda, Hiromu Ohara, and Tomonori Gido

R&D Center, Konica Minolta M&G Inc.,
2970 Ishikawa-machi, Hachiouji-shi,
Tokyo 192-8505, Japan
{chika.Honda, hiromu.oohara, tomonori.gido}@konicaminlota.jp
http://www.konicaminlta.com

Abstract. A digital full-filed mammography system using phase-contrast technique has been developed. The system consists of a dedicated mammography unit, a computed radiography unit with a sampling rate of 43.75 microns, and a photothermographic printer with a printing rate of 25 microns for photothermographic film with the maximum optical density of 4.0. The sharpness of the output image is improved with an edge effect due to phase contrast and magnification. The image noise is reduced by an air-gap method with no bucky. In this paper, the image qualities of the phase-contrast mammography are described for full-filed mammography and spot-compression at 1.5x magnification.

1 Introduction

In 1895, Röntgen discovered an x ray, however, the wave nature has been out of attention in x-ray medical imaging till 1991 when Somenkov and co-workers reported that refraction of x rays can increase contrast of x-ray images [1] ; this is "phase-contrast imaging". The principle of phase-contrast imaging is illustrated in Fig.1.

The phase-contrast imaging has been intensively studied employing x rays from synchrotron and micro-focus x-ray tubes in 1990's, and realized recently in mammography for clinical use. Utilization of this technique in full-field digital mammography is attempted for a goal to improve the image quality so as to be equal to or better than that of screen/film (SF) mammography. It has been reported that the phase-contrast mammography (PCM) system provides better detectability of micro-calcifications and masses in diagnostic images than SF mammography [2] .

Using the PCM system, we empirically assessed improvement of image-sharpness with an edge effect due to phase contrast, and magnification for full-filed mammography and spot compression at 1.5x magnification. Additionally, the image noises were measured for full-filed digital phase-contrast mammography comparing with conventional contact digital mammography.

Susan M. Astley et al. (Eds.): IWDM 2006, LNCS 4046, pp. 281–288, 2006.

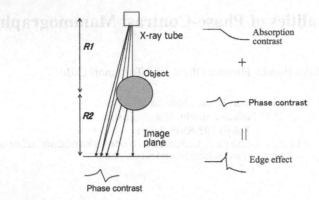

Fig. 1. Edge effect takes places with superimposition of phase contrast on an absorption contrast image. Note that the image plane should be away from the object in phase-contrast imaging.

2   Method

2.1   PCM System

The PCM system consists of a mammography unit, a computed radiography (CR) unit, and a photothermographic printer as shown in Fig.2. The mammography unit for phase-contrast imaging has a nominal 100 μm focal spot in a configuration of a 0.65 m distance from the focal spot to the object holder (R_1) and 0.49 m for the distance from the object holder to the storage phosphor plate holder (R_2) with no anti-scatter x-ray grid. Because the phase-contrast imaging is set at 1.75x magnification for full-field mammography, the storage phosphor plate used was 14x17 inches in size. For spot compression at 1.5x magnification, R_1 is 0.43 m, and R_2 is 0.71 m, resulting in a magnification ratio of 2.65 in image-acquisition. Note that the distance of $R_1 + R_2$, SID, is 1.14 m, equal to that for full-field digital PCM.

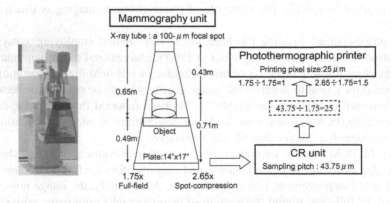

Fig. 2. Schematic diagram of a digital phase contrast mammography system

After phase-contrast imaging, the storage phosphor plate is scanned by a laser spot with a sampling rate of 43.75 μm in the CR unit. The size of the acquired image is reduced by 1.75x to the original object size for printing of full-filed mammography with a photothermographic printer, which printed the images with a printing rate of 25 μm on 8x10-inch dry films. The image magnified by 2.65x in acquisition is reduced also by 1.75x for1.5-magnified print image (2.65/1.75=1.5).

2.2 Experimental

The presampling modulation transfer function (MTF) was obtained from the Fourier transform of the line spread function (LSF), measured by 10-micron wide slit made of 2mm-thick tungsten slit mounted on the breast table for evaluation of increase of image-sharpness in magnification. The measurements of the LSF were performed at a 28kVp, Mo/Mo combination for contact mammography, 1.75x and 2.65x magnifications. LSF data were obtained using the angled-slit technique. The slit was slightly tilted to the cross line to the chest wall edge of the table.

In order to assess an edge effect due to phase contrast, a plastic fiber with an 8.5-mm diameter was radiographed for contact mammography, 1.75x magnification and 2.65x magnification. And then, x-ray intensity profiles for three images were obtained and analyzed with Fourier transformation. We obtained frequency responses indicating improvement of image sharpness by the edge effect due to phase contrast and by magnification.

One-dimensional noise power spectra (NPS) were measured from uniformly exposed images obtained with a 28kVp, Mo/Mo and 42mAs x-ray beam with 4-cm of added Lucite filtration mounted on the breast table. Contact mammography was performed with bucky, and PCM was without bucky.

3 Results

3.1 Increase of MTF Due to Magnification in the PCM System

In magnification, MTF value increases due to a rescaling effect [3] , and decreases with blur due to geometric unsharpness. The experimental results shown in Fig.3

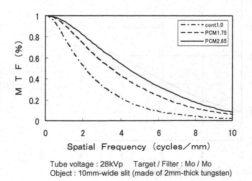

Tube voltage : 28kVp   Target / Filter : Mo / Mo
Object : 10mm-wide slit (made of 2mm-thick tungsten)

Fig. 3. PresamplingMTF'sfor digital contact mammography, 1.75x and 2.65x magnification

suggest that the magnification by 1.75x and 2.65x improves image sharpness from contact imaging.

3.2 Assessment of Edge Effect Due to Phase Contrast

The signal intensity profiles of the images for a plastic tube are shown in Fig.4. The edge effect due to phase contrast is clearly observed in the x-ray profiles of both 1.75x and 2.65x magnified images, although the edge of the object image in contact imaging is rounded. The x-ray intensity profiles were Fourier transformed to frequency responses along spatial frequency. The ratios of frequency responses were obtained for 1.75x and 2.65x magnified images with division by frequency response of the contact image at each corresponding spatial frequency. The results shown in Fig. 5 suggest that the image sharpness increases along with spatial frequency due to the edge effect. Note that the increases in Fig.5 include the image sharpness due to re-scaling effect accompanied with geometric unsharpness in magnification.

Using the results shown in Fig.5 and the MTF values for contact mammography shown in Fig.3, improvement of image sharpness for PCM images of full-field

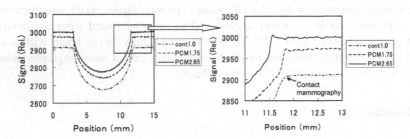

Fig. 4. X-ray intensity profiles of a 8.5-mm plastic fiber for contact mammography, and PCM at 1.75x and 2.65x magnification. The edge effect is clearlyobserved.

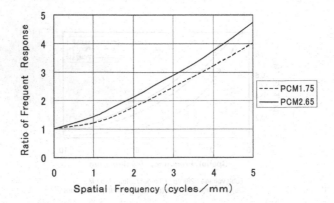

Fig. 5. Ratios of frequency responses for 1.75xand 2.65xphase contrast images on a conventional contact image for an tube

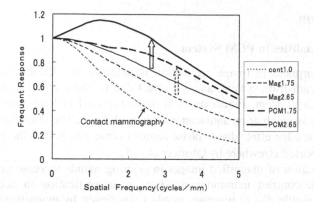

Fig. 6. Improvement of image sharpness by magnification and an edge effect due to phase contrast in magnification at 1.75x and 2.65x. The arrows indicate improvement of sharpness caused by the edge effect.

mammography and spot-magnification is illustrated in Fig.6. The edge effect due to phase contrast is conspicuous in the result for PCM 2.65, which exceeds over unity.

3.3 Image Noise

NPS's of contact mammography and PCM for full-field mammography at the same dose on breast table are shown in Fig. 7. The NPS for PCM is lower than the conventional contact mammography. Note that specifications of the photostimulable phosphor plate used here for contact CR and PCM are different to each other; i.e., design of MTF for PCM is lower than that for contact CR, and the NPS for PCM is lower than the contact CR.

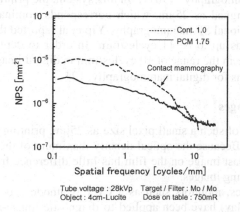

Tube voltage : 28kVp   Target / Filter : Mo / Mo
Object : 4cm-Lucite   Dose on table : 750mR

Fig. 7. NPS (Noise Power Spectra) for conventional contact mammography and full-field digital PCM

4 Discussion

4.1 Image Qualities in PCM System

The image sharpness in image acquisition is determined with three elements, i.e., MTF of the acquisition system, an edge effect due to phase contrast, and air-gap effect in the PCM system. Freedman et al. have reported that the air-gap eliminates scattered x ray as much as an anti-scatter x-ray grid [4] . The improvement of image sharpness of the edge effect due to phase contrast corresponds with the previous simulated result reported elsewhere by Ohara et al. [5] .

Demagnification of magnified images in printing avoids increase of image noise, although phase-contrast mammography here is magnification in acquisition 6 . Radiographic mottle due to quantum mottle is increased by magnification in the absence of concurrent increase of x-ray dose to an object because of the reduction in number for the x-ray photon hitting a unit area of the x-ray detector. It is easily understood that reduction of the magnified image to the original size of the object in printing would gain the increase of the mottle Additionally, the anti-scatter x-ray grid eliminates the primary x-ray so that image noise of contact mammography is higher than phase-contrast mammography without bucky.

4.2 Pixel Size in Output Images

Cowen et al. reported that the minimum detectable size of microcalcification in SF mammography is 200 µm after their literature review [7] , whereas the spatial resolution is one of the strengths of conventional SF mammography, because its spatial resolution is up to 20 cycles/mm, corresponding to a 25-µm pixel size in digital devices [8] . Higashida et al. reported that a pixel size of 100 µm in the detection of small microcalcifications will be problematic for CR mammography [9] . Improvement in the detection of subtle microcalcifications has been achieved with a 50-µm pixel size in CR mammography [10] . In this system, the printing rate in the output device has been designed as 25µm, which corresponds nominally with the spatial resolution of conventional SF mammography. Yip et al reported that spatial resolution of mammogram needs up to be 11 cycles/mm. In order to depict such fine images without aliasing noise in the range of 10 cycles/mm in digital images, the pixel size of 25 µm is advantageous for digital mammography [2] .

4.3 Hard Copy Images

In order to make use of such a small pixel size as 25µm, printing on dry-film is beneficial in this system. Because the optical density maximum of the film is designed up to 4.0, the digital breast image on the film has little difference from conventional SF breast images in reading images.

For thoracic images, monitors such as a CRT (Cathode Ray Tube) and an LCD (Liquid Crystal Display) have been applied to diagnostic image-reading for long. As seen in Fig.8, breast images should be depicted up to 11 cycles/mm [8] , and then for monitor reading of the breast images, new technologies in the monitors are required in addition to make the pixel-sizes smaller, although a pixel size of 150-200 µm for the monitors would be sufficient for reading of thoracic images.

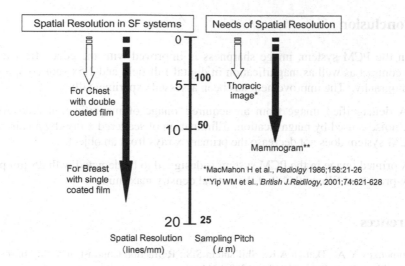

Fig. 8. Comparison of spatial resolution between thoracic imageand mammogram

4.4 Clinical Experiences

The PCM systems have been already installed in many medical facilities in Japan, and used for screening and examination of breast cancer. In the PCM system, phase-contrast imaging is magnification, however there is no further extension of exposure time than that for conventional SF systems. For example, the average exposure time for 249 exposures (Mo filter: 209, Rh filter: 40) a month in a hospital was 1.29 sec for the average compressed width of 37.2 mm. This average exposure time is shorter than the 1.38 sec for SF mammography which was reported as an average exposure time in a 1992 survey in the United States [11] . In the SF system, low-intensity reciprocal failure of silver halide materials causes the exposure time to be longer, especially beyond 2 sec for dense breasts [12] , whereas CR obeys the low-intensity reciprocity effect in the exposure time regions of seconds.

Because a 14"x17" plate is used with a sampling ratio at 43.75 μm, the data volume is 128 MB per exposure,i.e.,70 mega-pixels per image acquisition. The transfer of the image data in the full-field digital PCM system requires a period of time depending on the processing speed of the computer used; however, we do not suffer any delay in examination. An examination for one patient with four view images in mediolateral (MLO) and craniocaudal (CC) views takes 7-15 min with the full-field digital PCM system: the four shots for two MLO views and two CC views takes 4 min with the interval between patients being 3 min. As a result, to screen 200 patients, the time necessary would be about 2.5 h. This is an equivalent time to SF mammography.

The mammography unit of the PCM system seems that the bulky attachment for a phosphor plate under the object holder should be equipped, and would hinder positioning of patient' breasts for mammography in a CC view (Fig. 2). However, in our clinical experience, it has been revealed that a plastic protecting plate against the body of a patient helps the patient to relax by leaning on it in the CC-view position.

5 Conclusion

5-1. In the PCM system, image sharpness is improved with the edge effect due to phase contrast as well as magnification in digital full-field and 1.5x spot compression mammography. The improvement has been assessed experimentally.

5-2. A demagnified image from an acquired image of magnification recovers the image-noise caused by magnification. Elimination of scattered x rays by an air gap in the PCM system does not decrease the primary x rays from an object.

5-3. A printed image in the PCM system is designed to be depicted with 25-μm pixels on dry-processed film with 4.0 of the optical density maximum.

References

1. Somenkov V.A., Tkalich A.K., Shil'shtein S.S.: Refraction Contrast in X-Ray Introscopy. Sov. Phys. Tech. Phys. 36 (1991)1309-1311
2. Tanaka T., Honda C., Matsuo S. et al.: The First Trial of Phase Contrast Imaging for Digital Full-Field Mammography Using a Practical Molybdenum X-ray Tube. Invest. Radiol. 40 (2005)385-396
3. Shaw C.C., Lemack M.S., Rong J.X. et al.: Optimization MTF and DQE in magnification radiology – Theoretical analysis. Phys. Med. Imag. Proc.SPIE. 3977 (2000)466-475
4. Freedman M.T., B-Lo S.C., Honda C. et al.: Phase Contrast Mammography Using Molybdenum X-Ray: Clinical Implications in Detectability Improvement. Yaffe MJ, Antonuk LE (Ed.), Phys. Med. Imag. Proc.SPIE. 5030 (2003)533-540
5. Ohara H., Honda C., Ishisaka A. et al.: The improvement of x-ray image sharpness in x-ray phase imaging. Konica Minolta Tech. Rep. 1 (2004)131-134 (Japanese)
6. Funke M., Breiter N., Hermann K.P. et al.: Storage Phosphor Direct Magnification Mammography in Comparison with Conventional Screen-Film Mammography - a Phantom Study. Br. J. Radiol. 71 (1998)528-534
7. Cowen A.R., Launders J.H., Jadav M. et al.: Visibility of Microcalcifications in Computed and Screen-Film Mammography. Phys. Med. Bio. 42 (1997)1533-1548
8. Yip W.M., Pang S.Y., Yim W.S. et al.: ROC Curve Analysis of Lesion Detectability on Phantoms: Comparison of Digital Spot Mammography with Conventional Spot Mammography. British J. Radiol. 74 (2001)621-628
9. Higasida Y., Moribe N., Morita K et al.: Detection of Subtle Microcalcifications: Comparison of Computed Radiography and Screen-Film Mammography. Radiology 183 (1992)483-486
10. Ideguchi T., Higashida Y., Kawaji Y. et al.: New CR System with Pixel Size of 50 μm for Digital Mammography: Physical Imaging Property and Detection of Subtle Microcalcifications." Radiation Medicine 22(2004)218-224
11. Conway B.J., Suleiman O.H., Rueter, F. et al: National survey of mammographic facilities in 1985, 1988, and 1992. Radiology, 191 (1994) 323-330.
12. Kimme-Smith C., Bassett L.W., Gold, R.H. et al: Increased radiation dose at mammography due to prolonged exposure, delayed processing, and increase film darkening. Radiology 178 (1991) 387-391

Application of the Multiple Image Radiography Method to Breast Imaging

Christopher Parham[1], Etta Pisano[1], Chad Livasy[2], Laura Faulconer[1],
Miles Wernick[3], Jovan Brankov[3], Miklos Kiss[4], Dean Connor[5],
Jeddy Chen[5], Ann Wu[5], Zhong Zhong[5], and Dean Chapman[6]

[1] Department of Radiology and Biomedical Engineering, UNC Biomedical Research
Imaging Center and UNC-Lineberger Comprehensive Cancer Center,
Chapel Hill, NC 27599, USA
[2] Department of Pathology and Lab Medicine, University of North Carolina,
Chapel Hill, NC 27599, USA
[3] Illinois Institute of Technology, Department of Electrical and Computer Engineering,
3301 South Dearborn Street, Chicago, IL 60616, USA
[4] Department of Medical Physics, University of Wisconsin, Madison,
Wisconsin 53706, USA
[5] National Synchrotron Light Source, Brookhaven National Laboratory,
Upton, NY 11973, USA
[6] Department of Anatomy and Cell Biology, University of Saskatchewan,
Saskatoon, SK S7N 5E5 Canada

Abstract. The Multiple Image Radiography (MIR) method is new imaging
modality that extends the capability of conventional absorption based
radiography by adding the additional contrast mechanisms of x-ray refraction
and ultra-small angle scatter. In order to design a clinically based MIR system,
the MIR specific x-ray properties in breast tissue must be analyzed to determine
which are diagnostically useful. Developing MIR as an imaging modality also
requires developing new phantoms that incorporate x-ray refraction and ultra-
small angle scatter in addition to traditional x-ray absorption. Three breast
cancer specimens were imaged using MIR to demonstrate its MIR specific x-
ray properties. An uncompressed anthropomorphic breast phantom with an
imbedded low absorption contrast acrylic sphere was imaged to provide a
physical model of how the unique properties of MIR can be utilized to improve
upon conventional mammography and illustrate how these can be used to
design a clinically useful imaging system.

1   Introduction

The Multiple Image Radiography (MIR) method is a new imaging modality able to
generate images based on an object's x-ray absorption, refraction, and ultra-small
angle scatter [1, 2]. MIR is an improvement of a previously described method called
Diffraction Enhanced Imaging (DEI) [3-11]. DEI utilizes the Bragg peak of perfect
crystal diffraction to convert angular changes into intensity changes, providing a large
change in intensity for a small change in angle. The use of DEI for breast imaging

was first described by Pisano et al [12], and has been shown in multiple subsequent studies to generate improved contrast when compared to conventional radiography[13-15]. Previous studies investigating DEI specific contrast mechanisms in breast tissue have demonstrated considerable gains in contrast, up to 33 fold when compared to a conventional radiograph [16, 17]. MIR improves upon DEI by providing an ultra-small angle scatter image, produces more accurate absorption and refraction images, and has been shown to have good noise performance from photon limited data [2]. All DEI and MIR experiments to date have been performed using a synchrotron, which provides high flux x-rays over a wide energy range. The requirement of a monochromatic, collimated x-ray beam incident on the sample or object makes the design of a non-synchrotron based DEI or MIR system an engineering challenge. Initial studies using MIR with photon-limited data indicates that this method would be useful when using non-synchrotron x-ray sources.

2 Multiple Image Radiography

A detailed mathematical description of the MIR method has been presented previously by Wernick et al [1, 2]. MIR uses the reflectivity curve of a silicon analyzer crystal, presented in Figure 1, to generate parametric images representing the x-ray absorption, refraction, and ultra-small angle scatter of an object. For example, if the intrinsic rocking curve of a background region is used as a reference, then changes that decrease the area under the curve can be interpreted as x-ray absorption since photon absorption will decrease the maximum intensity. For a purely refractive event, the centroid of the rocking curve will be shifted, but the width and height of the rocking curve will remain constant. Interactions that lead to ultra-small angle scattering will scatter photons across the angular distribution of the rocking curve, causing the rocking curve to widen. Assuming that photons are not scattered outside the acceptance window of the rocking curve, scattering events will not affect the area under the curve. MIR analyzes these events and calculates the contributions of each on a pixel by pixel basis, producing three separate images from the same data set.

3 Experimental DEI Setup at the National Synchrotron Light Source

Experiments were carried out using the X15A beamline at the National Synchrotron Light Source (NSLS), Brookhaven National Laboratory, Upton, New York. A complete description of the DEI system at the NSLS has been previously described by Zhong et al [18]. In order to understand the parameters being analyzed, a brief description of the system is in order. The bending magnet source at the X15A beamline produces high flux x-rays from 10 to 60 keV. A double crystal silicon monochromator is used to select a particular energy from the incident x-ray beam. MIR images are obtained by placing a silicon analyzer crystal behind the object which is tuned to select a particular angle. The analyzer can be thought of as an angular notch filter with a resolution on the order of tenths of microradians, which facilitates the measurement of x-ray refraction and ultra-small angle scatter. Individual images are obtained by scanning the analyzer over a given angular distribution, and those images are used to generate parametric images representing the object's x-ray absorption, refraction, and ultra-small angle scatter. The width of the rocking curve changes with beam energy, so both the angular range and sampling distribution must be adjusted accordingly.

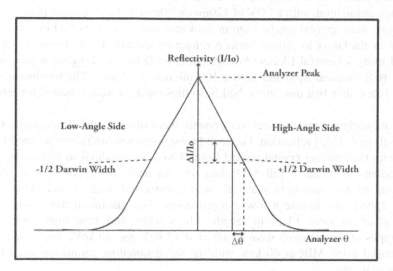

Fig. 1. Graphical depiction of an analyzer crystal rocking curve showing a large change in intensity for a given change in angle

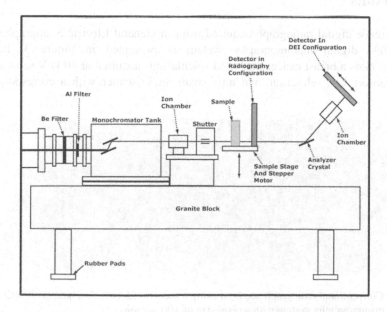

Fig. 2. Experimental setup at the X15A beamline, National Synchrotron Light Source (NSLS)

4 Methods

Three breast cancer specimens and one breast phantom were selected for imaging at the NSLS X15A beamline after receiving Institutional Review Board approval. A Photonic Science VHR-150 x-ray camera (Robersbridge, East Sussex, UK) was used for image acquisition, with a FOV of 120mm x 80mm and a 30 micron pixel size. The specimens were approximately 2 cm in thickness and were immersed in a water tank 4.5 cm in thickness to reduce surface refraction effects. Each specimen was also imaged using a General Electric Senographe 2000D full field digital mammography system (GE Medical Systems) with a 100 micron pixel size. The resolution of this system is less than that used at the NSLS, so these images were acquired for reference only.

The monochromator and analyzer crystals were tuned to the Bragg angle for the silicon 40 keV, [333] reflection. For each breast specimen (n=3), images (n=21) were taken with the analyzer crystal rotated from -4 to 4 microradians in increments of 0.4 microradians to obtain a full MIR data set. An anthropomorphic breast phantom composed of fat equivalent materials was constructed with an imbedded 3.0mm acrylic sphere to simulate a low contrast mass. The maximum dimensions of the breast phantom were 13cm in length, 11cm wide, and 6cm high. Synchrotron radiographs of the phantom were acquired at 18 keV and 40 keV. The phantom was also imaged using MIR at 40 keV with the same sampling parameters used for the breast specimens.

5 Results

A reference digital radiograph acquired using a General Electric Senographe 2000D full field digital mammography system is presented in Figure 3. Figure 4 demonstrates a breast cancer mass and spiculations acquired at 40 keV separated into x-ray absorption, refraction, and ultra-small angle scatter with a corresponding 40

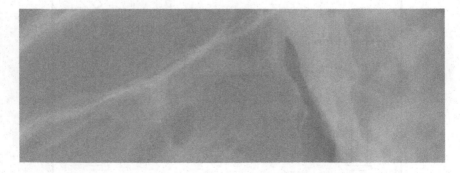

Fig. 3. Conventional radiograph acquired using a General Electric Senographe 2000D full field digital mammography system with a pixel size of 100 microns

keV synchrotron radiograph. Figures 5 and 6 illustrate an anthropomorphic breast phantom imaged both at conventional mammography energies of 18 keV and at 40 keV. The ability to visualize a low absorption contrast 3.0mm acrylic sphere simulating a mass is demonstrated in Figure 7.

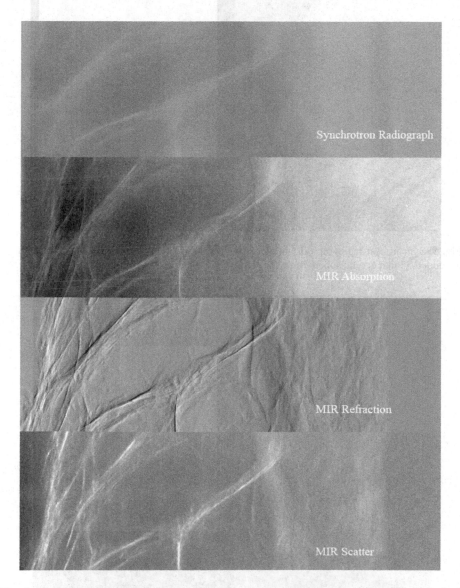

Fig. 4. Multiple Image Radiography analysis of a breast cancer mass and spiculations acquired at 40 keV with an angular sampling range of -4 to 4 microradians and theta increment of 0.4 microradians. A corresponding 40 keV synchrotron radiograph is provided for comparison. Contrast was adjusted to maximize visualization of the mass and spiculations in each image.

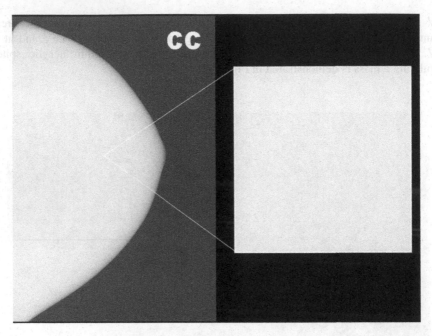

Fig. 5. Synchrotron radiograph of an uncompressed anthropomorphic breast phantom with an imbedded 3.0mm acrylic sphere imaged at 18 keV

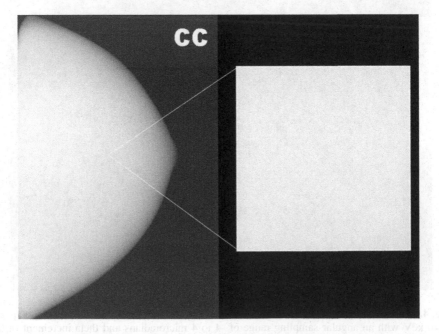

Fig. 6. Synchrotron radiograph of an uncompressed anthropomorphic breast phantom with an imbedded 3.0mm acrylic sphere imaged at 40 keV

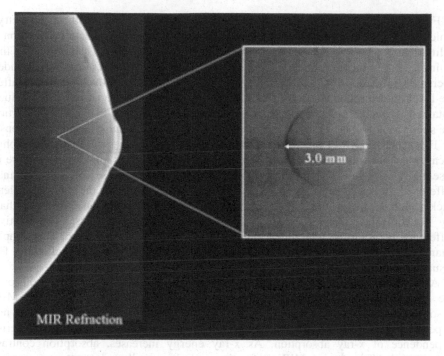

Fig. 7. Multiple Image Radiography refraction image acquired at 40 keV demonstrating visualization of a 3.0mm acrylic sphere

6 Discussion

One fundamental limitation of conventional mammography is the difficulty in visualizing low contrast objects immersed in highly absorbing background of adipose tissue. In conventional radiography, neoplastic lesions increase in size and density with time, eventually becoming large and dense enough to attenuate enough photons to be visualized against the surrounding adipose tissue. Since breast cancer mortality is directly related to the size and progression of a lesion, reducing the time between the generation of a malignant lesion and detection is a goal of all new breast imaging modalities.

MIR improves upon conventional radiography by utilizing multiple x-ray contrast mechanisms to help differentiate between benign and malignant structures. Adipose tissue may have an x-ray attenuation similar to a small malignant lesion, but they do not have the same refraction signatures. Adipose tissue has very little refraction and ultra-small angle scatter contrast, but the small cylindrical speculations of a breast cancer lesion has high refraction and ultra-small angle scatter contrast. Breast cancer masses, as demonstrated in Figure 4, also generate considerable x-ray refraction and ultra-small angle scatter contrast. At 40 keV, absorption contrast in soft tissue is minimal, increasing the overall contrast gradient between the lesion of interest and the background tissue.

Further gains in refraction contrast for spiculations come from their geometry, which is ideal for the refraction of x-rays. For a collimated x-ray beam incident on a cylindrical object, refraction contrast will be the greatest at the top and bottom of the cylinder, with minimal refraction contrast at the center. As the diameter of a cylinder decreases, refraction contrast will remain due to the geometry of the object, even after the level of absorption contrast fades into the background. Index of refraction values obtained across multiple breast cancer specimens indicates that the material properties are similar, and the increase in contrast should be observed in most cancer specimens.

The same properties are demonstrated using an uncompressed anthropomorphic breast phantom with a low contrast 3.0mm acrylic sphere. This low contrast sphere is essentially invisible using conventional radiography because of the nominal difference in x-ray attenuation of the sphere in relation to the fat equivalent background. However, the refractive properties of the sphere are much different than the fat equivalent material, which has very low refraction contrast. The relative difference between the two allows for excellent contrast of the sphere. This simple phantom illustrates the utility of MIR for breast imaging, potentially allowing for visualization of malignant structures at earlier stages of development.

A critical aspect of the breast specimens and breast phantom is the importance of the refraction and ultra-small angle scatter image in relation to both the MIR absorption image and the synchrotron radiographs. Refraction and scatter do not depend on the photoelectric effect, and thus do not suffer from the dramatic energy dependence of x-ray absorption. As x-ray energy increases, absorption contrast decreases as $1/E^3$, whereas MIR's refraction and ultra-small angle scattering contrast decreases by $1/E$. Primary utilization of x-ray refraction and ultra-small angle scatter for image contrast allows for the use of higher energy x-rays, decreasing the necessary photon flux and absorbed dose.

7 Conclusion

Multiple Image Radiography is a new imaging modality that could lead to significant improvements in breast imaging when compared to conventional radiography. The MIR experiments presented in this study demonstrate improved visualization in both breast cancer specimens and in refraction based imaging phantoms. The good noise performance of MIR from photon limited data combined with the ability to use higher x-ray energies for refraction and ultra-small angle scatter contrast makes this method promising for use in the development of a non-synchrotron based MIR breast imaging device.

Acknowledgement

This research, and the use of the X15A beamline at the National Synchrotron Light Source, Brookhaven National Laboratory was supported by the U.S. Department of Energy contract No. DE-AC02-98CH10886, by the Brookhaven National Laboratory LDRD 05-057, and by NIH grant R01 AR48292.

References

1. Wernick, M.N., Wirjadi, O., Chapman, D., Zhong, Z., Oltulu, O., Yang, Y.Y.: Preliminary investigation of a multiple-image radiography method. IEEE International Symposium on Biomedical Imaging (2002) 129-132
2. Wernick, M.N., Wirjadi, O., Chapman, D., Zhong, Z., Galatsanos, N.P., Yang, Y.Y., Brankov, J.G., Oltulu, O., Anastasio, M.A., Muehleman, C.: Multiple-image radiography. Physics in Medicine and Biology **48** (2003) 3875-3895
3. Ibison, M., Cheung, K.C., Siu, K., Hall, C.J., Lewis, R.A., Hufton, A., Wilkinson, S.J., Rogers, K.D., Round, A.: Diffraction-enhanced imaging at the UK synchrotron radiation source. Nuclear Instruments & Methods in Physics Research Section a-Accelerators Spectrometers Detectors and Associated Equipment **548** (2004) 181-186
4. Menk, R.H., Rigon, L., Arfelli, F.: Diffraction-enhanced X-ray medical imaging at the ELETTRA synchrotron light source. Nuclear Instruments & Methods in Physics Research Section a-Accelerators Spectrometers Detectors and Associated Equipment **548** (2004) 213-220
5. Chapman, D., Thomlinson, W., Johnston, R.E., Washburn, D., Pisano, E., Gmur, N., Zhong, Z., Menk, R., Arfelli, F., Sayers, D.: Diffraction enhanced x-ray imaging. Physics in Medicine and Biology **42** (1997) 2015-2025
6. Chapman, D., Pisano, E., Thomlinson, W., Zhong, Z., Johnson, R., Washburn, D., Sayers, D., Malinowska, K.: Medical Applications of Diffraction Enhanced Imaging. Breast Disease **10** (1998) 197-207
7. Dilmanian, F.A., Wu, X.Y., Parsons, E.C., Ren, B., Button, T.M., Chapman, L.D., Huang, X., Marcovici, S., Menk, R., Nickoloff, E.L., Petersen, M.J., Roque, C.T., Thomlinson, W.C., Zhong, Z.: The tomography beamline at the National Synchrotron Light Source. Physica Medica **13** (1997) 13-18
8. Kiss, M.Z., Sayers, D.E., Zhong, Z.: Measurement of image contrast using diffraction enhanced imaging. Physics in Medicine and Biology **48** (2003) 325-340
9. Pagot, E., Fiedler, S., Cloetens, P., Bravin, A., Coan, P., Fezzaa, K., Baruchel, J., Hartwig, J.: Quantitative comparison between two phase contrast techniques: diffraction enhanced imaging and phase propagation imaging. Physics in Medicine and Biology **50** (2005) 709-724
10. Bravin, A.: Exploiting the x-ray refraction contrast with an analyser: the state of the art. Journal of Physics D-Applied Physics **36** (2003) A24-A29
11. Lewis, R.A., Hall, C.J., Hufton, A.P., Arfelli, F., Evans, A.J., Evans, S.H.: X-ray diffraction-enhanced imaging (DEI). Radiology **221** (2001) 165-165
12. Pisano, E.D., Johnston, R.E., Chapman, D., Geradts, J., Iacocca, M.V., Livasy, C.A., Washburn, D.B., Sayers, D.E., Zhong, Z., Kiss, M.Z., Thomlinson, W.C.: Human breast cancer specimens: Diffraction-enhance imaging with histologic correlation - Improved conspicuity of lesion detail compared with digital radiography. Radiology **214** (2000) 895-901
13. Fiedler, S., Bravin, A., Keyrilainen, J., Fernandez, M., Suortti, P., Thomlinson, W., Tenhunen, M., Virkkunen, P., Karjalainen-Lindsberg, M.L.: Imaging lobular breast carcinoma: comparison of synchrotron radiation DEI-CT technique with clinical CT, mammography and histology. Physics in Medicine and Biology **49** (2004) 175-188
14. Kiss, M.Z., Sayers, D.E., Zhong, Z., Parham, C., Pisano, E.D.: Improved image contrast of calcifications in breast tissue specimens using diffraction enhanced imaging. Physics in Medicine and Biology **49** (2004) 3427-3439

15. Keryiläinen, J., Fernández, M., Fiedler, S., Bravin, A., Karjalainen-Lindsberg, M., Virkkunen, P., Elo, E., Tenhunen, M., Suortti, P., Thomlinson, W.: Visualization of calcifications and thin collagen strands in human breast tumour specimens by the diffraction-enhanced imaging technique: a comparison with conventional mammography and histology. European Journal of Radiology **53** (2005) 226-237
16. Hasnah, M.O., Zhong, Z., Oltulu, O., Pisano, E., Johnston, R.E., Sayers, D., Thomlinson, W., Chapman, D.: Diffraction enhanced imaging contrast mechanisms in breast cancer specimens. Medical Physics **29** (2002) 2216-2221
17. Hasnah, M.O., Parham, C., Pisano, E.D., Zhong, Z., Oltulu, O., Chapman, D.: Mass density images from the diffraction enhanced imaging technique. Medical Physics **32** (2005) 549-552
18. Zhong, Z., Thomlinson, W., Chapman, D., Sayers, D.: Implementation of diffraction-enhanced imaging experiments: at the NSLS and APS. Nuclear Instruments and Methods in Physics Research A **450** (2000) 556-567

Correlating Cone-Beam CT and Large-Section Histology Image Sets: Initial Results Using a Surgical Lumpectomy Specimen

James G. Mainprize[1], Shaista Okhai[1], Gina M. Clarke[1,2], Michael P. Kempston[1], Shawnee Eidt[1], and Martin J. Yaffe[1,2]

[1] Imaging Research, Sunnybrook Health Sciences Centre, 2075 Bayview Ave, Toronto, Ontario, Canada, M4N 3M5
[2] Department of Medical Biophysics, University of Toronto, Toronto, Canada

Abstract. Radiographic signs indicating the presence of a malignancy are a result of the morphology and composition of the lesion. Assessment of the size, distribution, extent and location of disease are crucial in guiding patient management. Often mammographic estimates of size and extent are underestimated. Radiologic/pathologic correlation between features is often by indirect classification methods rather than a direct, whole-volume, one-to-one spatial correlation between radiologic and pathologic images. As an initial step toward understanding how tumour morphology and composition yields a mammographic sign, we have begun work on correlating whole-mount histology sections to cone-beam computed tomography (CBCT) images of the same specimen. Preliminary results for a lumpectomy sample containing a 3.5 cm invasive ductal carcinoma qualitatively show a remarkable correspondence between CBCT slices and histology sections. Ultimately, the 3D CBCT data could be used to predict mammographic features, which could then be correlated precisely to the anatomy of the tumour.

1 Introduction

Mammography is used to detect lesions that are suspicious for cancer as well as to attempt to characterize those lesions and estimate the extent of disease. Unfortunately, limitations of the mammographic image frequently yield sub-optimal results. The mammographic assessment often underestimates disease extent and presence[1]. Often, the two-dimensional (2D) nature of mammographic images can lead to the appearance of areas of irregularity created by the overlap of normal breast structures[2]. As well, lesions may be hidden by the overlying or underlying tissue structures.. As a result, the radiological features in the 2D image can result in either false positives (mimicked lesions) or false negatives (hidden lesions).

Of important interest is the spatial correlation of the tumour to radiographic signs[3]. A better understanding of how different tumour morphologies and compositions lead to particular radiographic signs may improve assessment methods of the size, distribution, extent and location of disease that are crucial to guiding patient management.

Susan M. Astley et al. (Eds.): IWDM 2006, LNCS 4046, pp. 299–306, 2006.
© Springer-Verlag Berlin Heidelberg 2006

Extensive work has been done in correlating the radiographic signs (e.g. lesion margin, morphology, microcalcifications and architectural distortion) indirectly to the histopathologic findings (glandular differentiation, mitotic index, nuclear grade, architectural pattern)[4,5]. In general, these correlations are inferred at a classification level rather than by a whole-volume spatial correlation between radiologic and pathologic images. Direct visual correlation between the radiological and histological information is often very difficult.

Common clinical histopathology methods limit direct correlation between mammographic signs and tissue anatomy. Conformation of a lumpectomy is lost following excision. In our work we attempt to overcome this limitation by immobilizing the sample in a gel, thus approximating its *in vivo* conformation.

The second limitation to direct correlation of histology to radiographic appearance is the limited size of the tissue samples used to create a histology slide . A widely-used method developed by Egan [6] involves slicing the specimen, using radiographs of each slice to assist in determining tumour location and circumference, and then selecting *small* areas from each slice that include tumour, as well as some areas of normal tissue, for paraffin blocks. Only *parts* of the tumour and margin are excised, resulting in sampling of only a tiny fraction of the complete lesion volume. Without histological images of the entire lesion, it is not feasible to precisely correlate these images to radiographic data.

By trying to maintain the *in vivo* conformation and by imaging the intact resection with cone beam CT, a more accurate picture of the disease foci, the extent of disease, and the adequacy of the margin of resected normal tissue surrounding the disease, is obtained.

The first step toward direct spatial correlation of radiology and pathology is to implement a combined protocol that allows (near) complete characterization of the three-dimensional (3D) structure of an excised lesion through both radiographic and histological techniques.

To this end, we are currently developing methods in which the whole resected specimen is oriented spatially in a conformational gel and imaged with cone-beam computed tomography (CBCT) to obtain an x-ray volume dataset. The specimen is then cut into large slices, parallel to the CBCT images obtained, and prepared for histological staining of the entire lesion and surrounding breast tissue. Ultimately we believe this technique will improve our understanding of lesion architecture and our ability to optimize *in vivo* imaging.

2 Method

After obtaining institutional ethics review board approval, a lumpectomy sample with a 3.5 cm diameter node-negative invasive ductal carcinoma was obtained from a 47-year-old female.

Upon excision of the lumpectomy specimen, the lateral surface was marked with tissue-marking dye. To maintain spatial conformation, the specimen was immediately embedded in a 3.5% w/v agar gel.

Cone-beam CT images were acquired on a custom-built tabletop system (Fig. 1) consisting of a mammographic x-ray tube (GE DMR v. 2, GE Healthcare, Milwaukee,

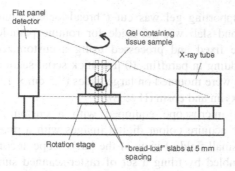

Fig. 1. Sketch of the cone-beam CT geometry layout (not to scale). An example of the locations of two bread-loaf slabs is shown, indicating that the slabs were cut parallel to the vertical axis of the system.

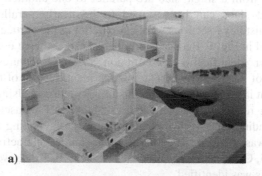

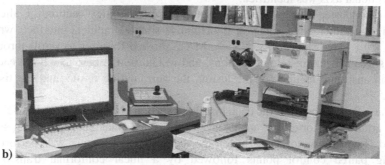

Fig. 2. a) Following CT imaging, the tissue sample embedded in agar was cut into 5mm-thick slabs (breadloafed). Alternate slabs were sent to clinical pathology for a routine work-up. b) The microscope with motorized stage and image display workstation.

WI) and a flat-panel imager (GE Senographe 2000D). An x-ray technique of 40 kV Rh target/Rh filter was used to obtain adequate penetration. Ninety-three (93) projection images were acquired at an interval of two degrees (2°). Reconstructed image volumes were set to a voxel size of $300{\times}600{\times}300$ μm^3 for a total volume size of $512{\times}288{\times}320$ voxels.

The agar-based supporting gel was cut ("bread-loafed") into 5 mm thick slabs (Fig. 2a). Every second slab was set aside for routine pathology processing. The remaining slabs were fixed and processed using a customized protocol[7]. After infiltration and embedding in paraffin, 10 μm thick serial sections were cut from the wax blocks. Sections were mounted on large slides (7.5 cm × 12.5 cm) and manually stained with haematoxylin and eosin (H & E).

A Zeiss Axiomat microscope equipped with a custom-built scanning stage (Fig. 2b) was used to acquire colour digital images with a pixel dimension of 1.87 μm. Because of the small field of view of the microscope, a composite image of the large slide was assembled by tiling a set of raster-scanned sub-images. The image acquisition software used was Clemex Lite v 3.5 (Clemex Technologies Inc, Montreal, Canada).

Alignment of the histology sections to the CT dataset was possible because all histology sections from a single slab are parallel to one another. Similarly, sections cut from different slabs can be assumed to be nearly parallel to one another. Additionally, the histology sections were cut parallel to the vertical axis of the CBCT system as indicated in Fig. 1. Because no fiducial markers were used, registration was performed by user identification of common anatomic features. The registration process consisted of 3 steps. The first step is the identification of the "cross-sectional axis" - the axis that is normal to all of the histology sections. Using a single histology section containing relatively distinct features, the CBCT dataset was reoriented to locate a corresponding slice with the same features. Navigating through the CBCT volume dataset was performed with an open-source interactive volume viewer (Microview 1.1.15, GE Healthcare). The axes of the CBCT data were rotated until the cross-sectional axis was identified.

The second step was to identify corresponding histology section/CT slice pairs through a user-interactive selection algorithm. A simple graphical interface, written in Matlab 7.0.1 (The Mathworks, Natick, MA), allowed the user to scroll through the CBCT slices and the histology sections, and to choose the best match for each slice based on anatomic features of the lesion, the surrounding tissue, and the tissue/gel margin.

Because the mounting of the each histology section is somewhat random, and some tearing artefacts distorted the appearance, a third and final 2D registration step was required. Registration of each histology section/CT slice pair was performed by selecting paired control points followed by a linear conformal transformation (translation, rotation and scaling) of the histology sections.

3 Results

The distortions in the specimen between the agar-embedding stage and the final slide preparation appear to be minimal. A total of 28 sections were cut, 22 of which contained the tumour. All of those with the tumour were imaged, as well as 3 of the sections without tumour. An example of one slide is shown in Fig. 3.

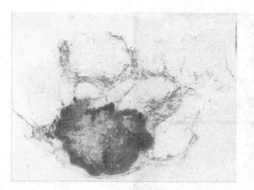

Fig. 3. Cross-section of a 3.5cm invasive ductal carcinoma of nuclear grade III. The irregular margins and radiating spicules of proliferating cells are characteristic of IDC.

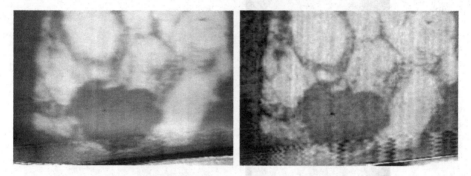

Fig. 4. Reconstruction slices through the lesion using an algebraic reconstruction technique (left) and filtered back-projection (right). The grey scale has been inverted to aide in comparison to the histology section in Fig. 3. The slices shown were manually aligned to the approximate orientation of the histology section in Fig. 3.

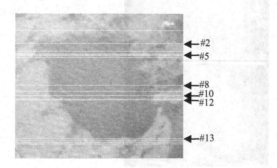

Fig. 5. A transverse slice (parallel to the rotation stage in Fig. 1) through the lesion showing the locations of 16 pathology slides (white lines). The numbered lines correspond to the slides in Fig. 6.

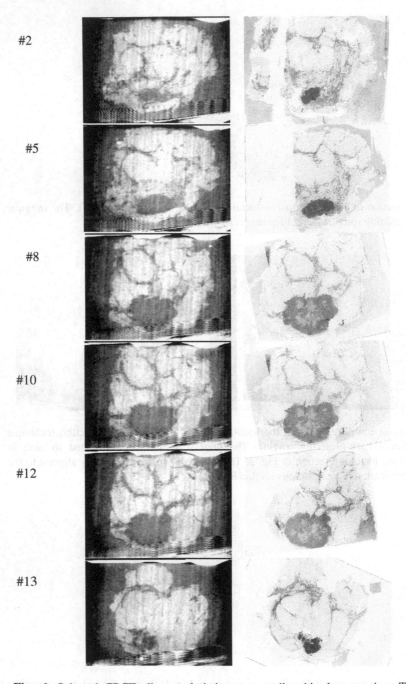

Fig. 6. Selected CBCT slices and their corresponding histology section. The histology sections were scaled, rotated and translated to align to the CBCT slices.

Tissue architecture and cellular details are well preserved using our method of large whole-mount tissue preparation. Adequate contrast between the darker, purple-coloured nuclei (haematoxylin stain), and the pink-coloured stroma (eosin counterstain), assists in comparing the histology images with the CBCT images. The irregularity of tumour cell proliferation is demonstrated by the large amounts of disorganized dark nuclei. Margin evaluation reveals a close posterior margin (Fig. 3). The architectural pattern and nuclear grade is indicative of a Grade III invasive ductal carcinoma (IDC).

The CBCT reconstructions show excellent fat and fibroglandular tissue contrast, and the lesion can be clearly delineated. The CBCT dataset was rotated and aligned to the histology sample based on the appearance of the tissue along the margins of the lesion (compare Fig. 3 and Fig. 4). Following rotation, the resampled CBCT data had voxel sizes of $320 \times 570 \times 300$ μm^3.

The irregular borders and high-density properties of the tumour mass are easy to identify; the spicules of dense tissue radiating from the mass into adjacent mammary tissue correlate well with the dark nuclear stained projections of infiltrating carcinoma seen in the histology image. Microcalcifications can be identified in several slices through the lesion (one is seen in the centre of the lesion in Fig. 4).

Sixteen histology section/CT slice pairs were aligned. Fig. 5 shows a transverse CBCT slice (perpendicular to the histology sections, and parallel to the rotation stage in Fig. 1) with lines indicating the location of each histology section. The two large gaps correspond to the slabs sent away for routine clinical pathology assessment. Fig. 6 shows six selected image pairs corresponding to those sections indicated in Fig. 5. Qualitatively, the margins of the lesion show strong correspondence between both modalities. The branching structure of normal fibroglandular tissue also appears to match well.

Shrinkage of the tissue sample was estimated by averaging the scale-factor calculated for each histological section in the third step (2D slice registration). Assuming uniform shrinkage, the linear dimensions of the lesion were reduced to 77% ± 2% of the original dimensions as captured in the CT dataset.

4   Discussion

As our initial results indicate, by successfully obtaining whole slices of the tissue for histological visualisation we are better able to correlate pathologic and radiologic features. Cellular detail is clearly seen, allowing pathologic classification to be carried out using the images.

It is possible that the fidelity of CT/histological correlation could be improved by implementing an additional 3D registration technique following the user-assisted registration. Future investigations will include the development of a robust fiducial marker. Use of a fiducial marker is highly desirable but problematic. Using a physical marker such as threads or suture inserted into the agar is currently not practical because this marker is dislodged when slabs are cut or processed. The marker may potentially damage the sectioning blade. Alternatively, injecting a tissue dye/radio-opaque solution, using a needle, in the agar surrounding the embedded tissue sample is promising, but potential problems include excessive dye diffusion (reducing localization) as well as tearing artefacts at the needle sites.

Our initial findings of positive correlation between the CBCT image slices and large histology sections are promising. Ongoing work in acquiring correlated CBCT and histology data from various tumour types will help build knowledge of the correlation between physiological and radiographical information. Furthermore, additional studies will involve simulating mammographic images obtained from the CBCT data providing further insight into the biology underlying the features observed on mammography.

References

1. Coombs, J.H., Hubbard, E., Hudson, K., Wunderlich, C., VanMeter, S., Bell, J.L., Gwin, J.L.: Ductal Carcinoma in Situ of the Breast: The correlation of pathologic and mammographic features with extent of disease. Am. Surg. 63 (1997) 1079-1083
2. Rafferty, E.A., Kopans, D.B., Wu, T., Moore, R.H.: Tomosynthesis: A new tool for breast cancer detection. Breast Cancer Res Treat 94 (2005) S2
3. Tot, T., Tabar, L., Dean, P.B.: The pressing need for better histologic-mammographic correlation of the many variations in normal breast anatomy. Virchows Arch. 437 (2000) 338-344
4. Nelson, T., Boone, J., Seibert, J., Kuhn, B., Kwan, A., Yang, K.: Visualization and identification of breast glandular tissue in breast CT volume data. Med Phys 32 (2005) 1897-1898
5. Feder, J.M., de Paredes, E.S., Hogge, J.P., Wilken, J.J.: Unusual breast lesions – A radiologic-pathologic correlation. Radiographics 19 (1999) S11-S26
6. Egan, R.L.: Multicentric breast carcinomas; clinical-radiographic-pathologic whole organ studies and 10-year survival. Cancer 49 (1982) 1123-1130
7. Clarke, G., Eidt, S., Peressotti, C., Zubovits, J., Mawdsley, G., Morgan, T., Rico, D., Yaffe, M.: Development of Three-Dimensional Digital Breast Histopathology Imaging. IWDM 2004 (2005) 484-489

Calcification Descriptor and Relevance Feedback Learning Algorithms for Content-Based Mammogram Retrieval

Chia-Hung Wei and Chang-Tsun Li

Department of Computer Science
University of Warwick
Coventry, CV4 7AL, United Kingdom
{rogerwei, ctli}@dcs.warwick.ac.uk

Abstract. In recent years a large number of digital mammograms have been generated in hospitals and breast screening centers. To assist diagnosis through indexing those mammogram databases, we proposed a content-based image retrieval framework along with a novel feature extraction technique for describing the degree of calcification phenomenon revealed in the mammograms and six relevance feedback learning algorithms, which fall in the category of *query point movement*, for improving system performance. The results show that the proposed system can reach a precision rate of 0.716 after five rounds of relevance feedback have been performed.

1 Introduction

Content-based image retrieval (CBIR) refers to the retrieval of images whose contents are similar to a query example, using information derived from the images themselves, rather then relying on accompanying text indices or external annotation [1]. One of the key challenges in CBIR is bridging the gap between low-level representations and high-level semantics. The semantic gap exists because low-level features are formulated in the system design process while high-level queries are used at the starting point of the retrieval process [2]. Relevance feedback is developed for bridging the semantic gap and improving the effectiveness of image retrieval systems [3]. With relevance feedback, CBIR systems can analyze the relevant images using a learning algorithm and return refined search results.

Content-based image retrieval has been proposed by the medical community for inclusion into picture archiving and communication systems (PACS) [4]. The idea of PACS is to integrate imaging modalities and interfaces with hospital and departmental information systems in order to manage the storage and distribution of images to radiologists, physicians, specialists, clinics, and imaging centres [5]. A crucial requirement of PACS is to provide an efficient search function for accessing images that are relevant to the query example. The contents of medical images provide useful information, which can be used to search for other images containing similar content.

In recent years an enormous number of digital mammograms have been generated in hospitals and breast screening centres. As hospitals and breast screening centres are

Susan M. Astley et al. (Eds.): IWDM 2006, LNCS 4046, pp. 307–314, 2006.
© Springer-Verlag Berlin Heidelberg 2006

connected together through PACS, content-based approaches can be applied to efficiently retrieve mammograms from distributed databases. However, content-based retrieval approaches are usually developed for specific contents of medical images. How existing retrieval approaches for other modalities can be effectively adopted for retrieving desired images from mammogram databases is not obvious. Given this motivation, along with a proposed general CBIR framework for the retrieval of mammograms with calcification phenomenon, this work develops a novel calcification detection method and six learning algorithms for coding the relevance feedback from the user.

2 Overview of the Proposed CBIR Framework

The proposed content-based retrieval framework as shown in Figure 1 can be divided into *off-line feature extraction* and *on-line image retrieval*. In the component of off-line feature extraction, the contents of the images in the database are extracted and described with a feature vector, also called a descriptor. The feature vectors of the images constitute a feature dataset stored in the database. In the component of on-line image retrieval, the user can submit a query example to the retrieval system to search for desired images. The system represents this example with a feature vector. The similarities between the feature vectors of the query example and those of the media in the feature dataset are then computed and ranked. Retrieval is conducted by applying an indexing scheme to provide an efficient way of searching the image database. Finally,

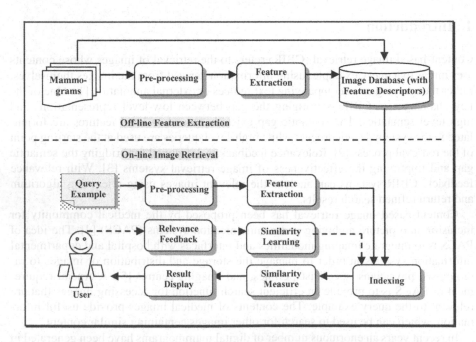

Fig. 1. The proposed framework for content-based mammogram retrieval

the system ranks the search results and returns the results that are most similar to the query example. If the user is not satisfied with the search results, the user can provide relevance feedback to the retrieval system in order to search further. To supply relevance feedback, the user simply identifies the positive image that is relevant to the query. The system subsequently recalculates the feature of the user's feedback using a learning algorithm and then returns refined results. This relevance feedback process can be iterated until the user is satisfied with the results or unwilling to offer any more feedbacks.

3   Pre-processing and Feature Extraction

A mammogram, like most medical images, usually contains a rich variety of information, including breast tissues, fat, and other noise. Calcifications are hard calcium deposits in breast tissues and are important clues of breast cancer revealed in mammograms [6]. Finding out the particular characteristics of calcifications is a key to effective extraction of calcification features in mammograms.

3.1   Pre-processing

The contrast between the areas of calcifications and their backgrounds is usually limited and, depending on the imaging equipments and the image capturing conditions, the dynamic range of gray scale of mammograms may vary significantly. To compensate these issues, we first perform histogram equalization on all the mammograms in the database. This pre-processing not only enhances the contrast but also normalize the gray scale of all the mammograms to the same dynamic range 0 to 255, smoothing way for feature extraction.

3.2   Calcification Detection

It is observed that calcifications usually appear as spots which are the brightest areas when compared to the other breast tissues, three spot detectors, D_1 - D_3 as shown in Figure 2, are applied to detect calcified spots of different sizes. Since the calcified spots are usually brighter than the backgrounds, to make good use of this *a priori* information so as not to pick up noise and misleading information, before the detector are applied, we first threshold the mammograms with the threshold T defined in Equation (1) as

$$T = \alpha \cdot \mu + (1 - \alpha) \cdot M \qquad (1)$$

where μ and M are the mean and maximal gray scales of the mammogram and α determines where between the mean and maximum the threshold T should lie. In this work we set α to 0.5, i.e., we take the average of the mean and maximum as the threshold. Since the mammograms have all been histogram equalized, M is always equal to 255. The spot detectors will skip those pixels with their gray scale lower than the threshold T by setting their corresponding responses to 0. Denoting the (i, j)th pixel of a mammogram g as $g(i, j)$, the response $r(i, j)$ of $g(i, j)$ to the kth spot detector D_k can be defined as

$$r(i,j) = \begin{cases} 0 & ,\text{if } g(i,j) < T \\ \sum_{x=1}^{X_k} \sum_{y=1}^{Y_k} D_k(x,y) \cdot g(i+x,j+y) & ,\text{if } g(i,j) \geq T \end{cases} \qquad (2)$$

where X_k and Y_k are the numbers of rows and columns of spot detector D_k. The strength of the response at each pixel is taken as the degree of calcification at that pixel. The effect of the thresholding is clearly shown in Figure 3. Figure 3(a) is an original mammogram before pre-processing (i.e., histogram equalization). Figure 3(b) shows the response map of the pre-processed mammogram to the spot detector D_1 without thresholding while Figure 3(b) illustrates the response map of the mammogram with thresholding. By comparing Figure 3(b) and (c), we can see that most of the non-useful information has been filtered out by the thresholding operation.

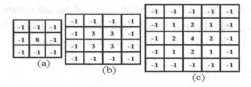

Fig. 2. (a) Detector D_1; (b) Detector D_2; (c) Detector D_3

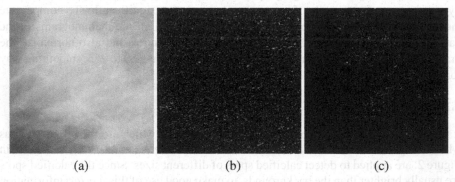

(a)   (b)   (c)

Fig. 3. (a) The original image. (b) Response map resulted from convolving *D1* with the histogram equalized mammogram *without* thresholding; (c) Response map resulted from convolving *D1* with the histogram equalized mammogram *with* thresholding.

3.3 Feature Extraction

Since the retrieval process is to be operated by comparing the features at image level rather than at pixel level, with the response (degree of calcification) at each pixel calculated, a feature describing the whole image has to be formulated as a function of responses of the pixels. Taking into account the facts that the brightest spots in the mammogram are most likely to be the position where calcification occurs and response to the spot detectors more strongly and that there are still some spurious and lower responses picked up (see Figure 3(c)), for each of the three response maps created by applying the three spot detectors to the mammogram according to Equation (2), we take the mean of the top 0.05% pixel responses as the calcification degree at image level and denote them as f_1, f_2 and f_3. The Euclidean distance f of the three calcification degrees as formulated in Equation (3) is then taken as the feature to describe the degree of calcification for the mammogram.

$$f = \sqrt{\sum_{j=1}^{3} f_j^2} \tag{3}$$

All the mammograms in the database are subjected to this feature extraction process in an off-line manner as shown in the upper part of the proposed framework in Figure 1.

4 Learning Algorithms in Relevance Feedback

According to the proposed framework in Figure 1, when a new query example/ mammogram is presented to the system, feature as formulated previously is extracted in real-time and submitted to the indexing component in framework. According to the degree of feature similarity between the query example and the ones in the database, 25 most similar mammograms are retrieved. To increase the performance, the user is placed in a loop to provide the system relevance feedbacks for further search. The idea of *query point movement* as shown in Figure 4 is adopted to move the point of the refined query toward the region in the feature space that contains the relevant images specified by the user. From Figure 4, we can see that by moving from the feature point of the original query example $q(1)$ to the refined/recalculated point $q(2)$ in the feature space, the system get closer to the center of the region containing more relevant images and less irrelevant ones, wherein the chance of retrieving more relevant images is higher.

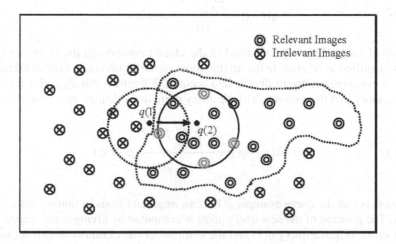

Fig. 4. The boundary of the region containing images which are relevant to the query example $q(1)$ is delineated by dotted line. As the blue points are identified as relevant images, the original query $q(1)$ will move to the ideal point $q(2)$, the centroid of the blue points.

Since *relevance* is somewhat subjective and, to some extent, user-dependent, the ways relevance feedback are incorporated is therefore worth investigating. In this work we propose six different algorithms, *LA1* to *LA6*, to learn the relevance feedbacks from the user in each round of the search and to determine the new query point for the next retrieval. To provide relevance feedbacks after being presented with the retrieved images of tth round of search, the user is allowed to identify an arbitrary number $n(t)$ of images as *relevant*. Let us denote the feature of the *pseudo query* to be used in the tth round of search by $q(t)$, $t >= 1$ and the feature of the kth image identified as relevant in the tth round of search by $f(t, k)$. So $q(1)$ is the feature of the original query example - a physical image. Apart from $q(1)$, *all the feature $q(t)$ is just a point, which does not correspond to any physical image*, in the feature space. This explains why we use the phrase 'pseudo query' earlier. The six proposed learning algorithms for calculating the refined pseudo query point $q(t+1)$ in the feature space can be described as follows.

$$LA1: \qquad q(t+1) = \frac{q(1) + \sum_{i=1}^{t}\sum_{j=1}^{n(i)} f(i, j)}{1 + \sum_{i=1}^{t} n(i)}, \quad t \geq 1 \tag{4}$$

With *LA1*, the new query point is calculated as the centroid of the clusters comprising the feature of the original query example and the features of those images identified as relevant in all the previous rounds. The characteristics of this algorithm are that all feedbacks are accumulated and taken into account and the influence of $q(1)$ diminishes as the retrieval process proceeds further and the size of the cluster increases.

$$LA2: \qquad q(t+1) = \frac{\sum_{j=1}^{n(t)} f(t, j)}{n(t)}, \quad t \geq 1 \tag{5}$$

The idea of *LA2* is to use the centroid of the cluster comprising the features of those images identified as relevant in the tth (the most recent) round only without taking $q(1)$ and the previous relevance feedbacks into account. Therefore, this algorithm has a very short 'memory' and the movement of the query point in the feature space can be radical.

$$LA3: \qquad q(t+1) = \frac{1}{2}q(1) + \frac{1}{2}\frac{\sum_{i=1}^{t}\sum_{j=1}^{n(i)} f(i, j)}{\sum_{i=1}^{t} n(i)}, \quad t \geq 1 \tag{6}$$

LA3 assumes that the query example $q(1)$ is an important basis in finding other similar images. The position of the new query point is computed by giving equal weight to the feature of the original query $q(1)$ and the centroid of the clusters comprising the features of those images identified as relevant in all the previous rounds of search.

$$LA4: \qquad q(t+1) = \frac{1}{2}q(1) + \frac{1}{2}\frac{\sum_{j=1}^{n(t)} f(t, j)}{n(t)}, \quad t \geq 1 \tag{7}$$

LA4 also recognizes the same importance of the query example $q(1)$. The position of the new query point is computed by giving equal weight to the feature of the original query $q(1)$ and the centroid of the features of the relevant images identified in the tth round of search. Note that the importance of $q(1)$ in both *LA3* and *LA4* remains constant (50%) throughout the retrieval process.

$$\text{LA5:} \qquad q(t+1) = e^{-\alpha t} \cdot q(1) + (1 - e^{-\alpha t}) \cdot \frac{\sum\limits_{i=1}^{t} \sum\limits_{j=1}^{n(i)} f(i,j)}{\sum\limits_{i=1}^{t} n(i)}, \quad t \ge 1 \qquad (8)$$

By giving variable weights $e^{-\alpha t}$ and $(1 - e^{-\alpha t})$ to the two terms in Equation (8), *LA5* reduces the influence of $q(1)$ and increases the significance of the centroid of the cluster comprising the features of the relevant images identified in all the previous rounds of search as the retrieving process proceeds further. Parameter α determines the rate at which the influences of the two terms changes. In this work, we set it to 1.

$$\text{LA6:} \qquad q(t+1) = e^{-\alpha t} \cdot q(1) + (1 - e^{-\alpha t}) \cdot \frac{\sum\limits_{j=1}^{n(t)} f(t,j)}{n(t)}, \quad t \ge 1 \qquad (9)$$

By the same token, *LA6* reduces the influence of $q(1)$ and increases the significance of the centroid of the clusters comprising the features of those relevant images identified in the tth round of search only.

5 Performance Evaluation

We have developed an interface of the proposed CBIR system with an example search result. This system allows the user to provide relevance feedbacks by identifying the relevant images. For each search the system returns 25 images on one page. There are 1000 200×200-pixel images, each containing the Region Of Interest (ROI) of one mammogram, in our database. 250 of the images reveal calcification phenomenon

Table 1. Results of performance evaluation in terms of mean precision rate

Learning Algorithm	Mean Precision Rate				
	Round 1	Round 2	Round 3	Round 4	Round 5
LA1	0.2	0.2	0.384	0.432	0.54
LA2	0.216	0.208	0.368	0.432	0.536
LA3	0.22	0.352	0.424	0.488	0.616
LA4	0.168	0.28	0.36	0.488	0.624
LA5	0.25	0.372	0.542	0.57	0.648
LA6	0.25	0.36	0.472	0.65	0.716

while the other 750 do not. Five images with calcification phenomenon were used as query examples to retrieve other similar images. Five rounds of relevance feedback were conducted for each query example. This procedure was repeated for the six learning algorithms, respectively.

Table 1 showes the retrieval performance of the system in terms of *number of positive images* using the six learning algorithms and the five query images, respectively. It is observed that the better performance of *LA5* and *LA6* suggest that allowing the influence of the original /physical query to attenuate *exponentially* seems to be a better approach.

6 Conclusions

A content-based mammogram retrieval system is proposed in this work. The main contributions of this work are the development of a novel feature extraction technique for describing the degree of the calcification phenomenon revealed in the mammograms and the proposal and study of six relevance feedback learning algorithms, which fall in the category of *query point movement*. The performance evaluation has shown that the six proposed learning algorithms can significantly increase the precision of the retrieval system from 0.168 up to 0.716 through five rounds of relevance feedbacks. Although we observed through our preliminary experiments that allowing the influence of the original/physical query to attenuate *exponentially* as the retrieval process evolves, further investigation is still necessary before more informed conclusions can be drawn.

References

1. El-Naqa, I., Yang, Y., Galatsanos, N. P., Nishikawa, R. M., Wernick, M. N.: A similarity learning approach to content-based image retrieval: Application to digital mammography. IEEE Transactions on Medical Imaging, Vol. 23, No. 10 (2004) 1233-1244.
2. Lew, M.S., Sebe, N., Eakins, J.P.: Challenges of Image and Video Retrieval. Proceedings of the International Conference on Image and Video Retrieval, (2002) 1-6.
3. Wei, C.-H., Li, C.-T., Wilson, R.: A Content-Based Approach to Medical Image Database Retrieval. In: Ma, Z. M. (Ed): Database Modeling for Industrial Data Management, Hershey, PA: Idea Group Publishing (2006) 258 – 291.
4. Lehmann, T. M., Guld, M. O., Keysers, D, Deselaers, T., Schubert, H., Wein B. B., Spitzer, K.: Similarity of medical images computed from global feature vectors for content-based retrieval. Lecture Notes in Artificial Intelligence (2004) 989-995.
5. Huang, H. K.: PACS, image management, and imaging informatics. In: Feng, D., Siu, W. C., Zhang, H. J. (Eds.): Multimedia information retrieval and management: Technological fundamentals and applications, New York: Springer (2003) 347-365.
6. Sampat, M. P., Markey, M. K., Bovik, A C.: Computer-aided detection and diagnosis in mammography. In: Bovik, A. (Ed): Handbook of image and video processing, London: Elsevier Academic Press (2005) 1195-1217.

Clinical Optimization of Filters in Direct a-Se FFDM (Full Field Digital Mammography) System*

Nachiko Uchiyama [1], Noriyuki Moriyama [1], Mayumi Kitagawa[1],
Shiho Gomi[1], and Yuichi Nagai[2]

[1] 5-1-1, Tsukiji, Chuo-ku, Tokyo, Japan, 104-0045 Department of Cancer Screening,
Research Center for Cancer Screening, National Cancer Center
nuchiyam@ncc.go.jp
[2] Tsukiji, Chuo-ku, Tokyo, Japan, 104-0045 Department of Radiology, Research Center for
Cancer Screening, National Cancer Center

Abstract. We evaluated three combinations of filters (Mo/Mo, Mo/ Rh, and W /Rh) in direct a-Se FFDM system to optimize radiation dose clinically. We measured CNR (Contrast to Noise Ratio) as physical characteristics changing radiation dose and phantom thickness in clinical range. In 20, 30, 40, and 50mm PMMA phantoms, Mo / Mo showed the best performances. On the other hand, in 60 and 70 mm, W/Rh 30kV showed best performance. In addition, in 40 and 50mm PMMA phantoms, W/Rh 30kV showed the second best performance. In direct a-Se FFDM system, W/Rh was valuable in minimizing radiation dose.

1 Introduction

Direct a-Se FFDM (Full Field Digital mammography) systems have been acquired in the clinical field[1-6] and recently, new image acquisition techniques such as tomosynthesis and breast CT (Computed Tomography) have also been developed. However, image quality should be prioritized clinically with a limit of radiation dose. In this paper, we evaluated optimization of filters and kV in direct a-Se FFDM system through physical characterization analysis and contrast-detail analysis changing radiation dose and phantom thickness in clinical range in an effort to minimize radiation dose without losing image quality.

2 Methods

Three combinations of filters in direct a-Se FFDM system were available and the pixel pitch of the system was 70 microns. We measured CNR (Contrast to Noise Ratio) as physical characterizations changing radiation dose and phantom thickness in clinical range (1.0-3.0mGy as AGD (Averaged Glandular Dose)). Combinations of filters were Mo/Mo, Mo/Rh, and W/Rh. kV ranged from 24kV to 34kv. The thickness of PMMA phantom was from 20 to 70mm. CNR was measured in accordance

---

* This study was supported by SIEMENS AG, Germany and SIEMENS-Asahi, Japan (K.Otsuka).

Susan M. Astley et al. (Eds.): IWDM 2006, LNCS 4046, pp. 315–323, 2006.
© Springer-Verlag Berlin Heidelberg 2006

with EUREF (European Reference Organization for Quality Assured Breast Screening and Diagnostic Services) guidelines[6]. CNR formula was as follows:

$$CNR = \frac{mean\ pixel\ value\ (signal\ )-mean\ pixel\ value\ (\ background\ )}{\sqrt{\dfrac{SD\ (signal)^2 + SD\ (background)^2}{2}}}$$

We also conducted a contrast- detail analysis utilizing CDMAM phantom (type 3.4: University Medical Centre Nijmegen St Radbaud, Netherland) and PMMA phantom. The total thickness of PMMA phantom and CDMAM phantom were 30, 40, and 60mm and AGD were 1.0, 2.0, and 3.0mGy. Combinations of filters were Mo/Mo, Mo/ Rh, and W/Rh. kV ranged from 24kV to 34kv.Four observers (three radiological technologists and one radiologist) evaluated the images and contrast-detail curves were analyzed.

3 Results

CNR Analysis (Fig. 1, Fig. 2a, Fig. 3a, Fig. 4, Fig. 5a, Fig. 6)
In 20 and 30mm thickness, Mo/Mo 28kV showed the better performances compared to other combinations of filters and kV and secondarily, Mo/Mo 24kV and Mo/Mo

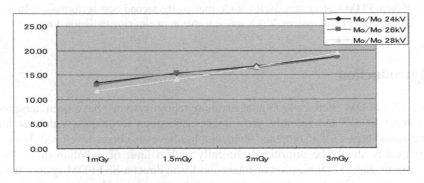

Fig. 1. CNR Analysis: 20mm Thick PMMA Phantom

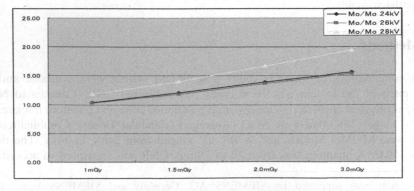

Fig. 2a. CNR Analysis: 30mm Thick PMMA Phantom

AGD 1mGy

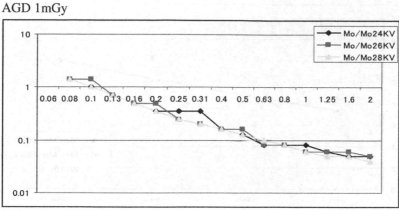

AGD2mGy

AGD 3mGy

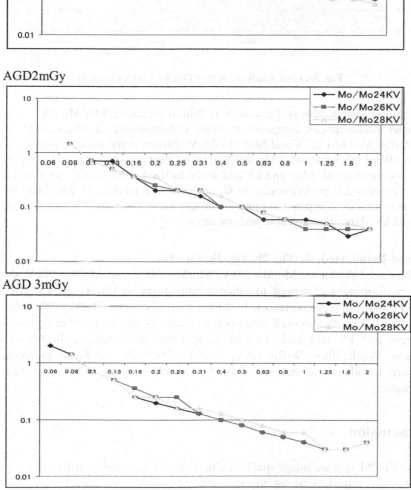

Fig. 2b. Contrast-Detail Analysis by CDMAM: 30mm Thick

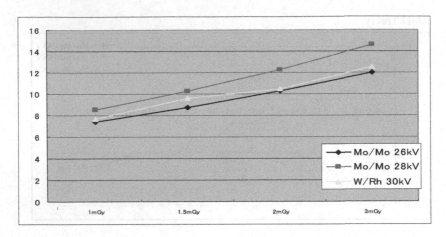

Fig. 3a. CNR Analysis: 40mm Thick PMMA Phantom

26kV showed comparable performances. In 30mm thickness, Mo/ Mo 28kV showed the better performances compared to other combinations of filters and kV and secondarily, Mo/ Mo 28kV and Mo/ Mo 26kV showed comparable performances. In 40 and 50mm thickness, Mo/ Mo 28kV showed best performance and compared to other combinations of filter and kV and secondarily, Mo/Mo 26kV and W/Rh 30kV showed comparable performances. In 60 and 70mm thickness, W/Rh 30kV showed better performance compared to other combinations of filter and kV and secondarily, W/Rh 32 kV showed comparable performances .

Contrast-Detail Analysis (Fig. 2b, Fig. 3b, Fig. 5b)
In 30mm total thickness, Mo/Mo 28kV, Mo/Mo 24kV and Mo/Mo 26kV showed better performances compared to other combinations of filters and kV and each showed comparable performances. In 40mm total thickness, Mo/Mo 28kV, Mo/Mo 26kV, and W/ Rh30kVshowed better performances compared to other combinations of filters and kV and each showed comparable performances. In 60mm total thickness, W/Rh 30kV, W/Rh 32kV, Mo/Mo 28kV showed better performances compared to other combinations of filters and kV and each showed comparable performances.

4 Discussion

In a-Se FFDM system, image qualities can differ in accordance with radiation dose and phantom thickness owing to characteristics of detectors and combinations of filters physiologically in CNR. In cases with relatively thin breasts, Mo/Mo 28kV showed the best performance on the other hand, in the case with relatively thick breasts, W/Rh 30 kV showed the best performance and W/Rh 32kVwould be the

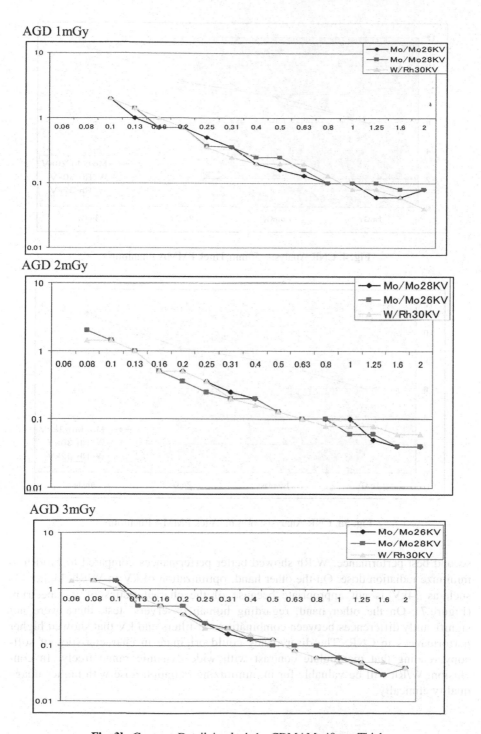

Fig. 3b. Contrast-Detail Analysis by CDMAM: 40mm Thick

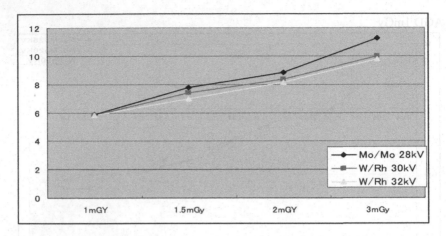

Fig. 4. CNR Analysis: 50mm Thick PMMA Phantom

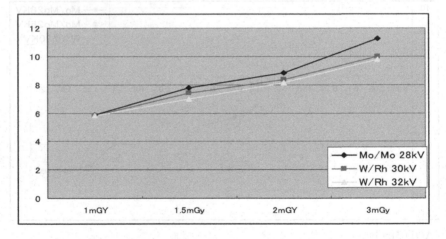

Fig. 5a. CNR Analysis: 60mm Thick PMMA Phantom

second best performance. W/Rh showed better performances compared to Mo/Rh to minimize radiation dose. On the other hand, optimization of kV in W/Rh, higher kV such as 34kV is not appropriate because of the characteristics of its spectrum (Figure.7). On the other hand, regarding human observers' test, there were not significantly differences between combinations of filters and kV that showed higher performances in CNR. The discrepancy could originate in characteristics of soft-copy reading that manipulate contrast with wide dynamic range freely. In con-clusion, W/Rh will be valuable for in minimizing radiation dose with higher image quality clinically.

AGD 1mGy

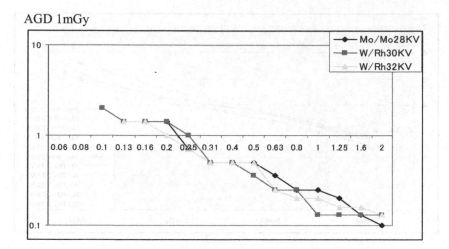

AGD 2mGy

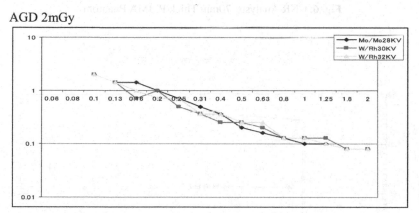

AGD 3mGy

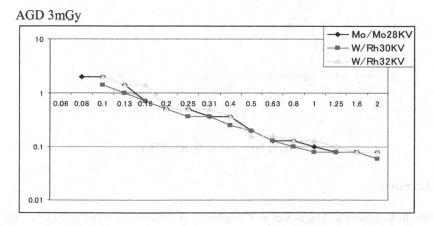

Fig. 5b. Contrast-Detail Analysis by CDMAM: 60mm Thick

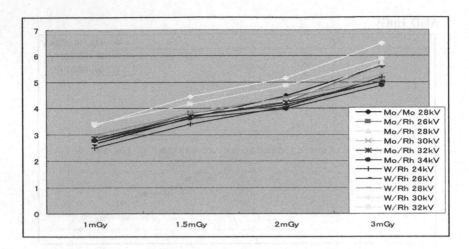

Fig. 6. CNR Analysis: 70mm Thick PMMA Phantom

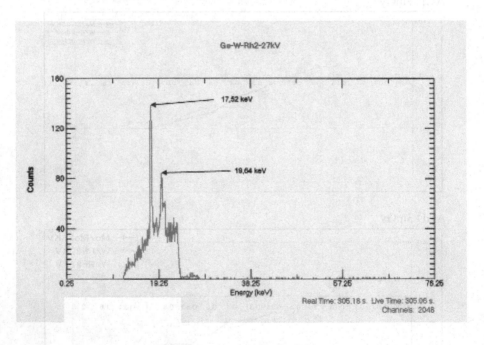

Fig. 7. Spectrum of W/Rh 27KV

References

1. Rivetti S, danielli C, Maggi S et al: Comparison of Different Commercial FFDM units by means of Physical Characterization and Contrast-Detail analysis. RSNA2004.
2. Lo J, Samei E, Jesneck J et al: Radiographic technique optimization for Amorphous Selenium FFDM System: Phantom and Patient Results. RSNA2004.

3. Schulz-Wendtland R, Wenkel E, Lell M, et al: Digital Luminance Mammography (CR) versus Full Field Digital Mammography: A Phantom Study. RSNA2004.
4. Alli K, Bloomquist, Sam Zhongmin Shen, Gordon Mawsley, Stewart Bright and Martin Yaffe: Acceptance Testing of digital Mammography Units for the ACRIN / DMIST Study. IWDM2002 85-89.
5. Saunders R. S., Samei E, Jesneck J. L. et al: Physical characterization of a prototype selenium-based full field digital mammography detector. Med. Phys. 32: 588-599, 2005.
6. The European protocol for the Quality Control of the physical and technical aspects of mammography screening; Addendum on Digital Mammography. version 1.0 November 2003. 19

Study on Cascade Classification in Abnormal Shadow Detection for Mammograms

Mitsutaka Nemoto[1], Akinobu Shimizu[1], Hidefumi Kobatake[1],
Hideya Takeo[2], and Shigeru Nawano[3]

[1] Tokyo University of Agriculture and Technology, Naka-cho 2-24-16, Koganei
184-8588 Tokyo, Japan
{nemo-m, simiz, kobatake}@tuat.ac.jp
[2] Kanagawa Institute of Technology, Shomo-ogino 798, Atsugi
243-0292 Kanagawa, Japan
takeo@ele.kanagawa-it.ac.jp
[3] National Cancer Center Hospital East, Kashiwanoha 6-5-1, Kashiwa
277-8577 Chiba, Japan
snawano@east.ncc.go.jp

Abstract. Classifier plays an important role in a system detecting abnormal shadows from mammograms. In this paper, we propose the novel classification system that cascades four weak classifiers and a classifier ensemble to improve both computational cost and classification accuracy. The first several weak classifiers eliminate a large number of false positives in a short time which are easy to distinguish from abnormal regions, and the final classifier ensemble focuses on the remaining candidate regions difficult to classify, which results in high accuracy. We also show the experimental results using 2,564 mammograms.

1 Introduction

Currently, breast cancer is one of the most serious cancers for women in the world and the amount of patients will increases year by year. Mammogram screening for breast cancer has become popular because it is effective in detecting breast cancer at an early stage. However, the burden on radiologists who have to deal with read a large number of mammograms in a very short time has increased tremendously. In order to decrease the burden, computer-aided diagnosis (CAD) systems have been developed. CAD systems for mammograms have the potential to be used as a second reader to increase the reliability of mass screening.

We have been developing the mammogram CAD systems [1]-[3]. For example, Kobatake *et al.* [1] proposed a tumor enhancement filter called "Iris filter" to boost the detection accuracy of faint tumors with low gradient of density. Furuya *et al.* [2] focused on the features for classification and selected the sub-optimal feature set from large feature database to discriminate abnormal shadows from normal tissues on mammograms. We also presented an improvement of the CAD system based on the classifier ensemble by AdaBoost combined with feature selection [3].

Susan M. Astley et al. (Eds.): IWDM 2006, LNCS 4046, pp. 324–331, 2006.

Recently a method for combining increasingly more complex classifiers in a "cascade" has been used for classification problem in the field of image pattern recognition. It allows false-positive regions on the image to be removed while spending more computation on regions to be detected. Viola *et al.* [4] applied the detection system with the cascade to the domain of face detection. However, there is no research report which introduces the cascade into mammographic mass detection system.

In this paper, we propose the novel classification system that has a cascade of four weak classifiers and one classifier ensemble trained by AdaBoost to improve classification accuracy. The weak classifiers eliminate a large number of false positive regions in a short time without removing any abnormal regions. And the final classifier ensemble analyses the details of remaining small number of the candidates difficult to classify, which takes time but achieves high accuracy.

2 Outline of the Proposed System

Fig.1 shows the flowchart of the proposed system. The details of each procedure are as follows.

1) Enhancement of tumors: First, the system enhances mass like regions by applying an adaptive ring filter [5] to the original mammogram. Here, the adaptive ring filter is a filter that evaluates to what degree the density gradient vector is concentrated to the point of interest. Consequently a circular convex region such as a mass is enhanced.
2) Extraction of suspicious regions: Next, it detects at most four local maximum points from the enhanced image. After, the boundary of each suspicious region (SR) is defined by SNAKES [6] in the neighborhood of each selected local maximum point on the enhanced image.
3) Cascade classification: This process consists of five layers of classifiers. Each of the first four layers (H_1~H_4) consists of a weak classifier and analyses the SRs to eliminate a large number of false SRs without removing SRs corresponding to true lesions. In the last layer (H_5), remaining SRs are analyzed by a ensemble of nine weak classifiers trained by AdaBoost with feature selection [3]. Here, all weak classifiers in the proposed system are based on the Mahalanobis distance D_i from an input feature vector x to an average vector of class i, which is defined as follows:

$$D_i = (x - m_i)^T \Sigma_i^{-1}(x - m_i)$$
(1)

where m_i and Σ_i are the average vector and the covariance matrix of the feature vectors of class i, respectively. The classification process calculates following ratio γ of two distances:

$$\gamma = \frac{D_{normal}}{D_{abnormal}}$$
(2)

If the ratio is greater than threshold T, the SR is classified as an abnormal mass region. And others are classified as normal shadows.

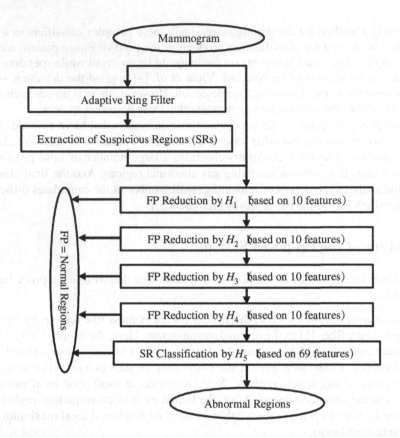

Fig. 1. Outline of the proposed abnormal shadow detection system. Note that the eliminated SRs by upper layers will not be analyzed by the subsequent layers.

Each weak classifier of all layers employs 10 features which are selected based on "plus 4–take away 3" algorithm [7] from the large scale feature database including over 1,000 features. The database consists of 25 shape based features, 960 density features, and other 23 features. So the total number of features is 1,008 [8]. The shape based features are composed of circularity, spreadness, area of SR, and other statistical values which relate to distance from a geometry center of SR to its boundary. The density features have 4 categories; the first order statistical values of density (e.g. mean, variance, entropy, etc) the second order statistical features measured by using co-occurrence matrix, the contrast based features calculated according to the density values of inside and outside SRs or the density correlation between SR and artificial mass models, and others. These density features are calculated from original SRs and five kinds of SRs processed by Sobel filter and Daubechies wavelet.

The "plus 4–take away 3" algorithm applies sequential forward selection four times followed by three steps of sequential backward selection and repeats the cycle of forward and backward selection until the required number of features is obtained. In this study, features used in the first four layers are selected so that the specificity is minimized when the true positive rate is 100.0%. And the feature sets used in the last layer are selected based on the area under ROC curve (Az).

3 Experimental Results

The performance of the proposed cascade classifiers was validated by use of a total of 10,092 SRs including 683 abnormal and 9,409 normal shadows. These SRs were extracted from 2,564 mammogram images whose size is 2,370×1,770 pixels with 0.1mm/pixel resolution and 10-bit accuracy. These mammograms were taken at the seven hospitals in Japan and the imaging system used are FCR-9000, FCR-5000, and FCR-AC3 of Fuji Photo Films Co., Ltd. The ground truth for the validation was determined by biopsy proven. Details of image database are shown in Table 1.

In these experiments, 10-fold cross validation methods was adopted to estimate errors, where dataset was divided in the ratio of 9 (for training) : 1 (for test) while preventing SRs of a patient from dividing into both training and test dataset. A computer with a 3.0 GHz Xeon processor and 3.5 GB memory was used in the experiments. The operating system was Windows XP Professional.

Table 2 and Fig. 2 present the comparison between classification accuracy of the proposed system and those of two classification systems each of which uses a classifier ensemble in order to vilify the cascade scheme. One of the systems for the comparison test has a classifier ensemble configured with nine weak classifiers where the number is the same as that of weak classifiers in H_5. Another system has a classifier ensemble consisting of 13 weak classifiers which is the same number as the total of weak classifier in the proposed system.

Comparing these classification systems, the proposed system in a cascade structure showed the best classification accuracy, where Az=0.972 and number of false positives (FPs) per mammogram=0.490 with 95% sensitivity. The FROC curve of the proposed (bold black curve in Fig. 2) is superior to other curves everywhere in the graph. After applying statistical test [9], [10], we found significant differences between the Az of the cascade system and those of two systems ($p<0.05$).

Table 1. Details of the mammogram database taken in the seven hospitals

Hospital	Number of patients	Number of images	Number of abnormal masses
Hospital A	51	112	38
Hospital B	252	1008	229
Hospital C	88	200	79
Hospital D	125	308	115
Hospital E	183	436	154
Hospital F	50	268	52
Hospital G	67	232	56
Total	816	2564	723

Table 2. Classification accuracies of the three systems (Az and number of false positives (FPs) per image)

	Az	sensitivity=0.80	FPs/image 0.90	0.95
cascade scheme	0.972±0.005	0.157±0.049	0.293±0.074	0.490±0.119
9 classifiers ensemble	0.962±0.008	0.205±0.081	0.390±0.109	0.662±0.173
13 classifiers ensemble	0.966±0.007	0.174±0.067	0.342±0.097	0.588±0.131

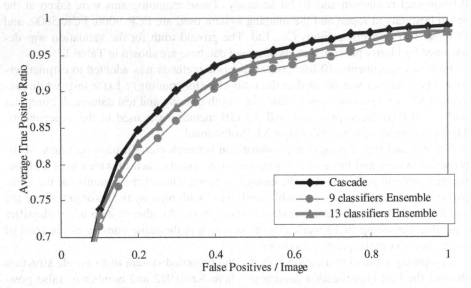

Fig. 2. FROC curves of the three classification systems. Each plot in this figure shows an average of the true positive ratios by 10 fold cross validation computed at each number of false positives.

The most powerful reason why the proposed classification system presents the best accuracy is that a large number of FPs were eliminated by the first four layers (H_1~H_4) of the cascade process. In this experiment, the first four layers could remove 466.3 FPs on average (from 1009.2 to 542.9) without removing SRs corresponding to true lesions. The result by each layer is summarized in Table 3 and examples of the removed FPs are shown on Fig. 3. Due to the reduction of the FPs, the last layer (H_5) could focus on the remaining SRs which included true positives and about half of the FPs detected by the extraction process. Consequently diversity of the FPs was greatly reduced, which resulted in high accuracy of the classification process. For further discussion, we computed the correlation coefficients between the output from the proposed system and those of the two systems used in the comparison test. The correlations were 0.545 and 0.555 respectively, while the correlation between the two systems was 0.994. The result told us that the proposed cascade classifier had different characteristic from the two classifiers, because of the difference in the training images for ensemble learning.

Table 3. Simulated computational cost and actual comutation time

(a) Proposed system

layers	#(features)	#(SRs)	simulated cost*	actual cost (sec.)	
H_1	10	1009.2	$10092.0a$	236.6	
H_2	10	751.6	$7516.0a$	263.6	
H_3	10	674.9	$6794.0a$	129.9	
H_4	9	591.9	$5327.1a$	86.5	
H_5	65	542.9	$35288.5a$	796.7	
Total	104		$64972.6a$	1513.3	= 5.90scc./image

(b) Two systems for comparison test

#(classifiers)	#(features)	#(SRs)	simulated cost*	actual cost (sec.)	
9	67	1009.2	$67616.4a$	1844.2	= 7.19sec./image
13	89	1009.2	$89818.8a$	1850.9	= 7.22sec./image

*simulated cost = #(feature) $\times$ #(SRs) $\times$ a(= average computation cost for one feature)

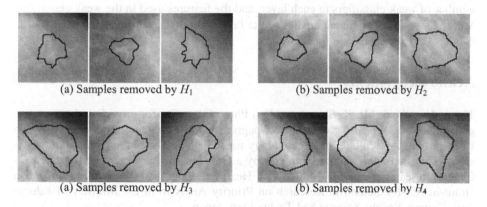

(a) Samples removed by H_1 (b) Samples removed by H_2

(a) Samples removed by H_3 (b) Samples removed by H_4

Fig. 3. Examples of removed FPs by each layer of the proposed cascade process

In the proposed cascade system, some SRs were analyzed by all layers and all of the 104 features in 13 classifiers were computed for them. We have simulated the computational cost of the three systems in the Table 3, where the average computation cost for calculating a feature was denoted by a. From this table, we found that the proposed cascade achieved the lowest computational amount among them, because about half of the SRs (456.3) were eliminated by the first four weak classifiers whose costs were low. To confirm the findings, we also measured the actual calculation time of features used in the systems. The results are also shown in the rightmost column in the Table 3 and we could see that proposed system by cascade scheme was the fastest system, where total computation time was 1513.3 seconds (5.90 sec/image). The difference between the simulated computational cost and actual cost is due to the variance of the computational costs of features.

4 Conclusion

In this paper, we proposed the novel abnormal shadow detection system from mammograms which has a cascade of four classifiers and a classifier ensemble to improve the classification performance. Experimental results with 10-fold cross validation showed that the classification performance by the proposed system was superior to that of the system which consists of classifier ensemble. The average Az was 0.972, and average number of false positive was 0.490/image when the true positive fraction was fixed at 95 %. The Az value of the proposed system was significantly larger than those of the two systems which consist of an ensemble used in the comparison test ($p<0.05$). A positive reason for the good result is the effective reduction of false positives without removing any true lesions. Consequently the last layer focused on the classification of the remaining SRs, which resulted in high accuracy. In addition, we found the proposed system had the smallest computation cost among the three systems evaluated in the comparison test.

In future studies, we plan to modify the weak classifier learning process to improve the system performance and we will optimize the number of layers in the cascade, the number of weak classifiers in each layer, and the features used in the weak classifiers. Moreover analysis of characteristics of the false positives and validation using a large database are also remained for future.

Acknowledgements

The authors thank Mr. K. Shimura of Fuji Photo Films Co. for providing the mammogram database. We also thank our colleagues in the Shimizu Laboratory of Tokyo University of Agriculture and Technology for their many helpful advices and discussions. This study was supported in part by a Grant-in-Aid for Scientific Research for Cancer Research from the Ministry of Health, Labour and Welfare, Japan and a Grant-in-Aid for Scientific Research on Priority Areas from the Ministry of Education, Culture, Sports, Science and Technology, Japan.

References

1. H. Kobatake, M. Murakami, H. Takeo, S. Nawano.: Computerized detection of malignant tumor on mammograms, IEEE Trans. Med. Imag., Vol. 18, No. 5, (1999) 369-378
2. S. Furuya, J. Wei, Y. Hagihara, A. Shimizu, H. Kobatake, S. Nawano.: Improvement of performance to discriminate malignant tumors from normal tissue on mammograms by feature selection and evaluation of feature selection criteria, *Syst. and Comp. in Japan*, vol. 35, no. 5, (2004) 72-84
3. M. Nemoto, A. Shimizu, H. Kobatake, H. Takeo, S. Nawano.: Classifier ensemble for mammography CAD system combining feature selection with ensemble learning, in Proc. 19th CARS, (2005) 1047-1051
4. P. Viola, M. Jones.: Rapid object detection using a boosted cascade of a simple feature, IEEE Computer Society Conf. on Computer Vision and Pattern Recognition (CVPR), vol.1, (2001) 511-518

5. J. Wei, Y. Hagihara, H. Kobatake.: Detection of cancerous tumors on chest X-ray images – Candidate detection filter and its application, Proc. ICIP, no.27AP4.2, (1999)
6. M. Kass, A. Witkin, and D. Terzopoulos.: SNAKES: Active contour models, in Proc. 1st ICNN'87, (1987) 259-268
7. P. Pudli, F. J. Ferri, J. Novovicova, and J. Kittler.: Floating search methods for feature selection with nonmonotomic criterion functions, in *Proc. IEEE Int. Conf. on Pattern Recognition*, (1994), 279-283
8. M. Nemoto, A. Shimizu, Y. Hagihara, H. Kobatake, H. Takeo, S. Nawano.: Improvement of tumor detection performance in mammograms by feature selection from a large number of features and proposal of fast feature selection method, *Syst. and Comp. in Japan* (to appear)
9. J. L. Doppman, M. Girton, and M. Vermess.: The risk of hepatic artery embolization in the presence of obstructive jaundice, *Radiology*, vol. 143, (1982) 37-43
10. J. A. Hanley, and B. J. McNeil.: A method of comparing the areas under receiver operating characteristic curves derived from the same cases, *Radiology*, vol. 148, (1983) 839-843

Classifying Masses as Benign or Malignant Based on Co-occurrence Matrix Textures: A Comparison Study of Different Gray Level Quantizations

Gobert N. Lee, Takeshi Hara, and Hiroshi Fujita

Department of Intelligent Image Information, Division of Regeneration and
Advanced Medical Sciences, Graduate School of Medicine,
Gifu University, Gifu City, 501-1194, Japan

Abstract. In this paper, co-occurrence matrix based texture features
are used to classify masses as benign or malignant. As (digitized) mammograms have high depth resolution (4096 gray levels in this study)
and the size of a co-occurrence matrix depends on Q, the number of
gray levels used for image intensity (depth) quantization, computation
using co-occurrence matrices derived from mammograms can be expensive. Re-quantization using a lower value of Q is routinely performed
but the effect of such procedure has not been sufficiently investigated.
This paper investigates the effect of re-quantization using different Q.
Four feature pools are formed with features measured on co-occurrence
matrices with $Q \in \{400\}$, $Q \in \{100\}$, $Q \in \{50\}$ and $Q \in \{400, 100, 50\}$.
Classification results are obtained from each pool separately with the use
of a genetic algorithm and the Fisher's linear discriminant classifier. For
$Q \in \{400, 100, 50\}$, the best feature subsets selected by the genetic algorithm and of size $k = 6, 7, 8$ have a leave-one-out area under the receiver
operating characteristic (ROC) curve of 0.92, 0.93 and 0.94, respectively.
Pairwise comparisons of the area index show that the differences in classification results for $Q \in \{400, 100, 50\}$ and $Q \in \{50\}$ are significant
($p < 0.06$) for all k while that for $Q \in \{400, 100, 50\}$ and $Q \in \{400\}$ or
$Q \in \{100\}$ are not significant.

1 Background

In computer-aided breast cancer diagnosis, one of the major signs of abnormality
is the presence of masses. Benign masses tend to have well defined boundaries
and are usually circular or oval in shape while malignant masses tend to have
fuzzy boundaries and are irregular in shape. This results in the presentation
of different textures. The capability in quantifying these textures can be very
useful in discriminating a benign mass from a malignant mass. One of the popular
techniques in texture features extraction is based on co-occurrence matrix [5].

A co-occurrence matrix $P_{ij} = Prob(i, j|d, \theta)$ is the joint probability of two
pixels in an image at a distance d in a direction θ take on values i and j separately. The size of a co-occurrence matrix, however, does not depend on d

Susan M. Astley et al. (Eds.): IWDM 2006, LNCS 4046, pp. 332–339, 2006.

nor θ, but on Q, the number of gray levels used for image depth (intensity) quantization. This can be a problem for high depth resolution images such as mammograms as the derived co-occurrence matrices are large and, therefore, sparse. Statistics measures become meaningless and data storage and computation can be expensive. In order to reduce the size of a co-occurrence matrix, gray level re-quantization is routinely performed. However, the effect of gray level re-quantization on co-occurrence matrix based features has not been sufficiently investigated. The employment of Q values of 128 [2] and 256 [1] [10] have been reported in the literature. The decision on a proper Q value is complicated but is probably dependent on the nature of the images, the attributes of the features subsequently measured, the task of the measured features and others. This study aims to investigate the role of Q in a restricted scenario.

In this study, four feature pools are constructed. The first three feature pools include the same set of features measured on co-occurrence matrices derived with $Q \in \{400\}$, $Q \in \{100\}$, or $Q \in \{50\}$. The fourth feature pool is the union set of the first three feature pools, that is, $Q \in \{400, 100, 50\}$. The Q values investigated are based on values of Q reported in the literature and the desire of a low Q value as a high Q value leads to a large co-occurrence matrix. In addition to the co-occurrence matrix derived features, 12 energy features and 8 gradient features are also included in each of the four feature pools. A genetic algorithm [6] is used to select the best feature subsets from a feature pool for classifying masses as benign or malignant. The classification performances of the four feature pools are compared and the effect of different Q values is observed.

2 Method and Materials

2.1 Data

A data set of 71 screening mammograms was employed in this study. Of the 71 mammograms, 43 contain malignant masses and 28 contain benign masses. The mammograms were randomly selected from the archives. All the malignant masses were biopsy proven and the benign had a three years elapse time showing no sign of malignancy. The size of the malignant lesions ranges from less than 1 cm to about 2 to 3 cm. Only one mass from each woman was included in the database. In addition, a benign mass was included only if no malignant lesions were found in the same or contralateral mammogram.

The selected mammograms were digitized using a *Lumiscan 150* (Lumisys) laser digitizer with a 4096 gray levels image depth resolution and a 50 μm spatial resolution. All the selected mammograms were annotated by a radiologist experienced in mammography. According to the radiologist's annotation, regions-of-interest (ROIs) with a centered or near-centered mass were extracted. The size of the ROIs is, typically, 1024 $\times$ 1024 pixels at full spatial and depth resolutions.

2.2 Method

Texture features based on co-occurrence matrix and first-order statistics were derived from the central mass region and the mass border region. Details of the texture features extraction were reported previously [7]. For the completeness of this paper, a brief description of the features is included in the following.

2.2.1 Texture Features

For each mass, the mass border was defined using two methods, the threshold method (B_t) and the polygon method (B_p). For each version of the mass borders, an 80 pixels wide ribbon around the mass border was extracted. The rubber band straightening transform proposed by Sahiner et al.[11] was used to obtain a regular array from the ribbon. A number of half overlapping blocks of size 40×40 pixels were then defined on the transformed ribbon. For each block, co-occurrence matrices with parameters $\theta = 0, \pi/2$; $d = 11, 15, 21, 25, 31$ were constructed and the inverse difference moment (IDM)

$$IDM = \sum \sum_{|i-j|=h} \frac{1}{1+h^2} P(i,j),$$

where $h = 0, 1, 2, \ldots, Q-1$ was computed. For a fixed distance d, the histogram of IDM values for $\theta = 0$ and $\theta = \pi/2$ were generated separately and the first four moments (M_1, M_2, M_3 and M_4) of the two histograms account for eight features (40 features when all 5 distances $d = 11, 15, 21, 25, 31$ were considered). Finally, the 80 features (the above 40 features $\times$ 2 mass borders) were measured once on each group of co-occurrence matrices with a Q value of 400, 100, or 50.

For the comparison of the effect of different Q, four feature pools were constructed. The above 80 features measured on co-occurrence matrices with $Q = 400$, $Q = 100$ and $Q = 50$ contributed to the first three feature pools. The union set of the three feature pools contributed to the fourth feature pool. In addition to the co-occurrence matrix features, 12 energy based features and 8 gradient based features were measured on each mass. Each of the four feature pools were augmented by the same 20 additional features. A summary of the 260 features (240 co-occurrence matrix based and 20 additional features) is given in Table 1.

2.2.2 Feature Selection and Classifier

From each feature pool, a genetic algorithm [6] was employed to select the best k feature subset for masses classification where $k = 2, 3, \ldots, 12$. The genetic algorithm was designed to find the (sub)optimal feature subset of a given size k from a feature pool. The chromosome was defined as a sequence of natural numbers of length k, that is, the values of the genes were the feature indices. Initial population was set to be 1000. The fitness function was defined as the performance of a feature subset as indicated by the area under the receiver operating characteristic (ROC) curve [9]. In updating a generation, chromosomes with a fitness below average were replaced by new chromosomes created by two

Table 1. Summary of the 260 features. Table entries are feature indices. Each co-occurrence matrix feature is specified by 5 parameters: Q, d, θ, M_x and B_t or B_p (Section 2.2).

12 energy features					8 gradient features				
	M_1	M_2	M_3	M_4		M_1	M_2	M_3	M_4
Mass center (25 × 25)	1	2	3	4	radial	13	14	15	16
border region (7 × 21)	5	6	7	8	tangential	17	18	19	20
border region (21 × 7)	9	10	11	12					

240 Co-occurrence matrix based features										
			Border region by threshold method B_t				Border region by polygon method B_p			
Q	d	θ	M_1	M_2	M_3	M_4	M_1	M_2	M_3	M_4
400	31	0	21	22	23	24	29	30	31	32
		$\pi/2$	25	26	27	28	33	34	35	36
	25	0	37	38	39	40	45	46	47	48
		$\pi/2$	41	42	43	44	49	50	51	52
	21	0	53	54	55	56	61	62	63	64
		$\pi/2$	57	58	59	60	65	66	67	68
	15	0	69	70	71	72	77	78	79	80
		$\pi/2$	73	74	75	76	81	82	83	84
	11	0	85	86	87	88	93	94	95	96
		$\pi/2$	89	90	91	92	97	98	99	100
100	31	0	101	102	103	104	109	110	111	112
		$\pi/2$	105	106	107	108	113	114	115	116
	25	0	117	118	119	120	125	126	127	128
		$\pi/2$	121	122	123	124	129	130	131	132
	21	0	133	134	135	136	141	142	143	144
		$\pi/2$	137	138	139	140	145	146	147	148
	15	0	149	150	151	152	157	158	159	160
		$\pi/2$	153	154	155	156	161	162	163	164
	11	0	165	166	167	168	173	174	175	176
		$\pi/2$	169	170	171	172	177	178	179	180
50	31	0	181	182	183	184	189	190	191	192
		$\pi/2$	185	186	187	188	193	194	195	196
	25	0	197	198	199	200	205	206	207	208
		$\pi/2$	201	202	203	204	209	210	211	212
	21	0	213	214	215	216	221	222	223	224
		$\pi/2$	217	218	219	220	225	226	227	228
	15	0	229	230	231	232	237	238	239	240
		$\pi/2$	233	234	235	236	241	242	243	244
	11	0	245	246	247	248	253	254	255	256
		$\pi/2$	249	250	251	252	257	258	259	260

chromosomes (parents) based on point cross-over. A mutation rate of 0.1 was set. The population was allowed to evolve for 500 generations and the (sub)optimal feature subset was given by the chromosome with the highest fitness score. A Fisher's linear discriminant function was then used as the classifier and the classification results were once again evaluated using the ROC methodology.

2.2.3 Statistical Significance Estimation

Note that for a fixed k value, many different combinations of k out of 100 (first 3 feature pools) or 260 (the fourth feature pool) were explored by the genetic algorithm. Due to this multiple testing scenario, the apparent superiority of the feature subset selected by the genetic algorithm could have been due to chance at work. Hence, statistical significance of the classification performances of the best feature sets was evaluated. For each fixed k value, the statistical significance was estimated by generating the empirical null distribution using the bootstrap resampling technique [8]. The empirical distribution consists of 500 data points. That is, 500 bootstrap samples were generated from the original data set of 71. Each bootstrap samples subsequently employed the genetic algorithm and the Fisher's linear discriminant function described in the above in arriving a sample classification score which makes up one data point of the bootstrap null distribution.

2.3   Area Under the ROC Curve: Nomenclature and Computation

The area under the ROC curve was used as a fitness measure in the genetic algorithm and a measure in evaluating the classification performance. The area was computed using the trapezoidal rule which is equivalent to the Wilcoxon statistics [3]. The symbol A_z, popular for reporting the area under the ROC curve calculated using a binormal distribution model, is not suitable in this study as non-parametric approach was used in computing the area. Throughout this paper, the symbol A_{roc} is used to refer to the area under the ROC curve, regardless of the technique used for the area estimation. Some of the A_{roc} values and their statistical analyses were computed using MedCalc for Windows, version 8.1.1.0 (MedCalc Software, Mariakerke, Belgium) and the ROCKIT software (Kurt Rossmann Lab., University of Chicago).

3   Results

3.1   Feature Subsets of Interest

As the optimal number of features, k, was not known *a priori* and the genetic algorithm was designed with a input parameter specifying the desired number of output features, a range of k was considered. Due to the relatively small sample size, the range of k to be considered was capped at 12. Visual inspection of the 1-dimensional feature plots shows that each of the features alone does not have sufficient discriminative power. Hence, $k > 1$ was adopted. For a fixed k, many different combinations of k features were inspected by the genetic algorithm.

Only the fourth feature pool with $Q \in \{400, 100, 50\}$ was employed in this section as it contains all available features. Using the entire data set for both training and testing, the resubstitution A_{roc} guided the genetic algorithm in finding the (sub)optimal feature subset. Figure 1 shows both the resubstitution and the leave-one-out classification results for each of k where $k = 2, 3, \ldots, 12$. (Note that for a fixed k, the best resubstitution A_{roc} and the best leave-one-out A_{roc} do not necessarily originated from the same feature subset.) Statistical significance (Section 2.2) of the resubsitution A_{roc} values were calculated. All the resubstitution A_{roc} values were found significant at a 0.05 level and for $k >= 4$, the A_{roc} values were significant at a 0.01 level.

In opting for a best k or best range of k, feature subsets resulting in a high classification performance are desirable. However, caution must be taken that as the number of features increases, the classifier performance will increase up to a certain point. Beyond this point, further increase in the number of features will lead to a decrease in the classifier's performance. An examination of Figure 1 reveals that both the resubstitution and the leave-one-out A_{roc} have high values

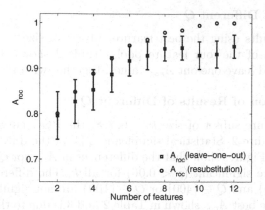

Fig. 1. A_{roc} values of the best feature subsets for a fixed number of features k. The feature subsets were selected by the genetic algorithm from the fourth feature pool ($Q \in \{400, 100, 50\}$). Error bars indicate one standard deviation.

Table 2. Classification results of the best feature subsets with size $k = 6, 7, 8$ from each of the four feature pools. *Note that for a fixed k, if the feature subset for the best resubstitution A_{roc} is not the same as that of the best leave-one-out A_{roc} scores, the two scores are entered in different rows and only the feature subset for the best leave-one-out A_{roc} is given.*

k	Best A_{roc} (resubstitution)	Best A_{roc} (Leave-one-out)	Feature subset associated with the best A_{roc} (Leave-one-out)
	\multicolumn{3}{l}{$Q \in \{400, 100, 50\}$, hence feature pool $\in \{1, \ldots, 260\}$ (see Table 1)}
6	0.950		
		0.918	55, 73, 109, 125, 171, 202
7	0.963		
		0.928	2,55,73,109,125,171,202
8	0.980	0.943	2,45,55,72,109,153, 169, 201
			or 2, 55, 72, 109, 125, 153, 169, 201
	\multicolumn{3}{l}{$Q \in \{400\}$, hence feature pool $\in \{1, \ldots, 100\}$ (see Table 1)}
6	0.926	0.883	12, 32, 55, 58, 75, 90
7	0.942	0.914	12, 32, 41, 42, 54, 60, 89
8	0.954		
		0.896	2, 3, 12, 30, 55, 58, 74, 90
			or 2, 3, 12, 31, 55, 58, 74, 90
	\multicolumn{3}{l}{$Q \in \{100\}$, hence feature pool $\in \{1, \ldots, 20, 101, \ldots, 180\}$ (see Table 1)}
6	0.932		
		0.884	2, 6, 109, 121, 125, 135
7	0.948	0.906	109, 121, 125, 128, 136, 154, 171
8	0.958	0.916	109, 110, 121, 125, 127, 135, 155, 172
	\multicolumn{3}{l}{$Q \in \{50\}$, hence feature pool $\in \{1, \ldots, 20, 181, \ldots, 260\}$ (see Table 1)}
6	0.913		
		0.860	13, 189, 202, 216, 235, 252
7	0.936	0.868	13, 192, 201, 216, 233, 245, 250
8	0.945	0.885	2, 6, 190, 197, 201, 206, 214, 255

(> 0.900) for $k >= 6$. However, for $k > 8$, the increase in A_{roc} is not significant. Hence, only the best feature subsets of size $k = 6, 7, 8$ are deemed to be of interest in this study. The feature subsets are given in Table 2 in the next Section.

3.2   Results of Different Q

Classification results using the best feature subsets of size $k = 6, 7, 8$ were obtained from each of the four feature pools. Table 2 shows the corresponding resubstitution and leave-one-out A_{roc} values, together with the feature subsets.

3.3   Comparison of Results of Different Q

For the best feature subset of size $k = 6, 7, 8$, the ROC curves of different Q are plotted in Figure 2. Statistical significances [4] of the difference in A_{roc} are given in Table 3. Figures show that the differences in A_{roc} for $Q \in \{400, 100, 50\}$ and $Q \in \{50\}$ are significant ($p < 0.06$) for all k. The differences in A_{roc} for $Q \in \{400, 100, 50\}$ and $Q \in \{400\}$ or $Q \in \{100\}$ are not significant. The slight discrepancy in the best A_{roc} shown in Table 2 and 3 is due to the use of different computation programs.

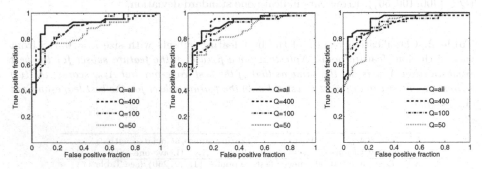

Fig. 2. ROC curves of different Q for the best feature subsets with k number of features. (Left) $k = 6$, (middle) $k = 7$ and (right) $k = 8$.

Table 3. Pairwise comparison of area under the ROC curves for $Q = 400$, $Q = 100$, $Q = 50$ and $Q = all$, i.e. $Q = 400, 100, 50$

k	Q	Best A_{roc} (leave-one-out)	ROC curves (pairwise comparison with Q =all)			
			Δ area	Standard error	95 % CI	p-value (one-tailed)
6	all	0.916				
	400	0.886	0.030	0.035	(-0.038, 0.098)	0.195
	100	0.885	0.032	0.031	(-0.028, 0.092)	0.152
	50	0.859	0.057	0.035	(-0.011, 0.126)	0.050
7	all	0.928				
	400	0.914	0.014	0.035	(-0.055, 0.084)	0.350
	100	0.905	0.022	0.025	(-0.027, 0.071)	0.185
	50	0.868	0.060	0.037	(-0.012, 0.132)	0.052
8	all	0.944				
	400	0.897	0.047	0.034	(-0.021, 0.114)	0.088
	100	0.917	0.027	0.023	(-0.019, 0.073)	0.128
	50	0.887	0.056	0.037	(-0.017, 0.129)	0.062

4 Conclusion

The results show that using 260 texture features, A_{roc} was found to be 0.92, 0.93 and 0.94 for the best feature subsets with 6, 7 and 8 number of features and $Q \in \{400, 100, 50\}$. Repeated trials with $Q \in \{400\}$, $Q \in \{100\}$ and $Q \in \{50\}$ all demonstrate a strictly lower A_{roc} for a given k. The differences in the classification results were found significant ($p < 0.06$) when using a single low Q value ($Q = 50$) for all number of features considered. For higher values of Q, the differences in the classification results were found not significant for all number of features considered. This result, in general, aligns with the Q values employed and reported in the literature.

Acknowledgments

This research was in part supported by a Grant-in-Aid for Scientific Research from the Ministry of Education, Culture, Sports, Science and Technology and a Grant-in-Aid for Cancer Research from the Ministry of Health, Labour and Welfare. The author GNL currently receives a Postdoctoral Fellowship from the Japan Society for the Promotion of Science.

References

1. Chan, H-P et al.: Phys. Med. Biol. **40** (1995) 857-876.
2. Gupta S. and Markey M.K.: Med. Phys.**32** (6) (2005) 1598-1606.
3. Hanley, J. A. and McNeil, B. J.: Radiology **143**(1) (1982) 29-36.
4. Hanley, J. A. and McNeil, B. J.: Radiology **148**(3) (1983) 839-843.
5. Haralick, R.M. et al.: IEEE Trans. Sys., Man, Cyb. **SMC-3**(6) (1973) 610-621.
6. Holland, J.: Adaptation in natural and artificial systems, MIT Press, (1975).
7. Lee, G. N. and Bottema M. J.: Proc. 5th IWDM (2001) 259-263.
8. Lee, G. N. and Bottema, M. J.: Proc. WDIM, APRS,(2003) 105-109.
9. Metz C.: Sem. Nucl. Med. **8** (1978) 283-298.
10. Mudigonda N.R. et al.: IEEE Trans. on Med. Img., **19**(10) (2000) 1032-1043.
11. Sahiner, S. et al.: Med. Phys. **25**(4) (1998) 516-526.

A Ranklet-Based CAD for Digital Mammography

Enrico Angelini[1], Renato Campanini[1], Emiro Iampieri[1], Nico Lanconelli[1],
Matteo Masotti[1], Todor Petkov[1], and Matteo Roffilli[2]

[1] Physics Department, University of Bologna, and INFN, Bologna,
Viale Berti-Pichat 6/2, 40127 Bologna, Italy
[2] Computer Science Department, University of Bologna,
Mura Anteo Zamboni 7, 40127 Bologna, Italy
nico.lanconelli@bo.infn.it

Abstract. A novel approach to the detection of masses and clustered microcalcification is presented. Lesion detection is considered as a two-class pattern recognition problem. In order to get an effective and stable representation, the detection scheme codifies the image by using a ranklet transform. The vectors of ranklet coefficients obtained are classified by means of an SVM classifier. Our approach has two main advantages. First it does not need any feature selected by the trainer. Second, it is quite stable, with respect to the image histogram. That allows us to tune the detection parameters in one database and use the trained CAD on other databases without needing any adjustment. In this paper, training is accomplished on images coming from different databases (both digitized and digital). Test results are calculated on images coming from a few FFDM Giotto Image MD clinical units. The sensitivity of our CAD system is about 85% with a false-positive rate of 0.5 marks per image.

1 Introduction

Two of the most frequent problems encountered in developing CAD systems for mammography are the following. First, the automatic detection of breast lesions can be hampered by the wide diversity of their shape, size and subtlety. Detection methods often rely on a feature extraction step: here, lesions are isolated by means of a set of characteristics. Due to the great variety of lesions, it is extremely difficult to get a common set of features effective for every kind of lesion. This is particularly true for masses, since they can vary considerably in optical density, shape, position, size and characteristics at the edge. A second difficulty arises from that the detection algorithms are often unstable, with respect to the dynamic range of the image histogram. As a matter of fact, the CAD algorithms have to be repeatedly tuned, when images coming from different systems are considered. A suitable Look Up Table (LUT) can accomplish a sort of "normalization" to the images before the CAD analysis. In this way, the same detection scheme can be applied to images coming from different detectors and acquired in different exposure conditions. Unfortunately, it is not so easy to gain a proper LUT, which can maximize the performance of the CAD for any acquisition condition.

Susan M. Astley et al. (Eds.): IWDM 2006, LNCS 4046, pp. 340–346, 2006.

In this paper, we present a detection system, which does not rely on any feature extraction step and which is stable with respect to the image histogram. The first attribute stems from using an SVM classifier, whilst the second derive from the ranklet representation. The algorithm automatically learns to detect the lesions by the examples presented to it. In this way, there is no *a priori* knowledge provided by the trainer: the only thing the system needs is a set of positive examples and a set of negative examples. The detection scheme codifies the image with a ranklet representation; the great amount of information handled by the algorithm is classified by means of a Support Vector Machine (SVM) classifier. SVMs have already been applied to CAD issues in mammography since 2001 [1]. An approach based on SVM classifier, without using extracted features, has been investigated both for masses and microcalcification detection [2,3,4]. Here, we present a novel use of ranklets, as an effective representation for the image crops to be classified. Ranklets are nonparametric, multiresolution and orientation selective features modeled on Haar wavelets first introduced in 2002 [5]. The first attempt to use ranklets as data representation for recognition problems was for face detection problems. Current comparative researches between wavelets and ranklets on CAD systems seem to demonstrate that ranklets are able to achieve better performances when applied to represents tumoral masses.

In this study, we validate our detection scheme with images coming from a few FFDM units: the systems used were "Giotto IMAGE MD" produced by IMS, Italy. They are based on amorphous Selenium flat panel digital detector manufactured by ANRAD Corporation, Canada. The active area of the imager is 17.4 cm × 23.9 cm with a pixel pitch of 85 micrometers; images have 2048 × 2816 pixels with 13 bit gray-level resolution. In order to have a large number of training images, we trained the CAD system both on digital images coming by the FFDM units and on digitized images coming the USF DDSM database available on the net [6].

2 Methods

The ranklet-based CAD is characterized by not requiring extracted features for detecting the breast lesions. The algorithm automatically extracts the needed information during the training phase. The CAD system has been trained to detect both clustered microcalcifications and masses. Figure 1 shows a chart of our detection scheme.

2.1 The Detection Scheme

The CAD detection scheme consists of two separate algorithms; one able to detect masses and another one for detecting clustered microcalcifications. The first step of the mass detection algorithm consists in a pre-selection of the suspect regions within the breast. This is achieved by means of adaptive local gray-level thresholding. All the selected pixels are then analyzed by an ensemble of three different experts. Each expert is able to accomplish a multiscale detection, in order to find out masses with size ranging from 3 mm to 35 mm. The searching performed by each expert is based on the SVM classification of the ranklet representation of all the crops centered on the pixels selected in the first step. Finally, a region is marked as suspect mass by using a *voting* strategy on the committee of the three experts. An ensemble of experts improves the overall performance of individual experts, if the individual experts commit mistakes on different objects. Basically, a region is considered suspect only if at least two of the three experts detect that region.

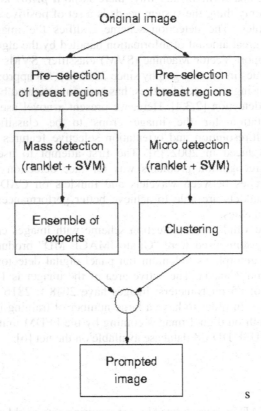

Original image

Pre–selection of breast regions	Pre–selection of breast regions
Mass detection (ranklet + SVM)	Micro detection (ranklet + SVM)
Ensemble of experts	Clustering

Prompted image

s

Fig. 1. Chart of the ranklet-based detection scheme

The first step of the microcalcification detection method consists in a pre-selection of the regions containing bright spots. This is achieved by means of a statistical test calculated on a linear-filtered image. Pixels passing that test are then provided to a detector similar to the experts used for the masses. Here, a ranklet representation of the crops centered on the points extracted in the first step is obtained. After that, the crops are judged as positive or not, by using an SVM classifier. The main difference of the featureless detection between masses and microcalcifications is that in the first case a multiscale searching is used, whereas in the second case crops of fixed size are considered. The single adjacent pixels classified as suspect are the grouped together and clusterized, if more than two signals in a 1 cm^2 area are detected.

Finally, signals discovered by the masses and clustered microcalcifications detectors are joined by means of a logical OR operator, and a maximum predetermined number of marks are presented as the final result. Signals are ranked by means of their distance from the separating hyperplane traced by SVM.

2.2 Image Dataset

The training dataset consists of a number of "positive" and "negative" crops. "Positive" crops were extracted from cancer images and are centered on the lesions (masses or single microcalcifications). "Negative" crops were extracted randomly from normal images (i.e. from images without lesions). We used about 850 positive crops for training the CAD system (600 single microcalcifications and 250 opacities). A more complete description of the training procedure can be found in [2].

The dataset used for testing CAD performance consists of more than 1000 images not used for training and coming from various "Giotto Image MD" FFDM systems. Images have a pixel size equal to 85 micrometers and a gray-level resolution of 13 bits; they have been collected both in the course of the clinical evaluation of the FFDM system and subsequently during the regular clinical examinations. The database includes about 900 normal images (without lesions) and 140 images with at least one lesion, such as tumor opacities or clustered microcalcifications. The location of the lesions have been marked by expert radiologists and collected together with the images. Digital mammograms were always available in four projections per patient. Each case is relative to one patient and comprises the four projections (two cranio-caudal and two medio-lateral views). Performances are estimated by means of FROC curves, both on a per-image and a per-case basis.

False-positives marks were calculated on 154 normal images coming from screening examinations and with a follow-up of at least 1 year. These normal images were extracted from randomly chosen patients. The true positive performance were evaluated on 140 cancer images coming from symptomatic patients and confirmed by biopsy. 30 cases show masses as only signs of cancer, whereas 37 cases show only clustered microcalcifications. Three patients show both masses and microcalcifications.

2.3 The Ranklet Representation

Given a set of $(x1, x2, ..., xN)$ pixels, the rank transform substitutes each pixel's intensity value with its relative order (rank) among all the other pixels. This is a nonparametric transform since, given an image with N pixels, it replaces the value of each pixel with the value of its order among all the other pixels. Ranklets are designed starting from the three 2D Haar wavelets and the rank transform. In analogy to the wavelet transform, ranklet coefficients can be computed at different orientations by applying vertical, horizontal and diagonal Haar wavelet supports to each image under analysis. As a result, the orientation selectivity feature of the ranklet representation follows.

Finally, the close correspondence between the Haar wavelet transform and the ranklet transform leads directly to the extension of the latter to its multiresolution formulation. This means that, as for the wavelet transform, it is possible to compute the ranklet transform of an image at different resolutions by means of a suitable stretch and shift of the Haar wavelet supports. At the same time, for each resolution, it is possible to characterize the image by means of orientation selective features such as the vertical, horizontal and diagonal ranklet coefficients. The multiresolution ranklet transform of an image is thus a set of triplets of vertical, horizontal and diagonal ranklet coefficients, each one corresponding to a specific stretch and shift of the Haar wavelet supports.

344   E. Angelini et al.

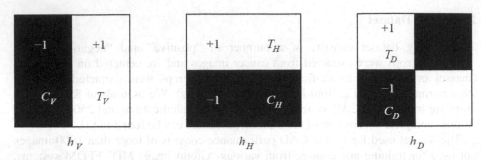

Fig. 2. The three Haar wavelet supports h_V, h_H and h_D. From left to right, the vertical, horizontal and diagonal Haar wavelet supports.

The ranklet transform is defined by first splitting the N pixels into two subsets T and C of size $N/2$, thus assigning half of the pixels to the subset T and half to the subset C. The two subsets T and C are defined being inspired by the Haar wavelet supports depicted in Fig. 2. In particular, for the vertical Haar wavelet support, the two subsets T_V and C_V are defined; similarly for the horizontal and diagonal ones. The definition of the aforementioned Haar wavelet supports forms the basis for the orientation-selective characteristic of the ranklet transform.

The second step consists in computing and normalizing in the range [-1, +1] the number of pixel pairs (p_m, p_n), with $p_m \in$ T and $p_n \in$ C, such that the intensity value of p_m is higher than the intensity value of p_n. This is done for each orientation, namely vertical, horizontal and diagonal.

The geometric interpretation of the so-called ranklet coefficient R_j is quite straightforward. Suppose that the image we are dealing with is characterized by a vertical edge, with the darker side on the left, where C_V is located, and the brighter side on the right, where T_V is located. R_V will be close to +1 as many pixels in T_V will have higher intensity values than the pixels in C_V. Conversely, R_V will be close to -1 if the dark and bright side are reversed. Horizontal edges or other patterns with no global left-right variation of intensity will give a value close to 0. Analogous considerations can be drawn for the other ranklet coefficients, R_H and R_D The use of the pixels' ranks, rather than their intensities, forms the basis for the non-parametric characteristic of the ranklet transform.

The close correspondence between the Haar wavelet transform and the ranklet transform leads directly to the extension of the latter to its multiresolution formulation. Similarly to what is done for the bidimensional Haar wavelet transform, the ranklet coefficients can be computed at different resolutions by simply stretching and shifting the Haar wavelet supports. The multiresolution ranklet transform of an image is thus a set of triplets of vertical, horizontal and diagonal ranklet coefficients, each one corresponding to a specific stretch and shift of the Haar wavelet supports. The possibility of computing ranklet coefficients at different resolutions forms the basis for the multiresolution characteristic of the ranklet transform.

3   Results

In order to have a remarkable number of training patterns, we accomplished the training of the CAD algorithm by using both digitized and digital images. Digitized examples were selected by cropping images from the USF DDSM database available on the net. Digital images coming from the Giotto FFDM units were used both for training and testing the CAD system. The use of images coming from various systems, without performing any normalization step has been practicable, thanks to the innate features of the ranklet transform.

The CAD system presents a sensitivity nearly equal to 85%, with a false-positive rate of 0.5 marks per image. The sensitivity has been calculated both on a per-case and on a per-image basis. In the first case, the true-positive rate is equal to the number of positive patients correctly detected over the total number of positive patients. In the latter case, results are equal to the ratio between the number of positive images correctly detected and the total number of cancer images. The false-positive rate has been computed on the normal images.

Fig. 3 shows the FROC curves of our CAD system on the test images. The distinct performance for the masses and microcalcifications algorithms for a specific point of the FROC curve is the following. The masses detector shows a per-case sensitivity equal to 76% with a false-positive rate of 0.3 false-positive marks per image, whilst microcalcifications detector demonstrates a true-positive per-case rate equal to 93% with a false-positive rate of 0.2 false-positives per image.

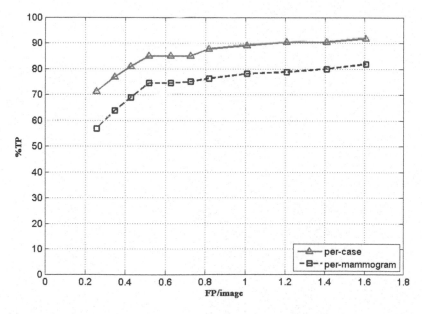

Fig. 3. FROC results of the ranklet-based CAD system on the test images. True-positive rate results are shown on a per-case and per-image basis.

References

1. Bazzani, A., Bevilacqua, A., Bollini, D., Brancaccio, R., Campanini, R., Lanconelli, N., Riccardi, A., Romani, D.: An SVM classifier to separate false signals from microcalcifications in digital mammograms. *Physics in Medicine and Biology,* 46 (6), (2001) 1651-1663.
2. Campanini, R., Dongiovanni, D., Iampieri, E., Lanconelli, N., Masotti, M., Palermo, G., Riccardi, A., Roffilli, M.: A novel featureless approach to mass detection in digital mammograms based on Support Vector Machines. *Physics in Medicine and Biology*, 49, (2004) 961-975.
3. El-Naqa, I., Yang, Y., Wernick, M.N., Galatsanos, N.P., Nishikawa. R.M.: A Support Vector Machine approach for detection of microcalcifications. *IEEE Trans. Med. Imag.* 21, (2002) 1552-1563.
4. Angelini, A., Campanini, R., Iampieri, E., Lanconelli, N., Masotti, M., Roffilli, M.: Testing the performances of different image representations for mass classification in digital mammograms. *International Journal of Modern Physics – C (Computational Physics and Physical Computation),* 17 (1), (2006) 113-131.
5. Smeraldi F.: Ranklets: Orientation selective non-parametric features applied to face detection. *Proc. of the 16th International Conference on Pattern Recognition,* 3, (2002) 379–382.
6. Heat, M., Bowyer, K., Kopans, D., Moore, R., Kegelmeyer, P.: The digital database for screening mammography. *Digital Mammography: IWDM2000 5th Int. Workshop on Digital Mammography*, Medical Physics Publishing, (2000) 212-218.

Detection of Microcalcifications in Digital Mammograms Based on Dual-Threshold

Yuan Wu[1], Qian Huang[1], YongHong Peng[2], and Wuchao Situ[1]

[1] South China University of Technology, Guangzhou, P.R. China
tuoge@tom.com
[2] University of Bradford, UK
y.h.peng@bradford.ac.uk

Abstract. Breast cancer is one of the main leading causes to women mortality in the world especially in the western countries. Since the causes are still unknown, breast cancer cannot be prevented completely even till now. Microcalcification clusters are primary indicators of malignant types of breast cancer, the detection is important to prevent and treat the disease. The microcalcifications appear in the small clusters of a few pixels with relatively high intensity and closed contours compared with their neighboring pixels. However, it is a challenge to detect all the microcalcifications since they appear as spots which are slightly brighter than their backgrounds. This paper presents an approach for detecting microcalcifications in digital mammograms employing a dual-threshold method. These microcalcifications can be located by our new method which is developed from LoG edge detection method. Two thresholds are proposed in our method based on two additional criterions. Experimental results show that the proposed method can locate the microcalcifications exactly in mammogram as well as restrain the contours produced by the noises.

1 Introduction

By far, breast cancer is the second leading cause to cancer death in women, exceeded only by lung cancer. Prevention in advance seems impossible since the causes to this disease are still unknown, but the early detection can increase the chance of cure and survival [1]. As the microcalcifications is nearly the only feature for the initial period of breast cancer except the body-touch checking, mammogram is the most reliable method for early detection of breast cancer while all the other methods, e. g. ultrasound and infrared, can not show the microcalcifications very well. The microcalcifications appear in the small clusters of a few pixels with relatively high intensity and closed contours compared with their neighboring pixels. Microcalcification clusters are primary indicators of malignant types of breast cancer, the detection is important to prevent and treat the disease. But it is still a hard work to detect all the microcalcifications due to the fact that mammogram presents poor contrast between microcalcifications and the tissues around them.

Susan M. Astley et al. (Eds.): IWDM 2006, LNCS 4046, pp. 347–354, 2006.

Still, many approaches have been proposed for detection of microcalcifications in mammograms, like neural network, wavelets, support vector machines, mathematical morphology, bayesian image analysis models, high order statistic, fuzzy logic, fractal models, etc. Davies and Dance [2] and Davies et al. [3, 4] used a local thresholding technique to segment clustered microcalcifications. The local threshold is selected at the valley of the local histogram. If the local histogram is unimodal, the sub-image will be interpolated from its neighboring sub-images, but the operation on histogram is usually hard to realized. Peitgen [5] proposed an approach for automatic detection of microcalcifications utilizing multi-scale analysis based on the Laplacian-of-Gaussian filter and the mathematical model describing microcalcifications as bright spots due to their sizes and contrast. Cheng et al. [6] proposed an approach to detecting microcalcifications based on fuzzy logic. Zheng et al. [7] used mixed feature-based neural network and [8] employed a neural network for a pixel-based classification. Some morphological methods can be found in the literature [1, 9].

Closed contours are often treated as the most important characteristic of the objects. In the application of object recognition, the closed contours of objects are the foundation of counting the objects' sizes, getting the objects' shapes and giving some further information. Our algorithm is based on the fact that all the microcalcifications have closed contours. In this paper we propose a dual-threshold method based on traditional LoG operator to locate all the microcalcifications in mammograms. The proposed algorithm consists of two main steps: 1. Convolving the original image with LoG filter to get all the zero-crossing points, then labeling all the closed contours which consist of zero-crossing points by a quick region filling method. 2. Determining whether the closed contours belong to the microcalcifications by two introduced thresholds. Most important, all the parameters in our algorithm need not be changed in the whole course if only the mammograms are taken from the same machine under the same conditions.

The rest of this paper is organized as follows: in the second section, the proposed approach is described in detail. In the third section, the experimental results are shown and discussed, Finally, in the fourth section, the conclusions are presented, some comments about future work are also mentioned.

2   Proposed Approach

In this section we will present how LoG operator works in our algorithm as well as some related information. Also, two criterions and the corresponding dual-threshold are introduced. The detailed implementation will be shown in the end of this section.

2.1   LoG Operator

LoG edge detecting method is a common method used in image processing [10, 11]. LoG(Laplacian of Gaussian) operator means smoothing the original image with Gaussian filter before a Laplacian operator, and Laplacian operator

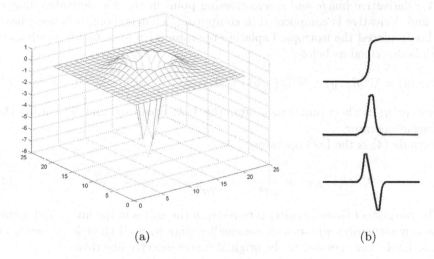

(a)   (b)

Fig. 1. (a) An example of two-dimensional LoG kernel and (b) the 1st, 2nd derivative of a one-dimensional step-edge signal

is a kind of 2nd derivative method to detect the edges. An example of two-dimensional LoG kernel can be seen in Fig. 1(a). Then Fig. 1(b) shows how to use the 1st and 2nd derivatives to detect the edges. In Fig. 1(b) the top one is a step-edge signal that indicates a sudden change in the gray level value, the middle one is a pulse that indicates a larger value in gradient image (1st derivative of the top one), and the bottom one (Laplacian operator) shows that the gray level value of an edge point turns to zero and the values of its two neighboring points turn to be positive and negative respectively. In fact, the gray level value of an edge point is not usually zero but close to zero. As a result, we judge an edge point by its two neighbors. If the values vary across zero from a neighbor to the other neighbor, there must be an edge point whose value is zero between the two neighbors. Concerning the two-dimensional image, Marr [12] proposed using Gaussian function to smooth the image before using the Laplacian operator in the LoG edge detecting method. The Gaussian function can be written as below:

$$G(x, y, \sigma) = \frac{1}{2\pi\sigma^2} \exp(-\frac{x^2 + y^2}{2\sigma^2}) \tag{1}$$

where, $G(x, y, \sigma)$ is a circular symmetry function, so the smooth effect to the image is linear.

We can suppose $f(x, y)$ as the original image, and $g(x, y)$ is the result image after the smoothing. The smoothing degree can be controlled by the parameter σ, namely larger σ can bring more smooth result.

$$g(x, y) = f(x, y) * G(x, y, \sigma) \tag{2}$$

According to the characteristic of vision, the edge point is located in which the gray level value changes greatly. This large change will produce a pulse in the 1st derivative image and a zero-crossing point in the 2nd derivative image. The 2nd derivative is complicated in computing, what is more, it is non-linear, so Marr replaced the isotropic Laplacian operator with formula (3) in advance, which is described as below:

$$r(x,y) = \nabla^2 g(x,y) = \nabla^2(f(x,y) * G(x,y,\sigma)) = f(x,y) * \nabla^2 G(x,y,\sigma) \qquad (3)$$

where $r(x,y)$ is the result image after the LoG operator, and ∇^2 means the Laplacian operator.

Formula (4) is the LoG operator.

$$\nabla^2 G(x,y,\sigma) = \frac{1}{\pi\sigma^4}(1 - \frac{x^2 + y^2}{2\sigma^2}) \cdot \exp(-\frac{x^2 + y^2}{2\sigma^2}) \qquad (4)$$

The purpose of Gaussian filter is to restrain the noises in the image and ignore some tiny structures whose sizes are smaller than σ. So if there is no noise, we can do Laplacian operator to the original image directly like this:

$$r(x,y) = \nabla^2 f(x,y) \qquad (5)$$

2.2 Maximum Difference Value of Zero-Crossing Point

Suppose (x_i, y_j) is a zero-crossing point in image $r(x,y)$, we define "maximum difference value of zero-crossing point" of (x_i, y_j) as $max_{zero}(x_i, y_j)$.

$$max_{zero}(x_i, y_j) = \max(|r(x_i, y_j) - r(x_i, y_{j-1})|, |r(x_i, y_j) - r(x_i, y_{j+1})|,$$
$$|r(x_i, y_j) - r(x_{i-1}, y_j)|, |r(x_i, y_j) - r(x_{i+1}, y_j)|) \qquad (6)$$

In fact, the value of $max_{zero}(x_i, y_j)$ can indicate whether a point is an obvious edge point. Larger $max_{zero}(x_i, y_j)$ indicates that point (x_i, y_j) is more likely to be an edge point, vice versa.

2.3 Dual-Threshold

We outline two thresholds T_1 and T_2 as dual-threshold to obtain the obvious contours. Concerning to zero-crossing point (x_i, y_j), if $max_{zero}(x_i, y_j)$ is larger than the threshold T_1, we can call this point as an "obvious edge point". In fact, a zero-crossing point is more possible to be an edge point if $max_{zero}(x_i, y_j)$ is larger.

After the LoG operation we can get a result image $r(x,y)$. The values of the points in image $r(x,y)$ may be positive, negative and zero. Then we must find all the zero-crossing points in image $r(x,y)$. For convenience we only check the right and down neighboring points of a point (x_i, y_j). If the values of the two neighbors are positive and negative respectively, then the point (x_i, y_j) is a zero-crossing point. Surely other rules and definitions of zero-crossing points in two-dimension images can be developed, however, they may bring different results and effects. We label all the zero-crossing points in image $r(x,y)$ as "1" and others as "0", then we get a new "0-1" image whose pixel values are composed of "0" and "1". In our method we keep all the closed contours composed of "1" in the "0-1" image first, then threshold T_2 mentioned in the next paragraph will be used to eliminate the false closed contours in the final result image.

For each closed contour in the "0-1" image we scan all the points on it to obtain all the "obvious edge point", then calculate the number (supposed as l) of "obvious edge point" and the total number (supposed as L) of points in this closed contour. If $l/L > T_2$, this closed contour will be kept in the final result image, otherwise we will eliminate it.

2.4 Implementation

The overall steps of our method are summarized as follows:

1. Do LoG operation to the original image, and find all the zero-crossing points.
2. Scan the result image of step 1 to obtain all the closed contours. In this step we use quick region filling method to obtain the closed contours from all kinds of structures.
3. Concerning each points on the closed contours, calculate their max_{zero} (x_i, y_j), then use threshold T_1 to decide whether it is an "obvious edge point".
4. Concerning each closed contours, calculate their numbers of "obvious edge point" and the total number of points on them, then use threshold T_2 to decide whether should we keep these closed contours or not.

In these steps we have three parameters that must be predetermined manually. The empirical parameters can affect the final result. In fact, σ is usually chosen as 1 or 2, T_1 ranges from 1 to 7 based on the noise level of the image and contrast between the microcalcifications and backgrounds while T_2 is set to 0.4 in most situations.

3   Experimental Results

A typical mammogram consisted of microcalcifications can be seen in Fig. 2. The digital mammogram database used in this paper is the mini-MIAS [13] (Mammographic Image Analysis Society) database which contains 322 digitized mammogram images. The images in the database are digitized at 50-micron pixel edge, which are then reduced to 200-micron pixel edge and clipped or padded so that every image has 1024×1024 pixels. The accompanying 'Ground Truth' contains details regarding the characters of the background tissue, class, severity, coordinates of the center of the abnormality and approximate radius of the circle enclosing it.

It should be noticed that all the parameters need not be changed in our experiments, and we set them as $\sigma = 1$, $T_1 = 6$ and $T_2 = 0.4$. Two testing images mdb148 and mdb186 are selected to show our results which can be seen in Fig. 3. In each row from left to right, they are the original image, the contours of microcalcifications and the result of adding contours to the original image. We

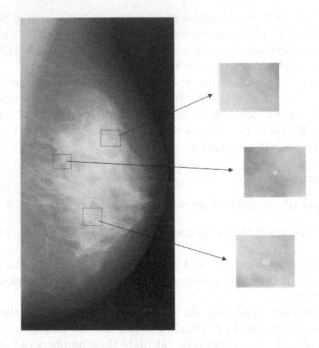

Fig. 2. A mammogram consisting of microcalcifications which have been marked and amplified

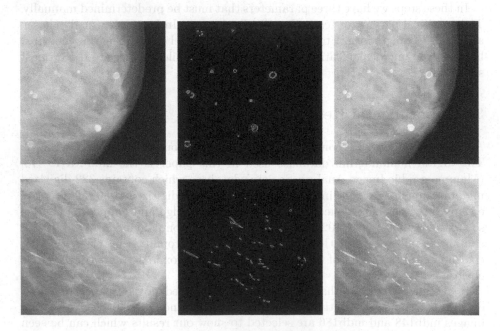

Fig. 3. The results of our algorithms

also test all the images from mini-MIAS database to verify our method which is supposed to be valuable in clinical CAD applications as the satisfying results.

The performance of the proposed algorithm was evaluated by a free-response receiver operating characteristic (FROC) in terms of TP (true-positive) fraction for a given number of FP (false-positive) clusters per image. Detection performance measured by FROC curve has been shown as in Fig. 4.

From the FROC curve we can see that our method has came up with a TP rate of 91% on the mini-MIAS database while the number of FP clusters per image is more than 4.

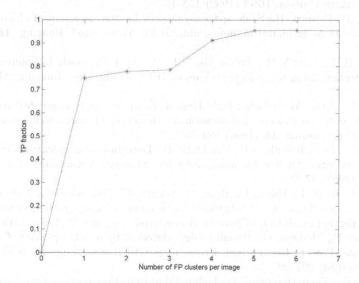

Fig. 4. Detection performance measured by FROC curve

4   Conclusion

This paper has presented a novel method to locate all the microcalcifications in digital mammograms. Traditional Log edge detecting method can not abstract the contours of objects integrally, especially when there are weak edges, noises and uneven background. The dual-threshold method we proposed can handle digital mammograms very well. The most important advantage is, the two thresholds in our method need not be changed in the whole course of testing all the images in mini-MIAS database. In fact, with certain hardware and environments we only need to set the two thresholds once at the beginning, then for all the images we use the constant parameters.

Our future work will focus on adding some new criterions to enhance the algorithm. Also, some new features should be added into our method to detect the tumors in the mammograms.

References

1. Dengler, J., Behrens, S. and Desaga, J.: Segmentation of microcalcifications in mammograms. IEEE Transactions on Medical Imaging. 12 (1993) 634–642
2. Davies, D.H., Dance, D.R.: Automatic computer detection of clustered calcifications in digital mammograms. Phys. Med. Biol. 35 (1990) 1111–1118
3. Davies, D.H., Dance, D.R., Jones, C.H.: Automatic detection of clusters of calcifiations. SPIE Med. Imaging IV: Image Process. 1233 (1990) 185–191
4. Davies, D.H., Dance, D.R., Jones, C.H.: Automatic detection of microcalcifiations in digital mammograms using local area thresholding techniques. SPIE Med. Imaging III: Image Process. 1092 (1989) 153–157
5. Netsch, T., Peitgen, H.: Scale space signatures for the detection of clustered microcalcifications in digital mammograms. IEEE Trans. Med. Imaging. 18 (1999) 774–786
6. Cheng, H.D., Lui, Y.M., Freimanis, R.I.: A novel approach to microcalcification detection using fuzzy logic technique. IEEE Trans. Med. Imaging. 17 (1998) 442–450
7. Zheng, B., Qian, W., Clarke, L.P.: Digital mammography: mixed feature neural network with spectral entropy decision for detection of microcalcification. IEEE Trans. Med. Imaging. 15 (1996) 589–597
8. Meersman, D., Scheunders, P., Van Dyck, D.: Detection of microcalcification using neural networks. Digital Mammography 96, Elsevier, Amsterdam, The Netherlands. (1996) 287–290
9. Astey, S., Hutt, I., Miller, P., Rose, P., Boggis, C., Adamson, S., Valentine, T., Davies, J. and Rmstrong, J.: Automation in mammography: computer vision and human perception. Int. J. of pattern Recog. And Art. Intt. 7 (1993) 1313–1338
10. Ulupinar, F., Medioni, G.: Refining edges detected by a LoG operator. Computer Vision and Pattern Recognition, Proceedings CVPR '88, Computer Society Conference. (1988) 202–207
11. Shen Liqin, Shen Dinggang, Qi Feihu: Edge detection on real time using LOG filter. Speech, Image Processing and Neural Networks, Proceedings, ISSIPNN '94, International Symposium. 1 (1994) 37–40
12. Marr, D., Hildreth, E.:Theory of edge detection. Proceedings lf the Royal Society. 1980 187–217
13. http://peipa.essex.ac.uk/ipa/pix/mias/

Feasibility and Acceptability of Stepwedge-Based Density Measurement

Michael Berks[1], Jennifer Diffey[2], Alan Hufton[2], and Susan Astley[1]

[1] Division of Imaging Science and Biomedical Engineering, Stopford Building,
University of Manchester, Oxford Road, Manchester M13 9PT
michael.berks@postgrad.manchester.ac.uk,
sue.astley@manchester.ac.uk
[2] North Western Medical Physics, Christie Hospital, Withington, Manchester M20 4BX
jenny.diffey@physics.cr.man.ac.uk,
alan.hufton@physics.cr.man.ac.uk

Abstract. A link between increased breast density, as visualised in mammograms, and increased risk of developing breast cancer has been established. Recently, a number of objective, quantitative methods for measuring breast density have been described. One such method requires a calibration object to be imaged alongside the breast. However, it is important that this should not interfere with the routine imaging process. In this paper, we investigate the amount of space in mammographic images which is not currently occupied by the breast or existing patient labels and markers, and which would therefore be available for imaging an additional calibration device. We do this with a view to estimating the likelihood of failure of the method, and also to determining whether, without detriment to the imaging process, a device could be permanently fixed to the breast support platform. We also examine the impact of markers attached to the compression plate on the visibility of breast tissue. The results show that our existing calibration device may be used successfully without interfering with the routine imaging process, although permanently fixing such a device may present problems in a small minority of cases, and we demonstrate that the number of cases which would fail can be reduced by using a smaller stepwedge.

1 Introduction

Currently, breast density measurement is not incorporated in risk prediction models used in Family History clinics [1], although the association of increased breast density with an increased risk of developing cancer is accepted [2, 3]. An improved estimate of individual risk would benefit women by enabling better informed decisions about strategies for detecting and preventing cancers. However, improvements such as the inclusion of breast density in risk prediction models must not only be reliable and accurate: they must also be practical, and should not interfere with the routine care the women receive.

To date, much of the work on the relationship of breast density to risk has been based on visual assessment of mammograms [4], although more recently a number of automated and semi-automated approaches have been developed in an attempt to

Susan M. Astley et al. (Eds.): IWDM 2006, LNCS 4046, pp. 355–361, 2006.

improve objectivity and accuracy [5, 6, 7, 8]. Some of these approaches rely on imaging calibrated density stepwedges on the mammogram [7, 8]. If such methods are to be used in the screening programme, it is important to ensure that they do not interfere with the routine screening process, and also that they can be successfully applied to the vast majority of women. Obesity is an increasing problem, and brings with it a greater number of women with larger breasts [9]. In these women particularly, there may not be much room to image additional devices during mammography.

In this paper, we investigate the amount of space in mammographic images which is not currently occupied by the breast or existing patient labels and markers, and which would therefore be available for imaging an additional calibration device, with a view to determining the likelihood of failure due to lack of room in the image, and also to investigating whether, without detriment to the imaging process, a device could be permanently fixed to the breast support platform. Our method for determining the volume of dense breast tissue also images markers attached to the compression plate to accurately measure breast thickness across the mammogram [7]. Here we examine the impact of these markers on the visibility of breast tissue.

2 Data

The dataset consists of mammographic films obtained from 66 women participating in a study of the effects of lifestyle on cancer risk [9]. Each woman had both craniocaudal (CC) and mediolateral oblique (MLO) views of both breasts, resulting in 264 films. Of these, 7 of the sets were obtained in 2002 and the remaining 59 in 2003. The majority of the films (180) were 18 by 24 cm (standard format), whilst the remaining 84 were 24 by 30 cm (large format), depending on the size of the breast. All films were digitised using a Kodak LS85 digitiser at a pixel size of 50 μm and with 12 bits (4096 grey levels) pixel depth. The pixel depth was later reduced to 8 bits (256 grey levels) to reduce the file size of the stored images. An example of the mammograms is shown in figure 1. Here, the name label has been obscured to protect the privacy of the woman, and appears as a grey rectangle at the edge of each image.

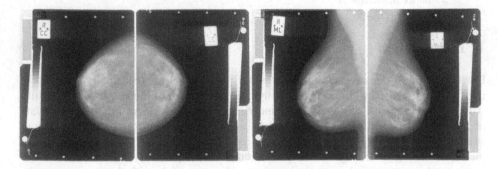

Fig. 1. The right and left, CC and MLO mammograms of a woman screened as part of the study of the effects of lifestyle on cancer risk . The (obscured) name label, side/view label, stepwedge and four pairs of markers are clearly visible in each image.

3   Analysis of Available Space

Each mammogram is identified by a name label containing identification and imaging data and a view label indicating the side (left or right) and the view (MLO or CC), thus to analyse the amount of free space in each mammogram, the area taken up by the two labels and the breast tissue was deducted from the overall size of the film. The digitised images were preprocessed to remove isolated noise pixels, then segmented using a semiautomatic process into regions corresponding to the breast, background and labels.

The area covered by breast tissue and the distance from the nipple to the edge of the image were calculated in all 264 mammograms. However, as there is very little variation in the area covered by name and view labels in the images, the area for each of these was calculated only in 20 standard format and 20 large format mammograms.

3.1   Results

The mean area of the image occupied by the name label is $17.8cm^2$ in standard format films and $17.7cm^2$ in large format films, whilst the label indicating radiographic projection and side occupies $6.0cm^2$ of the image area in the standard format and $6.0cm^2$ in the large format mammograms. In the standard format the mean areas occupied by the breast in the right CC, left CC, right MLO and left MLO views were $142.3cm^2$, $142.8cm^2$, $190.8cm^2$ and $191.4cm^2$ respectively, and in the large format, $294.9cm^2$, $301.9cm^2$, $371.4cm^2$ and $366.3cm^2$. The mean distances from the nipple to the edge of the film were 79mm, 79mm, 72mm, and 70mm, in standard format, and 82mm, 85mm, 64mm, and 66mm in the large format.

Table 1. The minimum available area and minimum distance between the nipple and the edge of the film

	Standard format films				Large format films			
	RCC	LCC	RML O	LML O	RC C	LC C	RML O	LM LO
Minimum available area in cm^2	205.1	194.6	152.1	164.9	233. 4	302. 0	202.0	115 .8
Min distance from nipple to edge (mm)	38	38	30	31	31	43	4	0

Table 1 shows the minimum nipple to edge distance, and the minimum free area for the four views, in both standard and large format films.

4   Impact of Compression Markers

The compression markers are small lead objects attached to an acetate sheet which is then placed on the breast compression plate during imaging. The markers are imaged on the mammogram, and the distance between pairs of markers on the image enables calculation of compressed breast thickness and tilt of the compression plate. Each view contains four pairs of markers: we refer to the markers nearest to the chest wall as the first pair of markers.

Ideally, the four pairs of markers should be imaged onto free space in the mammogram, as in figure 2 a. However, the markers may overlap tissue, as in figure 2 b and c, possibly covering clinical information in the image that may be useful for diagnosis. The markers may also be obscured by the name and view identification labels, thus impeding the calculation of breast thickness. Examples of this are shown in figure 2 d. We have analysed the frequency with which these cases occur.

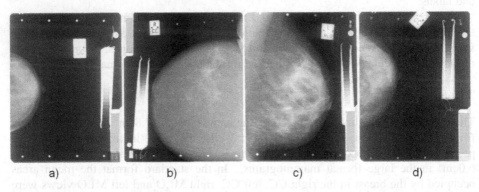

a)   b)   c)   d)

Fig. 2. Imaging the compression markers. a) All four pairs of markers are visible b) the lower marker of the 1st and 2nd pairs lie on breast tissue, the 1st upper and 3rd lower markers lie on the skinline c) the 1st upper marker lies on the pectoral muscle, the 1st lower marker lies on the infra-mammary fold d) the 3rd upper marker is covered by the view label, the 4th lower marker is covered by the sticker.

Markers were classified as being: in the background; overlying breast tissue; on the skinline; overlying the pectoral muscle (MLO views only); on the infra-mammary fold (MLO views only); covered by an identification label during imaging; covered by a sticker before digitisation; missing from the image.

4.1 Results

There was no observable difference in the classification of markers between the standard and large format films, so the results have been pooled for the 66 women. In the CC mammograms, the large majority of markers do not interfere with the imaging of the breast. Only 4 (out of 66) of the first pairs of markers, 2 of the second, 3 of the third and none of the fourth contained a marker overlying breast tissue in the right CC mammograms. Similarly, in the left CC mammograms, the respective counts are 4 of the first, 2 of the second, 1 of third and none of the fourth pairs. In the MLO mammograms, the results are very similar for the third and fourth marker pairs. However, the upper marker closest to the chest wall overlies the pectoral muscle in all cases it appeared on the film – 65 times in the right MLO films and 55 in the left. The second upper marker is also much more likely to coincide with other image features in the MLO views: 34 times on the right, and 27 on the left. It is, however, unlikely that these markers cover important clinical information because of their location.

In order to be used in the calculation of the thickness of the breast, the position of the markers must be measured accurately, and therefore they must not be obscured by the identification labels in the mammograms. This proves problematic in the third and fourth pairs of markers. For example, of the fourth pairs, only 42 of the right CC, 45 of the left CC, 47 of the right MLO and 39 of the left MLO have both markers fully visible. The category totals for each marker in each view are displayed in table 2.

Table 2. Categorised counts of markers pooled for the the upper (U) and lower (L) marker of the 1st to 4th pairs, in the right and left, CC and MLO mammograms

	RCC								LCC							
	1st pair		2nd pair		3rd pair		4th pair		1st pair		2nd pair		3rd pair		4th pair	
	U	L	U	L	U	L	U	L	U	L	U	L	U	L	U	L
Background	58	55	66	64	53	64	42	64	59	59	62	65	56	65	64	47
Breast	2	3	0	2	0	2	0	0	1	4	1	1	0	1	0	0
Skinline	5	1	0	0	0	0	0	0	1	3	0	0	0	0	0	0
Name/view label	0	0	0	0	11	0	9	2	0	0	2	0	10	0	1	4
Sticker	0	0	0	0	2	0	15	0	0	0	0	0	0	0	1	15
Missing	1	7	0	0	0	0	0	0	5	0	1	0	0	0	0	0

	RMLO								LMLO							
	1st pair		2nd pair		3rd pair		4th pair		1st pair		2nd pair		3rd pair		4th pair	
	U	L	U	L	U	L	U	L	U	L	U	L	U	L	U	L
Background	1	49	32	63	56	63	48	65	0	42	31	65	51	64	59	44
Breast	0	5	14	3	0	2	0	0	0	3	6	1	0	1	0	1
Skinline	0	1	20	0	0	0	0	0	0	4	21	0	0	1	0	0
Pectoral muscle	64	-	0	-	0	-	0	-	55	-	0	-	0	-	0	-
Infra-mammary	-	8	-	0	-	0	-	0	-	17	-	0	-	0	-	0
Name/view label	0	0	0	0	9	0	2	1	0	0	0	0	9	0	3	6
Sticker	0		0	0	1	0	14	0	0	0	0	0	0	0	1	15
Missing	1	3	0	0	0	1	2	0	11	0	8	0	6	0	3	0

5   Discussion and Conclusions

In the images obtained for this study, step wedges of dimensions (length by width) 125mm by 12mm and 175mm by 15mm were used. After magnification during imaging, the step wedge (and the shadow it casts) occupied a rectangle of approximately 135mm by 23mm in standard format films, and 188mm by 31mm in large format films. Ideally the wedge should be placed with its long axis parallel to the chest wall, and must not overlap the identification label. This requires a minimum rectangle of free space of approximately 140mm by 28mm in the standard format and 193mm by 36mm in the large format, running parallel to the long edge of the films.

It would be beneficial to permanently fix the stepwedge to the breast platform. The stepwedge imaged in this study was attached to the breast platform by a 'hook and eye' arrangement. However, this method proved unsatisfactory as in many cases the stepwedge slipped during imaging, particularly in MLO mammograms, where the compression plate is tilted. Permanently (or semi-permanently) fixing the stepwedge to the breast platform requires a sufficient rectangle of free background to lie in a consistent position in all films. The only suitable area is the top left corner of right side films and the bottom right corner of left side films. For the large format films, this area is marked by the larger dashed rectangle in each view in figure 3.

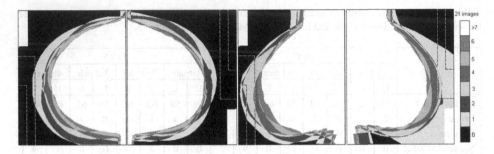

Fig. 3. Area occupied by breast tissue and name label in each of the RCC, LCC, RMLO and LMLO large format mammograms. The larger dashed rectangle represents the area ideally reserved for the stepwedge used to obtain the images in this paper, whilst the smaller rectangle depicts the area required for a new, smaller stepwedge [10].

Observing the minimum distances from nipple to film edge in table 1, we conclude that in the standard format films, the step wedge can be placed optimally in the mammograms obtained from all 45 women. However, in the large format, whilst the left CC views present no problem, a distance of less than 36mm was measured in 1 of the right CC mammograms, 4 of the right MLO mammograms and 4 of the left MLO mammograms (4 of the 21 women). The resulting overlap of these breasts into the area ideally reserved for the stepwedge is clearly seen in figure 3.

To overcome this problem, a new, smaller stepwedge has been developed which may be used in future trials [10]. This occupies less than a third of the area than the stepwedge used in the large format films in this study, with an imaged length of just 128mm and a width of 13mm. The minimum rectangle of free space required for the smaller stepwedge is marked by the smaller dashed rectangle in each view of figure 3. We can see that the smaller stepwedge may be placed optimally in all but 4 of the mammograms (3 of the 21 women), and in these cases there is still enough room in the image to place the step wedge, albeit not aligned optimally.

It is important to note that the women whose images were analysed were participating in a study of the effects of lifestyle on cancer risk [9]. To be selected for the study the women had to be 35 to 45 years old, and must have gained at least 10kg of weight since the age of 18. Since weight is related to the amount of fat in the breasts [9], we would expect these women to have larger breasts; thus they are not representative of the general population. This is portrayed by the fact that 32% (21 out of 66) of the women in the study required screening on large format films, whereas approximately only 9% of the women screened nationally require large format films [11]. In a general screening population, we predict that there would be very infrequent occurrences of failure due to women with very large breasts since in only three out of 66 cases the stepwedge could not be aligned optimally in our cohort.

We conclude that stepwedges may be used successfully in future trials, although permanently fixing such devices to the breast platform may cause problems in a very small minority of cases.

Compression markers do not significantly interfere with the routine imaging process. However many of the markers in this study were obscured, which restrict their use in calculating breast density. The large majority of the non-visible markers were covered either by the view label, or by a sticker attached the mammogram after imaging. Unlike the name label, the view label does not have a fixed position in the mammogram, so in future trials using compression makers it is recommended that care is taken to place the view label and sticker without covering the markers. The sticker can also be temporarily removed when digitising images and it is suggested this becomes practice in future methods.

References

1. Amir, E., Evans, D.G., Shepstone, A., Lallov, F., et al.: Evaluation of breast cancer risk assessment packages in the family history evaluation and screening programme. E. J. Med. Genet. (2003) 40 801-814
2. Boyd, N.F., Byng, J. W., Jong, R. A., Fishell, E.K., et al.: Quantitative classification of mammographic densities and breast cancer risk: results from the Canadian National Breast Screening Study. J Natl Cancer Inst. (1999) 87(9): 670-5
3. Wolfe, J.N.: Breast patterns as an index of risk for developing breast cancer. AJR Am J Roentgenol, (1976) 126(6):1130-7
4. Day, N., Warren, R.: Mammographic screening and mammographic patterns. Breast Cancer Res (2000) 2(4): 247-51
5. Pawluczyk, O., Augustine, B.J., Yaffe, M.J., Rico, D., Yang, J., Mawdsley, G.E.: A volumetric method for estimation of breast density on digitized screen-film mammograms. Med. Phys. (2003) 30:352-364
6. Highnam, R., Brady, M.: Mammographic Image Analysis. Dordrecht: Kluwer Academic Publishers (1999)
7. Hufton, A.P., Astley, S.M., Marchant, T.E., Patel, H.G.: A method for the quantification of dense breast tissue from digitised mammograms. Proceedings of the 7th IWDM, June 18-21 (2004) Durham, North Carolina
8. Shepherd, J.A., Herve, L., Landau, J., Fan, B., Kerlikowske, K., Cummings, SR.: Novel use of single x-ray absorptiometry for measuring breast density. Technol Cancer Res Treat (2005) 4(2): 173-82
9. Patel, H.G., Astley, S.M., Hufton, A.P., Harvie M., et al.: Automated breast tissue measurement of women at increased risk of breast cancer. Proceedings of the 8th International Workshop on Digital Mammography, June 19-21 (2006) Manchester, England
10. Diffey, J.: A new stepwedge for the volumetric measurement of breast density. Proceedings of the 8th International Workshop on Digital Mammography, June 19-21 (2006) Manchester, England
11. Young, K. C., Burch, A., Oduko, J. M.: Radiation doses received in the UK Breast Screening Program in 2001 and 2002. British Journal of Radiology (2005) 78:207-218

Use of the European Protocol to Optimise a Digital Mammography System

Kenneth C. Young, James J.H. Cook, and Jennifer M. Oduko

National Coordinating Centre for the Physics of Mammography
Royal Surrey County Hospital, Guildford GU2 7XX, UK
ken.young@nhs.net

Abstract. An experimental method of determining the optimal beam qualities and doses for digital mammography systems is described, and applied to a CR system. The mean glandular dose (MGD) and contrast-to-noise ratio (CNR) were measured using phantoms. For each thickness of phantom a range of kV and target/filter combinations were tested. Optimal beam quality was defined as that giving a target CNR for the lowest MGD. The target CNR was that necessary to achieve at least the minimum standard of image quality defined in European Guidance. An inverse relationship between CNR and threshold contrast was confirmed over a range of thicknesses of PMMA and different beam qualities and doses. Optimisation indicated that relatively high energy beam qualities (e.g. 31 kV Rh/Rh) should be used with a greater detector dose to compensate for the lower contrast when compared to using lower energy X-rays. The results also indicate that current AEC designs that aim for a fixed detector dose are not optimal.

1 Background

European guidelines provide quality control procedures and minimum standards of performance for digital mammography [1,2]. The image quality standards are based on contrast-detail measurements using the CDMAM phantom (version 3.4, UMC St. Radboud, Nijmegen University, Netherlands) [3]. The test on the automatic exposure control (AEC) involves the measurement of contrast-to-noise ratio (CNR) using a 0.2 mm thickness of Aluminium. The relationship between threshold contrasts and CNR values was measured here, and used as part of an optimisation process.

2 Methods

Measurements were made using a Fuji FCR Profect CS computed radiography (CR) system (Fuji Photo Film Co Ltd, Bedford, UK) used with a General Electric DMR+ mammography X-ray set (General Electric Medical Systems, Paris, France). The detector for the AEC on the X-ray set was always placed in the position closest to the chest wall edge. The same cassette and image plate were used for all measurements. The CR system was used with a "fixed" exposure data recogniser (EDR) setting and a

Susan M. Astley et al. (Eds.): IWDM 2006, LNCS 4046, pp. 362–369, 2006.

reading sensitivity (S value) of 120. Each CR image was saved as an unprocessed DICOM file for later analysis.

It is assumed in the European Guidelines that CNR and threshold contrast are related as given in Eq. 1,

$$\text{Threshold contrast} = \frac{\lambda}{CNR}, \tag{1}$$

where λ is a constant that is independent of dose, beam quality and the thickness of attenuating material. To test this relationship the dose, beam quality and attenuating material were systematically varied and CNR and threshold contrast measured. Three different thicknesses of attenuating material were used with the CDMAM test object [3]; 2cm, 4cm and 6cm of PMMA. In each case a 2cm thickness of PMMA was placed below the test phantom with the extra thicknesses on top. Squares of Aluminium (0.2mm thick) were placed on top of the two empty corners at the front of the CDMAM phantom. The phantom, with the additional PMMA layers indicated, was radiographed 8 times using each of the factors shown in Table 1. The mean glandular doses (MGD) for breasts of equivalent thickness were calculated for each set of exposure factors and are shown in Table 1 [1,4]. The CDMAM was assumed to have a thickness equivalent to 1 cm of PMMA. For each image the average pixel values for ROIs in the centre of each aluminium square, mean(Al), and in the adjacent background area, mean(bgd), were measured. The standard deviation of the pixel values in the background ROI, sd(bgd), and the aluminium ROI, sd(Al), were also determined. These data were used to calculate the CNR for each image as defined in the European protocol and shown in Eq. 2,

$$CNR = \frac{mean(bgd) - mean(Al)}{\sqrt{\dfrac{\left[sd(bgd)^2 + sd(Al)^2 \right]}{2}}} \tag{2}$$

Table 1. Exposure factors and thickness of PMMA used with CDMAM test object

Added thickness of PMMA (cm)	Equivalent breast thickness (mm)	kV target-filter	mAs	MGD (mGy)	CNR at corners	CNR at mid-line
2	32	25 Mo/Mo	51	0.90	9.67	11.4
2	32	28 Mo/Mo	16	0.44	6.84	8.07
2	32	28 Mo/Mo	25	0.69	8.56	10.1
4	60	26 Mo/Rh	71	0.94	5.47	6.45
4	60	26 Mo/Rh	280	3.72	10.5	12.4
4	60	34 Rh/Rh	22.5	0.75	5.37	6.34
4	60	34 Rh/Rh	40	1.33	7.18	8.47
6	90	30 Mo/Rh	237	3.99	5.81	6.86
6	90	34 Rh/Rh	63	1.60	4.51	5.32
6	90	34 Rh/Rh	160	4.06	6.82	8.05

Since the CNR was measured in the corner of the images the values were increased by 18% to reflect the value that would be found at the standard position on the mid-line. This corrected for the variation in detector dose (and therefore noise) at the different locations.

The threshold contrasts for each set of images of the CDMAM were scored by 3 observers and an automatic program [5]. The automatic program was used to predict the threshold contrast for a typical observer. The relationship between the threshold contrast and CNR was used to determine a target value for CNR (on the mid-line) necessary to meet the threshold contrast standards for the 0.1mm detail size in European guidance. The threshold contrast standards at this detail size were chosen as they are the most difficult to achieve.

2.1 Optimisation

PMMA blocks with an area of 180 x 240 mm and a total thickness ranging from 20 to 70 mm were used to simulate breasts of typical composition [4]. An aluminium square (10 mm x 10 mm) with a 0.2 mm thickness was placed on top of the 20 mm thick block, with one edge on the midline and 6cm from the chest wall edge. Additional layers of PMMA were added on top. For each thickness five tube voltage settings were used (25, 28, 31, 34 and 37 kV) with each of the target/filter combinations available (Mo/Mo, Mo/Rh, and Rh/Rh) and the mAs recorded. The MGDs to typical breasts (in the age range 50 to 65) with attenuation equivalent to each thickness of the PMMA were calculated as described in the European protocol and Dance et al [1,4]. Each exposure was designed to achieve a standard pixel value by using the AEC in automatic mAs mode.

The relationship between noise and pixel values in digital mammography systems has been previously shown to be approximated by

$$Relative\ noise = \frac{\sqrt{\dfrac{\left[sd(bgd)^2 + sd(Al)^2\right]}{2}}}{p} = k_t p^{-n} \tag{3}$$

where k_t is a constant, and p is the average background pixel value linearised with absorbed dose to the detector [6]. The value of n was found by fitting this equation to the experimental data. Eq. 4 was then used to calculate the dose required to achieve the target CNR, where k is a constant to be fitted

$$CNR = kD^n. \tag{4}$$

3 Results

3.1 CNR and Threshold Contrast

Eq. 1 was found to fit the experimental data within experimental error for both human and machine readings and at all relevant detail sizes. This is shown for human and automatic reading for the 0.1 mm and 0.25 mm detail sizes in Figs. 1 and 2. The correlation coefficient (R) is also shown with each graph and was highest for the

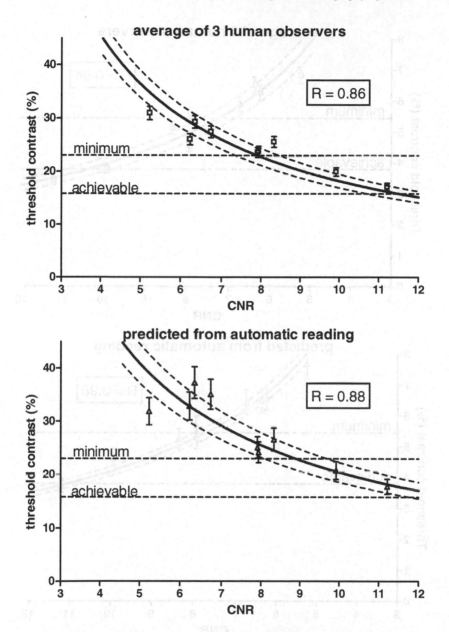

Fig. 1. CNR and threshold contrast for 0.1mm details. The upper graph shows the average threshold contrasts for 3 observers and the lower graph shows the predicted threshold contrast using automated reading. The fitted curve is in the form of Eq. 1 along with 95% confidence limits shown as dashed curves. Error bars are 1 sem. Also shown are the minimum and achievable standards in the European protocol.

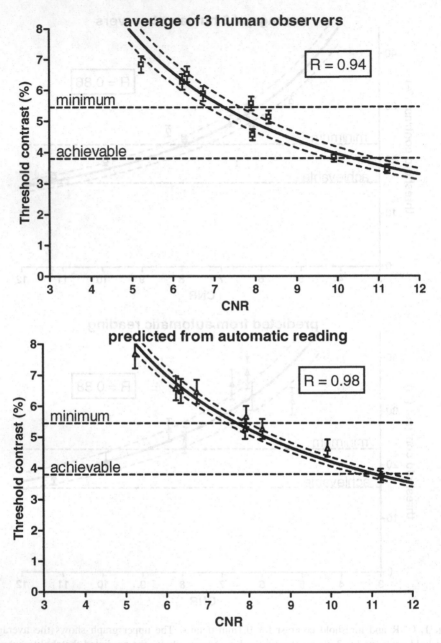

Fig. 2. CNR and threshold contrast for 0.25 mm details. The upper graph shows the average threshold contrasts for 3 observers and the lower graph shows the predicted threshold contrast using automated reading. The fitted curve is in the form of Eq. 1 along with 95% confidence limits shown as dashed curves. Error bars are 1 sem. Also shown are the minimum and achievable standards in the European protocol.

automatic reading of the 0.25mm detail size. Based on the data in Fig. 1 a target CNR of 8.5 was selected for optimisation purposes.

3.2 Optimisation

The MGDs required to achieve a CNR of 8.5 for different kV, target/filter combinations were compared at each thickness of PMMA to determine the optimal combination. Fig. 3 shows the results for a thickness of 60mm. At all thicknesses above 20mm the Rh/Rh target/filter combination was optimal and the choice of kV had relatively little effect but was in each case 31 kV as shown in Table 2. The doses indicated should be regarded as a minimum, and slightly higher may be desirable. Note that the linearised pixel value (p) rises with increasing breast thickness. This compensates for the loss in contrast due to beam hardening and increased scatter at greater thicknesses. The use of 31 kV Rh/Rh rather than 28 kV Mo/Mo achieves a dose saving of over

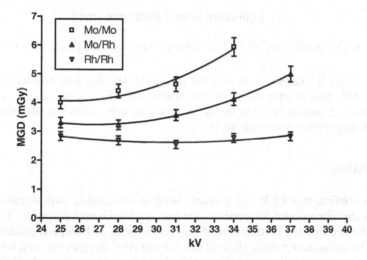

Fig. 3. The mean glandular dose (MGD) corresponding to a CNR of 8.5 for different kV, target/filter combinations using a 60 mm thickness of PMMA

Table 2. Optimal factors and doses required to achieve a target CNR of 8.5. Also shown are the corresponding doses using 28 kV Mo/Mo. Errors are 1 sem.

PMMA Thickness (mm)	Optimal factors to achieve a CNR of 8.5			MGD for a CNR of 8.5 using 28 kV Mo/Mo (mGy)	Acceptable dose limit in European protocol (mGy)
	kV target/filter	p value	MGD (mGy)		
20	28 kV Mo/Mo	49	0.28 ± 0.02	0.28 ± 0.02	< 1.0
40	31 kV Rh/Rh	66	0.89 ± 0.05	1.07 ± 0.06	< 2.0
50	31 kV Rh/Rh	78	1.55 ± 0.09	2.03 ± 0.12	< 3.0
60	31 kV Rh/Rh	87	2.60 ± 0.15	4.54 ± 0.27	< 4.5
70	31 kV Rh/Rh	105	4.65 ± 0.29	8.11 ± 0.49	< 6.5

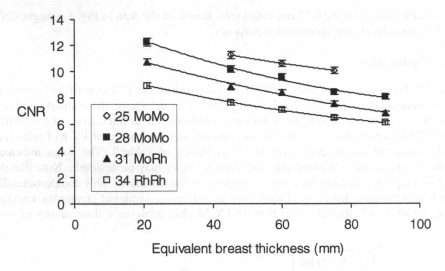

Fig. 4. The variation in CNR for four beam qualities and fixed pixel value of 60

40% at the larger thicknesses even with the increased detector dose required to reach the target CNR. This is quite different from traditional AECs which aim for constant detector dose (i.e. constant p). The impact of this approach on CNR is illustrated for a range of kV target/filter combinations in Fig. 4.

4 Discussion

The results confirm that CNR has a simple inverse relationship with threshold contrast and is therefore useful for optimisation and quality control purposes. They also provide evidence that the assumption of this relationship in European guidance was justified. The optimisation study showed that current AEC designs that aim for a fixed detector dose are not optimal, and that relatively high energy spectra should be used with sufficient detector doses at all breast thicknesses that the target CNR is achieved. The optimisation procedure described should be readily applicable to other types of digital mammography system.

It should be noted that the optimisation criteria employed here is different to that used previously for film screen systems. The reason for this is that in film/screen imaging the appropriate dose to the detector is that required to achieve the correct optical density on the processed film. As a result the main effect of using a higher X-ray energy with a film/screen system is to reduce patient dose at the expense of a loss in image contrast [7]. This has limited the use of higher energy X-rays to the small proportion of women with the greatest thickness on compression where a relatively small contrast loss may be acceptable for a large dose saving. In a review of radiation doses in the NHS Breast Screening Programme it was found that only 1.4% of exposures used either a Rh/Rh or a W/Rh target/filter combination with film screen systems [8]. However, the optimisation process is different with a digital system as the dose to the detector can be widely varied, in addition to the spectrum, without exposures going beyond the useful dynamic range of the system. Hence it is desirable to make greater use of higher energy spectra with digital systems provided sufficient detector dose is used.

References

1. Van Engen R., Young K.C., Bosmans H. and Thijssen M.: The European protocol for the quality control of the physical and technical aspects of mammography screening. Part B: Digital mammography. In: European Guidelines for Breast Cancer Screening, 4th Edition. Luxembourg: European Commission, 2006 (In press and available in draft on line at www.euref.org)
2. Young, K.C., Johnson, B., Bosmans, H., Van Engen, R.: Development of minimum standards for image quality and dose in digital mammography. In: Proceedings of the 7th International Workshop on Digital Mammography (2005) 149-154
3. Bijkerk, K.R., Thijssen, M.A.O., Arnoldussen, Th.J.M.: Modification of the CDMAM contrast-detail phantom for image quality of Full Field Digital Mammography systems. In: M. Yaffe (ed.): Proceedings of IWDM 2000. Medical Physics Publishing, Madison, WI , Toronto, (2000) 633-640
4. Dance, D.R., Skinner, C.L., Young, K.C., Beckett, J.R., C.J. Kotre.: Additional factors for the estimation of mean glandular breast dose using the UK mammography dosimetry protocol. Phys. Med. Biol. 45 (2000) 3225-3240
5. Young, K.C., Cook, J.J.H., Oduko, J.M., H. Bosmans.: Comparison of software and human observers in reading images of the CDMAM test object to assess digital mammography systems. In Proc SPIE Medical Imaging 2006. (In Press)
6. Young, K.C., Oduko, J.M., Bosmans H., Nijs K., Martinez L.: Optimal beam quality selection in digital mammography. Br J Radiol (In Press)
7. Young K.C., Ramsdale M.L., Rust A., Cooke J.: Effect of automatic kV selection on dose and contrast in mammography. Br. J. Radiol. 70 (1997) 1036-1042
8. Young, K.C., Burch A., Oduko J.M.: Radiation doses in the UK Breast Screening Programme in 2001 and 2002. Br. J. Radiol. 78 (2005) 207–218

Automated Detection Method for Architectural Distortion with Spiculation Based on Distribution Assessment of Mammary Gland on Mammogram

Takeshi Hara[1], Takanari Makita[1], Tomoko Matsubara[2], Hiroshi Fujita[1],
Yoriko Inenaga[3], Tokiko Endo[4], and Takuji Iwase[5]

[1] Division of Regeneration and Advanced, Graduate School of Medicine, Gifu University
1-1 Yanagido, Gifu-shi, Gifu, 501-1193 Japan
{hara, makita, fujita}@info.gifu-u.ac.jp
[2] School of Information Culture, Nagoya Bunri University
365 Maeda, Inazawa-cho, Inazawa-shi, Aichi, 492-8520 Japan
tomoko@nagoya-bunri.ac.jp
[3] Konica Minolta Medical & Graphic, Inc
2970 Ishikawa-cho, Hachiouji-shi, Tokyo, 192-8505 Japan
y.inenaga@konicaminolta.jp
[4] National Hospital Organization Nagoya Medical Center
4-1-1 Sannomaru, Naka-ku, Nagoya-shi, Aichi, 460-0001 Japan
endot@nnh.hosp.go.jp
[5] The Cancer Institute Hospital of JFCR
3-10-6 Ariake, Koto-ku, Tokyo, 135-8550 Japan
takiwase@nifty.com

Abstract. The clustered microcalcifications and mass are the important findings in interpreting breast cancer, architectural distortion on mammograms as well. We have developed the detection algorithm for distorted area based on concentration of mammary gland. The purpose of this study is to suggest the improvement of extraction method of mammary gland in order to achieve higher sensitivity. The mean curvature, and the combination of shape index and curvedness were performed for extracting of mammary gland in our previous methods. In our new method, the dynamic-range compression was added as the pre-processing before extracting mammary gland by mean curvature. The detection rate at initial pick-up stage was improved by this improvement. It was concluded that our detection method would be effective.

1 Background

Clustered microcalcifications and mass are the important findings in interpreting breast cancer, along with architectural distortion on mammograms. CAD techniques for detecting mass and clustered microcalcifications are well-documented and their performance continually improves. Whereas it was reported that fewer than one half of the cases of architectural distortion were detected by the two commercially available CAD systems[1]. In addition, a few CAD schemes have been specifically designed for detecting architectural distortion[2,3].

Susan M. Astley et al. (Eds.): IWDM 2006, LNCS 4046, pp. 370–375, 2006.
© Springer-Verlag Berlin Heidelberg 2006

The distorted areas of clinical images are mainly classified into two typical types: either retraction or spiculation. The contour of normal mammary glandular tissue on the breast border tends to be smooth. On the other hand, the contour of the tissue in retraction area is depressed. The distributions of the mammary gland are approximated by linear structures. Those directions are toward the nipple within the normal breast, whereas the directions are toward the spiculation areas within the abnormal one.

We have been developing the automated detection algorithms by using the top-hat processing for retraction[4] and the concentration index for spiculation[5], and mammary glands[6]. The high sensitivities of these algorithms indicate the system's potential usefulness. However, it was found that the extraction accuracy of mammary gland was not good enough in the visual evaluation in detecting spiculation. The purpose of this study is to suggest the improvement of extraction method of mammary gland in order to achieve higher sensitivity.

2 Method

Our previous method for detecting spiculation consists of five steps: 1) input of digital data, 2) extraction of mammary gland structure, 3) extraction of suspect area by concentration index, 4) elimination of false positives by discriminant analysis, and 5) annotation of architectural distortion (see Fig. 1).

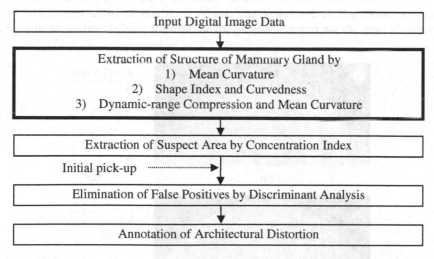

Fig. 1. Flowchart of extraction method for architectural distortion with spiculation

First, digital mammograms are obtained from screen-film mammograms that are digitized to a 0.05-mm pixel size with 12-bit resolution by using the Konica laser digitizer (LD-5500). All of them are subsampled to an effective pixel size of 0.2 mm for detection of architectural distortions. The border of the breast on the mammogram is automatically extracted for the segmentation of the breast area. The smallest rectangle containing the breast region is then cut off. Secondly, the structure of mammary gland is extracted in terms of the shape index and curvedness. The digital mammograms can be represented in the three-dimensional space where the Z-axis is the density (pixel value of the 2-D image). In this space, the density distribution is approximated by a curved surface. The density distribution of the linear structures in the mammary gland is described by a downward-curved surface. The shape index classifies the shape of a curved surface. For example, five well-known shape classes have the following shape index values: cup, rut, saddle, ridge, and cap. The curvedness characterizes the flatness, or scale, of the shape indicated by the shape index. Thirdly, the concentration index is calculated in order to extract the suspect area. This index means that the component magnitude of the line element directed to the center of the local area is weighted by the inverse of the distance from the center and summed over this area.

The summation is normalized by the sum of the length of the line element weight by the inverse of the distance so that the effect of the number of line elements. This index is high in the distorted area, because the linear structures of the mammary gland are toward the suspect area. Fourthly, the discriminant analysis is performed in order to eliminate false positives. Nine features are employed in this analysis. Five and four features are calculated in the suspect area and in the power spectrum, respectively. The residual candidates are finally determined as "true" architectural distortions and then indicate by circles in the concerned digitized mammogram on the computer display.

In this study, we investigate the extraction accuracy of mammary gland by three methods: 1) shape index and curvedness which are used in our previous method, 2) mean curvature, and 3) dynamic-range compression and mean curvature. The mean curvature's sign shows either a downward or upward curved surface at any given

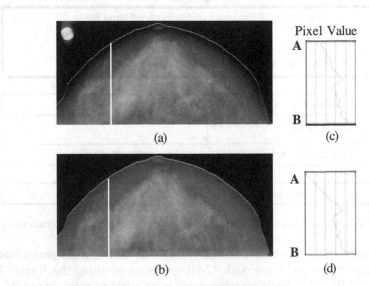

Fig. 2. Dynamic-range Compression. (a) An original image. (c) Processed image of (a). (b) and (d) are profiles of line AB of (a) and (c), respectively.

point. The dynamic-range compression compresses the pixel value nonlinearity. It is possible to eliminate the background density contributed from the breast thickness near breast border without changing contrast by this method. Figure 3 shows dynamic-range compression process.

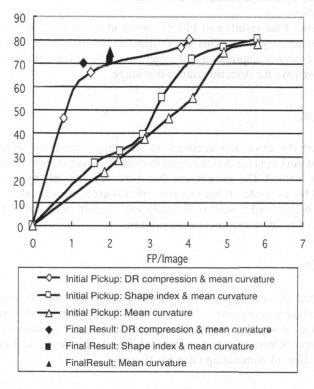

Fig. 3. Final results and FROC curves at initial pick-up of three methods

3 Results

First, we assessed the three methods in the synthetic images. We made some original synthetic images for this study. These synthetic images consist of many lines radiating in all directions. The lines were made based on Gaussian function. The lines are different in lengths, thickness and contrasts. The density changes and noises were added to background density.

When we compared the extraction results using the three methods, the results are comparable expect in the synthetic image with density change. It is not possible to detect any lines in density change area by only mean curvature. On the other hand, it is possible to detect some lines in that area by shape index and curvedness method, and dynamic-range compression and mean curvature method. The shape of detected line by mean curvature is better than one by the combination of shape index and curvedness.

Next, the three methods were tested in clinical images. Our image database of architectural distortions consists of 99 cases. The spiculation type that is detection target in this study is 56 cases within this database. To our knowledge, it is the maximum database with architectural distortions on mammography in the world. An experienced radiologist verified the diagnostic sketches and comments in details of all cases used in our studies.

Figure 3 shows final results and FROC curves at initial pick-up of three methods for extracting mammary gland. This shows that the best performance is the combination of dynamic-range compression and mean curvature at the initial pick-up stage. It is possible to improve the detection rate at this stage.

4 Discussion

We investigated the extraction accuracy of mammary gland by three methods. It showed the best performance that the combination of dynamic-range compression and mean curvature method. The spiculations that were detected only by this method were located around breast border. It became possible to detect them because the mammary glands around breast border were sufficiently extracted because the background density was removed by dynamic-range compression.

5 Conclusions

It was concluded that our approach was effective because the detection rate at the initial pick-up stage was improved. Nevertheless, many true positives were eliminated at the final stage. It was thought that the features of the false positives changed because of the improvement of detection method. For the future work, it is necessary to improve the method of eliminating false positives.

Acknowledgments

This research was in part supported by a Grant-in-Aid for Scientific Research for future CAD (http://www.future-cad.org) from the Ministry of Education, Culture, Sports, Science and Technology and a Grant-in-Aid for Cancer Research from the Ministry of Health, Labour and Welfare.

References

1. Baker, J.A., Rosen, E.L., Lo, J.Y., et al.: Computer-aided detection (CAD) in screening Mammography: Sensitivity of commercial CAD systems for detection architectural distortion. AJR, 181 (2003) 1083-1088
2. Ayres, F.J., Rangayyan, R.M.: Detection of architectural distortion in mammograms using phase portraits. Medical Imaging 2004: Image Processing, Proc. of SPIE 2004, 5370 (2004) 587-597

3. Tourassi, G.D., Floyd, Jr. G.E.: Performance evaluation of information-theoretic CAD scheme for the detection of mammographic architectural distortion. Medical Imaging 2004: Image Processing, Proc. of SPIE 2004, 5370 (2004) 59-65
4. Matsubara, T., Yamazaki, D., Hara, T., et al.: Automated detection of architectural distortions on mammograms. Proc of 6th International Workshop on Digital Mammography (2002) 350-352
5. Matsubara, T., Fukuoka, D., Yagi, N., et al.: Detection method for architectural distortion based on analysis of structure of mammary gland on mammograms. Proc. of CARS2005 (2005) 1036-1040
6. Nagata C, Matsubara T, Fujita H., et al. : Associations of mammographic density with dietary factors in Japanese women, Cancer Epidemiology Biomarkers & Prevention, 14 (2005), 2877-2880

Web Services for the DDSM and Digital Mammography Research

Chris Rose, Daniele Turi, Alan Williams,
Katy Wolstencroft, and Chris Taylor

Imaging Science and Biomedical Engineering,
The University of Manchester,
Manchester, M13 9PT, United Kingdom
http://www.medicine.manchester.ac.uk/isbe/

Abstract. The Digital Database for Screening Mammography (DDSM) is an invaluable resource for digital mammography research. However, there are two particular shortcomings that can pose a significant barrier to many of those who may want to use the resource: 1) the actual mammographic image data is encoded using a non-standard lossless variant of the JPEG image format; 2) although detailed metadata is provided, it is not in a form that permits it to be searched, manipulated or reasoned over by standard tools. This paper describes web services that will allow both humans and computers to query for, and obtain, mammograms from the DDSM in a standard and well-supported image file format. Further, this paper describes how these and other services can be used within grid-based workflows, allowing digital mammography researchers to make use of distributed computing facilities.

1 Background

The DDSM [6] provides high-resolution digitised mammograms, expert ground-truth and metadata (including the date of study and digitisation, the Breast Imaging Reporting and Data System (BI-RADS) [1] breast density and assessment categories, a subtlety rating, the type of pathology and detailed categorisation of the nature of the perceived abnormality using the BI-RADS lexicon). The DDSM is available free of charge by File Transfer Protocol (FTP).

While the DDSM does provide software to decode their mammograms[1], the default distribution of this software does not build under modern compilers without modification, a step that may prove difficult to those with insufficient experience of C/C++ software development for UNIX-like operating systems. Furthermore, even when properly compiled, the DDSM software outputs the image data as a stream of raw bytes; one then has to normalise these according to the model of digitiser used to image the original films and then create an image file that is readable by one's image analysis software environment. An introduction to web services is given in Section 1.1. Section 2.1 describes a web service that allows digital mammograms from the DDSM to be obtained

---

[1] In particular the DDSM's `jpeg` program.

Susan M. Astley et al. (Eds.): IWDM 2006, LNCS 4046, pp. 376–383, 2006.

in a standardised and well-supported lossless file format. Section 2.2 describes a service that allows groundtruth images to be obtained in the same file format.

While a web-based query tool is provided by the DDSM, it is useful only to human users or automated tools that have been specifically designed with the DDSM in mind. If the metadata were in a more useful format, it could easily be exposed for both human and computer use. Section 2.3 describes a formal ontology that has been developed to describe the DDSM resource and a web-based user interface to allow users to query the ontology.

Section 2.4 describes how web services can be used together within *workflows* to run full experiments and how a full record of how such experiments were performed can be recorded by capturing provenance events. Section 2.5 details a supporting website for the work described in this paper.

1.1 An Introduction to Web Services

The concept of web services may best be explained with a simple example of a hypothetical scientist named Bob who lives in Manchester, UK. Bob has a CAD algorithm that other scientists want to use. Traditionally, Bob would package his CAD algorithm into some form that is easily installed and run by other scientists. He would then deliver it to those scientists via Internet download or on physical media (e.g. CD-ROM). However, Bob might not be able to let other scientists run his software on their computers because:

- Bob may not have planned to share his software and may have made assumptions in its design that limits its portability;
- users might need an expensive license to use a required proprietary library;
- the software may need access to a resource (e.g. a large database) that resides at Bob's lab;
- Bob might frequently update his software, so making each update available to all his users might be troublesome;
- packaging the software for easy installation might be too time-consuming for a busy research scientist.

Bob might decide that it is easier to allow other scientists to run his software on his computer, accessing it via the Internet. This can be achieved by exposing his software as a web service. Using an appropriate piece of client software that implements the Simple Object Access Protocol (SOAP) standard [5], other scientists can run Bob's CAD algorithm on their data. In this way, Bob's CAD algorithm can be used by remote scientists as if it were installed on their computers, or integrated into software as if it is a library containing the required functionality.

The "interface" to a web service—the location of the computer that provides the service and a specification of its inputs and output and their data types—is described using the Web Service Description Language (WSDL) [2]. The URL of a service's WSDL file is all that is needed for a SOAP client to be able to use the service[2].

---

[2] The WSDL files for the services described in this paper can be obtained from the website described in Section 2.5.

The web services proposed in this paper open up the possibility of performing digital mammography research using grid-based workflows. In this context, a *grid* is an *ad hoc* collection of computing services offered by a number of (typically) different computers via a network (typically the Internet) and a *workflow* specifies how the services provided by the grid are orchestrated in order for some task to be performed. Section 2.4 describes workflows in more detail.

2   Method

2.1   Digital Mammogram Web Service

To create a web service that makes available mammograms from the DDSM, we developed a command-line program that, given the name of a particular DDSM mammogram (e.g. D_0160_1.RIGHT_MLO), downloads the associated .LJPEG file from the DDSM's FTP server, decodes the raw image data, normalises it according to the digtiser used and finally converts it to a PNG file [4]. This format is ideal for encoding mammograms as it is standardised, guarantees lossless compression and is widely supported by common software tools and libraries[3]. (In future, other lossless image formats may be more suitable—such as JPEG-LS and JPEG 2000—but as of this writing these formats are not widely supported.)

Downloading and converting the images takes a few minutes on a desktop computer with a fast connection to the Internet and so the program caches some of the converted mammograms locally so that future requests can be efficiently serviced. Our program is exposed as a service via SOAP [5]. DDSM mammograms can be obtained from this service using any SOAP client.

2.2   Groundtruth Web Service

To enable the evaluation of algorithms run on the DDSM mammograms delivered by the service described in Section 2.1, there is a need to be able to obtain the corresponding groundtruth images. We have developed a web service that allows DDSM groundtruth images to be generated and delivered in a suitable image format. Our approach to developing this service was the same as that described in Section 2.1. We first developed a command-line program that, given the name of a particular DDSM mammogram (e.g. D_0160_1.RIGHT_MLO) and an abnormality number[4], downloads the corresponding .OVERLAY file (which contains a description of the shape of the radiologist-annotated abnormalities for the image using a chain code). The DDSM groundtruth metadata defines two possible types of region: a *'boundary'* and a *'core'*, though *'core'* regions may be absent (see [6] for details). Our program then creates a image with the same number of rows and columns as the corresponding digital mammogram—i.e. there is a one-one correspondence between every pixel in a digital mammogram and the

---

[3] We encode DDSM mammograms as 16 bits/pixel grey-level images.
[4] Mammograms may contain more than one abnormality. The abnormality number is captured by the ontology that is described in Section 2.3.

pixel at the same location in its groundtruth image—and this image is populated with pixel values that indicate the class of each pixel. A value of zero represents normal tissue or the non-breast region, a value of 128 represents a pixel within a *'boundary'* region of the abnormality and a value of 255 represents a pixel within a *'core'* region of the abnormality. The resulting groundtruth image is saved as a PNG image. While downloading the .OVERLAY file and creating a groundtruth image takes approximately a minute, the resulting PNG files are very small (approximately 14 kb) due to the high correlation between successive scan lines in the images, and we therefore keep all generated images to efficiently service future requests. This program is then exposed as a web service via SOAP.

2.3   DDSM Ontology and Metadata Query Service

Being able to obtain mammograms and groundtruth is not particularly useful without knowing which mammograms have what characteristics. To this end, we have developed a formal *ontology* of the mammograms, groundtruth and metadata (e.g. abnormalities, patient information). An ontology is a description of the concepts and relationships that exist in some knowledge domain. The formal representation of metadata within ontologies (using technologies such as the Web Ontology Language (OWL) [9]) allows domain knowledge to be used alongside explicit labelling to infer implicit relationships and hence deliver more useful results. As a simple example, if an ontology were to state that a stellate lesion is a type of mass, then a query for masses could return—in addition to items explicitly labelled as masses—items that were labelled as stellate lesions; i.e. the domain knowledge captured in the formal ontology allows it to be inferred that items labelled as stellate lesions must also be returned.

Previous Work. The most relevant work on ontologies for digital mammography was done by the Medical Imaging with Advanced Knowledge Technologies (MIAKT) project, which developed a fairly complete ontology for breast cancer imaging studies called the Breast Cancer Imaging Ontology. This multi-level ontology incorporated classes for both X-ray and MRI breast imaging, for abnormal findings and medical assessments [3]. The project also used the DDSM images as exemplar breast X-ray image data [7]. In contrast, the ontology that we have developed is more narrowly confined to the DDSM database, as justified below.

Our DDSM Ontology. Within the DDSM, information about the mammograms is specified in an .ICS file and, for each image that contains abnormalities, an .OVERLAY file. The .ICS file contains information common to the case e.g. the patient's age, and also information necessary to interpret the four mammograms e.g. the number of pixels per scan line. The .OVERLAY file contains information particular to the abnormality, or abnormalities, that have been interpreted within a particular mammogram e.g. the left CC mammogram.

The ontology that has been developed for the DDSM allows the description of the information within the .ICS and the .OVERLAY files. The ontology is written in OWL [9]. A decision was made that the ontology would only describe the information specified within the DDSM, in particular it would not attempt to be a general model of mammograms, mammogram interpretation or breast cancer—as the MIAKT project developed—as we are interested only in making the DDSM database easily available.

For an individual case, an OWL ontology is populated with RDF (Resource Description Framework [8]) instances. The instance ontology combines the information within the .ICS and .OVERLAY files into a single semantic structure. This allows the easy searching of the instance ontology when it is loaded into an RDF repository.

Within the DDSM ontology, the *'case'* class specifies information that applies to a patient's visit and their four images. It has four relationships to *'views'* corresponding to the four mammograms. *'Views'* are subclassed into either abnormal or normal views. The information about the image is held within the

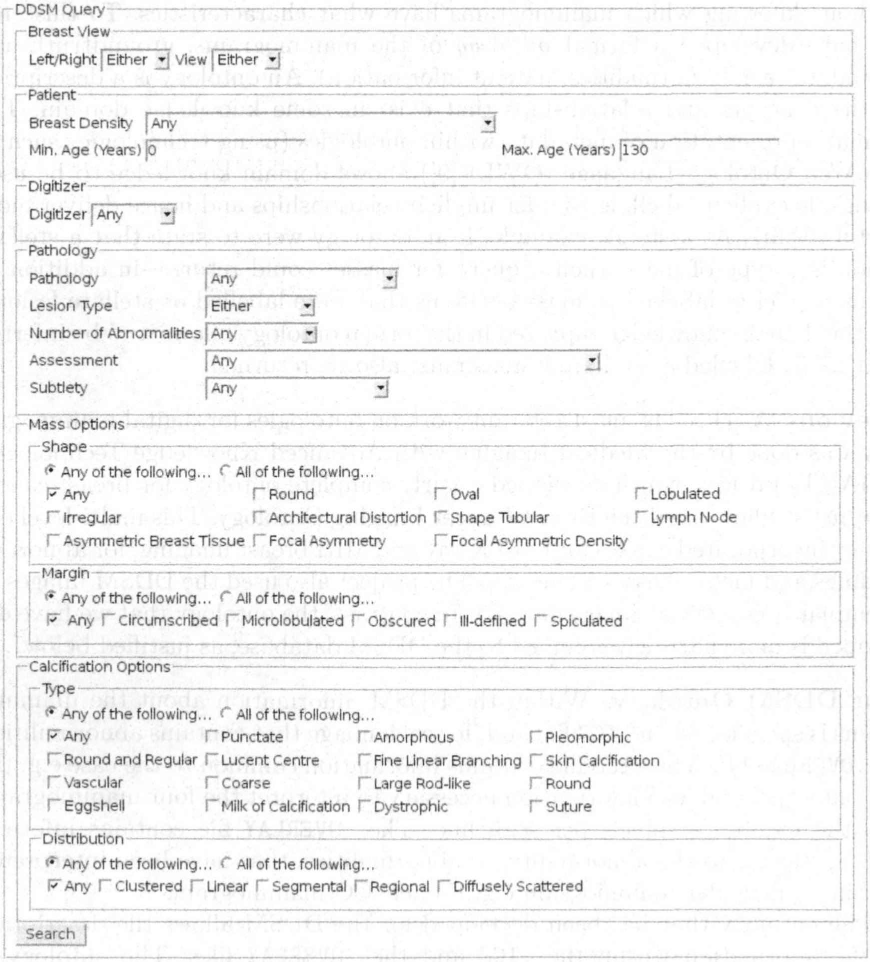

Fig. 1. The DDSM metadata query form

'view' superclass. If the 'view' is an 'abnormal view' then it has relationships to one or more 'abnormalities'.

An 'abnormality' contains information such as the assessment and subtlety. It also has specific information about the calcification or mass intrepretation of the abnormality. In addition, the bounding curves of the abnormality and any cores within it are specified.

We have automatically populated an RDF store with instances of the classes in our ontology by processing the DDSM metadata files. We are currently developing a web-based user interface that will allow users to query the RDF store for images and groundtruth in a user-friendly manner. Figure 1 shows the form used to create queries.

2.4   Workflow Enactment and Provenance Capture

A workflow describes how a number of services can be combined to perform some useful task. The Taverna workbench program—a Java application that originated in the bioinformatics research community—allows users to create and run workflows within a graphical user interface [10]. Taverna displays workflows as directed graphs, where nodes represent inputs, services or outputs and arcs represent the flow of data and control (see Figure 2 for an example). Workflows can be saved and easily exchanged between colleagues. Taverna allows users to run, pause, monitor and debug workflows in a manner similar to modern software development environments. Workflow results can be directly displayed within Taverna.

Aside from allowing researchers to make use of distributed computing resources, Taverna can capture *provenance events*—e.g. when a particular workflow was started and with which inputs—allowing the workbench to operate as an automated laboratory log book. This also allows researchers to obtain

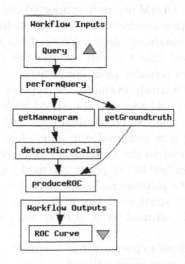

Fig. 2. A simple Taverna workflow

answers to questions like *'which images were used as inputs to the workflow I ran on 24 January 2006?'.*

2.5 Supporting Website

Those who wish to use the services described in this paper are directed to http://www.digital-mammography-services.net. This website will provide the most up-to-date documentation of the available services and provide links to the WSDL files that specify the web services described in this paper. We invite the community to make useful software and data available via services and are keen to document these at the above website.

3 Results

Our work is at a relatively early stage, but we already have useful services and infrastructure. The most significant contributions are the digital mammogram and groundtruth "getter" services, the DDSM ontology, the web-based query facility and the supporting website. We hope these will be useful to the digital mammography research community. While we are using the Taverna workbench software to integrate our services into simple grid-based workflows, our general approach—publishing our software as SOAP services—does not require clients to use Taverna; any SOAP client can be used.

4 Discussion

We have described three web services which allow both humans and computers to query a formal ontology of the DDSM data and obtain digital mammograms and groundtruth from the DDSM in a well-supported standard image format. We have also described how these services could be used within grid-based workflows. As Section 1 described, obtaining mammograms from the DDSM is currently non-trivial and it is hoped that the web services described in this paper will make using this important resource more convenient.

It is difficult to quantitatively evaluate the type of work that is described in this paper. While we could measure the speed with which requests can be processed, or the number that can be handled concurrently, such measurements do little to tell us if we have achieved our aims of developing and deploying infrastructure that is useful to the community. This will become apparent in time as the resources described in this paper are used (or otherwise) and if other researchers contribute their software and data in the form of web services for use by the community. In this spirit we welcome criticism and suggestions and are able to offer advice on an informal basis to those interested in developing their own web services.

Future work will focus on exposing other useful algorithms as web services (e.g. a CAD task such as microcalcification detection, a receiver operating characteristic (ROC) analysis service) and on maintaining the website described in

Section 2.5. Given these services, it will be possible to run a simple but typical digital mammography CAD experiment using web services (i.e. obtain mammograms → process each image using the CAD algorithm → obtain ground-truth → produce an ROC curve). By publishing the workflow, others in the community would be able to replicate the experiment exactly or swap one service (e.g. the CAD task) for their own to be able to fairly compare algorithms.

References

1. The ACR Breast Imaging Reporting and Data System (BI-RADS). American College Radiology, 1998. Third Edition.
2. Erik Christensen, Francisco Curbera, Greg Meredith, and Sanjiva Weerawarana. Web Services Description Language (WSDL) 1.1. W3C Note, World Wide Web Consortium, March 2001. (A W3C Recommendation for WSDL 2.0 is currently pending.).
3. S. Dasmahapatra, B. Hu, P. Lewis, and N. Shadbolt. Ontology-Based Medical Image Annotation with Description Logics. In *15th IEEE International Conference on Tools with Artificial Intelligence*, Sacramento, CA, USA, 2003.
4. David Duce. Portable Network Graphics (PNG) Specification (Second Edition). W3C Recommendation, World Wide Web Consortium, November 2004.
5. Martin Gudgin, Marc Hadley, Noah Mendelsohn, Jean-Jaques Moreau, and Henrik Frystyk Nielsen. SOAP Version 1.2 Parts 1–2. W3C Recommendation, World Wide Web Consortium, June 2003.
6. M. Heath, K. Bowyer, D. Kopans, R. Moore, and P. Kegelmeyer Jr. The Digital Database for Screening Mammography. In M. J. Yaffe, editor, *Digital Mammography: IWDM 2000, 5th International Workshop*, pages 212–218, Madison, Wisconsin, USA, December 2001. Medical Physics Publishing.
7. B. Hu, S. Dasmahapatra, D. Dupplaw, P. Lewis, and N. Shadbolt. Managing Patient Record Instances Using DL-Enabled Formal Concept Analysis. In *14th International Conference, EKAW 2004*, Whittlebury Hall, UK,, October 2004.
8. Frank Manola and Eric Miller. RDF Primer. W3C Recommendation, World Wide Web Consortium, February 2004.
9. Deborah L. McGuinness and Frank van Harmelen. OWL Web Ontology Language Overview. W3C Recommendation, World Wide Web Consortium, February 2004.
10. Tom Oinn, Tom Greenwood, Matthew Addis, M. Nedim Alpdemir, Justin Ferris, Kevin Glover, Carole Goble, Antoon Goderis, Duncan Hull, Darren Marvin, Peter Li, Phillip Lord, Matthew R. Pocock, Martin Senger, Robert Stevens, Anil Wipat, and Chris Wroe. Taverna: Lessons in creating a workflow environment for the life sciences. *Concurrency and Computation: Practice and Experience Grid Workflow Special Issue (Accepted)*, 2005.

GPCALMA: An Italian Mammographic Database of Digitized Images for Research

Adele Lauria[1], Raffaella Massafra[2], Sabina Sonia Tangaro[2], Roberto Bellotti[2,3],
MariaEvelina Fantacci[4], Pasquale Delogu[4], Ernesto Lopez Torres[5],
Piergiorgio Cerello[6], Francesco Fauci[7], Rosario Magro[7], and Ubaldo Bottigli[8]

[1] Università di Napoli "Federico II", Dipartimento di Scienze Fisiche, and
Istituto Nazionale di Fisica Nucleare, Sezione di Napoli, via Cinthia, I-80126 Napoli, Italy
adele.lauria@na.infn.it
[2] Università di Bari and Istituto Nazionale di Fisica Nucleare, Sezione di Bari, Italy
[3] TIRES, Center of Innovative Technologies for Signal Detection and Processing, Bari, Italy
[4] Università di Pisa, Pisa, and INFN, Sezione di Pisa, Italy
[5] CEADEN, Habana, Cuba
[6] INFN, Sezione di Torino, Torino, Italy
[7] Università di Palermo, Palermo, and INFN, Sezione di Catania, Italy
[8] Università di Siena, Siena, and Istituto Nazionale di Fisica Nucleare, Sezione di Cagliari

Abstract. In this work the implementation of a database of digitized mammograms is described. The digitized images were collected since 1999 by a community of physicists in collaboration with radiologists in several Italian hospitals, as a first step in order to develop and implement a Computer Aided Detection (CAD) system. 3369 mammograms were collected from 967 patients; they were classified according to the type and the morphology of the lesions, the type of the breast tissue and the type of pathologies. A dedicated Graphical User Interface was developed for mammography visualization and processing, in order to support the medical diagnosis directly on a high-resolution screen. The database has been the starting point for the development of other medical imaging applications such as a breast CAD, currently being upgraded and optimized for the use in conjunction of the GRID technology in the framework of the INFN-funded MAGIC-5 project.

1 Introduction

A medical images dataset is considered the starting point for important epidemiological and statistical studies and also to develop and test algorithms for CAD systems, but also for teaching and training of medical students and as an archive of rare cases. In 1995 Osuch et al. proposed a mammography database for a national mammography inspection and to monitor patients through a centralized system [1]. Technological improvements in digitizing scanners make now possible to digitize radiographic films with no significant loss of information. At the moment many large datasets of digitized mammograms are available on the web [2,3]. Other databases, also "GRID compliant", are described in the literature [4-6]. The development of a CAD system is strictly tied to the collection of a large dataset of selected images.

Susan M. Astley et al. (Eds.): IWDM 2006, LNCS 4046, pp. 384–391, 2006.

In this work a full description of the GPCALMA (*Grid Platform for Computer Aided Library in Mammography*) database is given.

2 Method

Images were acquired in various mammographic centers using different mammographic screen/film systems and settings (all with molybdenum anode) and in the framework of different applications, including both clinical routine carried out on symptomatic women, and screening programs addressed to asymptomatic women. Moreover, many images come from an archive of particularly meaningful clinical cases collected in the previous years at the Bari hospital. Unfortunately at the moment of the digitization the information about acquisition settings were no more available, thus making impossible normalization procedures. A workstation, composed of a PC running the Linux operating system and a film scanner, was installed at each site involved in the program. Digitized images are stored in a dedicated hard disk, which presently stores the whole GPCALMA database of mammographies. All the mammograms of the database were digitized using the same digitizer model and under the same conditions in order to avoid fake features caused by variations in the digitization step. A CCD scanner was used, choosing [7] a pixel size of 85 μm and a 12 bit depth. The typical scan time is 20s. The acquisition software provided with the scanner was modified to scan and save images in a special format (called CALMA format) consisting of a long vector of numbers corresponding to the pixel intensities and two other numbers representing the image dimension. These numbers are used to transform the vector in a matrix: each pixel of the image can be represented by a triplet (x, y, I), where x is the row number, y is the column number and I is the intensity of the pixel, ranging from 0 (black) to 4095 (white). Such workstations have been continuously operative in various collaboration sites for several years without problems. In sites where clinical studies were performed, the PC was connected to a high resolution and high luminosity B/W LCD monitor.

3 Description of the Database

The database is composed of 3369 mammographic images, each including data and clinical information. Images were collected from 967 patients. The age distribution is reported in figure 1. Each patient has from one to six views, according to the distribution shown in figure 2. The repartition of the database in left/right breast images is 1835 (51%) and 1734 (49%) respectively, while for the craniocaudal/oblique/lateral views is 1601 (48%), 1456 (43%) and 312 (9%) respectively. The image size is 2067 x 2657 pixels, 85μm of pitch, 12 bit/pixel (4096 grey levels); each image file is about 8 Mbytes. All the mammographic images with other information related to the patient (follow up, age of patients and interesting cases) were collected in the Italian hospitals involved in the collaboration from 1997 to 2002. The geographic provenience of the images is shown in figure 3.

Prior to being processed all images were anonymized. All the images of the database containing one (or more) lesions were characterized according to the kind of

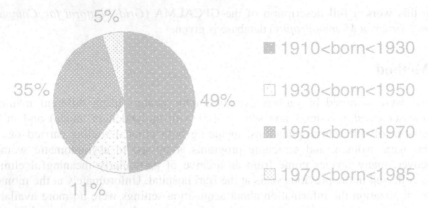

Fig. 1. Distribution of the birth-date of the analyzed patients

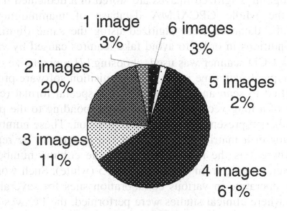

Fig. 2. Number of cases with 1-6 views

lesions (massive or microcalcification), its grade of malignancy, the kind of texture of the breast, etc.

In this study there are the images from 306 (32%) patients who were defined *normal* when there was no evidence of any lesion, in many cases proven by three years of radiological follow up. The remaining images proceed from 661 (68%) "abnormal" patients: when a suspicious lesion was found by the radiologist in these images, it was classified as *suspicious*; *benign* or *malignant*. For many malignant lesions there are also available cytological or histological results. In any case, detailed radiological annotations of the abnormalities are included in the database as notes. The relative distribution of grade of malignancy of the lesions is: 560 (35%) suspicious lesions, 468 (29%) benign lesions and 592 (37%) malignant lesions. In the table 1 are reported the histotypes related only to some patients.

We consider abnormal images the ones which contain at least one mass or one microcalcification, as diagnosed by an expert radiologist. In the database there are1062 images containing at least one Region Of Interest (ROI) with a massive

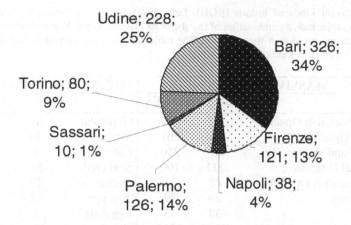

Fig. 3. Geographic provenience of the images within the MAGIC-5 project

Table 1. Kind of histoypes classified in the database

Invasive Lobular Carcinoma	17	Fibrosis	6
Lobular Carcinoma	5	Fibroadenoma	7
Ductal Carcinoma	3	Cystica fibrose mastopatia	2
Ductal Invasive Carcinoma	124	Sclerosing Adenosis	2
Ductal in Situ Carcinoma	16	Epitheial Hyperplasia	3
Intraductal Carcinoma	11	Adenosis	5
Papilloma Intaductal	1	Tubular Carcinoma	10
Dysplasia	2	Muciparo Carcinoma	5
		Total	219

lesion and 304 images containing at least one ROI with microcalcifications. In total there are 1296 (38%) abnormal images containing at least one lesion (massive or microcalcification or both) and 2073 (62%) normal images with no lesions; each image can also contain more than one lesion, so the total number of ROIs is 1620 (1236 massive and 384 microcalcification).

Each of these main classes of lesions (microcalcification clusters and massive lesions) are further classified according to the morphological characteristics of the lesion. For our database, we adopted the scheme of Lattanzio and Guerrieri [8], which has been recognized as a satisfactory reference framework by the national panel of radiologists, with more than 20 years of experience in mammography, who identified and localized each lesion according to such a classification.

Each abnormal image comes with a description of the lesion as shown in table 2, in which is reported the partition of the ROIs for different kind of massive lesions and microcalcifications, with the corresponding number of images from which each kind of lesions comes.

The location and size of a mass is defined by a radiologist-drawn circle, characterized by center coordinates $\{X_{rad}; Y_{rad}\}$ and radius $\{R_{rad}\}$, which fully contains

Table 2. Different kinds of lesions (ROIs). Left: different kinds of masses present in the database; others include a combination of the above mentioned kinds. Right: different kinds of microcalcifications present in the database. The table includes the corresponding number of images from which each kind of lesions comes.

MASSIVE LESIONS			MICROCALCIFICATIONS		
	ROIs	IMAGES		ROIs	IMAGES
Irregular Roundish Opacity	406	369	Glandular	163	124
Spiculated Opacity	294	261	Mixed	99	73
Regular Roundish Opacity	289	210	Lobular	9	8
Parenchimal Distorsion	111	109	Scattered	57	45
Blurred Roundish Opacity	47	41	Ductal	10	10
Fibroadenoma	29	29	Teacup	37	37
Others	58	43	Eggshell	6	4
Total	*1236*	*1062*	Tubular	3	3
			Total	*384*	*304*

the mass. The radius size of the masses ranges from 3.1 mm to 47.2 mm with a mean size of 11.7 mm, while the radius size of the clusters of microcalcification ranges from 1 mm to 72.8 mm with a mean size of 11.9 mm.

Another important parameter to characterize the image is the breast tissue type. Collaborating radiologists were asked to identify the breast texture for a full images characterization. As far as the breast background is concerned in the GPCALMA database, we adopt a tissue classification recognized as a standard by many Italian radiologists [9][10]:

i)   Fibro-adipose tissue indicates a fat breast with little fibrous connective tissue;
ii) Glandular tissue: indicates the presence of prominent duct patterns;
iii) Dense tissue: indicates a dense breast parenchyma.

The breast background classification is based only on the appearance of the parenchyma, without any reference to skin, vascularity, presence/absence of masses, calcifications, lymphnodes, nor to parity, history of breast disease, age and family history. Figure 4 reports the background composition of the database. Most of the images are glandular-like: the detection of pathological structures in this kind of images is a quite hard task, since the target is surrounded by a "noisy" environment.

The database presents some limitations. The first is that images are collected from different centers and were acquired with different mammograms under different conditions, so the grey level scales are quite uniform only for the images coming from the same center. Besides that, images were collected in different clinical and screening conditions, so they do not represent a typical distribution of the mammographic masses and microcalcifications in terms of ratio of benign to malignant cases from an epidemiological point of view. Moreover it was not possible to classify the lesions according to their visibility grade because different radiologists view the images, and the classification should have been radiologist's dependent. In any case, this database represent the larger Italian one in terms of digitized mammograms and it has been

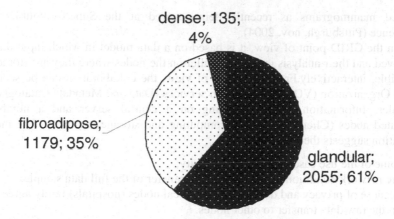

Fig. 4. Breast tissue composition of the database

successfully utilized not only for the development and the test of the GPCALMA Computer Aided Detection System [7] also in conjunction of the GRID technology [11]. In fact it has been also the basis of an experimental study about the peculiarities of monitor refertation [12], it has been used to test the performance of different CAD systems as second readers [13]. Moreover, it has been successfully used [14] for developing a CAD system for microcalcification cluster identification in a pan-European distributed database of mammograms in the preliminary (when the abnormal cases in the new database were still too few to be used) training step of the neural based classification analysis.

4 Discussion

The database collected in the course of this study represents a useful archive of digitized mammographic images. According to the rules established within the GPCALMA collaboration, it can be a valuable tool to the scientific community for different tasks such as training and testing of Neural Network based classification tools, for retrieval use and for statistics and epidemiology studies.

Like in a screening program, data are collected from geographically remote sites. The growth of the database and the distributed nature of the collaboration raises a problem, since images are generally not replicated between remote sites. The approach used to solve the problem of remote access was to use techniques developed for GRID computing. The need for acquiring and analyzing data stored in different locations requires the use of GRID Services for the management of distributed computing resources and data. GRID technologies allow remote image analysis and interactive online diagnosis, with a relevant reduction of the delays presently associated to the diagnosis in screening programs. A Virtual Organization (VO) has been deployed, so that authorized users can share data and resources and implement screening, tele-training and tele-diagnosis for mammograms. A small-scale prototype of the required GRID functionality was already implemented for the analysis of digitized mammograms as recently demonstrated at the SuperComputing 2004 Conference (Pittsburgh, nov. 2004).

From the GRID point of view, it is based on a data model in which input data are not moved and their analysis is run in parallel on the nodes where they are stored and, if possible, interactively.From this point of view, the collaboration can be seen as a Virtual Organization (VO), with common services (Data and Metadata Catalogue, Job Scheduler, Information System) running on a central server and a number of distributed nodes (Clients) providing computing and storage resources. The medical application suggests these constrains:

1. some of the use cases require interactivity;
2. the network conditions do not allow the transfer of the full data sample;
3. because of privacy and data ownership, local nodes (hospitals) rarely agree on the raw data transfer to other nodes.

Integration of tools for remote disk storage access into the CAD system has successfully been tested: a prototype that makes possible to share data between the different sites of the research and to run CAD from remote sites has been built [11]. The next step would be to transfer the prototype into a clinical environment, involving radiologists collaborating in the project, to implement tele-diagnosis and tele-screening.

Acknowledgement

This work was made in the framework of the MAGIC-5 collaboration. We thank the medical staff involved in this study: prof. M. Bazzocchi (Udine), prof. R. Ienzi (Palermo), prof. V. Lattanzio (Bari), prof. G.B. Meloni (Sassari), prof. M. Rosselli del Turco (Firenze), prof. A. Sodano (Napoli), prof. E. Zanon (Torino).

References

1. Osuch, J.R., Anthony, M., Bassett, L.W., DeBor, M., D'Orsi, C., Hendrick, R.E., Linver, M. and Smith, R.: A proposal for a national mammography database: content, purpose, and value AJR 164 (1995)1329-1334
2. URL: http://marathon.csee.usf.edu/Mammography/Database.html. Accessed 28/12/2005
3. URL: http://peipa.essex.ac.uk/ Accessed 28/12/2005
4. Nunes, F.L.S., Schiabel, H., Rodrigo, H. and Benatti, R.H.: A computer system to record and retrieve information from a mammographic images database by Internet World Congress on Medical Physics and Biomedical Engineering (2003) 24-29
5. McClatchey, R., Manset, D., Hauer, T., Estrella, F., Saiz, P., Rogulin, D. and Buncic, P. The MammoGrid project Grids architecture CHEP '03 (2003), San Diego
6. Ertas, G., Gulcur, H.Ö., Aribal, E. and Semiz, A.: Development of a secure mammogram database MEDNET 2001 (2001) abstract n. 54
7. Fantacci, M.E., et al. 2002 Search of microcalcifications clusters with the CALMA CAD Station Proc. SPIE 4684 (2002) 1301-1310
8. Lattanzio, V. and Guerrieri, A.: The mammography report *Radiologia* Medica 96 (1998) 283-8

9. J.N. Wolfe, "Risk for breast cancer development determined by mammographic parenchymal pattern", Cancer 37, 2486-2492 (1976).

10. Lattanzio, V. and Simonetti, G. "Mammography – Guide to interpretation, reporting and auditing mammographic images Re.Co.R.M.", Spriger-Verlag ISBN 3-540-20018-5.

11. Bagnasco, S., et al: GPCALMA: a GRID based tool for mammographic screening, Methods of Information in Medicine 44(2) (2005) 244-48.

12. Lauria A., Drogo M., Fantacci M.E., Gallo R., Gilardi C., Masala G.L., Palmiero R. and Zanon E.: Comparison between different monitors to be used in the reading of digital mammographic images Proc. SPIE 5034 (2003) 448-452.

13. Lauria A., et al: Diagnostic performance of radiologists with and without different CAD systems for mammography Proc. SPIE 5034 (2003) 244-248.

14. Delogu P., Fantacci M.E., Preite Martinez A., Retico A., Stefanini A. and Tata A.: A Scalable System for Microcalcification Cluster Automated Detection in a Distributed Mammographic Database; Nuclear Science Symposium Conference Record, 2005 IEEE Volume 3, October 23 - 29, (2005)1530 – 1534.

Development of Breast Ultrasound CAD System for Screening

Daisuke Fukuoka[1], Yuji Ikedo[2], Takeshi Hara[2], Hiroshi Fujita[2], Etsuo Takada[3],
Tokiko Endo[4], and Takako Morita[5]

[1] Technology Education, Faculty of Education, Gifu University, Japan
[2] Department of Intelligent Image Information, Division of Regeneration and
Advanced Medical Science, Graduate School of Medicine, Gifu University, Japan
[3] Division of Medical Ultrasonics, Center of Optical Medicine, Dokkyo University
School of Medicine, Japan
[4] Department of Radiology, National Hospital Organization Nagoya Medical Center,
Japan
[5] Department of Mammary Gland, Chunichi Hospital, Japan

Abstract. Mass screening of breast cancer utilizing mammography
(MMG) has been widely carried out. However, MMG might not be able
to depict small impalpable masses in dense breast tissue clearly. We have
developed a computer-aided detection (CAD) scheme in whole breast ultrasound (US) system for mass screening which has been developed by
ALOKA CO., LTD., Japan. Our CAD scheme and image processing
techniques have the following three benefits.

1. Indication of mass candidates by our CAD scheme.
2. Visualization of breast US images in two views of B-planes (CC View
   and ML View) and C-plane.
3. Comparison of left and right breast images as in MMG.

The performance of the CAD scheme in detecting malignant masses on
an initial study has a true positive fraction of 0.91 (10/11) at a 0.69
(633/924) false positive per image. Although mass screening utilizing
US was not appropriate because images acquired by conventional hand
probe were poor in reproduction, the problem could be solved in our
system.

1 Introduction

Among Japanese women, breast cancer has the highest incident rate of all cancers. In Japan, breast cancer screening using mammography has been establised
for women over 40 years of age with the recommendation of the government.
When interpreting mammograms, small impalpable masses might be overlooked
when dense breast tissue obscures these small masses, and younger Japanese
women tend to have dense breast tissue. Ultrasonography can depict these masses
even if they have dense breasts. Hence, breast mass screening by ultrasonography
has started in some regions in Japan. However, it is difficult for inexperienced radiologists to interpret ultrasound (US) images because the quality of US images

Susan M. Astley et al. (Eds.): IWDM 2006, LNCS 4046, pp. 392–398, 2006.

is poorer than that of mammograms. In addition, the large volume of screening US images can be a burden to radiologists. Computer-aided detection (CAD) systems on US images can reduce oversights of masses and provide valuable second opinions to radiologists.

Many CAD schemes for detection and classification breast masses have been reported. Giger et al. have reported an automatic lesion detection technique using a radial gradient index filtering[KD1, MK1]. They have also investigated breast mass classification using a Bayesian neural network and computer-extracted lesion features[KD1, KD2]. Chang et al. have proposed a method that finds suspicious frames among whole breast US images using watershed segmentation[RC1]. We have developed a CAD scheme based on active contour and balloon models in 2-D and 3-D spaces[DF1, TH1]. However, these automated mass detection methods require substantial computation time in analysing. In addition, some systems also need a radiologist to indicate the mass position on a US image manually. Extracting a mass region from segmented regions is difficult, because US images are noisy when compared with mammograms. Boundaries between two regions are obscure due to speckle noise. Moreover, in a mass with a disappearance posterior echo, it is very difficult to determine the extension of a region accurately.

In this study, we investigated CAD system for the detecting masses based on the orientation of edges.

2   Materials

The ultrasound images were acquired by a whole breast mechanical scanner ASU-1004 (ALOKA Co.). This system has 6cm linear transducer with a frequency of 6-10 MHz. The scanner can scan 16 x 16cm of the breast area automatically by three separate path scans. These path data overlaps 1cm width as shown in Fig. 1 and it has B-plane images with 0.125-2mm intervals.

In this study, a whole breast image usually consist of 84 slices (image size:694 x 400 pixels, 256 graylevels, slice interval:2mm) . Our database is consist of 11 whole breast files(924 slices) diagnosed by experienced radiologists. The distribution of database is 11 malignant masses (65 slices), 3 fibroadenomas (8 slices) and 8 cysts (53 slices).

3   Methods

3.1   Image Integration

Whole breast images are prepared by integrating with three path images. The composite image $f_i(x, y)$ is calculated as

$$f_i(x,y) = \begin{cases} g_i(x, y + \Delta y_i) & ((x,y) \in g_i, (x,y) \notin g_{i-1}) \\ g_{i-1}(x, y) & ((x,y) \in g_{i-1}, (x,y) \notin g_i) \ (i=2,3) \\ \alpha g_i(x, y + \Delta y_i) + (1-\alpha) g_{i-1}(x, y) & ((x,y) \in otherwise) \end{cases}$$

$$(1)$$

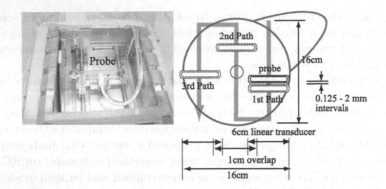

Fig. 1. Whole breast mechanical scanner, ASU-1004. 6cm linear transducer with a frequency of 6-10 MHz.

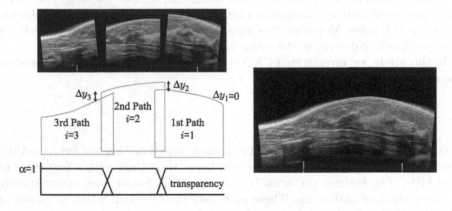

Fig. 2. Composite image constructed from the three path images

$$i = \begin{cases} 1 & \text{1st path image} \\ 2 & \text{2nd path image} \\ 3 & \text{3rd path image} \end{cases}$$

where Δy_i represents the adjustment value for fit postion. α is transparency. A composited image using this method is shown in Fig.2.

3.2   Preprocessing

US images are always noisy and brightness of these images varies with the variation of the gain. Consequently, the result of a CAD system is affected by these noises and the changes in this brightness. Therefore, noise reduction and image intensity normalization are important.

The following steps address these issues. (1)Efficient median filter for ellimination of impulse noises. (2)A hysteresis smoothig algorithm[RE1] was applied to the image for ellimination of minor fluctuations.

3.3   Extraction of Free-Echo Masses

Free-echo masses are depicted in the lowest intensity region in the mammary gland. Hence, candidate regions of free-echo masses were extracted by intensity thresholding. Free-echo masses are mostly cysts. The shape of a typical cyst is horizontally long ellipse form because this mass consists of a sac of liquid. Therefore, we reduced the false positive regions among the candidate regions using the following features and thresholds: size of region $S < 100$; roundness $R < 0.5$; depth-width ratio $DW \geq 2.0$.

3.4   Extraction of Low-Echo Masses

The breast US image consisting of five main kinds of tissue is shown in Fig.3(a). Fig.3(b) gives an example of a normal image which consists of mainly horizontal edges. Fig.3(c) gives an example of an abnormal image. This image includes not only horizontal edges but also vertical edges around the border of a mass.

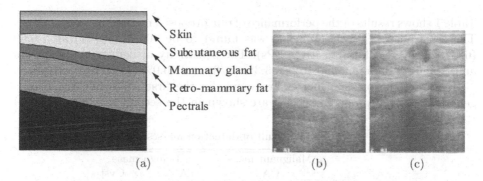

(a)   (b)   (c)

Fig. 3. Breast US image. The illustration of a breats US image is shown in (a). The normal breast US image is shown in (b). The abnormal breast US image with malignant mass is shown in (c).

Our detection masses method extract the vertical edges by the popular Canny edge detector[JC1]. The gradient direction θ classfing edges into vertical and horizonal edges are calculated as

$$\theta = arg(\frac{\partial g}{\partial x}, \frac{\partial g}{\partial y}) + \frac{\pi}{2}$$

where $arg(x, y)$ is the angle from the x axis to the point (x, y). The input image g was caluated by Canny detector. Fig 4(b) and (c) show the edges of Fig.4(a) detected by a Canny operator with $\sigma = 5.0$.

3.5   Segmentation Region

The ROI was segmented by the watershed algorithm[LV1]. This algorithm is one of the seed-based region growing techniques that uses gradient magnitude as a threshold value. This technique is easily affected by noises because of the use of

396   D. Fukuoka et al.

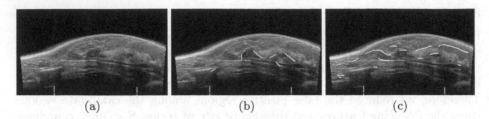

Fig. 4. Example image of detected edges using the Canny edge detector. (a) Original image. (b) Image with vertical edge lines. (c) Image with horizonatal edge lines.

the gradient magnitude. The preprocessing procedure has a significant effect on the segmentation results.

4 Results

Table 1 shows results of the performance of our proposed method in our database. The sensitivity (TP) of carcinoma was found to be 90.9% (10/11) at a 0.69 (633/924 images) false positives(FPs). The sensitivity of benign fibroadenoma and benign cyst were found to be 33.3% (1/3) and 50.0% (4/8), respectively.

In Fig.5, The original images are shown in the first row while the results generated by the proposed scheme are shown in the second row. Fig.5(a), (b)

Table 1. Result of detection masses

| | Malignant mass | Benign mass | |
	CA	FA	Cyst
TP (per mass)	90.9% (10/11)	33.3% (1/3)	50.0% (4/8)
TP (per slice)	66.2% (43/65)	25.0% (2/8)	56.6% (30/53)
FP rate (FP/slice)	0.69 (633/924)		

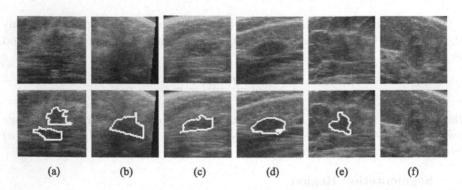

Fig. 5. Results of detection. (a), (b) and (f) have malignant masses (CA), (c) has a benign mass (FA) , (d) and (e) doesn't have any masses.

and (f) have malignant masses (CA), (c) has a benign mass (FA) , (d) and (e) do not have any masses. The candidate masses in (a)-(c) are true-positive detections except the one in the lower region of (a). which is not a mass but a posterior shadow and is a false-positive detection. The detected regions shown in (d) and (e) are rib and fat, respectively. These are also false-positive detections.

5   Conclusion

We developed a fully automatic computer-aided detection system for breast masses on US images scanned by whole breast scanner for mass screening.

Our proposed system has two detection processes for free- and low-echo breast masses. One is based on the intensity thresholding, the other one is based on the gradient analysis. Our scheme can detect a wide variety of masses effectively. On an initial study, it indicates that this method will aid radiologists on screening ultarasonograms.

Our Viewer of the CAD system can display bilateral breasts of B-plane (CC View and ML View) and C-plane. An example of reconstructed B-Plane and C-plane images are shown in Fig.6. This visualization technique is effective for comparison of left and right breast as in MMG.

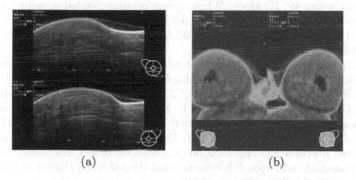

(a)   (b)

Fig. 6. Viewer of the CAD system. It can display bilateral breasts of B-planes (CC View and ML View) and C-plane.

In the future, it is necessary to employ a larger database in order to establish the reliability and accuracy of the method. This automatic mass detection scheme is fundamental to an ultrasonographic CAD system in classifying breast masses on C-plane images and 3-D images.

Acknowledgements

This work is supported in part by a grant for the Knowledge Cluster Gifu-Ogaki from Ministry of Education, Culture, Sports, Science and Technology, JAPAN. This research was partially supported by the Ministry of Education,

Science, Sports and Culture, Grant-in-Aid for Young Scientists (B),16790749 and Scientific Research on Priority Areas. This work was supported in part by cancer research funds from Ministry of Health and Welfare, JAPAN. The authors are grateful to ALOKA CO., LTD., JAPAN and TAK CO., LTD., JAPAN for their assistance of this study.

References

[KH1] K. Horsch and M. L. Giger and L. A. Venta and C. J. Vyborny: Automatic segmentation of breast lesions on ultrasound, Med. Phys., 28, 1652-1659, (2001)

[KD1] K. Drukker and M. L. Giger and K. Horsch and M. A. Kupinski and C. J. Vyborny: Computerized lesion detection on breast ultrasound, Med. Phys., 29, 1438-1446, (2002)

[KD2] K. Drukker and M. L. Giger and and C. J. Vyborny and E. B. Mendelson: Computerized detection and classification of cancer on breast ultrasound, Acad. Radiol., 11, 526-535, (2004)

[MK1] M. A. Kupinski and M. L. Giger: Automated seeded lesion segmentation on digital mammograms, IEEE Trans. Med. Imaging, 17, 510-517, (1998)

[KH2] K. Horsch and M. L. Giger and L. A. Venta and C. J. Vyborny: Computerized diagnosis of breast lesions on ultrasound, Med. Phys., 29, 157-164, (2002)

[RC1] R. F. Chang and K. C. Chang-Chien and H. J. Chen and D. R. Chen and E. Takada and W. K. Moon: Whole breast computer-aided screening using freehand ultrasound, Computer Assisted Radiology and Surgery, H. U. Lemke and K. Inamrua and K. Doi and M. W. Vannier and A. G. Farman, Proc. CARS 2005, 1075-1080, (2005)

[YH1] Y. L. Huang and D. R. Chen: Watershed segmentation for breast tumor in 2-D sonography, Ultrasound in Medicine & Biology, 30, 625-632, (2004)

[DC1] D. R. Chen and R. F. Chang and C. J. Chen and M. F. Ho and S. J. Kuo and S. T. Chen and S. J. Huang and W. K. Moon: Classification of breast ultrasound images using fractal feature, Journal of Clinical Imaging, 29, 235-245, (2005)

[DF1] D. Fukuoka and T. Hara and H. Fujita and T. Endo and Y. Kato: Automated dtection and classification of masses on breast ultrasonograms and its 3D imaging technique, 5th International Workshop on Digital Mammography, Proc. IWDM 2000, 182-188, (2001)

[TH1] T. Hara , D. Fukuoka , H. Fujita , T. Endo and Y. Kato: Development of CAD system for 3D breast ultrasound images, 6th International Workshop on Digital Mammography, Proc. IWDM 2002, 368-371, (2002)

[RE1] R.W.Ehrich: A symmetric hysterisis smoothing algorithm that preserves principal features, CGIP8,121-126,(1978)

[JC1] J.F.Canny: A computational approach to edge detection, IEEE Trans. Pattern Anal. Mach. Intell. 9, 679-698, (1986)

[LV1] L. Vincent and P. Soille: Watersheds in Digital Spaces: An efficient algorithm based on immersion simulations, IEEE Trans. Pattern Anal. Mach. Intell., 13, 583-598, (1991)

Linking Image Structures with Medical Ontology Information

Da Qi[1], Erika R.E. Denton[2], and Reyer Zwiggelaar[1]

[1] Department of Computer Science,
University of Wales,
Aberystwyth SY23 3DB, UK
[2] Norfolk and Norwich University Hospital,
Norwich NR4 7UY, UK
ddq04@aber.ac.uk, rrz@aber.ac.uk

Abstract. Medical ontologies are being developed with some of these specifically for mammographic computer aided diagnosis (CAD) systems. However, to provide full functionality for such mammographic CAD systems it is essential that the ontology information is fully linked to the image information. This linking can be through problem specific image attributes. However, such an approach tends to be non-generic. Here, we propose a framework that will use generic image structures and the topology that links the image structures. In the process we describe a comparison approach which takes the classes, attributes and semantics into account.

1 Introduction

A large number of medical ontologies have been developed in recent years [1, 2, 3, 4, 5, 6]. Recently, mammographic ontologies have been developed, with an emphasis on triple assessment [7], computer aided diagnosis systems [8] and abnormality detection by expert radiologists [8]. A typical example of the high level structure of such an ontology is shown in Fig. 1. At a lower level (details can be found in Fig. 2) the ontology indicates attributes of the abnormality (e.g. size and shape descriptors), but also include associated findings of additional abnormalities (e.g. the association between calcifications and masses or deformity). The final part of a mammographic ontology consists of semantic aspects, which include a) a description of how the values of the attributes, in combination with specific abnormality classes, lead to classification of the abnormality [9], b) spatial relationships and associations between abnormality classes [10], c) synonyms for abnormality classes and attributes [11], d) spatial relationships between abnormalities and image location [12]. The specific values of the attributes and the association between the various abnormalities in combination with some suitable logic will determine the classification of the mammographic images. A typical five point score scale would be: 1. normal, 2. benign, 3. indeterminate (probably benign is also used), 4. probably malignant, and 5. definitely malignant. Such classification will determine the subsequent process.

In breast screening programmes [13, 14, 9] the emphasis in detecting abnormalities is on image information [15, 16, 11]. However, very little work has been done to

Susan M. Astley et al. (Eds.): IWDM 2006, LNCS 4046, pp. 399–406, 2006.

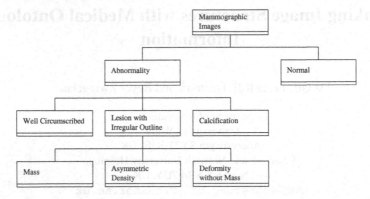

Fig. 1. High level structure of the mammographic ontology

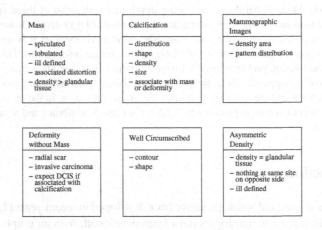

Fig. 2. Attribute details of the mammographic ontology

date to provide a clear link between the mammographic ontologies and generic image structures present in mammographic images. This is a theoretical investigation into the topological representation of medical ontologies and how these are linked to the available image information. More specifically, the investigation provides direct mapping between a radiologists mammographic ontology and image structures. The comparison is provided at all levels of the ontology, covering classes, attributes and semantics. This is closely related to the work on image topologies [17], ontologies [18, 19] and mereotopology [20, 10]. It is expected that such semantic enrichment will lead to an improved image understanding. This work is based on collaboration with expert breast-screening radiologists and is expected to be incorporated within future CAD, eLearning and image retrieval systems.

The layout of the remainder of the paper will be as follows. In Sec. 2 an image formation model is developed, which forms the basis for a mammographic image model. Subsequently, a string comparison approach is described to provide a mapping between the mammographic ontology and image model. Results, application areas and potential future research direction are discussed in Secs 3 and 4. The paper concludes with conclusions.

2   Methods

2.1   Image Information

Work on image topologies [17], ontologies [18] and mereotopology [10] has indicated the underlying structure within images which constitutes fundamental generic structures such as lines and regions and a set of rules to describe the relationship between these generic structures. An image might be regarded as a high dimensional object which is made up of a large number of lower dimensional (anatomical) structures and a set of connectivity rules. The lower dimensional structures are represented by a small set of generic classes and here the anatomical structures are specific *instances* of these classes. The relationships between the anatomical structures can be described by term such as *part-of* and *location-of*, which indicates a bottom-up approach (the inverse relationship *has-part* and *has-location* can also be used). Additional semantic relationships that are being incorporated include *is-a*, *attribute-of*, *instance-of*, *overlap*, *acronym-of*, *synonym-of*, and *value-of* aspects.

2.2   Mammographic Image Information

The image model described above can be made *mammography* specific by adding an additional layer, which divides the mammographic image into distinct regions. This effect is shown in Fig. 3, which has divided the mammographic image in a breast and other regions (it should be noted that mammographic abnormalities can be present in pectoral muscle area, but this is seen as outside the remit of this investigation, although a simple solution would be to treat the pectoral muscle area as independent in which case the same approach as followed for the breast region can be used).

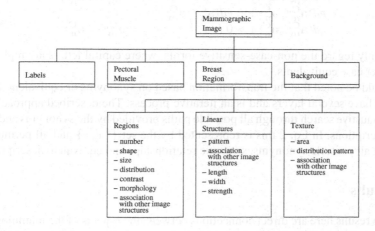

Fig. 3. Incorporation of the generic image structures into a mammographic image representation

2.3 Linking Medical Ontology and Image Information

A bottom-up approach is used to provide a mapping between the ontology and image information. To link the mammographic ontology and the image topology the attributes (and semantic relationships) of both can be matched to indicate which image structures are essential for the detection of specific mammographic abnormalities. The comparison of a set of attributes and semantic relationships is based on class similarity metrics and synonyms or equivalent descriptions.

One of the important aspects within the used methodology is the generation of a list of semantic relationships, synonyms or equivalent descriptions between mammographic anatomic structures, mammographic abnormalities, generic image structures, and their attributes. This list is populated from a range of mammographic [16, 11] and image processing [21, 22] sources. For some of the mammographic classes and attributes there are in excess of four synonyms or alternative descriptions, which indicates the large variation in lexicon usage within mammographic radiology and screening.

The comparison of a set of attributes (including the class they belong to and the associated semantic relationships) is based on string similarity metrics, which takes *synonyms* fully into account. To be specific, the similarity between two attributes $C_u : a_m^{C_u}$ and $C_v : a_n^{C_v}$ (C_u and C_v represent two different classes and m and n the mth and n^{th} attributes of those two classes, respectively) is given by [23]

$$sm_a(a_m^{C_u}, a_n^{C_v}) = \max\left(0, \frac{\min(|a_m^{C_u}|, |a_n^{C_v}|) - ed^s(a_m^{C_u}, a_n^{C_v})}{\min(|a_m^{C_u}|, |a_n^{C_v}|)}\right) \quad (1)$$

where $|....|$ determines the length of a string and

$$ed^s(a_m^{C_u}, a_n^{C_v}) = \min(ed(a_m^{C_u}, a_n^{C_v}), ed(a_m^{C_u}, \{^s a_n^{C_v}\})) \quad (2)$$

where $ed()$ is a string edit distance, which effectively counts the deletions, insertions and substitutions to match two strings. $\{^s a_n^{C_v}\}$ is the set of synonyms for $a_n^{C_v}$. It should be noted that:

$$\begin{aligned}
ed(a_m^{C_u}, a_n^{C_v}) &= 0 & \Longleftrightarrow\quad a_m^{C_u} = a_n^{C_v} \\
ed(a_m^{C_u}, a_n^{C_v}) &= ed(a_n^{C_v}, a_m^{C_u}) & \\
ed(a_m^{C_u}, a_n^{C_v}) &> 0 & \Longleftrightarrow\quad a_m^{C_u} \neq a_n^{C_v}
\end{aligned} \quad (3)$$

and we only regard the non-case-sensitive forms, where capital letters are replaced by their lower case equivalents.

It should be noted that the transformation based on synonyms or equivalent descriptions can have several layers and is an iterative process. The described approach relies on an exhaustive search through all possible paths provided by the synonyms and equivalent descriptions. In Eq. 2 this is represented by the set $\{^s a_n^{C_v}\}$ and all permutations including all possible synonyms, semantic relationships and equivalent descriptions.

3 Results

The main results here are direct connections between the aspects of the mammographic ontology and generic image structures. A summary of these results can be found in

Tab. 1. This shows that for all but one of the mammographic ontology attributes are matched to image structures and their specific attributes. These results provide a logical mapping, but a full model would need to include a set of images, so the association with other images, and specific values for the attributes in both domains is incorporated.

Table 1. Mapping between the mammographic ontology and generic image structures. Here the class names are indicated by unique acronyms of the classes in Figs 1 and 3.

Mammographic Ontology		Image Structures	
M:	spiculated	**LS:**	pattern
M:	lobulated	**R:**	shape
M:	ill defined	**R:**	morphology
M:	associated distortion	**R:**	association
M:	density > glandular tissue	**R:**	contrast
C:	distribution	**R:**	distribution
C:	shape	**R:**	shape
C:	density	**R:**	contrast
C:	size	**R:**	size
C:	association mass/deformity	**R:**	association
MI:	density area	**T:**	area
MI:	pattern distribution	**T:**	distribution pattern
DM:	radial scar	**LS:**	association
DM:	invasive carcinoma	**LS/R:**	association
DM:	DCIS if with **C**	**R:**	association
WC:	contour	**R:**	morphology
WC:	shape	**R:**	shape
AD:	density = glandular tissue	**R:**	contrast
AD:	nothing same site other side		
AD:	ill defined	**R:**	morphology

It should be noted that we have not put any cost on the number of synonyms that are used to obtain a path from the ontology to the image structures. This also means that a path can vary from a direct connection to several steps. A few typical examples are shown in Tab. 2. This shows that an almost direct connection is possible, but that several steps also occur in providing a link between the mammographic ontology and an image structure.

4 Discussion

The described approach provides a direct path from the image structures and their attributes to the final mammographic classification. It should be clear from Tab. 1 that the reverse paths are not always unique. However, the inclusion of specific values for the attributes and the association with other attributes provides a solution to this problem. As such this approach will provide a semantic enablement of CAD systems. In addition, it will give a direct basis for comparison between expert radiologists and CAD systems.

The work by Taylor et al. [24] might be seen as a pre-cursor to the presented work, but the main difference is that they only covered micro-calcifications as mammographic

Table 2. Mapping between specific parts of the mammographic ontology and generic image structures, including the path. Here the class names are indicated by unique acronyms of the classes in Figs 1 and 3.

Mammographic Ontology	path	Image Structures
C: size	**C** *has-attribute* size ∧ **C** *is-a* region ⇒ Region *has-attribute* size	**R**: size
M: spiculated	**M** *has-attribute* spiculated ∧ spiculated *has-synonym* (Spicules *has-attribute* radiating pattern ∧ !*has-part* mass) ⇒ Spicules *has-attribute* radiating pattern ∧ Spicule *is-a* Linear Structure ∧ radiating pattern *instance-of* pattern ⇒ Linear Structures *has-attribute* pattern	**LS**: pattern
AD: density = glandular tissue	**AD** *has-attribute* density *has-value* glandular tissue ∧ **AD** *is-a* region ∧ density *has-synonym* local greylevel value ∧ glandular tissue *has-synonym* non-local greylevel value ⇒ Region *has-attribute* local greylevel value *has- value* non-local greylevel value ∧ local greylevel value *has-value* non-local greylevel value *has-synonym* comparison local and non-local greylevel value ∧ contrast *has-synonym* comparison local and non-local greylevel value ⇒ Region *has-attribute* contrast	**R**: contrast

abnormalities and linked some of the attributes of this type of abnormality to non-generic image metrics.

From the results it is clear that a mapping between the mammographic ontology and generic image structures is possible as long as only a single mammographic image is considered. However, some of the mammographic ontology aspects clearly relate to a comparison with additional mammographic images. The extension to multiple images forms one of the future research aspects.

This mapping can also be used to select specific computer vision approaches for the segmentation of regions [25, 26], the detection of linear structures [27, 28] and texture classification [29, 30] as there is a clear indication which attributes and semantic relationships are essential for these image structures and specific abnormalities.

So far, we have only used simple semantic rules, and more specific notions within spatial relations [10] could be incorporated in future work. In addition, it might be essential to further develop the *association* attributes within the image structures and provide clear links to final generic image structures.

An initial evaluation of the proposed mapping between mammographic and image information is seen as beyond the scope of the current paper and forms part of our future research directions. There are a number of distinct stages to this evaluation, which will incorporate: a) detailed annotation, classification and assignment of relevant mammographic ontology attribute values for a mammographic image database by a number of expert radiologists, b) assignment of relevant image ontology attribute values for the detailed annotations by computer vision experts, c) the links between the attributes provided by the mammographic and computer vision experts will be investigated, d) the same attributes and their variation will be used to investigate the classification potential, and finally e) the attributes provided by expert radiologists will be used on their own to investigate the potential these attributes have in manual classification by alternative expert radiologists. The final evaluation will be based on the full implementation of the automatic detection of basic image structures and the determination of the values of associated attributes. This will form the basis for a mammographic CAD system when the image evidence is used to provide specific mammographic ontology information.

5   Conclusions

We have investigated the link between a mammographic ontology and generic image structures. Using a string comparison approach, incorporating classes, attributes and semantic relationships it has been shown that almost all mammographic ontology attributes, and hence the mammographic ontology classes, can be linked to generic image structures. Such mapping means a direct connection between image structures and mammographic classification, which can potentially provide semantic enablement of CAD systems. Although a mammographic examplar is used, the developed technique provides a generic approach to link image structures to medical ontology information.

References

1. A. Rector. Clinical terminology: why is it so hard? *Methods of Information in Medicine*, 38:239–252, 1999.
2. Workshop on Ontologies in Medicine. *October 8-9*. 2003.
3. Computers in Biology and Medicine. *Medical Ontologies, special issue*. 2005.
4. OntoWeb. http://www.ontowcb.org/. *accessed 06/10/05*.
5. OpenGALEN. http://www.opengalen.org/. *accessed 10/10/05*.
6. SNOMED. http://www.snomed.org/. *accessed 10/10/05*.
7. S. Dasmahapatra, D. Dupplaw, B. Hu, P. Lewis, and N. Shadbolt. Ontology-mediated distributed decision support for breast cancer. *Lecture Notes in Artificial Intelligence*, 3581: 221–225, 2005.
8. E. Manley, D. Qi, E.R.E. Denton, and R. Zwiggelaar. Development of a computer aided mammographic ontology from multiple sources. In 7th *International Workshop on Digital Mammography*, page to be published, 2004.
9. NHS Breast Screening Programme. http://www.cancerscreening.nhs.uk/breastscreen/index.html. *accessed 06/10/05*.
10. J.G. Stell. Part and complement: fundamental concepts in spatial relations. *Annals of Mathematics and Artificial Intelligence*, 41:1–17, 2004.
11. R.L. Birdwell, E.A. Morris, S.-C. Wang, and B.T. Parkinson. *PocketRadiologist - Breast Top 100 Diagnoses*. W.B. Saunders Company, 2003.
12. S. Caulkin, S. Astley, J. Asquith, and C. Boggis. Sites of occurrence of malignancies in mammograms. 4th *International Workshop on Digital Mammography*, Nijmegen, The Netherlands:279–282, 1998.

13. J. Patnick. *NHS Breast Screening Programme, Review.* 1994.
14. F.J. Gilbert et al. *Computer Aided Detection in Mammography.* NHS Cancer Screening Programmes, 2001.
15. L. Tabar and P.B. Dean. *The Mammographic Teaching Atlas.* Georg Thieme Verlag, Stuttgart, 1985.
16. L. Tabar, T. Tot, and P.B. Dean. *Breast Cancer - The Art and Science of Early Detection with Mammography.* Georg Thieme Verlag, Stuttgart, 2005.
17. V.A. Kovalevsky. Finite topology as applied to image analysis. *Computer Vision, Graphics and Image Processing,* 46:141–161, 1989.
18. T. Bittner and S. Winter. On ontology in image analysis. *Lecture Notes in Computer Science,* 1737:168–191, 1999.
19. D. Do and A. Tam. Formal semantic models for images and image understanding. *Proceedings of the Fourth International Conference on Computational Semiotics for Games and New Media,* 2004.
20. A. Galton. Multidimensional mereotopology. *Proceedings of the Ninth International Conference on Principles of Knowledge Representation and Reasoning,* pages 45–54, 2004.
21. R.M. Haralick and L.S. Shapiro. *Computer Vision,* volume 1. Addision Wesley, Reading, MA, 1992.
22. M. Sonka, V. Hlavac, and R. Boyle. *Image Processing, Analysis and Machine Vision.* Chapman and Hall Publishing, 1993.
23. M. Ehrig and S. Staab. Qom - quick ontology mapping. *International Semantic Web Conference,* 2004.
24. P. Taylor, E. Alberdi, R. Lee, J. Fox, M. Sordo, and A. Todd-Pokropek. Incorporating image processing in a clinical decision support system. *Lecture Notes in Computer Science,* 2082:134–140, 2001.
25. N.R. Pal and S.K. Pal. A review on image segmentation techniques. *Pattern Recognition,* 26(9):1277–1294, 1993.
26. Y.J Zhang. A survey on evaluation methods for image segmentation. *Pattern Recognition,* 29:1335–1346, 1996.
27. L.J. Quackenbush. A review of techniques for extracting linear features from imagery. *Photogrammetric Engineering and Remote Sensing,* 70:1383–1392, 2004.
28. R. Zwiggelaar, S.M. Astley, C.R.M. Boggis, and C.J. Taylor. Linear structures in mammographic images: Detection and classification. *IEEE Transactions on Medical Imaging,* 23:1077–1086, 2004.
29. T.R. Reed and J.M.H. Dubuf. A review of recent texture segmentation and feature-extraction techniques. *Computer Vision, Graphics and Image Processing,* 57(3):359–372, 1993.
30. J. Zhang and T. Tan. Brief review of invariant texture analysis methods. *Pattern Recognition,* 35:735–42, 2002.

Comparison Between Wolfe, Boyd, BI-RADS and Tabár Based Mammographic Risk Assessment

Izzati Muhimmah[1], Arnau Oliver[2], Erika R.E. Denton[3], Josep Pont[4], Elsa Pérez[4], and Reyer Zwiggelaar[1]

[1] Department of Computer Science, University of Wales Aberystwyth, UK
iim04@aber.ac.uk, rrz@aber.ac.uk
[2] Dept. of Electronics, Informatics & Automatics, University of Girona, Spain
[3] Department of Breast Imaging, Norwich and Norfolk University Hospital, UK
[4] University Hospital Dr. Josep Trueta of Girona, Spain

Abstract. Mammographic risk assessment provides an indication of the likelihood of women developing breast cancer. A number of mammographic image based classification methods have been developed, such as Wolfe, Boyd, BI-RADS and Tabár based assessment. We provide a comparative study of these four approaches. Results on the full MIAS database are presented, which indicate strong correlation (Spearman's > 0.9) between Wolfe, Boyd and BI-RADS based classification, whilst the correlation with Tabár based classification is less straight forward (Spearman's < 0.5, but low correlations mainly caused by one of the classes).

1 Introduction

Mammographic risk assessment metrics commonly used are those based on Wolfe [1], Boyd [2], Tabár [3], or BI-RADS [4] (see Figure 1 for examples). These four metrics can be grouped into two approaches of assessment. Boyd's measures the percentage area of dense breast tissue. By way of contrast, Wolfe, BI-RADS, and Tabár all include patterns and texture information in estimating the classification. The main aim of this study is to investigate how these four metrics are correlated. Brisson *et al.* [5] studied correlation between Wolfe and Boyd metrics. Gram *et al.* [6] reported correlation between Tabár and Wolfe based classification on Tromsö screening mammograms. Gram *et al.* [7] reported a study about correlation between Wolfe, Boyd and Tabár metrics. To our knowledge, this is the first study to investigate the correlation between Wolfe, Boyd, Tabár and BI-RADS classification on a well known publicly available database [8].

1.1 Mammographic Risk Assessment Metrics

Mammographic risk assessment is often related to breast density estimation, and this is claimed to be a robust risk indicator. Moreover, Byrne *et al.* claimed that mammographic density is the strongest risk factor for breast cancer [9]. It should be noted that density estimation can also be used to evaluate how likely abnormalities are hidden from the observer [10].

Susan M. Astley et al. (Eds.): IWDM 2006, LNCS 4046, pp. 407–415, 2006.
© Springer-Verlag Berlin Heidelberg 2006

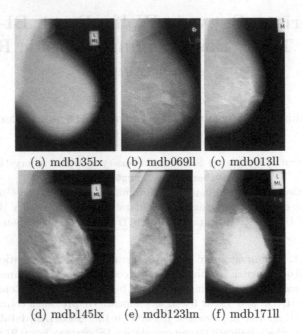

(a) mdb135lx   (b) mdb069ll   (c) mdb013ll

(d) mdb145lx   (e) mdb123lm   (f) mdb171ll

Fig. 1. Example mammograms, where: (a) SCC: 0%, W: N1, T: Pattern II, B: I (b) SCC: 0 − 10%, W: N1, T: Pattern III, B: I (c) SCC: 11 − 25%, W: P1, T: Pattern III, B: II (d) SCC: 26 − 50%, W: P2, T: Pattern I, B: III (e) SCC: 51 − 75%, W: P2, T: Pattern IV, B: III and (f) SCC: > 75%, W: DY, T: Pattern V, B: IV

Wolfe [1] proposed four categories of mammographic risk: N1 is defined as a mammogram that is composed mainly of fat and a few fibrous tissue strands; P1 shows a prominent duct pattern and a beaded appearance can be found either in the subareolar area or the upper axillary quadrant; P2 indicates severe involvement of a prominent duct pattern which may occupy from one-half up to all of the volume of the parenchyma and often the connective tissue hyperplasia produces coalescence of ducts in some areas; DY features a general increase in density of the parenchyma (which might be homogeneous) and there may or maynot be a minor component of prominent ducts. These four groups had an incidence of developing breast cancer of 0.1, 0.4, 1.7 and 2.2, respectively [1].

Boyd *et al.* [2] introduced a quantitative classification of mammographic densities. It is based on the proportion of dense breast tissue relative to the breast areas. The classification is known as Six Class Categories (SCC) where the density proportions are: Class1: 0%, Class2: $\langle 0 - 10\% \rangle$, Class3: $[10 - 25\%)$, Class4: $[25 - 50\%)$, Class5: $[50 - 75\%)$, and Class6: $[75 - 100\%]$. The increase in the level of breast tissue density has been associated with increase in the risk of developing breast cancer, specifically the relative risk for SCC 3 to 6 are 1.9, 2.2, 4.6, and 7.1, respectively [2].

Tabár *et al.* [3] describes breast composition of four building blocks: nodular density, linear density, homogeneous fibrous tissue, and radiolucent adipose tissues which also define mammographic risk classification. Pattern I: mammograms are composed of 25%, 16%, 35%, and 24% of the four building blocks, respectively; Pattern II has approximate compositions as: 2%, 14%, 2%, and 82%; Pattern III is quite similar in composition to Pattern II, except that the retroareolar prominent ducts are often associated with periductal fibrosis; Pattern IV is dominated by prominent nodular and linear densities, with compositions of 49%, 19%, 15%, and 17%; Pattern V is dominated by extensive fibrosis and is composed as 2%, 2%, 89%, and 7% of the building blocks. Tabár *et al.* defined Patterns I-III corresponding to lower breast cancer risk, whilst Patterns IV-V relate to higher risk [3].

There are four BI-RADS [4] categories, which are: BI-RADS I: the breast is almost entirely fatty; BI-RADS II: there is some fibroglandular tissue; BI-RADS III: the breast is heterogeneously dense; BI-RADS IV: the breast is extremely dense. Lam *et al.* reported associations between BI-RAD II-IV and breast carcinoma (adjusted for weight) in postmenopausal women which were 1.6, 2.3, and 4.5, respectively [11].

2   Material and Methods

To investigate the correlation between the four mammographic risk assessment metrics, 321 images (case mdb295ll has not been included for historical reasons) from the MIAS database [8] were classified by three experienced breast screening radiologists (ED, JP, ES). All the mammograms were digitised (8-bits) with a scanning microdensitometer (Joyce-Loebl, SCANDIG3) to 50 micron × 50 micron resolution. The grey-scale response of the instrument is linear in the optical density range 0-3.2OD [8]. It should be noted that the mammograms were displayed on a standard PC monitor, which cannot be used for diagnostic purposes but is sufficient for mammographic risk assessment.

All results are shown in the form of confusion matrices. We have also computed the Spearman's correlation (r_S) between the metrics (using SPSS version 13 for Windows) and linear-weighted kappa values (κ) [12] (it should be noted that κ only tends to make sense when an equal number of classes is compared, but κ is provided for all cases for completeness).

2.1   Correlation Between Metrics

This part of the evaluation is based on assessment by one (ED) of the expert radiologists. All 321 images were classified according to Wolfe (N1, P1, P2, and DY), Boyd (Class 1-6), Tabár (Pattern I-V), and BI-RADS (I-IV). The images were displayed according to MIAS's numbering. It should be noted that Tabár and BI-RADS methods are not routinely used by the radiologist and all classifications for each mammogram were obtained at the same time (both these aspects might introduce bias).

2.2   Intra and Inter Observer Variation

To address the reproducibility, we compared the radiologist (ED) ratings to the same radiologist's previous assessments of Wolfe and Boyd's SCC. It should be noted that for this intra-observer results, the data was assessed twice with the initial assessments two years before those described in section 2.1. In addition, the number of cases for *Rating 1* $n = 319$ and for *Rating 2* $n = 320$, which were due to a technical problem in displaying the cases mdb321lm and/or mdb322rm.

We also compared the BI-RADS ratings by one radiologist (ED) with assessment by two other experts (JP,EP). It should be noted that there was a slight difference in protocol for JP and EP in that images were presented in left-right pairs, instead of individual images as was the case for ED.

3   Results and Discussions

3.1   Correlation Between Metrics

The confusion matrices for all assessment by radiologist (ED) are shown in Tables 1- 6.

Table 1. Expert radiologist (ED) classification according to Boyd and Wolfe

		Wolfe			
		N1	P1	P2	DY
Boyd	SCC1	6	0	0	0
	SCC2	55	5	0	0
	SCC3	1	44	1	0
	SCC4	0	41	34	0
	SCC5	0	2	72	16
	SCC6	0	0	0	44

Table 1 shows that Boyd's Class 1 and 6 are all grouped as Wolfe's N1 and DY, respectively. The distribution of Class 2-5 are mainly mapped into lower risk according to Wolfe. The correlation for these two measures was $r_S = 0.928$ ($\kappa = 0.2033$). This is in line with a study reported by Brisson *et al.* [5] which showed a correlation of $r_S = 0.81$ ($P = 0.0001$). Moreover, they concluded that Wolfe's classification was redundant when percentage density was available in breast cancer risk assessment, which is supported by the results presented in Table 1.

Table 2. Expert radiologist (ED) classification according to BI-RADS and Wolfe

		Wolfe			
		N1	P1	P2	DY
BI-RADS	I	58	1	0	0
	II	4	80	2	0
	III	0	11	104	27
	IV	0	0	1	33

Table 2 shows a high agreement between Wolfe and BI-RADS measures, with a correlation of $r_S = 0.929$ ($\kappa = 0.8645$).

Table 3 shows that Tabár's Pattern V is all grouped as Wolfe's DY. The correlation for these two measures was $r_S = 0.454$ ($\kappa = 0.204$). By excluding Pattern I, Tabár and Wolfe show high correlation $r_S = 0.93$ ($\kappa = 0.8378$). Gram *et al.* reported result on this agreement was $\kappa = 0.23$ [6]. They also showed that Tabár's Pattern I corresponds to Wolfe's DY in 45.6% of the mammograms and Pattern II to V has a unique mapping into Wolfe N1 to DY, respectively [6]. The recently published study by Gram *et al.* [7] reported moderate agreement between Wolfe and Tabár metric ($\kappa = 0.51$) and here the mappings between Tabár and Wolfe based classifications were similar to our result. Some examples of images which have Tabár's Pattern I and various Wolfe's classes can be seen in Figure 2, which clearly shows the variation for Tabár's Pattern I.

Table 3. Expert radiologist (ED) classification according to Tabár and Wolfe

		Wolfe			
		N1	P1	P2	DY
Tabár	I	0	61	56	2
	II	52	1	0	0
	III	10	30	0	0
	IV	0	0	51	30
	V	0	0	0	28

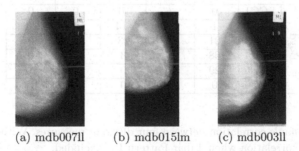

(a) mdb007ll   (b) mdb015lm   (c) mdb003ll

Fig. 2. Example mammograms which were rated as Tabár's Pattern I and various Wolfe's classes: (a) *P1*, (b) *P2*, (c) *DY*

Table 4 shows the agreement between BI-RADS and Tabár measures, with a correlation of $r_S = 0.408$ ($\kappa = 0.1347$). However, as shown above, when ignoring the Tabár's Pattern I results the correlation increases to $r_S = 0.96$ ($\kappa = 0.9145$).

Table 5 shows a high agreement between BI-RADS and Boyd measures, with a correlation of $r_S = 0.908$ ($\kappa = 0.1792$).

Table 6 shows agreement between Boyd and Tabár measures, with a correlation of $r_S = 0.459$ ($\kappa = 0.2127$). However, as shown above, when excluding the Tabár's Pattern I results the correlation increases to $r_S = 0.93$ ($\kappa = 0.5679$).

Table 4. Expert radiologist (ED) classification according to Tabár and BI-RADS

| | | BI-RADS | | | |
		I	II	III	IV
Tabár	I	0	54	65	0
	II	50	3	0	0
	III	9	29	2	0
	IV	0	0	75	6
	V	0	0	0	28

Table 5. Expert radiologist (ED) classification according to Boyd and BI-RADS

| | | BI-RADS | | | |
		I	II	III	IV
Boyd	SCC1	6	0	0	0
	SCC2	53	7	0	0
	SCC3	0	46	0	0
	SCC4	0	33	42	0
	SCC5	0	0	84	6
	SCC6	0	0	16	28

Table 6. Expert radiologist (ED) classification according to Boyd and Tabár

| | | Tabár | | | | |
		I	II	III	IV	V
Boyd	SCC1	0	6	0	0	0
	SCC2	1	45	14	0	0
	SCC3	21	2	23	0	0
	SCC4	68	0	3	4	0
	SCC5	29	0	0	60	1
	SCC6	0	0	0	17	27

Table 7. Spearman's correlation between four different measures. Within brackets are the Spearman's correlation when Tabár Pattern I is excluded.

	Boyd	Tabár	BI-RADS
Wolfe	0.928	0.454 (0.93)	0.929
Boyd		0.459 (0.93)	0.908
Tabár			0.408 (0.96)

Correlations are significant at the level of 0.01 (2-tailed).

A summary of the correlation between the four measures (from Tables 1- 6) can be found in Table 7. This shows that Wolfe - Boyd and Wolfe - BI-RADS have similar high correlation values, followed by the Boyd - BI-RADS correlation. It should be noted that such correlation does not necessarily imply that the metrics are based on the same information and this needs further investigation. In contrast, Tabár's does not correlate with the other measures. It is pointed out by Gram *et al.* that Tabár's classification captures something more than just density measurements and its relation to breast cancer risk needs further investigation [7].

3.2   Intra Observer Variation

We present the intra-reproducibility of our radiologist (ED) on Wolfe's and Boyd's SCC metrics in Table 8 and Table 9, respectively. Intra-radiologist agreement on Wolfe's classification were $r_S = 0.81$ ($\kappa = 0.5999$) and $r_S = 0.85$ ($\kappa = 0.6606$) for the two previous assessments compared to the most recent (*Rating 3*) assessment. For SCC, the intra-radiologist agreement were $r_S = 0.89$ ($\kappa = 0.6989$) and $r_S = 0.90$ ($\kappa = 0.7181$). These indicate a moderate to good agreement. It should be noted that for both metrics the most recent assessment shows a clear shift to higher risk classes when compared to previous assessment.

Part of our future research will concentrate on extending these intra-observer aspects.

Table 8. Intra-observer (ED) reproducibility for Wolfe based assessment

		Rating 3							Rating 3			
		N1	P1	P2	DY				N1	P1	P2	DY
Rating 1	N1	62	59	8	0		Rating 2	N1	62	60	5	0
	P1	0	8	9	0			P1	0	17	18	0
	P2	0	25	88	40			P2	0	15	81	25
	DY	0	0	0	20			DY	0	0	2	35

(a) $\kappa = 0.5999$ (b) $\kappa = 0.6606$

Table 9. Intra-observer (ED) reproducibility for Boyd's SCC based assessment

		Rating 3									Rating 3					
		SCC1	SCC2	SCC3	SCC4	SCC5	SCC6				SCC1	SCC2	SCC3	SCC4	SCC5	SCC6
Rating 1	SCC1	3	8	0	0	0	0		Rating 2	SCC1	1	5	0	0	0	0
	SCC2	3	48	13	3	0	0			SCC2	5	52	10	2	0	0
	SCC3	0	4	28	25	10	0			SCC3	0	3	33	31	6	0
	SCC4	0	0	5	44	35	0			SCC4	0	0	3	39	40	1
	SCC5	0	0	0	1	45	27			SCC5	0	0	0	2	42	19
	SCC6	0	0	0	0	0	17			SCC6	0	0	0	0	2	24

(a) $\kappa = 0.6989$ (b) $\kappa = 0.7181$

3.3   Inter Observer Variation

To evaluate the inter-observer variations, we compared BI-RAD bases assessment by three radiologists. The results are presented in Table 10. The agreement between ED and two other radiologists were $r_S = 0.85$ ($\kappa = 0.5699$) and $r_S = 0.82$ ($\kappa = 0.6381$), respectively, whilst agreement between JP and

ES was $r_S = 0.82$ ($\kappa = 0.7139$). It should be noted the results of radiologist 1 (ED) tends toward higher BI-RADS classes when compared to the other radiologist.

Future research will concentrate on extending these inter-observer variation evaluation, ensuring we cover the full range of metrics and a similar protocol.

Table 10. Inter-observer reproducibility for BI-RADS based assessment

		Radiologist 1					Radiologist 1					Radiologist 2		
		I	II	III	IV		I	II	III	IV		I	II	III	IV
Rad. 2	I	57	66	6	0	I	57	29	0	0	I	83	3	0	0
	II	2	20	57	0	II	2	48	62	0	II	38	57	17	0
	III	0	0	62	7	III	0	9	64	7	III	8	19	46	7
	IV	0	0	17	27	IV	0	0	16	27	IV	0	0	6	37

(a) $\kappa = 0.5699$ (b) $\kappa = 0.6381$ (c) $\kappa = 0.7139$

4 Conclusion

We have investigated the correlations between four different mammographic risk assessments on the MIAS database. The results show strong correlations among Wolfe/BI-RADS/Boyd metrics. However, Tabár based assessment is less correlated to the other three metrics. In addition, intra- and inter-observer variation results have been presented and discussed.

Acknowledgments

I. Muhimmah would like to gratefully acknowledge funding from the Islamic Development Bank and the University of Wales Aberystwyth that enabled the presented research. A. Oliver would like to acknowledge MEC grant number TIN2005-08792-C03-01.

References

1. Wolfe, J.N.: Risk for breast cancer development determined by mammographic parenchymal pattern. Cancer **37** (1976) 2486–2492
2. Boyd, N., Byng, J., Jong, R., Fishell, E., Little, L., Miller, A., Lockwood, G., Tritchler, D., Yaffe, M.J.: Quantitative classification of mammographic densities and breast cancer risk: results from the Canadian national breast screening study. Journal of the National Cancer Institute **87** (1995) 670–675
3. Tabár, L., Tot, T., Dean, P.B.: Breast Cancer: The Art and Science of Early Detection with Mammography. Georg Thieme Verlag (2005)
4. ACR: Breast Imaging Reporting and Data System (BI-RADS) 2nd edition. Reston: American College of Radiology (1995)
5. Brisson, J., Diorio, C., Mâsse, B.: Wolfe's parenchymal pattern and percentage of the breast with mammographic densities: redundant or complementary classifications? Cancer Epidemiol Biomarkers Prev **12** (2003) 728–732

6. Gram, I.T., Funkhouser, E., Tabár, L.: The Tabár classification of mammographic parenchymal patterns. European Journal of Radiology **24** (1997) 131–136

7. Gram, I.T., Bremmes, Y., Ursin, G., Maskarinec, G., Bjurstam, N., Lund, E.: Percentage density, Wolfe's and Tabár's mammographic patterns: agreement and association with risk factors for breast cancer. Breast Cancer Research **7** (2005) R854–R861

8. Suckling, J., Parker, J., Dance, D., Astley, S., Hutt, I., Boggis, C., Ricketts, I., Stamatakis, E., Cerneaz, N., Kok, S., Taylor, P., Betal, D., Savage, J.: The mammographic image analysis society digital mammogram database. Excerpta Medica. International Congress Series **1069** (1994) 375–378

9. Byrne, C., Schairer, C., Wolfe, J., Parekh, N., Salane, M., Brinton, L.A., Hoover, R., Haile, R.: Mammographic features and breast cancer risk: Effects with time, age, and menopause status. Journal of National Cancer Institute **87** (1995) 1622–1629

10. Egan, R., Mosteller, R.: Breast cancer mammography patterns. Cancer **40** (1977) 2087–2090

11. Lam, P.B., Vacek, P.M., Geller, B.M., Muss, H.B.: The association of increased weight, body mass index, and tissue density with the risk of breast carcinoma in Vermont. Cancer **89** (2000) 369–375

12. Lowry, R.: KAPPA Calculator [http://faculty.vassar.edu/lowry/kappa.html]. (Accessed 7/3/06)

Initial Results of the Daily Quality Control of Medical Screen Devices Using a Dynamic Pattern in a Digital Mammography Environment

J. Jacobs, T. Deprez, G. Marchal, and H. Bosmans

University Hospitals Leuven, Radiology Department,
Herestraat 49, 3000 Leuven, Belgium

Abstract. In digital mammography it is of utmost importance that the quality of screen devices is checked on a regularly basis. The EUREF guidelines propose to do this daily using the AAPMtg18-QC pattern. In this paper we report our initial results with the use of an alternative, recently developed, dynamic pattern ("MoniQA") and a scoring scheme.

As soon as the observers are familiar with the procedure, the measurements are very stable and we could not observe big variations in the quality of the monitor. In order to control the intrinsic quality of the monitor, the number of quality control checks could thus be reduced. The global working condition (such as the ambient light level) is controlled as well with the proposed procedure and this may be of great interest, especially during the start-up of digital mammography (screening) units: it is very informative to trace the influences of different light sources (such as (occasional) viewing boxes).

1 Introduction

For an optimal visualisation of medical images on screen devices it is of utmost importance that the quality of these monitors can be guaranteed. This is especially the case for digital mammography and even more if they are being used for screening purposes. Therefore the European Guidelines for Quality Assurance in Breast Screening (EUREF) [1] propose a quality control procedure, both for long-term as well as for constancy checking (daily quality control, DQC). Their guidelines are based upon the results of the AAPMtg18 [2]. Another well-known and often used protocol is the DIN protocol [3], which uses the SMPTE-pattern [4] and the DIN-IEC pattern. Daily quality control is performed by scoring dedicated patterns (Fig. 1a, b and c) to check the different, important parameters of display devices (luminance, resolution, geometric distortion and general image quality). These patterns are quite complex, making their evaluation difficult. They are also static and by that over time the results of the evaluations will be biased due to a learning effect. Recently a new type of patterns, dynamic patterns, have been introduced. These patterns are randomly created according to certain rules. An example is the "MoniQA pattern" (Fig. 1d and e). A previous study showed that this pattern can be used as a valid alternative for the DQC procedure as proposed by the European Guidelines (the AAPMtg18 DQC procedure)

Susan M. Astley et al. (Eds.): IWDM 2006, LNCS 4046, pp. 416–423, 2006.

and the DIN protocol. The study also showed that a protocol based on this MoniQA pattern results in a faster evaluation than the other two mentioned protocols [5].

The MoniQA pattern was used in present study. The pattern includes elements to check a medical screen device for luminance (using 4 sets of 5 random low contrast characters and a gradient bar with random low contrast characters), resolution (via line pair patterns at Nyquist and half-Nyquist frequency), geometric distortions (by drawing a standard grid and thin lines in the corners of the pattern to check the use of the full display area) and general image quality artefacts (including a high contrast element -the hourglass- to check for ghosting and blurring). All these items have to be evaluated separately and we have now combined the results into a global score.

In this study we report on the initial results of the application of this dynamic pattern in our digital mammography environment over a longer time period and on a series of workstations for general radiology modalities. A larger European trial is on-going.

2 Methods and Materials

Over a time period of eight months we performed daily quality control (DQC) on six dual-head workstations using the MoniQA pattern. With dedicated software, the results were sent automatically to a central computer in the medical physics group of our hospital for on-line quality control monitoring [6]. One of the tested workstations was dedicated for mammography (BARCO 5MP CRT monochrome). On this workstation, the DQC was done by a random person out of a group of 4 radiographers (so each observer did the test about once a week). On the other workstations (4 workstations with Siemens 1.3MP CRT monochrome monitors and 1 workstation with Siemens 1.3MP CRT colour monitors) always the same radiologist performed all controls. All observers started after one common teaching session of 15 minutes.

The results of the evaluations were monitored for each screen device. The total score was calculated as follows: an ideal screen that passes all tests gets 100 points; for each reported malfunction, points are subtracted according to the seriousness of the malfunction. I.e. it is not such a big issue if a least visible character of a random character set can not be read. Therefore we subtract less points than if there was a problem with a resolution pattern, for which we subtract 5 points. For a random low contrast character we subtract the difference of the grey scale value with the background.

The MoniQA Pattern had been applied on various monitors dedicated for digital mammography (Barco LCD, Barco CRT, Eizo LCD, Siemens LCD, Siemens CRT). We did acceptance checking of these systems and we noticed that quite often the MoniQA score for an accepted system was between 90 and 100 points. We have also applied this pattern on a large number of monitors for general radiology from different vendors (Barco, Eizo, Totoku, NEC) and of different types (CRT and LCD) and sizes (2MP and 3MP). The experience we had with all these systems gave us an indication to propose an acceptable level of 90 and an achievable level of 95. An ideal screen would then be 100 points.

Because some data were biased by incorrect evaluations that may lead to low overall scores (example human reading errors or typing errors), we applied simple correction rules to filter out the effect of some of these incorrect evaluations.

Example rule 1: if in the luminance test the best or second best visible character is not visible while the other characters are visible, then we propose to consider this as a mistyping error and therefore we may accept this apparently wrong answer as correct.
Example rule 2: is related to the use of static elements (i.e. resolution patterns or corner lines): some are marked incorrectly on discrete moments only and are otherwise marked correctly. This indicates that the observer had unintentionally misevaluated this element.

Another element which is very important to measure is the difference between the scores of the different monitors in the multi-monitor setup of a workstation. After some initial measurements, we decided to put the acceptable level for this difference, on 5 points. This gives a possible deviation margin of 10 points.

During our test period we also monitored the time needed to perform this test for each screen device. As the test is intended for daily application, this is an important performance parameter that is, moreover, directly linked with the acceptability of the procedure.

3   Results

We illustrate the overall findings with the data of 4 workstations: the workstation that is used in our mammography unit (A), one workstation used in an orthopaedic department (B), one used in a paediatrics department (C) and one colour monitor used for urography (D). The other two workstations in our test setup gave similar results as workstation B. Fig. 3, 4, 5 and 6 show the scores for these 4 workstations before and after application of the correction rules. The number of corrections that had to be performed for workstation A was 28 (on 166 evaluations). For workstations B, respectively C and D, we had to correct only 6/134, respectively 3/157 and 6/176 times. Workstations A and B (and the 4 other monitors) turned out to be very stable over time. In the results of workstation C we can see an obvious decrease in score, that is however, never sudden. The score of workstation D turned out to be bad from the beginning. In Fig. 2 we show the average time needed to perform a quality control with the MoniQA pattern for the 6 different workstations.

4   Discussion

There is a remarkably big difference between the original and the corrected scores of the digital mammography workstation (A). We didn't see this difference in the results of the other workstations. We think that this is due to the fact that for the first workstation more than one person performed the test and by that, each person did the test only about once a week. Due to this low frequency, these observers were not so well trained and this may explain the larger amount of mistakes. On the other workstations, almost always the same observer performed the check. In Fig. 2 we can also see that these more regular observers needed less time.

After correction, the results of workstation A and B were at least in the acceptable area, except for a very small number of occasions (A=4; B=0). The results are quite stable over a long time period. The scores of the evaluations didn't drop suddenly, but only after a certain time period we got a trend towards a worse monitor quality (C). Workstation D performed from the beginning very bad and this score was also constant over time.

Different additional features were discovered with the proposed daily quality control protocol over this time frame:

- the monitor of the digital mammography had been replaced and this replacement unit had been calibrated wrongly;
- it is an easy check for awful ambient light conditions;
- the DQC procedure was very informative (teaching and motivation aid) during the start-up of the digital mammography unit as it allowed to optimize the positioning of viewing boxes and triggered the awareness of our radiologists for the viewing conditions;
- during the acceptance testing of different systems dedicated for mammography, MoniQA proved to be a helpful tool to have a first impression on the overall quality of the screen device.

We noticed in our results that especially the luminance check in the MoniQA pattern turned out to be crucial.

It could be concluded that quality control on a daily basis may result in an overflow of irrelevant data. If we would do this test on a weekly basis we may be able to trace the same major effects. On the other hand a reduction of the test frequency may result in negligence and the familiarity of the observer with the check will go down, resulting in incorrect evaluations.

A compromise between an extensive test as the MoniQA pattern (or as the AAPMtg18 protocol or as the DIN6969-57 protocol) or a quicker evaluation on a daily basis, may be to run this extensive test only twice a week after an initial learning period. During the other days of the week a much simpler test focused towards checking the luminance of the system for the darker and the brighter grey scale values could then be performed. This would ensure to check the parameters which are more influenced by daily fluctuations. If this is done by a dynamic (random) pattern, it can be profited from the fact that results will not be biased by a learning effect.

There are definitely limitations to this study: the daily quality control procedure should be implemented on many more workstations and during a longer time period. At that moment better statistical methods can be applied to evaluate the stability of these medical screen devices. Present daily quality control procedure with the same software support is now run in different European centres. In our poster we hope to illustrate the results of a large number of workstations of different European partners.

Major future challenges include the further reduction of the test pattern to an even quicker (validated) procedure and to create the interest for quality control of the users.

420   J. Jacobs et al.

Acknowledgements

We would like to acknowledge the input of different European partners who are participating in the further validation of this study. This work was sponsored by the SENTINEL project, contract number 012909. This project was partially supported by the Euratom Research and development Programme and has received funding from the Community's Sixth Framework Programme.

References

1. Samei E, Badano A, Chakraborty D, Compton K, Cornelius C, Corrigan K, Flynn MJ, Hemminger B, Hangiandreou N, Johnson J, Moxley M, Pavlicek W, Roehrig H, Rutz L, Shepard J, Uzenoff R, Wang J, Willis C: Assessment of Display Performance for Medical Imaging Systems, Report of the American Association of Physicists in Medicine (AAPM) Task Group 18. Medical Physics Publishing, Madison, WI, AAPM On-Line Report No. 03, April 2005
2. European Guidelines for Quality Assurance in Mammography Screening, Addendum European Guidelines (3rd ed.), Digital Mammography, Euref, November 2003
3. DIN 6868-57-2001, Image quality assurance in x-ray diagnostics, Acceptance testing for image display devices. The German Standards Institution, Deutsches Institut für Normung e.V., February 2001
4. SMPTE RP 133-1991, Specifications for Medical Diagnostic Imaging Test Pattern for Television Monitors and Hard-Copy Recording Cameras
5. J.Jacobs, T.Deprez, F.Rogge, G.Marchal, H.Bosmans: Validation of a new dynamic pattern for daily quality control of medical screen devices. 91st Scientific Assembly and Annual Meeting of the RSNA, McCormick Place, Chicago, November 2005
6. J.Jacobs, T.Deprez, G.Marchal, H.Bosmans: MoniQA: A general approach to Monitor Quality Assurance. Proc. SPIE 6145, 2006

Figures

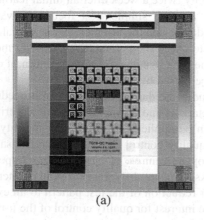
(a)

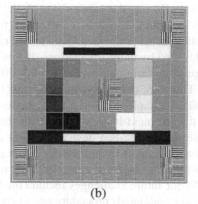
(b)

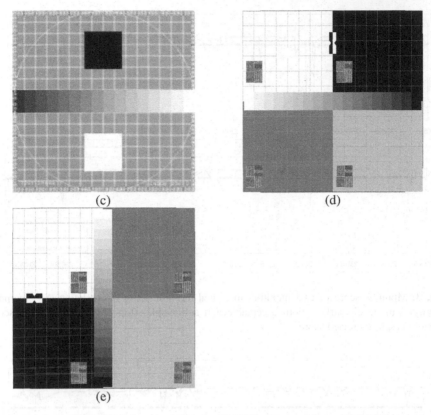

Fig. 1. (a) the AAPMtg18-QC pattern, (b) the SMPTE pattern, (c) the DIN-IEC pattern and (b) and (c) two instances of the MoniQA pattern used for daily quality control of monitors

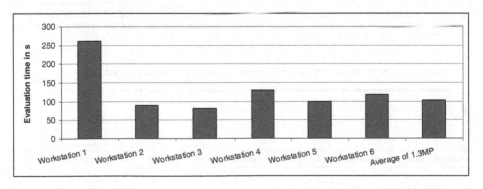

Fig. 2. Overview of the time needed to score the MoniQA pattern of one monitor. Workstation 1 is the workstation dedicated for mammography and the others are all workstations with 1.3MP monitors. The last bar indicates the average of the time needed for the workstations with 1.3MP monitors.

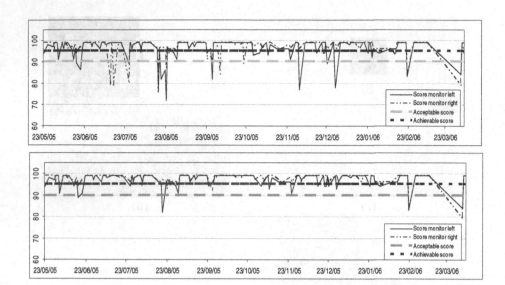

Fig. 3. MoniQA score of two monitors in a dual-monitor setup (workstation A – mammography) with level markers both acceptable and achievable. (top graph) uncorrected score; (bottom graph) corrected score.

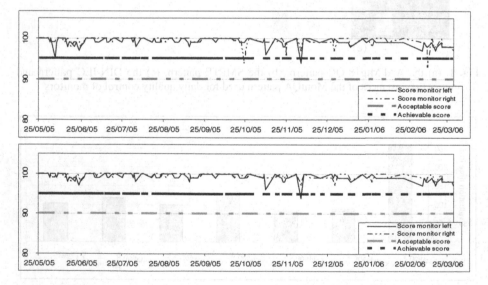

Fig. 4. MoniQA score of two monitors in a dual-monitor setup (workstation B - orthopaedics) with level markers both acceptable and achievable. (top graph) uncorrected score; (bottom graph) corrected score.

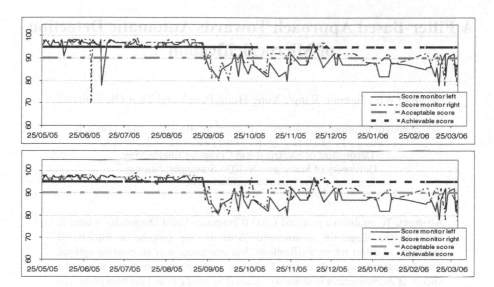

Fig. 5. MoniQA score of two monitors in a dual-monitor setup (workstation C - pediatrics) with level markers both acceptable and achievable. (top graph) uncorrected score; (bottom graph) corrected score.

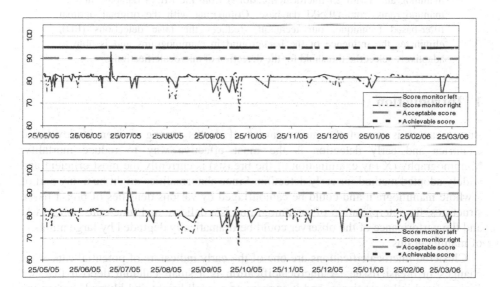

Fig. 6. MoniQA score of two monitors in a dual-monitor setup (workstation D - urography) with level markers both acceptable and achievable. (top graph) uncorrected score; (bottom graph) corrected score.

A Filter-Based Approach Towards Automatic Detection of Microcalcification

Zhi Qing Wu[1], Jianmin Jiang[1], Yong Hong Peng[1], and Thor Ole Gulsrud[2]

[1] School of Informatics, University of Bradford, Bradford, BD7 1DP, UK
{zwu3, j.jiang1, y.h.peng}@Bradford.ac.uk
[2] Department of Electrical and Computer Engineering,
University of Stavanger, N-4036 Stavanger, Norway
thor.gulsrud@uis.no

Abstract. To establish a practical CAD (Computer-Aided Diagnosis) system to facilitate the diagnosis of microcalcifications, we propose a filter-based technique to detect microcalcifications. Via examination of an existing optimal filter-based technique, it is found that its performance on highlighting the energy of mammograms is seriously affected by artefacts and the background of breast. As a result, four methods in pre and post-processing are described in this paper to improve the optimal filtering, leading to an adaptive selection of thresholds for input mammograms. These methods have been tested by using 30 mammograms (with 25 microcalcifications) from the MIAS database and 23 mammograms from DDSM database. Comparing with the original optimal filter-based technique, our technique reduces the false detections (FD), eliminates the influence of the background in mammograms and is able to adaptively select the threshold for the detection of microcalcifications.

1 Introduction

Breast cancer is one of the major causes of deaths among women in developed countries and early detection is the most effective way to reduce mortality. Mammography (X-ray examination of the breasts) is currently the most efficient and widely adopted method for early detection. Since abnormalities might be a tiny part of a whole mammogram and could be camouflaged by various densities of breast tissue structures, the interpretation of mammograms is a delicate and time-consuming task, and the performance of the observer could be dramatically degraded by large numbers of mammograms.

Clustered microcalcifications are one of the early indicators of potential cancerous changes in breast tissue. A microcalcification is a small calcium deposit that has accumulated in breast tissue, and it appears as a small bright and blurred spot on the mammogram. Typically, individual microcalcification ranges in size from 0.1-1.0 mm, which could be overlooked by an examining radiologist.

Some commercial CADs have been developed to help radiologists in diagnosis. According to recent researches on some typical commercial systems, they could achieve a True Positive (TP) rate of 85%-87% with a False Positive (FP) rate of about 0.2 detections per image for a single view [1], [2]. However, some researches [3] show the sensitivity of the commercial system may need further improvement

Susan M. Astley et al. (Eds.): IWDM 2006, LNCS 4046, pp. 424–432, 2006.

according to their experiments. Our experience of using an existing commercial CAD system is similar: too many prompts were activated every time a mammogram is being read in testing the system. In order to further improve TP rates and reduce FP rates, we are developing a microcalcification detection system, which adopts a latest optimal filter-based detection technique. In this paper, a technique composed of several new pre- and post-processing methods is proposed to address the issues of applying the optimal filter-based technique to more practical utilization and facilitate to apply data mining techniques for further classification.

The optimal filter-based technique [4], [5] is a texture feature extraction scheme. It extracts local frequencies in the mammogram where one of the textures has low signal energy and the other texture has high, and its filter is optimised with respect to the Fisher criterion. Reported results show a TP rate of 100%, with a 1.5 FP clusters per image [5], [6]. Different from other filters such as LoG (Laplacian-of-a-Gaussian) filter [7], [8], the optimal filter-based technique is based on the texture features: feature mean and variance.

This paper is organised as follows. The new pre- and post-processing methods are proposed in Sect. 2 and our experiment results are provided in Sect. 3. Discussion on the results and our future plan are presented in Sect. 4.

2 New Pre-processing and Post-processing Methods

Roughly speaking, a microcalcification detection system usually consists of two main procedures: microcalcification enhancement and microcalcification classification. In the first procedure, the signals that represent possible microcalcifications are enhanced and the signals that represent the normal tissue are suppressed. A threshold is applied to processed mammograms to segment the signals of possible microcalcifications from those of normal tissue. In the second procedure, the features of the possible microcalcifications are extracted, and trained by using different data mining technologies such as neural network [9] and SVM [10] to decide the property of the suspicious regions: normal, begin or cancer. Our new methods are proposed to improve the result of the first procedure and their relationships with the optimal filter-based technique are shown in Fig. 1.

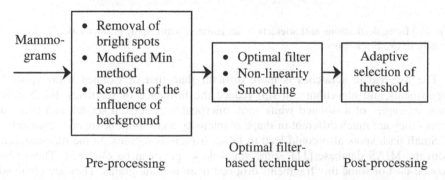

Fig. 1. Relationships between four new methods (3 methods for pre-processing and 1 for post-processing) and the optimal filter-based technique

Our target is to remove as many artefacts as possible without affecting the detection of microcalcifications and provide a good basis for microcalcification classification.

2.1 Reducing Artefacts Causing False Detections

The artefacts include both white spots and dark sports. The white spots can be divided into two types: isolated white spots that probably have been formed during producing X-ray film, and scratches that are some mechanical damages on the surface of X-ray film. Generally, the isolated white spots are apparently 20-30 grey levels (256 greyscale) brighter than their surroundings and seem "floating" on the surface of the mammogram. Besides, the size of isolated white spots is usual quite small (2-5 pixels).

A method is proposed to reduce the influence of these spots. It employs a sliding window (which size is 9 pixels by 9 pixels) to remove the white spots:

1. The sliding window scans the mammogram horizontally and vertically at the step length of 3 pixels. At each movement, only the pixels in the centre region (3 pixels by 3 pixels) of the window are considered.
2. If the intensity of some of these pixels (in the centre region) is more than 20 (256 greyscale) above the average intensity (say, m) of the pixels closely surrounding them, replace the intensities of these pixels in the centre region with m.

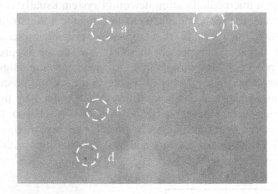

Fig. 2. Microcalcifications and artefacts a. an isolated white spot; b. microcalcifications; c. a scratch; d. two black spots

The removal of scratches is more difficult than that of isolated white spots. In experiments, our algorithm can still reduce the influence of scratches. Fig.2 shows some examples of a isolated white spot, microcalcifications, a scratch and two dark spots - they are much different in shape & intensity and should be treated separately.

Small dark spots also could lead to false suspicious regions. In the mammograms from the MIAS database [11], some small dark spots can be observed. These spots may be dust or some tiny fragments dropped from mammograms. They are obviously much darker than its surroundings and have no relationships with them. The Min method [6] in pre-processing is modified so that this kind of spots can be ignored in using the optimal filter.

The Min method was designed to remove the normal breast tissue so that only possible microcalcifications would be enhanced by the optimal filter. In the Min method, a mammogram was divided into blocks of size M by N and the minimum intensities of all blocks form a feature image. Interpolated the feature image and expanded its size to that of original mammogram. Finally, the estimation of normal tissue – the interpolated feature image - was subtracted from original image to remove the influence of normal tissue. We modified the subtraction step and ignored the pixels whose intensities are below the estimation of the normal tissue.

2.2 Removing the Influence of Background

The optimal filter works well in the regions without the background of breast (the area around the breast). If the optimal filter is applied to the cut mammogram with both breast and its background (containing pure noise), the whole background of breast will be marked as a suspicious region. The problem is probably due to the variation of intensities in background is much larger than that of intensities in the breast area of mammograms. We have tried using segmentation to remove the background but met two problems in applying segmentation:

- The threshold for segmentation need to be determined adaptively for different mammograms;
- After segmentation, large numbers of suspicious regions were generated along the edge of segmentation since the optimal filter is sensitive to fast changing signals.

To remove these false suspicious regions, a new method is designed before applying the optimal filter:

$$Y_2 = Y_1 * \sqrt{Feature_{image}} \tag{1}$$

Y_1 is the resulted image from Sect. 2.1 and $Feature_{image}$ is the interpolated feature image in Sect. 2.1. Y_2 is the result of the array multiplication between Y_1 and the square root of $Feature_{image}$. As the result, the variation of intensities in background is suppressed due to their intensities are much lower than breast tissue. The cube root of the interpolated feature image also has been evaluated but it may bring some false suspicious regions. The interpolated feature image can be treated as the smoothed result of the original mammogram, and it does not contain the artefacts and other impulse signals, which makes it most suitable for suppressing the noise from the background.

Fig.3 shows an example result of this procedure: the left image is a part of a mammogram, which contains some background, the middle is the result without suppressing the variation of intensities in background and the right is the result of applying our algorithm. The drawn circles in the middle and right images mark the position of microcalcifications. The influence of background in middle images is disappeared in the right image and the TP cluster stands out clearly.

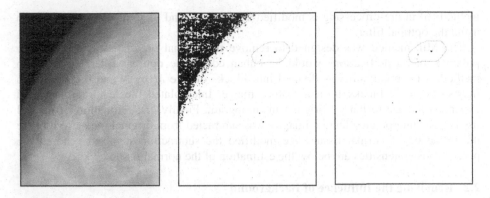

Fig. 3. Removing the Influence of Backgrounds. Left image: the original image; Middle image: the result of the optimal filter; Right image: the result of our technique.

2.3 Adaptively Setting Thresholds

Adaptively setting thresholds is very important for a practical system but is a big challenge in microcalcification detection: lower thresholds may bring too many suspicious regions and increase the burden of the next step, while larger thresholds may miss microcalcifications and lead to FN (False Negative) cases. The selection of thresholds usually depends on one's experience [12], [13] or is based on complex statistical models [14]. Since some advance technologies will be utilised in microcalcification classification, complex segmentation methods are not selected at this stage. Different schemes have been tried to predict the threshold in terms of some features of filter-processed images such as the features of their histograms and the features of clustering. According to our experience, a new scheme is designed for adaptively setting thresholds:

a. Divide a filter-processed mammogram into blocks, each of which is K pixels by L pixels;
b. A start threshold is set for each image – the intensities of about 0.3% pixels in the breast region of each mammogram are above the start threshold since all pixels belong to microcalcifications in each image are in these 0.3% pixels according to our experiments based on histogram.
c. The pixels whose intensities above the threshold will form tens of suspicious regions. The regions whose area is no more 3 pixels will not be considered. Count the number of suspicious regions for each block.
d. The threshold is gradually increased and the step c is repeated until the sum of blocks (containing no more than 1 suspicious region) is larger than X percent of total blocks.

The scheme is designed in terms of observed regular distribution patterns of microcalcifications. In our observations, microcalcifications usually take up a small part of the whole mammogram and they tend to exist in several clusters. Therefore, if a threshold results in hundreds of suspicious regions all over the whole mammograms, the threshold is too low and need to be increased. The parameter X is a control of the distribution of suspicious regions.

3 Experiments and Results

The data set for our experiments comes from two existing mammogram databases:

1. The Mammographic Image Analysis Society (MIAS) [13] has produced a digital mammography database, in which mammograms have been digitised to a resolution of 50μm and each pixel is represented by 8 bits grey depth. In our experiment, all 20 mammograms in the database, which contains radiologist's truth information on microcalcifications (i.e., the locality of the abnormality is given as the coordinate of its centre and an approximate radius of a circle enclosing the abnormality, 25 annotated clusters in total), are utilized and the other 10 normal mammograms are randomly picked from the database. These 30 images do not include the background of breast regions.
2. The Digital Database for Screening Mammography (DDSM) [15] is a benchmark database for CAD tools on screening mammograms. 23 mammograms randomly selected for our experiments: 7 of them have a spatial resolution of 50μm and the rest have a spatial resolution of 43.5μm. Their 12-bit grey-scale is mapped into 8-bit grey-scale in the following experiments. These mammograms are also supported with radiologist's truth information on microcalcification. 10 of these 23 images include some background of breast regions.

To avoid the influence of other artefacts such marks in mammograms, our experiments are based on the images, each of which is 1366 by 1058 pixels in size and cut from a selected mammogram. These images contain all microcalcifications in the original mammograms. A true cluster is considered detected if at least two findings are located in the associated truth circle and a cluster is defined as a group of three or more calcifications within 1 cm^2 area [12].

When the original optimal filter technique (with the Min method) and our technique are applied to the images from MIAS, the size of the optimal filter is 8 by 8 pixels and the size of smoothing filter is reduced to 4 pixels in the optimal filter-based technique to increase the sensitivity of detection. The original optimal filter technique achieved a TP rate of 100% with a FP rate of 1.9 false detections per image while our technique achieved the same TP rate with a FP rate of 1.7 false detections per image.

For the experiments based on the mammograms from DDSM, the original optimal filter technique marks all background as suspicious regions while our technique avoid the influence of the background and achieve a TP rate of 100% with a FP rate of 1.6 false detections per image.

The threshold for above experiments is determined by using the adaptive thresholding technique in Sect. 2.3: K and L are set to 100 pixels and X is set to 96%. Both K and L are set to 100 pixels since 100 pixels is equal to 5mm in images (from MIAS), which could facilitate the estimation the distance between suspicious regions. Initially, X is determined by using 3 images picked out from 53 selected mammograms. The signals to representing microcalcifications are quite weak in two of the three images.

After the above experiments have been finished, the relationship between $K\&L$ and X are studied. Table1 lists the values of X when our technique achieves 100% sensitivity in the detection of microcalcifications in all 53 images. While the values of $K\&L$ reduce from 100 to 60, the value and FP cluster rates only increase a bit.

Table 1. Relationship between $K\&L$ and X

$K \& L$ (pixels)	X	FP rate
100	96%	1.7
80	97%	1.7
60	98%	1.8

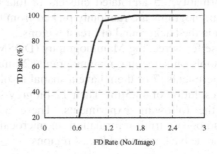

Fig. 4. FROC curve after adding our techniques

The Free-response Receiver Operating Characteristic (FROC) [16] curve of our system is generated by plotting true detection (TD) rates against the average number of false detections per image plotted in Fig. 4.

4 Discussion for Further Improvements

After the proposed methods are added into pre- and post-processing, the artefacts caused by small dark spots and the background of breast, have been removed completely. The proposed pre-processing algorithms do not reduce the TP rate and the selection of the threshold become adaptive. About 30% artefacts due to white spots still can be seen after applying the optimal filter. The reason for the incomplete removal is because these artefacts (probably caused by scratching) are a bit large in size and needs further consideration.

Due to the difference of selection of data set for experiments and algorithm procedures, it is difficult to compare our algorithms with other existing approaches accurately. In our above experiments, the features of clustered suspicious regions are not included in remove FP clusters. However, they are very effective in reducing FP rate: we have tried using a modified feature for measuring the compactness [13] of a cluster in reducing the FP cluster rate (3 images for setting parameters), a TP rate of 100% is achieved with 0.4 false detections per image for the rest 50 images. Apart from this feature, other features will be used in designing our algorithms for microcalcification classification. This paper only demonstrates the effectiveness of our pre- and post processing technique.

The automatic extraction of the breast region will be added into the system and the implementation of the filter-based technique will be converted from Matlab to Java. By reducing the consumption of computer memory, the Java system will enable us to do the experiments based on full mammograms. In the near future, an algorithm for vessel detection will be added into pre-processing and new microcalcification classification techniques will be developed.

References

1. Zheng, B., Hardesty, L. A., Poller, W. R., Sumkin, J. H. and Golla, S.: Mammography with computer-aided detection: reproducibility assessment - initial experience, vol. 228, no. 1, Radiology (2003) 58-62
2. Destounls, S. V., Dinitto, P., Logan-Young, W., Bonacclo, E., Zuley, M. L. and Willison, K. M.: Can computer-aided detection with double reading of screening mammograms help decrease the false-negative rate? initial experience, vol. 232, Radiology (2004) 578-584
3. Soo, M. S., Rosen, E. L., Xia, J. Q., Ghate, S. and Baker, J. A.: Computer-aided detection of amorphous calcifications, vol. 184, no. 3, American Journal of Roentgenology (2005) 887-892
4. Randen, T. and Husoy, J. H.: Texture segmentation using filters with optimized energy separation, vol. 8, no. 4, IEEE Transactions on Image Processing (1999) 571-582
5. Gulsrud, T. O. and Husoy, J. H.: Optimal filter-based detection of microcalcifications, vol. 48, no. 11, IEEE Transactions on Biomedical Engineering (2001) 1272-1281
6. Gulsrud, T. O. and Mestad, E.: Perprocessing techniques for improved segmentation of clustered microcalcifications in digital mammograms, in 2nd International GABOR Workshop in Vienna (2001)
7. Netsch, T. and Peitgen, H. O.: Scale-space signatures for the detection of clustered microcalcifications in digital Mammograms, vol. 18, no. 9, IEEE Transactions on Medical Imaging (1999) 774-786
8. Cheng, H. D., Wang, J. L. and Shi, X. J.: Microcalcification detection using fuzzy logic and scale space approaches, vol. 37, no. 2, Pattern Recognition (2004) 363-375
9. Bocchi, L., Coppini, G., Nori, J. and Valli, G.: "Detection of single and clustered micro calcifications in mammograms using fractals models and neural networks, vol. 26, no. 4, Medical Engineering & Physics (2004) 303-312
10. El-Naqa, I., Yang, Y., Wernick, M. N., Galatsanos, N. P. and Nishikawa, R. M.: A Support Vector Machine Approach for Detection of Microcalcifications, vol. 21, no. 12, IEEE Transactions on Medical Imaging (2002) 1552-1563
11. Suckling, J., et al.: The Mammographic Image Analysis Society digital mammogram database, in Proceedings of the 2nd International Workshop on Digital Mammography (1994) 375-378
12. Qian, W., Mao, F., Sun, X., Zhang, Y., Song, D. and Clarke, R. A.: An improved method of region grouping for microcalcification detection in digital mammograms, vol. 26, Computerized Medical Imaging and Graphics (2002) 361-368
13. Kallergi, M.: Computer-aided diagnosis of mammographic microcalcification clusters, vol. 31, no. 2, Medical Physics (2004) 314-326

14. Heine, J. J., Deans, S. R., Cullers, D. K., Stauduhar, R. and Clarke, L. P.: Multiresolution statistical analysis of high-resolution digital mammograms, vol. 16, no. 5, IEEE Transactions on Medical Imaging (1997) 503-515
15. Heath, M., Bowyer, K., Kopans, D., Kegelmeyer, P., Moore, R., Chang, K. and Munishkumaran, S.: Current status of the digital database for screening mammography, Digital Mammography (1998) 457–460
16. Chakraborty, D. P. and Winter, L. H. L.: Free-response methodology: Alternate analysis and a new observer-performance experiment, 174, Radiology (1990) 873–881

Texture Based Segmentation

Reyer Zwiggelaar[1] and Erika R.E. Denton[2]

[1] Department of Computer Science,
University of Wales,
Aberystwyth SY23 3DB, UK
rrz@aber.ac.uk
[2] Norfolk and Norwich University Hospital,
Norwich NR4 7UY, UK

Abstract. The ability of human observers to discriminate between textures is related to the contrast between key structural elements and their repeating patterns. Here we have developed an automatic texture classification approach based on this principle. Local contrast information is modelled and a hybrid metric, based on probability density distributions and transportation estimation, are used to classify unseen samples. Quantitative and qualitative evaluation, based on mammographic images and Wolfe classification, is presented and shows segmentation results in line with the various classes.

1 Introduction

Texture is one of the least understood areas in computer vision. Although no generic texture model has emerged so far a number of problem specific approaches have been developed successfully [1,2,3,4]. More recently, approaches have been investigated which aim to automatically determine a feature vector to be used for segmentation purposes [5,6] or provide a more fundamental approach to texture segmentation [7,8,9].

The work described here can be seen as such a more generic approach towards texture modelling. The principles behind this modelling are based on the notion that human observers are able to distinguish between textures if there is significant contrast difference between the main structural elements and the way those specific (sub-)structures form a repeating pattern. To achieve this we have investigated the modelling of the distribution of texture structural elements within specific grey-level bands. Subsequently, unseen texture regions can be compared with the developed models. The comparison can be based on various distance metrics.

In this paper we consider the segmentation of texture information within mammographic images. Here the main aim is to distinguish between a number of textures that appear in mammographic images (e.g. the various textures associated with Wolfe [10] or Tabar [11] based risk assessment) and use the extracted information to obtain segmentation of texture images. We have investigated the use of a *Hybrid Metric* which can be regarded as the non-integer approximation of the transportation cost approach. We provide both quantitative and qualitative assessment of the developed approach.

The layout of the paper is as follows. In Sec. 2 the local contrast based texture segmentation approach is presented, which covers the extraction of the local contrast information and the use of a novel *Hybrid Metric* to measure the similarity between

Susan M. Astley et al. (Eds.): IWDM 2006, LNCS 4046, pp. 433–440, 2006.

distributions. In Sec. 3 quantitative and qualitative results based on real textures are presented. The paper concludes with discussion and conclusions sections.

2   Methods

The aspects discussed in the section cover: a) the model describing the local contrast structures, b) the way that these are used to provide texture models, and c) the approach to evaluate the difference between local contrast structure models and new local areas within unseen images.

2.1   Local Contrast Structures

One of the motivations behind this research is that texture recognition is driven by the contrast between key structural elements. Images are decomposed into distinct grey-level bands. The binary images, $B(x, y)$, representing only distinct grey-level bands are determined by

$$B(x,y) = \begin{cases} 1 \text{ if } \delta_{low} <= I(x,y) < \delta_{high} \\ 0 \text{ otherwise} \end{cases} \tag{1}$$

where $I(x, y)$ is a grey-level image, and δ_{low} and δ_{high} are low and high threshold values.

It should be clear that the distinct structures that represent the textures are only present in very specific grey-level bands and that a specific position within the image can only become equal to 1 once if the high and low threshold values in Eq. 1 form a non-overlapping series (as will be the case throughout the presented work).

2.2   Modelling

Modelling the repeating key (sub-)structures that are essential to describe textures can be achieved by estimating local aspects using a set of binary images determined by Eq. 1, where the set is based on a sequence of n $(\delta_{low}, \delta_{high})$ values covering the full range of grey-level values within the images and $(\delta_{high} - \delta_{low})$ is constant (e.g. a possible $(\delta_{low}, \delta_{high})$ set would be $\{(0, 64), (64, 128), (128, 192), (192, 256)\}$, and some binary images based on such sets can be found in Fig. 1). Once such a set of images has been obtained a model of local structures needs to be obtained. To achieve this for a specific binary image in the set a region of interest (with size equal to $(2w+1) \times (2w+1)$) is extracted at each position in $B(x, y)$ with value equal to one. For each region of interest the segment containing the central position is extracted using simple four-connectivity. Using each position in the obtained segments provides a summation over $B(x, y)$ restricted by $\pm w$. After normalisation with respect to total occurrence, this results in a probability density distribution representing local structures within a specific grey-level range (as specified by Eq. 1). Such a probability density is denoted as $P_m(i, j)$, where the subscript indicates the level in the set of binary images for which the probability density is derived, $m \in [1, n]$, n represents the number of grey-level bands, and (i, j) covers the region of interest, i.e. $i, j \in [-w, w]$.

Subsequent to the modelling it becomes possible to determine if a new region of interest extracted from an image that was not part of the modelling data belongs to the

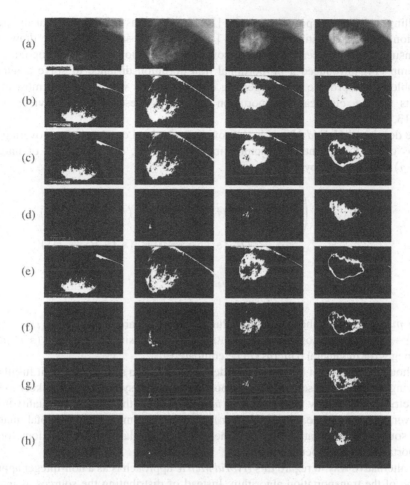

Fig. 1. Local contrast structures, with (a) original images and the other images determined by Eq. 1, where the $(\delta_{low}, \delta_{high})$ values are (b): $(64, 192)$, (c): $(64, 128)$, (d): $(128, 192)$, (e): $(64, 96)$, (f): $(96, 128)$, (g): $(128, 160)$, and (h): $(160, 192)$

modelled texture or not. The methodology is very similar to that described to obtain the local contrast structures model, with the exception that in this case it is only based on a single region of interest instead of all the relevant regions of interest within a whole image. The new region of interest is only compared with the relevant model which covers the grey-level value that occurs at the centre of the region of interest. Such a single region of interest based texture description is denoted as $R_m(i, j)$, where m indicates the level in the set of grey-level values within which the grey-level value of the centre position falls.

2.3 Hybrid Metric

The similarity between a new region of interest and the various local contrast texture models is determined by a *Hybrid Metric*, which is based on probability density modelling and the transportation metric [12,13,14]. It has been noted that the transportation metric has distinct advantages [13], but at the same time some drawbacks that ensure it is not generic enough to cover all applications [14]. Giannopoulos and Veltkamp [14] introduced a proportional transportation distance to solve a number of problems and provide a more generic distance metric which retained most of the benefits of the classical transportation metric as described in previous work [6,12,13,14,15,16,17].

The developed *Hybrid Metric* is to provide a weighted cost of the non-overlapping regions of the local contrast structures model, $P_m(i,j)$, and the region of interest, $R_m(i,j)$. This is given by

$$p_{hm}(x,y) = \left(\sum_{(i,j)} \sum_{(s,t)} (R_m(i,j) - min\{P_m(i,j), R_m(i,j)\}) \right.$$
$$(P_m(s,t) - min\{P_m(s,t), R_m(s,t)\}) \tag{2}$$
$$\left. k(i,j,s,t) \right)^{-1}$$

where $min\{.,.\}$ gives the minimum value of the two parameters and $k(i,j,s,t) = |i-s| + |j-t|$ is the cost for transportation between positions (i,j) and (s,t) in the two images (or in general patterns) to be compared.

It should be noted that the distance underlying Eq. 2 is a semi-metric as it fulfills the following properties: a) self-identity, b) positivity, and c) symmetry. It is likely to be a full metric, but as to now we do not have a full proof that the triangle inequality holds. However, this is only the case if the cost function k is a metric and the total quantity at the source and destination are the same, which is similar to the restrictions for the transportation distance being a metric.

An alternative way to regard this *Hybrid Metric* approach is as a non-integer approximation of the transportation algorithm. Instead of distributing the sources as integer quantities to the destinations, the *Hybrid Metric* approach distributes weighted values from all sources to all destinations.

2.4   Texture Likelihood Estimation

The metric used to compare local contrast structure representations results in a similarity estimation (see Eq. 2). The likelihood that pixels belong to a specific texture t are determined by an odds-ratio:

$$p_{hm}^{t}(x,y) = \frac{p_{hm}(x,y)|_{n_c=t}}{\sum_{n_c} p_{hm}(x,y)} \tag{3}$$

where n_c indicates the number of texture models that are being considered. In the experiments presented here combinations of four textures (representing the four Wolfe classes) were considered and hence the value of $n_c \in \{1, 2, 3, 4\}$.

3   Results

The evaluation involves the segmentation of images representing the various Wolfe classes [10]. The database consists of sixty images. The images in the database were all assigned a Wolfe classification by an expert radiologist and the distribution over the four Wolfe classes are 0.25, 0.10, 0.55 and 0.10 for N1, P1, P2 and DY, respectively.

An overview of example segmentation results can be found in Fig. 2.

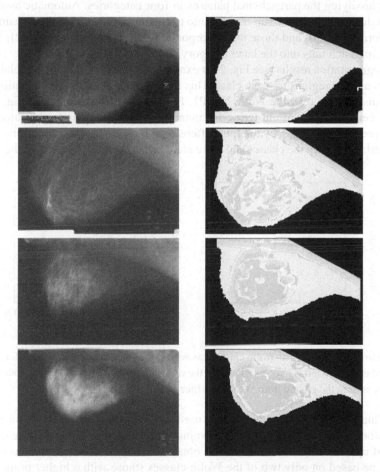

Fig. 2. Example segmentation results, where from top to bottom the four Wolfe classes are represented, with on the left the original mammograms and on the right the segmentation results

The segmentation results in Fig. 2 show a strong correlation between the various texture regions in the mammographic images and the segmented areas in the resulting images. However, there also seem to be some region boundary effects playing a significant role, which warrant further investigation. In addition, it should be noted that for most segmentation results the relative area is mainly occupied by two classes; there are a number of possible explanation for this, like the un-balanced distribution over the four Wolfe classes, and this needs further investigation (it is interesting to note that for BI-RADS breast density categories it is not uncommon to mainly use two out of the four available classes [18,19]).

3.1 Mammographic Risk Assessment

The origins of breast density classification are the work of Wolfe [10], who showed the relation between mammographic parenchymal patterns and the risk of developing breast cancer, classifying the parenchymal patterns in four categories. Automatic assessment of breast density/risk can be sub-divided into two groups, those that are just using grey-level information [20] and those that incorporate texture information [21,22]. The developed approach falls into the latter category.

The segmentation results (see Fig. 2 for examples) are used to obtain the relative size of the segmented regions for each class. This feature is used as our classification space and the distribution over the Wolfe N1, P1, P2 and DY is represented in Fig. 3. This shows a certain degree of clustering for mammograms belonging to the same Wolfe class (represented in Fig. 3 by the four different markers), but at the same time there is clear overlap between the classes and there are distinct outliers for some of the classes.

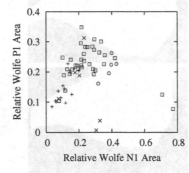 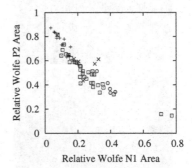

Fig. 3. Distribution of relative Wolfe class areas within the mammographic images for the used dataset, where on the left N1 versus P1 and on the right N1 versus P2 is shown. The four different markers represent the ground truth Wolfe classifications.

The data as represented in Fig. 3 can be used as a 4D feature space. Based on a k nearest neighbour classifier and a leave-one-woman-out methodology correct classification results of up to 72% (with $\kappa = 0.48$) are obtained. However, the correct classification tends to be based on only two of the Wolfe classes (those with a higher proportion in the used dataset) and as such do not represent satisfactory results and indicate a need for further investigation involving a larger dataset and a more even distribution of the Wolfe classes (and alternative metrics like BIRADS) for the training data.

4   Discussion

The developed *Hybrid Metric* is a generic approach for the comparison of distributions or patterns and as such will have a wide range of application areas. It would be of interest to investigate the use of this metric in applications such as image retrieval, image registration, pattern matching and general allocation cost estimation problems.

The developed approach to texture modelling might on the surface show similarities to the local binary pattern (LBP) based texture analysis [9]. However, the main differences are: a) grey-level bands are used to generate the binary images and hence the models, b) modelling is based on the binary images and no histogram information is extracted to summarise the information, c) models at each grey-level band can be directly compared, d) only one model per grey-level band exists, and e) the region of interest tends to be an order of magnitude larger than typically used for LBP.

The developed approach does also show similarities to USAN [23]. The first step in our process uses local binarised information based on grey-level bands. The grey-level bands in SUSAN are taken as +/- around the central pixel's grey-level value, whereas here we use distinct bands independent of the grey-level value of the central pixel. Further to this we would like to mention: a) SUSAN is measuring an area in the USAN whilst here we use statistical modelling of the local area as a fundamental step, b) the window size used here tends to be an order of magnitude larger than those used for SUSAN, c) our approach does not only model the central region but all univalue regions within the local area, and d) to our knowledge USAN or more advanced information like used here has not been used in this fashion for texture segmentation.

To provide further evaluation on a full range of (w, n) values it might be essential to develop a less algorithmic complex estimation of the transportation cost. The *Hybrid Metric* based approach already shows significant improvements over the classical transportation metric and this will be further investigated. Further might incorporate texture clique aspects [24,25], where the central segment within the region of interest could be sub-divided into a number of cliques.

5   Conclusions

We have investigated a novel texture segmentation methodology based on a concept of local contrast structures. In the process we have developed a hybrid transportation/probability metric to compare distributions, which is a generic metric with potential beyond the presented work. The evaluation on mammographic images shows overall good segmentation results and limitations on the current results have been discussed.

References

1. M.W. Haralick. Statistical and structural approaches to texture. *Proceedings of the IEEE*, 67(5):786–804, 1979.
2. R.W. Conners and C.A. Harlow. A theoretical comparison of texture algorithms. *IEEE Transactions on Pattern Analysis and Machine Intelligence*, 2(3):204–222, 1980.
3. A.P. Pentland. Fractal-based description of natural scenes. *IEEE Transactions on Pattern Analysis and Machine Intelligence*, 6(6):661–674, 1984.
4. T.R. Reed and J.M.H. Dubuf. A review of recent texture segmentation and feature-extraction techniques. *Computer Vision, Graphics and Image Processing*, 57(3):359–372, 1993.
5. C.C. Reyes-Aldasoro and A. Bhalerao. Volumetric texture description and discrimant feature selection for MRI. *Lecture Notes in Computer Science*, 2732:282–293, 2003.

6. R. Zwiggelaar. Texture based segmentation: automatic selection of co-occurrence matrices. In 17th *IEEE International Conference on Pattern Recognition*, pages 588–591, 2004.
7. M. Varma and A. Zisserman. Classifying images of materials: achieving viewpoint and illumination independence. *Lecture Notes in Computer Science*, 2352:255–271, 2002.
8. M. Chantler and L. Van Gool. Special issue on "texture analysis and synthesis". *International Journal of Computer Vision*, 62:5, 2005.
9. M. Pietikainen. Image analysis with local binary patterns. *Lecture Notes in Computer Science*, 3540:115–118, 2005.
10. J.N Wolfe. Risk for breast cancer development determined by mammographic parenchymal pattern. *Cancer*, 37(5):2486–2492, 1976.
11. I.T. Gram, E. Funkhouser, and L. Tabar. The tabar classification of mammographic parenchymal patterns. *European Journal of Radiology*, 24(2):131–136, 1997.
12. F.L. Hitchcock. The distribution of a product from several sources to numerous localities. *Journal of Mathematical Physics*, 20:224–230, 1941.
13. Y. Rubner, C. Tomasi, and L.J. Guibas. A metric for distributions with applications to image databases. In 6th *International Conference on Computer Vision*, pages 59–66, 1998.
14. P. Giannopoulos and R.C. Veltkamp. A pseudo-metric for weighted point sets. *Lecture Notes in Computer Science*, 2352:715–730, 2002.
15. A.S. Holmes, C.J. Rose, and C.J. Taylor. Measuring similarity between pixel signatures. *Image and Vision Computing*, 20(5-6):331–340, 2002.
16. S. Haker, L. Zhu, A. Tannenbaum, and S. Angenent. Optimal mass transport for registration and warping. *International Journal of Computer Vision*, 60(3):225–240, 2004.
17. F. Jing, M.J. Li, H.J. Zhang, and B. Zhang. An efficient and effective region-based image retrieval framework. *IEEE Transactions on Image Processing*, 13(5):699–709, 2004.
18. F.M. Hall. Mammographic density categories. *American Journal of Radiology*, 178:242–242, 2002.
19. L.A. Venta and R.E. Hendrick. Mammographic density categories - reply. *American Journal of Radiology*, 178:242–243, 2002.
20. N. Karssemeijer. Automated classification of parenchymal patterns in mammograms. *Phys. Med. Biol.*, 43:365–378, 1998.
21. J.W. Byng, M.J. Yaffe, G.A. Lockwood, L.E. Little, D.L. Tritchler, and N.F. Boyd. Automated analysis of mammographic densities and breast carcinoma risk. *Cancer*, 80(1):66–74, 1997.
22. R. Zwiggelaar and E.R.E. Denton. Optimal segmentation of mammographic images. In 7th *International Workshop on Digital Mammography*, to be published, 2004.
23. S.M. Smith and J.M. Brady. Susan – a new approach to low level image processing. *International Journal of Computer Vision*, 23(1):45–78, 1997.
24. S. Geman and D. Geman. Stochastic relaxation, Gibbs distribution, and the Bayesian restoration of images. *IEEE Transactions on Pattern Analysis and Machine Intelligence*, 6:721–741, 1984.
25. G.L. Gimel'farb. Texture modeling by multiple pairwise pixel interactions. *IEEE Transactions on Pattern Analysis and Machine Intelligence*, 18:1110–1114, 1996.

Image Quality of a Photon-Counting Mammography System Compared to Digital Mammography Based on Amorphous Silicon with CsI-Scintillator

Arne Fischmann and Günther Steidle

University of Tübingen, Department of Diagnostic Radiology
Hoppe-Seyler-Str. 3, 72072 Tübingen, Germany
arne.fischmann@med.uni-tuebingen.de

Abstract. To compare image quality and dose of a photon-counting multi-slit scanner (PC) and a system based on amorphous silicon (aSi), images of the CDMAM 3.4 were taken in standard mode. For 3cm PMMA, the PC used 29kV/11.7mAs, aSi used 27kV/ 50mAs. For 5cm PMMA, PC used 35kV /14.8mAs, aSi used 31kV/ 50 mAs. Exposure was manually increased for PC and lowered for aSi-system. Average glandular dose and an image quality index (IQI) were calculated over the diameter ranges 0.06 - 2.0mm and 0.1-1. In standard mode with 3cm PMMA, IQI for PC was 35% lower than for aSi at 80% lower dose. Increased dose of PC resulted in 13% lower IQI at 57% lower dose. With 5cm PMMA IQI in standard mode was 18 % lower with PC at a 69% lower dose. Increasing the dose of PC resulted a 7% lower IQI at 54% lower dose. In conclusion the PC-system might reduce dose by up to 54% at equivalent image quality, although maximal quality of aSi could not be reached.

1 Background

The aim of this study was to compare the image quality and dose of two full-field-digital-mammography (FFDM) systems based on different technologies: a photon-counting multi-slit scanner (PC) and a system based on amorphous silicon (aSi) with a CsI-scintillator. Both systems are available on the market. The aSi-System (Senographe 2000D, General Electric Medical Systems, Milwaukee, USA) is FDA-approved since 2000; the FDA-approval for the PC-system (Microdose, Sectra, Linköping SE) is pending.

2 Methods and Materials

Images of a contrast detail phantom (CDMAM 3.4, St. Randbout, NL) with 3 and 5cm PMMA-equivalent thickness were taken using the automatic exposure control of each system. For the PC-system imaging parameters at 3cm PMMA were 29kV and 11.7mAs in Standard mode. To increase dose, maximal values of 29kV, 16.1mAs as well as 32kV, 18.4mAs were added manually. For the aSi-system image parameters were 27kV, 50mAs (standard-mode); 25kV, 71mAs (contrast-mode); 28kV and

Susan M. Astley et al. (Eds.): IWDM 2006, LNCS 4046, pp. 441–446, 2006.

36mAs (dose-mode). To achieve a comparable dose, the aSi-System was manually lowered to 32kV, 16mAs and 28kV, 16mAs.

At 5cm PMMA, imaging parameters of the PC-system were 35kV and 14.8mAs, and were increased to 35kV, 17.9mAs and 38kV, 16.1mAs. The parameters for the aSi-System in standard mode were 31kV and 50 mAs; dose was manually lowered with 31kV and 11, 16 and 40mAs as well as 35kV and 18mAs. Other beam quality choices might have been made to reduce dose for the aSi system, but have not been tested.

The average glandular dose was calculated for both systems according to Dance [1]. For the PC system spatial dose-distribution is inhomogeneous with lower dose in peripheral than in central parts of the scanned sector, this was considered when calculating average glandular dose. At every parameter setting, 8 images were taken and evaluated with the CDCOM-program. An image quality index (IQI) was calculated over the diameter range 0.06 to 2.0mm (equation 1).

$$IQI= \frac{1}{N} \sum_{i=1}^{N} \frac{1}{D_i T_i} \qquad (1)$$

As all gold disks with large diameters, as well as none of the smallest gold disks were detected with both systems, we also calculated a modified IQI (mIQI) over the diameter-range 0.1 to 1mm. To our knowledge this mIQI is better suited to detect differences between the systems and is less influenced by random errors of the CDCOM-program.

3 Results

3cm PMMA-Phantom
IQI with the aSi-system in standard mode was 34.3 vs. 22.2 (35% difference) with the PC-system, at an average glandular dose of 1.52 mGy and 0.30 mGy (80% difference) respectively (see figure 1). When the dose of the PC-system was manually increased to the maximum of 0.66 mGy, IQI could be increased to 29.8, resulting in a 13% lower IQI at 57% lower dose. The IQI of the aSi-System could not be reached. If the dose of the aSi-system was manually lowered, IQI was 21.4 at 0.50mGy (aSi) vs. 22.2 at 0.30 mGy (PC) a 40% difference in dose at comparable image quality.

Using the diameter ranges of 0.1-1mm the modified image quality index (mIQI) of the aSi-System in standard mode was 42.9 vs. 27.3 with the PC-System or a difference of 36% at 80% lower dose (see figure 2). If the dose of the PC-system was manually increased, mIQI reached up to 36.8 or 90% of the level with aSi, at a 57% lower dose.

5cm PMMA-Phantom
With 5cm PMMA IQI in standard mode was 21.3 for the aSi-System vs. 17.5 for the PC-System at a glandular dose of 1.58 and 0.49 mGy respectively (see figure 3). This translates into a 69% lower dose at 18% lower IQI for a standard patient with 6cm compressed breast. Increasing the dose of the PC system resulted in IQI of 19.8 at

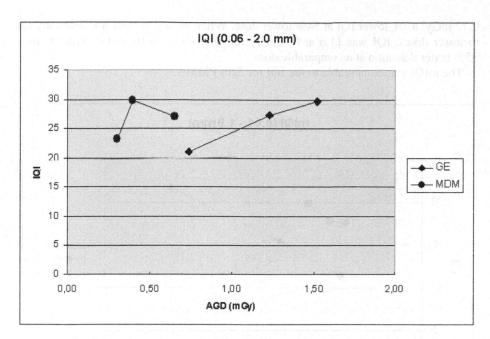

Fig. 1. Image Quality Index (IQI) of both systems at 3 cm PMMA-equivalent

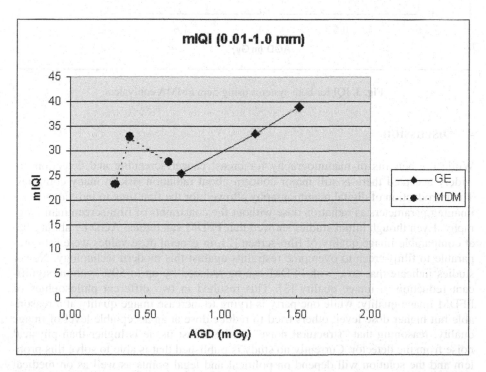

Fig. 2. Modified Image Quality Index (mIQI) over the reduced diameter range for 3cm PMMA

0.72 mGy, a 7% lower IQI at 54% lower dose. When the aSi-system was manually set to lower doses, IQI was 11.6 at 0.52mGy for aSi vs.17.5 at 0.49mGy with PC or a 35% better detection at a comparable dose.

The mIQI was comparable to the IQI for 5cm PMMA.

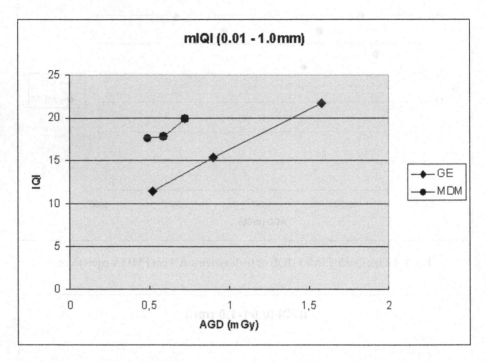

Fig. 3. IQI for both systems using 5cm PMMA equivalent

4 Discussion

While the benefits of mammography for breast cancer screening and detection are widely accepted there is still major concern about radiation risk in many countries. The introduction of digital mammography allowed for the first time to individually set imaging parameters as radiation dose without the constraints of film-screen mammography. Even though initial studies showed that FFDM can reduce AGD by about 30% at comparable image quality of film-screen [2], in general dose values were set comparable to film-screen to overcome restraints against this modern technology. Newer studies indicate that dose with FFDM can be reduced by up to 50% without significant reduction in image quality [3]. This resulted in two different philosophies of FFDM image quality: while one party is trying to increase image quality at a reasonable but higher dose level, others tried to reduce dose at an acceptable level of image quality, reasoning that "structural noise" of the breast tissue is higher than physical noise from the detector. Currently no study is published that is able to solve this problem and the solution will depend on political and legal points as well as on medical reasoning for one side. The PC-system that we compared in our study was able to reduce the dose by up to 54% at an equivalent IQI-value. In standard mode AGD with the PC-system for thin breasts (3cm PMMA) was 20% of that with the aSi-system at 60% of the IQI.

The dose of the PC-system is limited to a very low value; hence the standard IQI of the aSi-system could not be reached. A version of the PC system which is able to achieve a higher dose is available on the market but was not available for this study. As the direct comparison of image quality was done at a level that is optimal for the photon-counter but probably below the optimal beam quality level for the aSi-system, this is a clear limitation of our study. Also the aSi-System used was an older version, subsequently several changes have been applied to AEC, that might influence AGD in standard mode. In addition the AEC of the aSi-system is programmed to adjust imaging parameters to breast density, which can not be used in phantom imaging. It is therefore possible that in clinical images the differences between the systems might be smaller.

The ideal phantom for contrast detail analysis would be unlimited in all directions, a property certainly not available for the CDMAM. This causes difficulties in evaluation: both systems are able to detect all gold discs of the diameters 1 to 2mm, while the 0.06 and 0.08mm discs are not reliably detected (see figure 4). This causes the program to extrapolate the measurements causing inconclusive results. We tried to overcome this limitation by calculating a modified IQI (or mIQI) over the values 0.1 to 1mm. Evaluating this mIQI the difference in standard mode was smaller than with

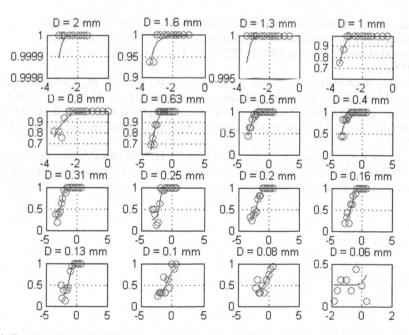

Fig. 4. Results of the CDCOM evaluation for 3cm PMMA with the aSi-System in standard mode. For the large discs of more than 0.63mm diameter as well as for very small discs of 0.06 mm the threshold level of 0.62 could not be reached.

the previous method of detection, as the large discs -that were detected in any case and therefore useless in differentiation- could not dilute differences present.

A critical point against the mIQI is that the detection of very small discs might be overlooked, which was not the case in our study: Only for 3cm PMMA in contrast mode the aSi-system was able to reach the threshold level of the CDCOM program for the 0.08mm disks, in all other parameter-settings the small discs were undetectable for both systems. For smaller discs, detection was possible but not reliably enough to reach the threshold level. This indicates that the aSi-system is able to detect objects below its spatial resolution, while the higher resolution of the PC-system does not translate into better detection of small objects.

5 Conclusion

The PC-system seems to reduce dose by up to 54% at equivalent image quality index (IQI). Standard image quality of aSi could not be reached with this version of the PC system. There is currently no scientific evidence how increasing IQI will translate into better detection and what is the optimal trade-off between image quality and radiation dose.

References

1. Dance D.R., Skinner C.L., Young K.C.; Beckett J.R., Kotre C.J. Additional factors for the estimation of mean glandular breast dose using the UK mammography dosimetry protocol. Phys Med Biol. 2000 Nov; 45(11): 3225-3240. D R Dance et al 2000 Phys. Med. Biol. 45 3225-3240
2. Hemdal, B., Andersson, I., Grahn, A., Håkansson, M., Ruschin, M., Thilander-Klang, A., Båth, M., Börjesson, S., Medin, J., Tingberg, A., Månsson, L. G., Mattsson, S. 2005 Can the average glandular dose in routine digital mammography screening be reduced? A pilot study using revised image quality criteria. Radiation Protection Dosimetry 114 (1-3): 383-388
3. Hermann, K.P., Obenauer, S., Funke, M., Grabbe, E.H. 2002 Magnification mammography: a comparison of full-field digital mammography and screen-film mammography for the detection of simulated small masses and microcalcifications. Eur. Radiol. 12: 2188-2191

Understanding Hessian-Based Density Scoring

Jakob Raundahl, Marco Loog, and Mads Nielsen

IT University of Copenhagen

Abstract. Numerous studies have investigated the relation between mammographic density and breast cancer risk. These studies indicate that women with high breast density have a four to six fold risk increase. An investigation of whether or not this relation is causal is important for, e.g., hormone replacement therapy (HRT), which has been shown to actually increase the density.

No gold standard for automatic assessment of mammographic density exists. Manual methods such as Wolfe patterns and BI-RADS are helpful for communication of diagnostic sensitivity, but they are both time consuming and crude. For serial, temporal analysis it is necessary to be able to detect more subtle changes.

In previous work, a method for measuring the effect of HRT w.r.t. changes in biological density in the breast is described. The method provides structural information orthogonal to intensity-based methods. Hessian-based features and a clustering of these is employed to divide a mammogram into four structurally different areas. Subsequently, based on the relative size of the areas, a density score is determined.

We have previously shown that this method can separate patients receiving HRT from patients receiving placebo. In this work, the focus is on deeper understanding of the methodology using tests on sets of artificial images of regular elongated structures.

1 Introduction

Numerous studies have investigated the relation between mammographic density and breast cancer risk, and women with high breast density appear to have a four to six fold increase in breast cancer risk, e.g. [9, 2, 1, 7]. Therefore *density* is an important feature embedded in a mammogram. Currently, however, the density is not used to asses risk in the standard clinical screening procedures.

The specific purpose of this work is to investigate the nature of the actual structural changes in the breast tissue caused by hormone replacement therapy (HRT) detected by our clustering technique. This Hessian-based method has been validated in a previous experiment, using two sets of mammograms of 50 patients from a double blind, placebo controlled HRT experiment [8]. The method was able to significantly separate the HRT patients from placebo patients ($p = 0.0002$) [5].

The method is interesting seen both from a practical, image analysis perspective, but also from a medical point of view, where is might provide insight into important anatomical changes relating to density alterations. In order to get this insight, we have to have an in depth understanding of the method used, which is

Susan M. Astley et al. (Eds.): IWDM 2006, LNCS 4046, pp. 447–452, 2006.

the focus of the study presented. To achieve understanding we do tests on sets of canonical images of regular stripe-like patterns of different frequency.

2   Methods

Detecting HRT Using Hessian-Based Pixel Classification

The breast tissue is manually segmented. Within this region of interest (ROI), for every pixel, features based on eigenvalues of Hessian at three scales are determined. The Hessian at scale s is defined by

$$
H_s(I) = \begin{bmatrix} \dfrac{\partial_s^2 I}{\partial_s x^2} & \dfrac{\partial_s^2 I}{\partial_s x \partial_s y} \\[2ex] \dfrac{\partial_s^2 I}{\partial_s y \partial_s x} & \dfrac{\partial_s^2 I}{\partial_s y^2} \end{bmatrix}
$$

where ∂_s denotes the Gaussian derivative at scale s [4]. The scales used are 1, 2 and 4 mm. The features used are given by the quotient:

$$
q_s = \frac{|e_1| - |e_2|}{|e_1| + |e_2| + \epsilon}
$$

where e_1 and e_2 are eigenvalues of the Hessian at scale s, $e_1 > e_2$ and ϵ is a number much smaller than 1 used to avoid instabilities associated with near zero division. This quotient relates to the elongatedness in an image at a certain location (x, y) at scale s. It is close to zero if image structure is "round" and closer to 1 or +1 for more elongated structures. It is invariant to rotation of the image and locally linear scaling of the intensities.

In a training phase, a large collection of randomly chosen pixels from the different images in the data set are used to generate a representative collection of features. These features are divided into four clusters using k-means clustering [6]. The means are stored and used for nearest mean classification [6].

In the testing phase this nearest mean classifier (NMC) is used to score each mammogram as follows:

- Extract Hessian-based features
- Classify each pixel in one of four classes using the NMC
- Determine relative areas of the classes
- Compute the score from these areas

The score is based on a linear combination of the relative areas of the classes in the breast tissue. The combination is determined using a linear classifier given the HRT group and the placebo group. We assume Gaussian distributions with equal covariance and use the resulting linear Fisher discriminant [6] to separate the placebo and the HRT groups. In the HRT experiment we found that using only two of the classes gave good results and adding information about the other two did not improve the separation significantly.

Feature and Classifier Evaluation Using Artificial Images

What do changes in these two clusters mean, and how can we get an understanding of which changes in tissue structure the HRT/Placebo classifier bases its decision on? To answer this question we analyse the clustering of some simple, regular, stripy images. An example of a set of analytical images that can be considered member of the "canonical" images of stripy/elongated structures are the sinusoids. A lot of different types could be used, but we found that images of the type $|sin\omega_1 x + sin\omega_2 y|$ served our purpose well. Adjusting ω_1 and ω_2 within some reasonable boundaries produces a collection of images of regularly varying scale and elongatedness.

For each image in this set we do pixel classification and record the percentage areas of each of the four classes. Doing this for N frequencies produces $N \times N$ sets of relative areas. For each of these sets, the ratio used to separate HRT and Placebo is computed. Then we have the HRT likelihood as function of frequency and we can look at the gradient vector field of these $N \times N$ scores to investigate which changes in frequency the classifier picks up. These frequencies also relate to the scale of the elongated structures, with lower frequencies giving larger scales.

3   Results

The best linear combination, using the Fisher discriminant to separate HRT and placebo, uses class one and class two and is illustrated in Fig. 1 in a scatter plot. The actual combination corresponds roughly to "$2 \times Area2 - Area1$".

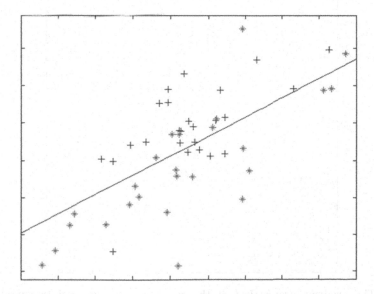

Fig. 1. Best linear separation of the HRT and Placebo groups using class one and two. +'s are HRT patients and *'s placebo.

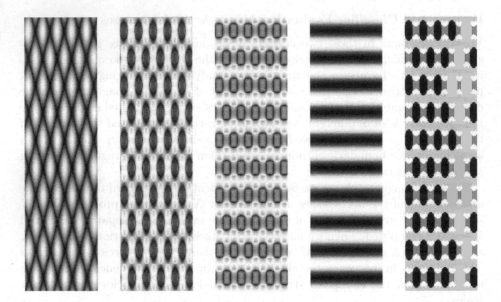

Fig. 2. From left to right: An example canonical image, Hessian-based feature at scale 5 pixels, 10 pixels, 20 pixels and the classification showing the four different classes. The two classes that was combined to separate HRT and Placebo are the black (class one) and the darkest grey (class 2).

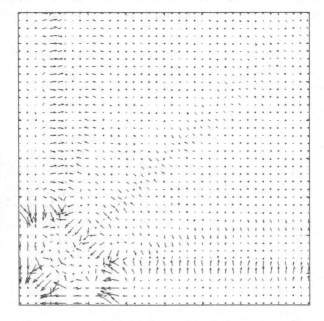

Fig. 3. The gradient vector field of the ratio of class one and two used in the HRT/Placebo classification shown as function of increasing wavelength

The actual construction of the pixel classifier is as follows. A million pixels are selected at random among the images in the data set as training data, after determining ROIs. Features are extracted from these pixels, the k-means algorithm is applied and the NMC is constructed from the labelled training data.

The wave lengths used in the analysis of sinusoids are from 2 to 100 pixels to provide a range suitable for the scales of the features (5, 10 and 20 pixels). In Fig. 2 an example image is shown together with the feature response and classification by the pixel classifier (the vertical wave length is 70 pixels and the horizontal 20). The test-images are constructed such that they have periodic boundaries and since the scale derivatives are computed in the Fourier domain we avoid artifacts along the boundaries of the feature images.

Getting the relative areas of the four clusters and computing the structural density as a combination of the first two areas allows the computation of the gradient vector field. The vector field for the set of sinusoid images described above is shown in Fig. 3.

4   Discussion

Unsupervised clustering of mammograms based on the quotient of Hessian eigenvalues at three scales can be used to differentiate between patients receiving HRT and patients receiving placebo. The Hessian eigen values have not been used in connection with density, but have been used to characterize vesselness in other medical applications [3].

We want to make longitudinal studies, but not wait 5-10 years to get the real digital images. A problem we often face when using digitized film mammograms is lack of gray-scale calibration. That is why a measure using features of the image, such as the Hessian eigenvalues, which is invariant under linear (or indeed just locally linear) grey-scale transformations is highly desirable.

Looking at the vector field in Fig. 3 we can make some comments on the classifier. From the behavior around the diagonal (not in the bottom left-hand corner), it appears that becoming more isotropic leads to an increased HRT likelihood. From the two other "rays" (horizontal and vertical), that go along the bottom and left borders of the image, it looks like tending towards a wave length of about 15 pixels (corresponds to 3 mm) from a larger or smaller wave length also increases the HRT likelihood. In the bottom left-hand corner things seem less clear. Overall, it looks as if becoming of higher frequency gives an increase in the measure.

These results provide a little insight into the important changes of elongatedness and, for that matter, density. Future work includes getting a more precise quantitative description of the changes and discussing these results with physicians to get a qualitative understanding of the changes detected in the HRT group. Future validation studies on more HRT data are also planned to improve the clinical validation of the measure.

References

1. N F Boyd, J W Byng, R A Jong, E K Fishell, L E Little, A B Miller, G A Lockwood, D L Trichler, and M J Yaffe. Quantitative classification of mammographic densities and breast cancer risk: Results from the canadian national breast screening study. *Academic Radiology*, 87(9):670–675, 1995.
2. N F Boyd, B O'Sullivan, J E Campbell, and et al. Mammographic signs as risk factors for breast cancer. *British Journal of Cancer*, 45:185–193, 1982.
3. A.F. Frangi, W.J. Niessen, K.L. Vincken, and M.A. Viergeve. Multiscale vessel enhancement filtering. In *Medical Image Computing and Computer-Assisted Intervention - MICCAI'98*, pages 130–137. Springer, 1998.
4. Tony Lindeberg. Scale-space: A framework for handling image structures at multiple scales. CERN School of Computing, September 1996.
5. Jakob Raundahl, Marco Loog, and Mads Nielsen. Mammographic density measured as changes in tissue structure caused by hrt. *SPIE Medical Imaging*, 2006.
6. F. van der Heiden, R.P.W. Duin, D. de Ridder, and D.M.J. Tax. *Classification, Parameter Estimation, State Estimation: An Engineering Approach Using MatLab*. Wiley, New York, 2004.
7. C H van Gils, J H C L Hendriks, R Holland, N Karssemeijer, J D M Otten, H Straatman, and A L M Verbeek. Changes in mammographic breast density and concomitant changes in breast cancer risk. *European Journal of Cancer Prevention*, 8:509–515, 1999.
8. L. Warming, P. Ravn, D. Spielman, P. Delmas, and C. Christiansen. Trimegestone in a low-dose, continuous-combined hormone therapy regimen prevents bone loss in osteopenic postmenopausal women. *Menopause*, 11(3):337–342, May-June 2004.
9. J N Wolfe. Risk for breast cancer development determined by mammographic parenchymal pattern. *Cancer*, 37(5):2486–2498, 1976.

Review of the Dose and Image Quality Characteristics of 3 FFDM Systems in Clinical Practice in a Screening Programme

Gillian Egan and Niall Phelan

BreastCheck, The National Breast Screening Programme, 36 Eccles St., Dublin 7, Ireland
gillian.egan@breastcheck.ie, niall.phelan@breastcheck.ie

Abstract. The purpose of this study was to review the dose and image characteristics of three different FFDM systems; Sectra MDM, GE SenoDS, Lorad Selenia. The dose and image quality characteristics were assessed in terms of both physics and clinical performance. A phantom study was carried out to look at the mean glandular dose delivered to breasts of varying thickness. The dose was also investigated by carrying out a clinical dose survey of a random sample of women on each of the three units. The CDMAM 3.4 was imaged on each unit with varying thicknesses of PMMA and the results correlated with the dose results at each equivalent thickness. The CNR of each unit at varying breast thicknesses was also calculated.

1 Background

The three systems investigated in the study were;

- ❑ Sectra Micro Dose Mammography
- ❑ GE SenoDS
- ❑ Lorad Selenia

All images were reviewed on a common PACS platform.

The dose characteristics of the systems were evaluated by measuring mean glandular dose and performing a clinical dose survey, which looked at a consecutive sample of women on each of the three units. The image quality was quantified using the CDMAM 3.4 phantom to generate contrast detail curves. The CNR of each system was also used as a performance indicator.

2 Method

Mean glandular dose was measured in accordance with the EUREF protocol (2005). To assess the dose delivered by each system, the factors selected by the x-ray set when imaging a range of thicknesses of PMMA 20 - 70mm were recorded. In each case the dose was measured using a RadCal 9010 and a 6cc ioisation chamber. The HVL at all clinical settings was also measured, allowing the entrance surface air kerma to be measured. The method described by Dance et al (2000) was used to calculate the mean glandular dose to the typical breast.

Susan M. Astley et al. (Eds.): IWDM 2006, LNCS 4046, pp. 453–459, 2006.
© Springer-Verlag Berlin Heidelberg 2006

Contrast detail measurements were made using the CDMAM phantom (version 3.4, Bijkerk, 2002). The CDMAM consists of a matrix of gold discs of thicknesses from 2μm to 0.03μm and diameters from 2mm to 0.06 mm on a 2 mm aluminium base encased in Perspex. In each square of the matrix are a pair of identical gold discs. One is in the centre and the other is in one of the four corners. In order to correlate the results of this test with the mean glandular dose results at varying breast thickness the CDMAM was setup with different thickness of PMMA equivalent to the 20-70mm used in the mean glandular dose measurement. Each arrangement was imaged using the x-ray unit's automatically selected factors normally set for clinical use for a breast of equivalent attenuation. The digital images had the contrast and density adjusted to optimally display the details in the test object, before scoring on softcopy display workstations. These results were used in conjunction with an excel spreadsheet to generate contrast detail curves.

CNR was calculated for each unit using the methodology as outlined in the EUREF protocol. The CNR measurements are referenced to the limiting value of the 0.1mm diameter column for 50mm PMMA thickness.

A clinical dose survey was carried out on each of the three units. A consecutive sample of women was chosen from each unit and their data was retrospectively collected. The views acquired, kV, mAs and target filter combinations chosen for each woman was recorded, as well as breast thickness, force applied and dose as measured by the unit. The data was analysed using the Breast Dose calculator, version 2.0 (Young 2004), provided for the NHSBSP dose survey.

3 Results

As expected the MGD delivered by the units was consistently lowest on the Sectra MDM and highest on the Lorad Selenia over a range of phantom thicknesses. MGD was measured using the factors automatically selected by each unit in clinical practice. These factors are displayed in Table 1 below. MGDs for each unit is shown in Figure 1 below.

Table 1. Automatically selected factors for each unit under varying thickness of PMMA

Breast Thickness (mm)	Sectra MDM	SenoDS	Lorad Selenia
21	26 W/Al	26 Mo/Mo	24 Mo/Mo
32	29 W/Al	26 Mo/Mo	26 Mo/Mo
45	32 W/Al	29 Rh/Rh	28 Mo/Mo
53	35 W/Al	29 Rh/Rh	29 Mo/Mo
60	35 W/Al	29 Rh/Rh	30 Mo/Mo
75	35 W/Al	31 Rh/Rh	32 Mo/Rh
90	28 W/Al	30 Rh/Rh	32 Mo/Rh

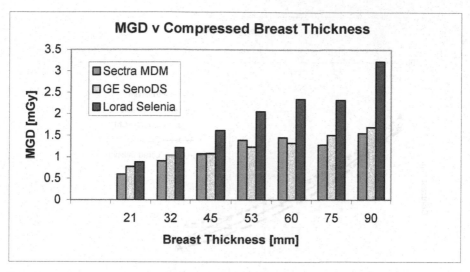

Fig. 1. Mean glandular dose delivered by each unit to compressed breast of varying thickness

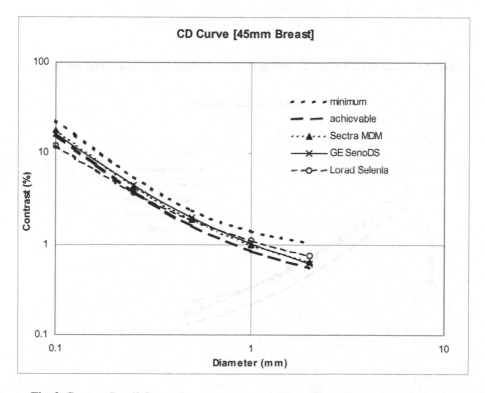

Fig. 2. Contrast Detail Curves for all 3 units using CDMAM equivalent to 45mm Breast

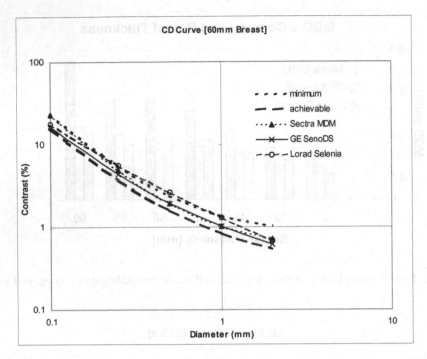

Fig. 3. Contrast Detail Curves for all 3 units using CDMAM equivalent to 60mm Breast

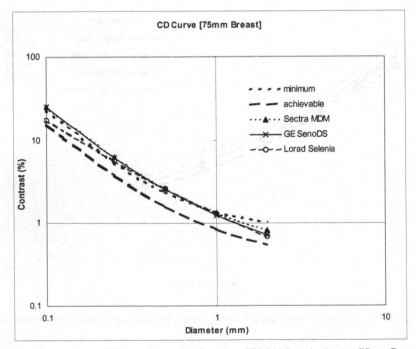

Fig. 4. Contrast Detail Curves for all 3 units using CDMAM equivalent to 75mm Breast

The CD curves were derived for all three units. All three units generated contrast detail curves that surpassed the achievable limit for small breast thicknesses. The GE outperformed the other two units at these small breast sizes. As the breast size increased above 45mm the contrast detail curves for all units moved between the minimum and achievable limit. Above 60mm while the units remained within limits at the high and low contrast detail size they all dipped below minimum for medium sized contrast detail. Displayed below in Figures 1,2 and 3 are the resultant curves for breasts of 45mm, 60mm and 75mm respectively. These thicknesses were chosen for display as they are representative of common thicknesses encountered in clinical practice.

The CNR for all three units was calculated. The percentage CNR at all thickness relative to the limiting value for the 0.1mm diameter column of the CDMAM for a 60mm breast are displayed in Table 2.

Table 2. Percentage Contrast on each unit at all breast thicknesses referenced to a limiting vlaue of the 0.1mm diameter column for a 60mm breast

| Breast Thickness (mm) | % CNR [EUREF] | | | |
	Sectra MDM	SenoDS	Lorad Selenia	Tolerance (%)
21	145	239	236	>115
32	138	200	202	>110
45	113	138	159	>105
53	110	131	151	>103
60	100	123	130	100
75	74	110	105	>95
90	68	99	87	>90

The results of the clincal dose survey gave good insight into the different parameter selections for the three units and the number of repeats or extra views required on each system. The range of doses on the Sectra unit is much lower than the GE SenoDS or Lorad Selenia. The Sectra MDM also displayed a much narrower spread of doses in clinial practice. Table 3 below summarises the main findings of the clinical dose survey.

Table 3. Summary of the main findings from the clinical dose survey

Sectra MDM	GE DenoDS	Lorad Selenia
Top 3 Auto Selections	Top 3 Auto Selections	Top 3 Auto Selections
35 W/Al (266)	29 Rh/Rh (267)	32 Mo/Rh (106)
28 W/Al (99)	27 Mo/Rh (51)	30 Mo/Mo (69)
32 W/Al (32)	31 Rh/Rh (20)	21 Mo/Mo (59)

Table 3. (*continued*)

Sectra MDM	GE DenoDS	Lorad Selenia
Average MGD (mGy)	Average MGD (mGy)	Average MGD (mGy)
CC 0.97	CC 2.13	CC 2.28
MLO 0.98	MLO 2.20	MLO 2.35
Screening Exam 1.97	Screening Exam 3.97	Screening Exam 4.79
Ave. Dose to 5-6cm Breast	Ave. Dose to 5-6cm Breast	Ave. Dose to 5-6cm Breast
0.97mGy	2.17mGy	2.37mGy
Extra Views	Extra Views	Extra Views
2 CC	6 CC	4 CC
9 MLO	7 MLO	7 MLO
11 Total	13 Total	11 Total

4 Discussion

The image quality and radiation dose characteristics of three distinct FFDM detector systems have been comprehensively evaluated in this study.

The Lorad Selenia unit consistently delivered the highest mean glandular dose at all breast thicknesses. Increased utilization of the Mo/Rh spectrum on this unit is likely to reduce the MGD delivered. The Sectra MDM delivered the lowest dose for most breast thicknesses with the exception of the mid range thickness where the MGD delivered by the MDM was comparable to that of the GE SenoDS.

The results of the clinical dose survey showed good correlation with the phantom MGD study. Again the Lorad Selenia delivered the highest average MGD per exam and the Sectra MDM the lowest. The average clinical dose to a 50-60mm breast also followed the same pattern. The clinical dose survey showed a slightly elevated number of extra views on the GE SenoDS unit. It is believed that this was as a result of the small field size, which necessitates extra views on above average sized breasts. This number would likely be higher still if women with larger breast thicknesses were not deliberately imaged on other units.

Finally, the clinical dose survey highlighted that the three units made very different automatic selections. The Sectra unit is inherently restricted to five kV target/filter combinations due to its setup. These are 26, 29, 32, 35 and 38kV all using a W/Al target /filter. 35 W/Al was by far the most commonly selected of these. The GE Seno DS offered a wider range of exposure factors. As was evidenced by the phantom MGD study, this unit begins to use the Rh/Rh spectrum at relatively low breast thickness. This choice of Rh/Rh contributed to a significant dose saving. The GE SenoDS most commonly selected 29Rh/Rh. Although the Lorad Selenia most commonly chose 32 Mo/Rh, overall this unit selected a Mo/Mo spectrum more often than a Mo/Rh. As discussed above the frequent selection of the Mo/Mo spectrum for this unit played a significant role in the relatively high doses it delivered. This unit requires some optimisation to utilize the Mo/Rh spectrum more frequently and as a result, reduce the dose.

As part of the image quality review, threshold contrast curves were generated for each unit over a range of thicknesses. A number of observations were made in relation to acquiring and reading the CDMAM images. Due to non-uniformity of the Sectra images, we initially found it difficult to read the CDMAM images from this unit. Because of this, we decided to image the phantom perpendicular to the chest wall in order to reduce the effect of poor image quality at the edges of the image field. However the general non-uniformity of the images also caused problems, which we overcame by taking a second set of images with the phantom positioned at 180 degrees to its original position. If a correct result was read on either image this was taken to be the overall result for that square. In general the Sectra MDM images proved more difficult to read due to the presence of noise in the images.

With regard to the GE SenoDS, it was noted that particular attention was necessary when positioning the phantom on the detector as the phantom is a close fit to the field of view. Where the phantom is not accurately centred in the field of view there may be discs missing from the resultant image.

As would be expected, all three units surpass or perform close to the achievable performance at breast thicknesses below 32mm. At these lower thicknesses, the GE SenoDS consistently outperforms the other units. For breast thickness between 45mm and 60mm all three units perform between the minimum and achievable limits with some crossover in the order of performance. CD curves on all units for breast thicknesses above the 60mm follow this trend and while they perform well at the extreme ends of the contrast detail spectrum they tend to drop performance in the mid range. Where the units are failing to meet the minimum tolerance there is the opportunity to increase their performance in this respect by increasing the dose, which is currently below the maximum allowed.

CNR measurements at varying PMMA thicknesses were made on each unit. A percentage contrast was calculated for each thickness with reference to the limiting threshold contrast for the 0.1mm diameter column for a 60mm breast (CDMAM plus 40mm PMMA). The GE Seno DS exceeded the recommended tolerance at all breast thicknesses. The Lorad Selenia also met the tolerances with the exception of the 90mm breast. The Sectra unit failed to meet the recommended tolerances for breast size above 75mm. It is felt that those thicknesses that failed on the Lorad and Sectra units could be brought into tolerance with some optimization of the units and also increased experience of reading the CDMAM phantom which influences the 100% value.

References

1. European Protocol for the Quality Control of the Physical and Technical Aspects of Mammography Screening, European Commission
2. Dance DR et al., Additional factors for the estimation of mean glandular breast dose using the UK mammography dosimetry protocol, 2000 Phys. Med. Biol.(45) 3225-3240
3. Bijkerk KR, Thijssen MAO, Arnoldussen THJM, Manual CDMAM-phantom, 2002
4. Young KC, Breast Dose surveys in the NHSBSP : Software and instruction manual, Version 2.0

Impact of Textured Background on Scoring
of Simulated CDMAM Phantom

Bénédicte Grosjean* and Serge Muller

Mammography Department, GE Healthcare
283 rue de la Minière – 78530 BUC – France

Abstract. CDMAM phantom scoring is widely used to assess the detectability performance of mammography systems. We propose to study the impact of structured background on this performance assessment, using simulated CDMAM phantom images with flat and textured backgrounds. Three dose levels have been investigated, ranging from -50% to +50% around the reference dose computed by the acquisition system. For textured backgrounds, the simulated projected breast corresponds to a 50mm thick, 60% glandular breast, with a texture generated by a power-law filtered noise model. Images have been scored by four image quality experts. For the smaller insert sizes, Image Quality Factor (IQF) scores obtained in textured backgrounds are lower than and well correlated with those obtained in flat backgrounds. IQF values increased with dose. For the larger insert sizes, detectability performance in textured background is even more degraded and is not as dose dependent as it is in flat backgrounds.

1 Introduction

The CDMAM phantom is widely used to evaluate the detectability performance of mammographic x-ray equipment. This contrast-detail phantom assesses the ability of a system to distinguish objects with very small contrast and small diameter. The task involved with scoring the CDMAM phantom consists of detecting disc-like inserts of various thicknesses and diameters in flat noisy background. However, such a detection task does not reflect the detection task done by radiologists in clinical conditions. One of the main limitations is the use of flat noisy backgrounds that are not representative of backgrounds associated with clinical breast imaging. The structure of clinical backgrounds is due to overlapping projection of the normal breast anatomical structures in 2D mammograms. In terms of detection performance, it has been shown [1, 2] that radiographic abnormalities detection is limited by both imaging system noise and anatomical noise. Observer experiments [3] demonstrated that the breast structure is often the main limiting factor for lesion detection performance. Bochud et al. [4] showed that for a small object, like microcalcifications, the observer performance is limited by the system noise and eventually by anatomical fluctuations depending on the amplitude of these fluctuations. For large objects, like a nodule, the effect of anatomical fluctuations was found more dominant than system noise.

---

* benedicte.grosjean@ge.com; Phone: +33 1 3070 9737; Fax: +33 1 3070 4140; http://www.gehealthcare.com

Susan M. Astley et al. (Eds.): IWDM 2006, LNCS 4046, pp. 460–467, 2006.
© Springer-Verlag Berlin Heidelberg 2006

Synthesizing images gives the opportunity to simulate CDMAM phantom images with spatially varying backgrounds in order to simulate real mammographic backgrounds for detection experiments. Moreover, in contrast with real phantoms, it enables to generate images with textured backgrounds for various texture realizations. Such a simulation tool would enable the assessment of mammography systems with different potential design options through textured CDMAM scoring, approaching a more clinically relevant detection task than with standard CDMAM phantom images.

The purpose of this work was to study the impact of structured background on the detectability performance, function of intensity values, assessed by the CDMAM phantom scoring.

2 Method

The CDMAM 3.4 phantom [5] consists of a matrix of 205 cells. Each cell contains two identical gold disks of given thickness and diameter. One is placed in the center and the other in a randomly chosen corner. The observer has to indicate the corner where the eccentric disk is located. The phantom covers a range of object diameters between 60μm and 2mm, and thicknesses between 0.03 and 2μm, including size and contrast ranges for microcalcifications. We simulated images of this contrast-detail phantom with flat and textured backgrounds (Figure 1) using the same acquisition conditions (Mo/Mo, 28kVp and 3 intensity values equal to 50, 100 and 160mAs) for a Senographe 2000D^{TM} system. We already validated [6] the simulation of the digital mammography system when applied to the simulation of standard CDMAM phantom images. In this study, a power-law model [7, 8] of the projected breast structure has been added [9] to the simulation tool in order to generate structured backgrounds. This power-law model of projected breast structure is based on the average power spectrum of real mammograms under an isotropic assumption. No phase information about mammographic images is included in this model since it makes the assumption of random phase. Nevertheless, detection experiments [11] showed that it can be used to investigate perceptual laws in mammography, leading to similar contrast-detail diagrams as in mammographic textured backgrounds.

For flat backgrounds, we simulated the image of the CDMAM phantom inserted between 2 PMMA plates of 20mm thickness. For textured backgrounds, we considered the projection of a breast with the same thickness than the CDMAM phantom assembly and with a power-law exponent equal to 3. This simulated breast was chosen 60% glandular in order to give the same grey level value than the CDMAM phantom assembly when imaged under the standard technique used to image the CDMAM phantom (Mo/Mo, 28kVp, 100mAs). Here the chosen glandularity would correspond to the glandularity derived from the breast thickness and the grey level measured in the most attenuating area of the breast by the automatic exposure of the mammography system [10]. The grey level ratio between the greatest and least attenuating areas of the breast was fixed based on typical grey level distribution in real mammograms.

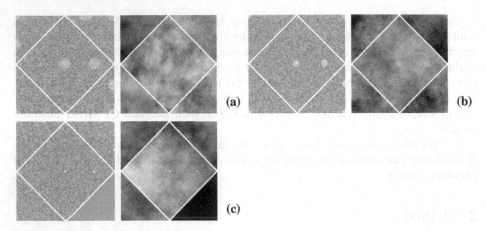

Fig. 1. Simulated images of CDMAM cells with flat (left) and textured (right) backgrounds, at Mo/Mo, 28kVp, 100 mAs. Each cell contains two identical inserts with a diameter of (a) 1.6mm, (b) 1mm, (c) 0.25mm, and a thickness of (a) 0.25µm, (b) 0.36µm, (c) 2µm.

For each acquisition condition and each type of background, four image realizations have been generated and rated by four image quality experts using the mammography-dedicated GE review workstation. The Image Quality Factor (IQF) was calculated on both image sets:

$$IQF = \frac{16}{\sum_{i=1}^{16} D_i \cdot T_{i,min}}, \tag{1}$$

where $T_{i,min}$ is the lowest thickness perceived in column i corresponding to an insert diameter D_i. We also defined the $IQF_{smaller\_inserts}$ and the $IQF_{larger\_inserts}$ as the IQF of the eight smaller (≤ 0.31mm), and eight larger (≥ 0.4mm) phantom insert sizes:

$$IQF_{smaller\,inserts} = \frac{8}{\sum_{i=1}^{8} D_i \cdot T_{i,min}} \quad \text{and} \quad IQF_{larger\,inserts} = \frac{8}{\sum_{i=9}^{16} D_i \cdot T_{i,min}}. \tag{2}$$

These definitions give higher scores for better detection performance. The three IQF values have then been normalized in order to have their variations in the same range for comparison purpose:

$$IQF_N = \frac{\sum_{i=1}^{16} D_i}{\sum_{i=1}^{16} D_i \cdot T_{i,min}}, IQF_{N,\,smaller\,inserts} = \frac{\sum_{i=1}^{8} D_i}{\sum_{i=1}^{8} D_i \cdot T_{i,min}} \quad \text{and} \quad IQF_{N,\,larger\,inserts} = \frac{\sum_{i=9}^{16} D_i}{\sum_{i=9}^{16} D_i \cdot T_{i,min}}. \tag{3}$$

3 Results

The values of the IQF_N, $IQF_{N, smaller\_inserts}$ and $IQF_{N, larger\_inserts}$ are shown for the four human readers and the three dose levels in Figure 2.

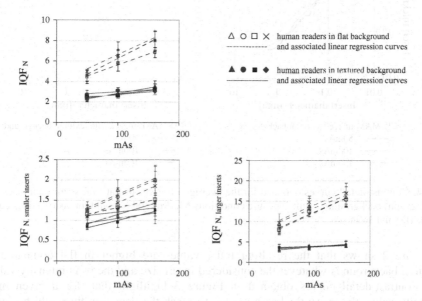

Fig. 2. IQF_N, $IQF_{N, smaller\_inserts}$ and $IQF_{N, larger\_inserts}$ values derived from the scoring of the 4 readers in flat and textured backgrounds (average over the 4 image realizations), with exposure conditions Mo/Mo, 28kVp and 3 intensity values (50, 100 and 160mAs)

Figure 3 and Figure 4 show contrast-detail curves obtained for the average observer in flat and textured backgrounds for the various intensity mAs values. For each given insert size, the curves indicate the minimal insert thickness needed to reach the detection threshold.

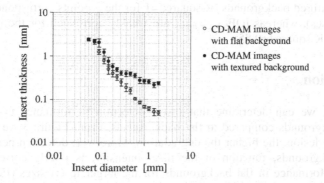

Fig. 3. Contrast-detail curves obtained for the average observer in flat and textured backgrounds, with exposure conditions Mo/Mo, 28kVp, 100mAs

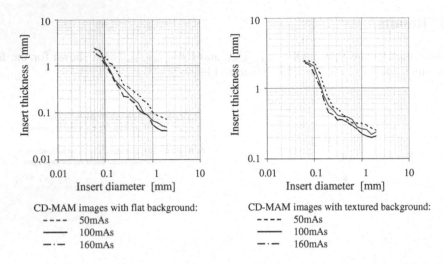

CD-MAM images with flat background:
- - - -   50mAs
———   100mAs
—·—   160mAs

CD-MAM images with textured background:
- - - -   50mAs
———   100mAs
—·—   160mAs

Fig. 4. Contrast-detail curves obtained for the average observer in flat (left graph) and textured (right graph) backgrounds, with exposure conditions Mo/Mo, 28kVp, and intensity values equal to 50, 100 and 160mAs

Figure 2 shows that the resulting IQF_N values are higher in flat compared to textured backgrounds whatever the considered insert size and the mAs intensity value. The contrast-detail curves obtained in Figure 3 highlight that, for a given mAs intensity value, the insert thickness needed to reach the detection threshold becomes much higher in textured backgrounds than in flat backgrounds as the insert size increases. Furthermore, IQF_N values (Figure 2) increase with increasing mAs values in both flat and textured backgrounds. This increasing variation trend is of the same order of magnitude for flat and textured backgrounds when considering the smaller inserts sizes (with a regression slope of $IQF_{N, \text{smaller inserts}}$ versus mAs equal to 0.006 and 0.003 respectively for flat and textured backgrounds). It is much higher for flat than for textured background for the larger inserts sizes (slope of $IQF_{N, \text{larger inserts}}$ versus mAs equal to 0.065 and 0.008 respectively). Regression analysis restricted to the smaller inserts indicates good correlation between $IQF_{N,\text{smaller inserts}}$ values obtained in flat and textured backgrounds (R-squared=1 for the 3 points corresponding to the 3 intensity values), whereas $IQF_{N,\text{larger inserts}}$ are weakly correlated for the inserts larger than 0.4mm (R-squared=0.85).

4 Discussion

As expected, we can determine that insert detection performance is degraded in textured backgrounds compared to flat backgrounds. From Figure 3 we can see that the larger the lesion, the higher the degradation. Moreover, detection performance in textured backgrounds, function of the mAs intensity, is poorly correlated to the detection performance in flat backgrounds for the larger insert sizes (Figure 2). For such insert sizes, it is believed that structure noise becomes predominant compared to noise sources induced by the image acquisition processes (quantum noise, scintillator point spread function, aliasing noise or detector noise) [4, 9, 11]. This can be explained by inspection of power spectra frequency distributions of real mammograms, up to frequencies of about 1cycle/mm [7]. The contribution of the breast structure relative to the other noise sources is more important in the low frequency range. Therefore, as the insert size increases, the mammographic structures amplitude becomes the limiting factor for detection. Taking into account structured backgrounds improves the relevance of the CDMAM phantom scoring, especially for the larger inserts sizes. However, the CDMAM phantom scoring in flat backgrounds remains meaningful for the smaller insert sizes, since we found a good correlation between results obtained in flat and in textured backgrounds. Thus, for comparison of system performance using the CDMAM phantom, we would recommend to restrict the scoring results analysis to the smaller inserts sizes of the phantom.

Furthermore, contrast-detail curves of Figure 4 show negative detection slopes in both flat and textured backgrounds. Burgess showed [11] that in mammographic and also power-law filtered noise backgrounds, for lesion sizes larger than about 1mm, the detection slope is positive, in opposite as intuitively expected. However, this result depends on the shape of the considered signal. Whereas positives slopes were found for shapes corresponding to projected spheres, slopes were negatives for flat-top disc shapes [12]. Thus, the unrealistic disc-like form of the phantom inserts prevents, for the larger insert sizes, from extrapolating the scoring results to clinical performance of large size lesion detection. Furthermore, during the scoring process we noticed that for inserts larger than about 1mm, human readers rely more on the insert edges than on the insert contrast. The simulation of more clinically relevant inserts with smoother edges and with a material composition closer to real microcalcifications would be an additional interesting improvement. The generation of artificial mammographic abnormalities has already been studied in the literature [13, 14]. In future work, it would be interesting to use such inserts as the input to generate simulated CDMAM phantom-like images with textured backgrounds and realistic inserts, in order to provide a contrast-detail test closer to the clinical task.

Van Metter [15] and Young [16] refined the interpretation method for CDMAM phantom scoring results. Indeed, the test suffers from several sources of variability, one of the most significant being the inter- and intra-observer variability. In our study, inter-observer variability and scoring reproducibility must be regarded carefully. The CDMAM phantom scoring procedure [5] applies correction rules, which tend to flatten the variations induced by the presence of texture. Even if the variability seems to be of the same order of magnitude for flat and textured backgrounds, more false positive and false negative detections were found for all the observers in textured backgrounds.

Finally, the opportunity to reduce dose while keeping an acceptable image quality has been described by some authors [4, 17, , 18, 19]. For inserts with contrast in the clinically relevant range 3-30%, the CDMAM provided overlapped curves for dose levels reduced within 40-50% from the reference [18]. These insert contrasts are related to the smaller insert sizes of the CDMAM phantom for the dose levels considered in the study. It has been shown that [19] decreasing dose significantly degrades the detection of microcalcifications, whereas it has minimal effect on the detection of masses. For optimization purposes, if the targeted clinical task consists of detecting the smallest microcalcifications, better performance would be obtained with higher dose. Moreover, when considering an actual microcalcification, its contrast is often linked to its size. Thus, for a given target size of the smallest microcalcification to be detected, larger microcalcifications will be more easily detectable since they usually lead to a higher contrast in the image. If the optimization task is restricted to mass detection, the dose level could be decreased preserving detection performance since breast structure impairs detection more than any other noise source.

5 Conclusion

CDMAM phantom scoring is very widely used to estimate the detectability performance of mammography x-ray equipment. However, the detection task induced by this contrast-detail phantom is not representative of the clinical task done by radiologists, mainly due to its flat background. We evaluated in this study the impact of structured background on the detectability performance assessed by the CDMAM phantom scoring.

We developed a simulation tool generating quantitative images of CDMAM phantom, depending on the exposure spectrum, and including a model of the projected breast structure based on the average power spectrum of real mammograms. We generated simulated CDMAM phantom images with flat and textured backgrounds for the standard exposure technique of the CDMAM phantom (Mo/Mo, 28kVp) and for three mAs intensity levels (50, 100 and 160mAs). Images have then been scored by four readers. Scoring results show that detection performance in textured backgrounds is degraded compared to flat backgrounds. This degradation increases with increasing insert size. We found that the IQF values obtained in textured and flat backgrounds, function of the mAs intensity level, are well correlated for the smaller insert sizes. This confirms the relevance of the scoring of the CDMAM phantom in flat background for the smaller insert sizes. However, the correlation was weak for the larger insert sizes, since breast structure becomes the limiting detection factor compared to other noise sources for such insert sizes. As a result, for comparison of system performance, the CDMAM phantom scoring analysis should be restricted to the smaller insert sizes.

Furthermore, the simulation tool developed in this study offers the potential to validate new design options with a more clinically relevant detection task than standard CDMAM phantom images.

References

1. G. Revesz, H.L. Kundel, and M.A.Graber, "The influence of structured noise on the detection of radiological abnormalities", *Invest. Radiol.*, 9(6), pp.479-486, 1974
2. J.P. Rolland, and H.H. Barrett, "Effect of random background inhomogeneity on observer detection performance", *J. Opt. Soc. Am.*, A(9), pp.649-658, 1992
3. A.E. Burgess, F.L. Jacobson, and P.F. Judy, "Human observer detection experiments with mammograms and power-law noise", *Med. Phys.*, 28(4), pp.419-437, 2001
4. F.O. Bochud, J.F. Valley, F.R. Verdun, C. Hessler, and P. Schnyder, "Estimation of the noisy component of anatomical backgrounds", *Med. Phys.*, 26(7), pp.1365-1370, 1999

5. K. Bijkerk, M. Thijssen, and Th. Arnoldussen, *Manual CDMAM-phantom type 3.4*, University Medical Centre, Nijmegen, The Netherlands, 2000

6. B. Grosjean, S. Muller, H. Souchay, R. Rico, X. Bouchevreau, "Automated scoring for CDMAM phantom from simulated images", *Proceedings of IWDM 2004*, 2004

7. A.E. Burgess, "Bach, breasts, and power-law processes", *Proceedings of SPIE*, Vol.4324, pp.103-113, 2001

8. J.J. Heine, and R.P. Velthuizen, "Spectral analysis of full filed digital mammography data", *Med. Phys.*, 29(5), pp.647-661, 2002

9. B. Grosjean, S. Muller, H. Souchay, "Lesion detection using an a-contrario detector in simulated digital mammograms", *Proceedings of SPIE*, to be published in 2006

10. N. Shramchenko, P. Blin, C. Mathey, and R. Klausz, "Optimized exposure control in digital mammography", *Proceedings of SPIE*, Vol.5368, pp.445-456, 2004

11. A.E. Burgess, F.L. Jacobson, and P.F. Judy, "Lesion detection in digital mammograms", *Proceedings of SPIE*, Vol.4320, pp.555-560, 2001

12. A.E. Burgess, "Evaluation of detection model performance in power-law noise", *Proceedings of SPIE*, Vol.4324, pp123-132, 2001

13. A.K. Carton, H. Bosmans, C. Van Ongeval, G. Souverijns, F. Rogge, A. Van Steen, and G. Marchal, "Development and validation of a simulation procedure to study the visibility of microcalcifications in digital mammograms", Med. Phys., Vol.30(8), pp2234-2240, 2003

14. M. Ruschin, A. Tingberg, M. Bath, A. Grahn, M. Hakansson, B. Hamdal, I. Andersson, "Using simple mathematical functions to simulate pathological structures – input for digital mammography clinical trial", *Radiat. Prot. Dosimetry*, Vol.114(1-3), pp.424-431, 2005

15. R. Van Metter, M.D. Health, L.M. Fletcher-Health, "Applying the European protocol for the quality control of the physical and technical aspect of mammography screening to digital systems", *Proceeding of SPIE*, to be published in 2006

16. K.C. Young, J.J. Cook, J.M. Oduko, H.T.Bosmans, "Comparison of software and human observers in reading images of the CDMAM test object to assess digital mammography systems", *Proceeding of SPIE*, to be published in 2006

17. R.P. Highnam, J.M. Brady, and B.J. Shepstone, "Mammographic image analysis", *Eur. J. Radiol.*, Vol.24(1), pp.20-32, 1997

18. G. Gennaro, L. Katz, H. Souchay, C. Alberelli, and C. di Maggio, "Are phantoms useful for predicting the potential of dose reduction in full-filed digital mammography?", *Phys. Med. Biol.*, 50, pp.1851-1870, 2005

19. A.S. Chawla, R.S. Saunders and E. Samei, "Effect of dose reduction on the detection of mammographic lesions based on mathematical observer models", *Proceedings of SPIE*, to be published in 2006.

Magnetic Resonance Electrical Impedance Mammography: A Pilot Study

Maria Kallergi[1], Ernest Wollin[2], John J. Heine[1],
Nataliya Kovalchuk[1], and Anand Manohar[1]

[1] H. Lee Moffitt Cancer Center & Research Institute, Cancer Control and Prevention, 12902
Magnolia Drive, Tampa, Florida, USA, 33620
{kallergi, heinejj, kovalcn, manohara}@moffitt.usf.edu
[2] Wollin Ventures, Inc., 5409 Overseas Highway, Marathon, FL 33050
Ewollin@attglobal.net

Abstract. A new breast imaging approach is proposed and implemented that combines Magnetic Resonance Mammography and Electrical Impedance Scanning. In this paper, we report the results of a pilot study that demonstrated the feasibility of this new breast imaging approach. We also discuss our initial experience with the MR imaging parameters and sequences that are critical in observing the desired signal.

1 Introduction

Magnetic Resonance Mammography (MRM) has been used since late 1980's in combination with conventional methods to improve breast cancer diagnosis [1]. MRM is currently becoming the standard of care for preoperative loco-regional staging of breast cancer, screening of high-risk patients, and problem solving [2],[3]. MRM is done with either specially designed, dedicated units that provide high spatial resolution due to specific imaging sequences or whole body scanners equipped with special coils that provide high temporal resolution based on dynamic enhancement properties. Either approach requires the injection of paramagnetic contrast agents and the use of fat suppression techniques and specific sequences for optimum imaging [4],[5]. Despite the advantages, MRM's dissemination in the clinic and particularly the broader community has been slow due to cost but also conflicting technical requirements.

Electrical Impedance Scanning (EIS) of the breast is a clinically established method for the characterization of breast pathology. The T-Scan 2000 (TransScan Medical, Inc., Ramsey, NJ) was the first system to receive FDA approval in 1999 and was recommended for use as an adjunct to mammography in patients who have equivocal mammographic finding with ACR BIRADS™ categories 3 or 4 [6]. The studies on this system, and older work as well, have clearly demonstrated that complex permittivity is a clinically valuable marker for breast cancer detection and diagnosis because cancer tissues have conductivity and dielectric properties remarkably different than normal breast tissues [7],[8].

We propose the simultaneous application of magnetic and electric fields that could lead to a new breast imaging methodology, the Magnetic Resonance Electrical Impedance Mammography (MREIM). The electric field generates an additional

Susan M. Astley et al. (Eds.): IWDM 2006, LNCS 4046, pp. 468–474, 2006.

magnetic field that is spatially dependent on the local conductivity properties of the sample. Hence, the resulting image provides information on both the magnetic resonance and complex permittivity properties of the breast. In theory, MREIM does not require and is not affected by fat suppression techniques or by the injection of paramagnetic contrast agents and can be performed simultaneously with either high spatial resolution or high temporal resolution MRM examinations at any clinically useful field strength. MREIM also differs from an earlier attempt to combine MRI and EIS, namely the Magnetic Resonance Electrical Impedance Tomography (MREIT), in that it is not based on direct electrical injection of current into the breast, it does not require surface electrodes, or tomographic imaging [9]. It still permits, however, real-time MR guided localization or core biopsy of suspicious findings [10].

2 Materials and Methods

In our pilot study, we established the theoretical basis of the new approach, performed a simulation study, and conducted tests with custom-made phantoms and various imaging parameters to demonstrate the feasibility of the new imaging approach. Our experimental data supported the simulation and theoretical work and have shown great promise for the development of a new technology. A brief description of the materials and methods used to demonstrate the feasibility of the MREIM is given below.

2.1 Simulation

A proton density spin echo imaging sequence was simulated to study the relationships between the driving frequency of the applied electric field, which will be referred to as the phase modulation frequency (PMF), the induced current distribution, and the associated effects on the image. The current simulation work to date represents idealizations because noise was not considered. The solutions for the magnetic field caused by the induced current were responsible for the image-perturbations.

A two-dimensional image of a disk was considered for the simulation, first unperturbed (no external current), and then perturbed (with current). The disk was not homogenous in its conductivity properties. The central region of the disk had 40-times the conductivity of the outer region, a relationship similar to the properties of breast cancer and normal breast tissue respectively.

2.2 Phantom Design

Conduction phantoms were developed using materials with magnetic resonance and conductivity properties equivalent to normal breast tissues and tumors. Specifically, materials simulating healthy breast fatty tissue should have T1 and T2 relaxation times around 370 ms and 53 ms respectively and electrical conductivity in the range of 0.02-0.07 S/m at a frequency of 1 kHz. Materials simulating breast tumors or glandular tissue should have T1 and T2 relaxation times around 1135 ms and 58 ms respectively with breast tumors having electrical conductivity 20-40 times higher than that of healthy breast tissue. In addition, phantoms were required to be chemically and physically stable over long periods of time.

Initially, fragrance free Neutrogena soap was selected as the material equivalent to healthy breast tissue. Its electrical conductivity was measured to be 0.03 S/m at

1 kHz. Two types of phantoms were constructed with the soap: (a) The first one contained a spherical cavity in the center of 1 cm in diameter filled with a soap/salt solution the conductivity of which was 1.2 S/m. (b) The spherical cavity in the second one was filled with a piece of fat-free hot dog with a conductivity of 2.17 S/m. A photograph of this phantom is shown in Fig. 1.

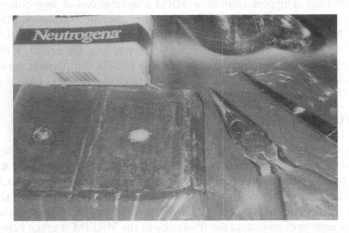

Fig. 1. Sliced MREIM phantom constructed of fragrance free Neutrogena soap showing the spherical piece of fat-free hotdog, 1 cm in diameter, simulating cancer

A third phantom was constructed using agar gel as the material equivalent to healthy breast tissue and a piece of fat-free hotdog as the cancer surrogate. Paramagnetic contrast agent, ProHance (gadoteridol injection) was added to the gel to adjust the T1 relaxation time. The T1 and T2 of the phantom were adjusted by varying the concentration of the agar gel and ProHance. The final gel solution consisted of 14g/100mL agar gel with 2.5 mM of ProHance. This was place in an electrically conductive carbon polyethylene bag that represented a skin surrogate. The conductivity of this phantom was measured to be 0.09 S/m. A picture of this phantom is shown in Fig. 2.

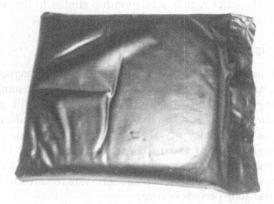

Fig. 2. MREIM phantom made of agar gel and ProHance solution in a polyethelene bag

All three phantoms were imaged under the same imaging conditions and parameters using the same setup. A series of three images was recorded in each run: one with the current off, one with the current on, and one with the current off again.

2.3 Experimental Setup and Imaging Parameters

The experimental setup included the following:

1. A Siemens Magnetom Symphony Maestro Class 1.5 Tesla system (Siemens Medical Solutions USA, Inc., Malvern, PA) was used for all experiments in the pilot study. The system was equipped with a breast coil and a breast biopsy system both from Invivo Corp. (Orlando, FL).

2. The stabilization/compression paddles in an MR breast coil (InVivo – Symphony Breast Biopsy Array) was modified to include Faraday-shield electrodes required to produce a current flux in the breast essentially orthogonal to the main magnetic H_0 field. The Faraday shield was constructed of a pair of copper sheets that were made out of rectangular bars. Two different sizes of copper foil sheets were tested: (a) One with dimensions of 5 cm × 7.5 cm consisting of bars that were 0.32 cm in width with a .016 cm spacing between them. (b) One with dimensions of 14 cm × 15 cm consisting of bars that were 0.2 cm in width with a 0.1 cm spacing between them (Electron Machine Corp., Umatilla, FL).

3. A time varying voltage generated with a frequency generator and power supply, connectors, multimeter, and a battery-operated oscilloscope were used for the application of the electric field. The total current density flowing through the phantom(s) reached 10 A/m^2 at frequencies in the range of 200 – 1000 Hz.

4. Gradient rephrased (GR), spin echo (SE), and echo planar (EP) sequences were tested in out pilot study for image acquisition. The sequence parameters were selected to satisfy the following requirements: (a) The temporal bandwidth per pixel (BW/Hz) had to be less than the phase modulation frequency to avoid volume averaging. (b) The "read" time had to be greater than the maximum digital sampling interval, which is half of the period of the total BW, to avoid Nyquist ghosting. (c) The "read" time had to be much greater than the period of the phase modulating frequency to reduce noise power and avoid volume averaging by reducing spectral broadening from temporal truncation of the phase modulating field. (d) The echo time (TE) was limited by T2 attenuation where "read" time was twice the TE. (e) The repetition time (TR) had to be greater than 1500 ms to permit T1 relaxation. (f) The weaker gradient should be orthogonal to both the main magnetic field H_0 and the current flux to maximize shift. (g) The acquisition plane had to be parasagittal to include the plane of spin displacement. The SE sequence with minimum TE set by (d) above approaching spin density contrast was selected as a basic sequence for our experiments.

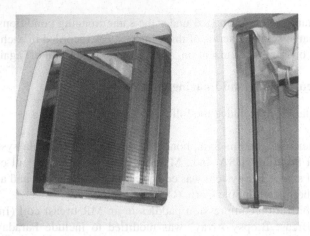

Fig. 3. Photograph of the stabilization/compression paddles of the MR breast coil. The left paddle of the coil was modified to include a Faraday shield made of a pair of copper sheets consisting of rectangular parallel bars. The copper sheets shown here were 14x15 cm. The phantoms were positioned between the two plates for imaging.

3   Results

Our pilot study focused on validating the theoretical frame of MREIM through simulation and phantom studies. The results from these tests are presented below.

3.1   Simulation

For the simulation study, a spin density image that has two concentric disks of different spin densities was considered. An example is shown in Fig. 4. Fig 4(a) shows a spin density image acquired with a spin density spin echo (SDSE) imaging sequence

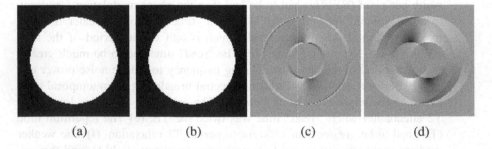

(a)   (b)   (c)   (d)

Fig. 4. Simulation results for an SDSE imaging process: (a) Image of a disk with no perturbation (current off) at a frequency resolution of 100 Hz/pixel; (b) Image of the disk with perturbation (current on – current density of 1 A/m²); (c) Difference image, i.e., difference between images (a) and (b) when driving frequency is 200 Hz; (d) Difference image when driving frequency is 1000 Hz

with no perturbation, i.e., no current, at frequency resolution (df) of 100 Hz/pixel. The difference in spin densities for outer and inner disk is considered to be very small; in this case it is one. This is the reason we don't see the disks well differentiated in the figures where there is no perturbation (current off). Fig 4(b) shows a simulation image when perturbation is applied, i.e., when the current is on; in this case the current density is 1 A/m^2. Fig 4(c) is the difference image between the current on/current off images when the driving frequency (Ω) is 200 Hz. Fig. 4(d) is the difference image when Ω is 1000 Hz. The drifting effect is greater when Ω is high with respect to the frequency resolution, e.g., Fig. 4(d). When Ω is too large the effect is lost and there is no signal.

3.2 Phantom Measurements

Our phantom tests showed that imaging with the soap with the soap/salt solution was unstable. This experiment yielded good results initially that were not reproducible and were extremely variable over time. Imaging with the agar phantom proved to be more stable and consistent. Representative SDSE images of the agar phantom are shown in Fig. 5 below. The desired signal under perturbation is observed in the difference images of Fig. 5 and it is in agreement with simulation and theory. One of the slices is shown here; similar results were obtained for other slices in the series.

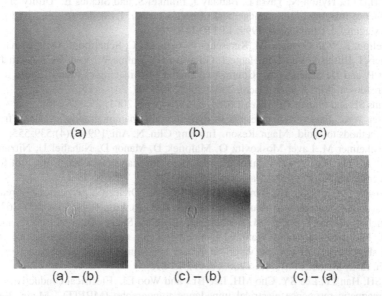

Fig. 5. Phantom image acquired with an SDSE sequence. Three images were acquired in the series: (a) Image of the phantom with current off, (b) Image of the phantom with current on, (c) Image of the phantom with current off. The second row shows the difference images, i.e., difference between images (a) and (b), (c) and (b), and (c) and (a). The first two images, i.e., (a)-(b) and (c)-(b) show the effect of the perturbation (current on) around the cancer surrogate. The aberration around the cancer surrogate is clearly seen in both images. This effect is not observed when the two "current off" images are subtracted.

4 Discussion and Conclusions

Our pilot study has confirmed the theoretical expectations for MREIM with promising and exciting results. The phantom data support our hypothesis that imaging of both the magnetic resonance and complex permittivity properties of the breast in the same clinical imaging configuration is possible. This has the potential of revolutionizing current magnetic resonance mammography practice because it does not require ionizing radiation, gadolinium contrast injection, or fat signal suppression.

This work has also identified major areas that need to be further explored and understood. Specifically, the type and quality of the phantom, the imaging sequence, and the experimental parameters play a defining role in the imaging process and, hence, the appearance or not of the signal of interest. The optimization of these elements is critical in further testing, validation, and clinical implementation of the proposed methodology.

References

1. Kaiser WA and Zeitler E. MR imaging of the breast: fast imaging sequences with and without Gd-DTPA. Preliminary observations. Radiology 1989; 170(3 Pt 1):681-686.
2. Esserman L, Hylton N, Yassa L, Barclay J, Frankel S, and Sickles E. Utility of magnetic resonance imaging in the management of breast cancer: Evidence for improved preoperative staging. J. Clin. Oncol. 1999; 17:110-119.
3. Schelfout K, Van Goethem M, Kersschot E, Colpaert C, Schelfhout AM, Leyman P, Verslegers I, Biltjes I, Van Den Haute J, Gillardin JP, Tjalma W, Van der Auwera JC, Buytaert P, and De Schepper A. Contrast-enhanced MR imaging of breast lesions and effect on treatment. Eur. J. Surg. Oncol. 2004; 30(5):501-507.
4. Harms SE and Flamig DP. Breast MRI. J. Clin. Imag. 2001; 25:227-246.
5. Kaiser WA. False-positive results in dynamic MR mammography. Causes, frequency, and methods to avoid. Magn. Reson. Imaging Clin. N. Am. 1994; 2(4):539-555.
6. Assenheimer M, Laver-Moskovitz O, Malonek D, Manor D, Nahaliel U, Nitzan R, and Saad A. The T-SCAN^{TM} technology: electrical impedance as a diagnostic tool for breast cancer detection. Physiol. Meas. 2001; 22:1-8.
7. Surowiec AJ, Stuchly SS, Barr JB, and Swarup A. Dielectric properties of breast carcinoma and the surrounding tissues. IEEE Trans. Biomed. Eng. 1988; 35(4):257-263.
8. Malich A, Bohm T, Facius M, Keinteich I, Fleck M, Sauner D, Anderson R, and Kaiser WA. Electrical impedance scanning as a new imaging modality in breast cancer detection – a short review of clinical value on breast application, limitations, and perspectives. Nucl. Instr. Methods Phys. Res. 2003; A497:75-81.
9. Oh SH, Han JY, Lee SY, Cho MH, Lee BL, and Woo EJ. Electrical conductivity imaging by magnetic resonance electrical impedance tomography (MREIT). Magn. Res. Med. 2003; 50:875-878.
10. Malich A, Bohm T, Facius M, Freesmeyer MG, Fleck M, Anderson R, and Kaiser WA. Differentiation of mammographically suspicious lesions: Evaluation of breast ultrasound, MRI mammography, and electrical impedance scanning as adjunctive technologies in breast cancer detection. Clin. Radiology 2001; 56:278-283.

Experimental Investigation of the Necessity for Extra Flat Field Corrections in Quality Control of Digital Mammography

Paula Pöyry[1], Federica Zanca[2], and Hilde Bosmans[2]

[1] Radiation and Nuclear Safety Authority - STUK, P.O. Box 14, FI-00881 Helsinki, Finland
paula.poyry@stuk.fi
[2] Leuven University Centre of Medical Physics in Radiology, Department of Radiology, University Hospitals, 3000 Leuven, Belgium
federica.zanca@uz.kuleuven.ac.be,
hilde.bosmans@uz.kuleuven.ac.be

Abstract. The purpose of this work was to investigate whether extra flat field corrections should be applied prior to the calculations of quality control quantities and whether there are necessary precautions regarding flat fielding in digital mammography. Effects from using one standard flat field correction for all imaging situations or absence of correction procedures were examined using homogenous PMMA slabs. Differences in field profiles for various exposure geometries and breast thicknesses were quantified. For three systems the maximal deviation of averaged pixel values (along a profile of ROIs parallel to the chest wall) varied from 1.3 % to 6.8 % over the whole image and from 0.6 % to 2.6 % if the analysis is limited to the central part. Extra flat field corrections are not necessary for most applications. If required, the corrections should be performed from images acquired with the same manual exposure and not after a time gap.

1 Introduction

In digital mammography, the degree of inhomogeneity in an image or changes in (average) pixel values over time depend on the characteristics of the x-ray tube, beam geometry, detector and the built-in correction algorithms [1, 2]. They are usually evaluated from images acquired from homogeneous slabs of material, the "flat field images". To reduce inhomogeneity in practice, direct radiography systems are being recalibrated with system-specific procedures on a routine basis.

While the remaining inhomogeneities after the calibration and any other time dependent variation may look acceptable in patient images, they may not be negligible for particular quality control studies (like calculation of contrast to noise ratio) or quantitative measurements that rely on pixel values or signal to noise ratios in series of successive images. For accurate measurements of these quantities, it has to be questioned whether these images should be made more homogenous or reproducible with additional correction procedures (such as, e.g "flat field corrections"). As we did not find (in the literature) any clear guidance on the necessity and requirements regarding such corrections, we performed a specific analysis for three digital mammography systems.

Susan M. Astley et al. (Eds.): IWDM 2006, LNCS 4046, pp. 475–481, 2006.
© Springer-Verlag Berlin Heidelberg 2006

The main questions addressed in this study were: How large are variations in mean pixel values for images acquired under conditions close to the vendor-specific calibration procedure and for other combinations of test object thicknesses and beam qualities? How reproducible are the profiles of mean pixel values in repeated series of images?

2 Materials and Methods

The study was performed on 3 digital mammography systems:

1. Siemens Novation DR (Erlangen, Germany). The detector is based on amorphous selenium technology and has a pixel size of 70 µm (image size 3328 × 4096 pixels). The system can be used with a Molybdenum (Mo) anode and a Mo filter (thickness 30 µm) or a Rhodium (Rh) filter (thickness 25 µm), or with a tungsten (W) anode with a Rh filter (thickness 50 µm).
2. Agfa DM1000 (Mortsel, Belgium). The detector is similar to the one of the Siemens Novation, but an x-ray tube of Lorad is used. The x-ray system has a Mo anode which can be used with a Mo filter (thickness 30 µm) or a Rh filter (thickness 25 µm).
3. Agfa CR MM3.0 phosphor plate with Agfa CR 85-X digitizer (Mortsel, Belgium), in combination with a Lorad Platinum IV mammographic unit. The detector has a pixel size of 50 µm (image size 3328 × 4096 pixels). The x-ray system is similar to the system used with the DM1000.

Flat field images were acquired from sets of homogenous PMMA (polymer-thylmethacrylate) slabs with a thickness of 1 cm each. Different exposure settings were used as explained in the paragraphs below. Raw images were exported to an off-line computer for analysis with ImageJ [3]. The same analysis was performed for all the images: the mean pixel values were calculated in square ROIs (2 cm × 2 cm), with a center to center distance of 100 pixels. We illustrate the quantitative analyses along two profiles (a profile parallel to the chest wall and 6 cm from the chest wall and a second profile perpendicular to the chest wall and centered in the image). The maximum deviations of these mean pixel values were calculated for all ROIs along a profile in the whole image and in the central part (50 % of the complete profile). Relative pixel values were calculated by dividing the mean pixel values by the mean pixel value from the ROI in the middle of the profile. For some comparisons, we normalized the measurement distances such that corresponding physical points coincide in the graph.

A preliminary experiment was performed on the Siemens Novation system: flat field images obtained under the calibration conditions (4 cm of PMMA is to be attached to the tube) [4] and the clinically used geometry, 4 cm of PMMA on top of the detector (with and without compression paddle in the beam), were compared.

2.1 Differences in Flat Field Images Acquired with Different PMMA Thicknesses and Beam Qualities

The effect of various PMMA thicknesses were examined from images of 2 cm, 4 cm, and 7 cm of PMMA using the clinically used anode/filter combinations and a tube voltage of 28 kV. In addition, with the Siemens Novation system the effect of radiation quality was tested using very low and high tube voltages (23 kV and 35 kV) and all three anode/filter combinations. The automatic exposure controller (AEC) was used to obtain clinically relevant tube current time products.

2.2 Reproducibility of Flat Fields from Repeated Images

Reproducibility was studied using manual settings. Images were performed with 4 cm of PMMA and the clinically used anode/filter combination and tube voltage. A tube loading close to typical values obtained in AEC mode was chosen. For the CR system, the same CR plate was always used.

3 Results

Figure 1 shows pixel value profiles parallel to the chest wall for the condition used during the standard calibration procedure and a clinical setting with and without compression paddle (CP). The maximal variation in mean pixel value in the flat field images acquired similarly as during the calibration is 1 %. It increases up to 3.5 % for the clinical setting (when PMMA is used on top of the detector, with compression paddle).

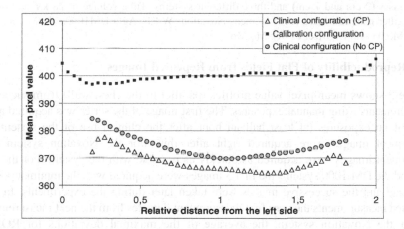

Fig. 1. Profiles measured parallel to the chest wall from the flat field images (W/Rh anode/ filter, 28 kV, 71 mAs) in calibration and clinical configurations (with and without compression paddle (CP))

3.1 Differences in Flat Field Images Acquired with Different PMMA Thicknesses and Beam Qualities

In Figure 2, mean pixel value profiles for 2 cm and 7 cm of PMMA thickness are shown for the 3 systems. In Table 1, maximal variations between values in the mean pixel value profiles are calculated for three different systems and PMMA thicknesses (2 cm, 4 cm and 7 cm). Variations are calculated for the complete profile and for the central part of it (50 %), both for profiles parallel to the chest wall and perpendicular to it.

For the Siemens Novation, system deviations in relative pixel values for different beam qualities were in average 1 %.

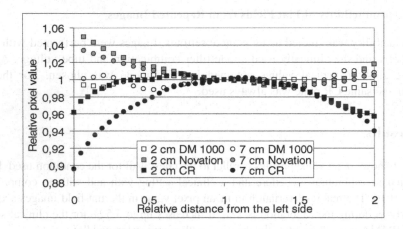

Fig. 2. Profiles measured parallel to the chest wall in flat field images for different PMMA thicknesses (2 cm and 7 cm) and three different systems. Tube voltage of 28 kV and clinical anode/filter materials were used: Siemens Novation: W/Rh, Agfa DM1000: Mo/Mo and Agfa CR MM3.0 (with Digitizer 85-X): Mo/Mo.

3.2 Reproducibility of Flat Fields from Repeated Images

Figure 3 shows mean pixel value profiles (parallel to the chest wall) from successive measurements using manual exposures. The first image of the series was acquired after a time of no exposures (at least half an hour after the clinical use of the system) and subsequent images were acquired right after this. For the Novation system all 5 subsequent images were acquired as quickly as possible with the system. For the Agfa CR and the DM 1000 systems the first 3 images were acquired with the minimal possible time gap and the successive images were taken later during the experiments. In these repeated measurements the very first measurement deviates from the next measurements.

For the Novation system, the average of the maximal deviations for ROIs on corresponding positions in 6 different exposures is 2.7 %. Taking into account only images 2 – 6, this deviation is only 0.7 %. This effect was seen in a repeated experiment on day 2 as well, and the numbers were 3.2 % and 1.0 %, respectively. The analysis of similar series of images acquired during all the tests on the same system showed occasionally sudden and more deviating profiles (this had been the ultimate trigger for this study).

Variations for values in repeated images for the DM 1000 and CR systems are bigger than for the Novation system. The average of maximal deviations for the same ROIs in 7 different exposures is 4.7 % for the DM 1000 and 5.8 % for the CR.

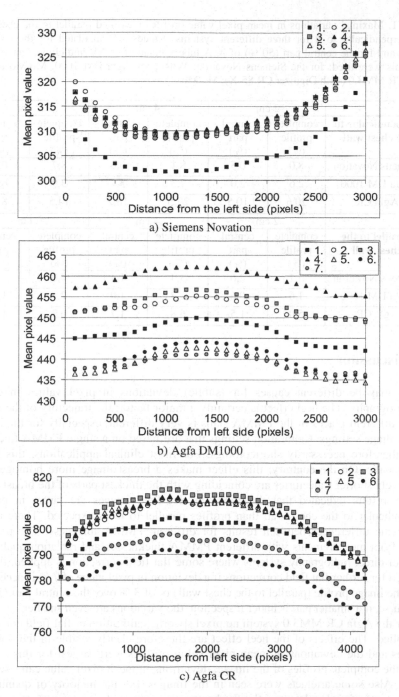

a) Siemens Novation

b) Agfa DM1000

c) Agfa CR

Fig. 3. a-c Profiles measured parallel to the chest wall from repeated flat field images of 4 cm PMMA. (a) Siemens Novation system: W/Rh anode/filter, 27 kV and 71 mAs (b) Agfa DM1000: Mo/Mo anode/filter, 28 kV and 65 mAs, (c) Agfa CR MM3.0 with Digitizer 85-X: Mo/Mo anode/filter, 25 kV and 64 mAs.

Table 1. Maximal variations in mean pixel value profiles measured parallel to the chest wall and perpendicular to it for three different systems. Values are calculated for the complete profile and for the central part (50 %) of it. A tube voltage of 28 kV and clinical anode/filter materials were used: for the Siemens Novation; W/Rh, for Agfa DM 1000; Mo/Mo and for Agfa CR MM3.0 (with Digitizer CR 85-X); Mo/Mo.

	2 cm		4 cm		7 cm	
Perpendicular to the chest wall	complete profile (%)	central part (%)	complete profile (%)	Central part (%)	complete profile (%)	central part (%)
Siemens Novation	8,0	0,5	8,1	0,6	8,7	0,7
Agfa DM 1000	2,6	2,0	7,3	3,7	3,9	0,4
Agfa CR	20,6	10,5	29,5	18,7	14,5	8,1
	2 cm		4 cm		7 cm	
Parallel to the chest wall	complete profile (%)	central part (%)	complete profile (%)	central part (%)	complete profile (%)	central part (%)
Siemens Novation	5,7	2,6	3,4	1,4	4,0	1,9
Agfa DM 1000	1,6	0,6	1,3	1,0	2,1	1,2
Agfa CR	5,0	1,5	6,8	1,7	6,3	1,8

4 Discussion

There may be different causes for (subtle) deviations in pixel values in digital mammography. The heel effect is certainly a major factor: the trajectory of the x-rays in the different places of the PMMA slabs is very different, especially for the lowest tube voltage settings. Calibration settings that are based on a single PMMA thickness have therefore necessarily shortcomings. For most clinical applications, this is not problematic. On the contrary: this effect makes a breast image more homogeneous (relatively shorter trajectories are coinciding with the thickest parts of the breast).

Our results indicated that deviations in flat field images are larger in profiles perpendicular to the chest wall than profiles parallel to it, as expected. There are no systematic differences between results for different PMMA thickness. The practical result from measurements with different PMMA thicknesses and radiation qualities is that, for direct radiography systems where some flat field correction is applied, there is no need for further flat field corrections if a deviation in pixel value of 7 % is acceptable over the image profile (parallel to the chest wall) or of 3 % over the central part (50 %). Of course, if a smaller part is under inspection, the variations are even smaller.

For the Agfa CR MM3.0 system no pixel specific calibration or flat field correction is applied. The effects of the heel effect are therefore clearly visible in the flat field images and the deviations in mean pixel value profiles were largest for this system. Over the complete profiles of the image, deviations in mean pixel value can rise up to 30 %. Also some artefacts were seen in the images. For the majority of quantitative assessments of such a detector, flat field corrections should be performed.

A surprising result was the deviating line profile for the first measurement of a series of flat images as compared to successive images for all detectors (a-Se detectors and CR plates). It remains to be investigated whether this effect is due to the digital detectors or the x-ray tube. In practice, a similar effect can be expected if there is just a different time window between exposures. This fact has to be considered during acceptance tests of the equipment where measurements of different images may have to be compared; other applications that combine pixel values from successive images (such as contrast enhanced mammography) may be influenced as well.

Deviations in repeated images means in practice that for contrast-to-noise calculations of these detectors, pixel values for different inserts in contrast-to-noise measurements should be taken from the same image (and preferably from the central area of the image). An extra flat field correction could be performed with an appropriate reference image (manual exposures fully incorporated in the measurement series, i.e. without any time gaps). In the majority of cases, the improvements will be very limited.

One limitation of this work is that we have no reproducibility data from many time points. It is possible that present observations are not fully representative for the system. In addition, we did not study the homogeneity of the standard deviations (noise) in full detail. Preliminary results showed that these effects are even smaller than the effects on pixel value. Another limitation of this study is that it should be performed on more systems of the same vendor and on systems from more other vendors.

We did not have the attempt to judge the performance of the routine flat field calibration for the clinical images.

5 Conclusions

For most applications, it is not necessary to perform an extra flat field correction. If requirements are very demanding extra correction can be considered. For the a-Se detectors, the flat field image should be acquired during the same imaging session, using the same beam quality and PMMA thickness. For the CR image, flat filed corrections are more indicated. For all systems, the very first image after a long period of down time of the system should not be used.

References

1. Handbook of Medical Imaging, Vol 1. Physics and Psychophysics, Edited by Beutel, J. et. al (SPIE, Bellingham, WA, 2000)
2. Saunders, R. S. Jr., Samei, E., Jesneck, J. L., Lo, J. L.: Physical characterization of a prototype selenium-based full field digital mammography detector. Med. Phys. Vol. 32, (2005) 588–599
3. Abramoff, M. D., Magelhaes, P.J., Ram, S.J.: Image processing with ImageJ. Biophotonics International, Vol. 11, (2004) 36–42
4. Mammomat Novation DR Users Manual, Siemens AG (2005)

Observer Evaluations of Wavelet Methods for the Enhancement and Compression of Digitized Mammograms

Maria Kallergi[1], John J. Heine[1], and Bradley J. Lucier[2]

[1] H. Lee Moffitt Cancer Center & Research Institute, Cancer Control and Prevention, 12902 Magnolia Drive, Tampa, Florida, USA, 33620
{kallergi, heinejj}@moffitt.usf.edu
[2] Department of Mathematics, Purdue University, West Lafayette, IN
Lucier@purdue.edu

Abstract. Two observer experiments were performed to evaluate the performance of wavelet enhancement and compression methodologies for digitized mammography. One experiment was based on the localization response operating characteristic (LROC) model. The other estimated detection and localization accuracy rates. The results of both studies showed that the two algorithms consistently improved radiologists' performance although not always in a statistically significant way. An important outcome of this work was that lossy wavelet compression was as successful in improving the quality of digitized mammograms as the wavelet enhancement technique. The compression algorithm not only did not degrade the readers' performance but it improved it consistently while achieving compression rates in the range of 14 to 2051:1. The proposed wavelet algorithms yielded superior results for digitized mammography relative to conventional processing methodologies. Wavelets are valuable and diverse tools that could make digitized screen/film mammography equivalent to its direct digital counterpart leading to a filmless mammography clinic with full inter- and intra-system integration and real-time telemammography.

1 Introduction

Wavelets have found several applications in medical imaging including mammography. Applications range from image compression to image enhancement, feature extraction and segmentation to image reconstruction.[1] Depending on the selected type of wavelet, the outcome even within the same application may be dramatically different. In addition, a single wavelet processing may yield multiple effects, e.g., enhancement and compression, enhancement and segmentation.

We have experimented with several wavelet methods for a variety of processes of digitized and digital mammograms.[2],[3],[4],[5],[6],[7]. In this paper, we will report the results from the wavelet-based enhancement [8] and compression [9] of the same set of digitized mammograms that were evaluated by the same radiologists in similar experiments. The results, significant on their own, are analyzed here simultaneously to obtain a better understanding of the effect of the wavelet analysis on the images as well as the observer.

Susan M. Astley et al. (Eds.): IWDM 2006, LNCS 4046, pp. 482–489, 2006.
© Springer-Verlag Berlin Heidelberg 2006

The work presented here is based on high-resolution digitized mammograms as opposed to direct digital mammograms. The reason for this lies in our past efforts and deep interest to find ways to integrate screen/film (SFM) with full field digital mammography (FFDM), a process that is currently facing serious impediments due to the advent of FFDM and the shift of interest, not unjustifiably, to the latter. However, film mammography is the current standard of practice worldwide with a major share in the international system market. Furthermore, mammography can no longer stay outside the filmless radiology department. Hence, methodologies that provide solutions to a filmless SFM are urgently needed.

2 Materials and Methods

2.1 Wavelet Enhancement Method

The purpose of enhancing digitized mammograms was to obtain high quality images that could be used for primary diagnosis from computer monitors (softcopy display and interpretation). For this application, we used multiresolution statistical analysis [4],[10] based on the orthogonal wavelet expansion of the original images and Fourier spectral characterization.[5] The 12-coefficient wavelet basis was used that is nearly symmetric with the mother wavelet having a large, almost symmetric, center lobe that resembles to some degree to the profile of the average calcification. More details of the method are given in Ref. [8].

2.2 Wavelet Compression Method

The images in this application were decomposed using a biorthogonal wavelet decomposition. Specifically, we used the biorthogonal, fifth-order accurate wavelets with piecewise constant duals of Cohen, Daubechies, and Feauveau, found on page 272 of Ref. [11]. The fifth-order wavelet was used for compression because it was found to give measurably smaller RMS errors at the same compression rates that the lower order wavelets. More details of the method are given in Ref. [9].

2.3 Evaluation Experiments

Two evaluation studies were performed for the two methodologies. First, a localization response operating characteristic (LROC) experiment was conducted. The LROC evaluation involved both signal likelihood and signal location tasks that, theoretically, offer a more complete analysis of observer performance. The LROC test was followed by a localization experiment that resembled the multiple alternative forced choice (MAFC) setup.[12] The results of both LROC evaluations are reported in detail elsewhere [8],[9] and will be briefly summarized here. The second evaluation test is the focus of this work.

The same database and readers were used for all tests. The set consisted of 500 single view mammograms, 250 of which were negative, 131 benign, and 119 cancer cases. A total of 375 findings were present in the benign and cancer cases, 182 of which were masses (98 benign and 84 cancer) and 193 calcification clusters (100 benign and 93 cancer). Negative cases were selected from negative mammograms with at least two years of negative follow-up. Negative views matched the abnormal ones (benign or malignant) in terms of breast parenchymal density and size. Films were digitized at 30 μm and 16 bits per pixel with an ImageClear R3000 scanner (DBA Inc., Melbourne, FL).

All digital images were reviewed on one or two high-resolution DR 110 monitors (Data-Ray Corp., Westminster, CO) with Md5/SBX boards (Dome, Waltham, MA) in an Ultra Sparc 2 workstation (Sun Microsystems, Santa Clara, CA). Each DR110 monitor provided a 2048×2560 pixel display with an 8-bit digital to analog (DAC) converter.

In the LROC studies, the 500 single-view mammograms were reviewed one at a time in three different formats (original, enhanced, compressed) randomly mixed by three expert mammographers. The observers reported the x,y coordinates of a detected lesion and rated the suspiciousness for each detected lesion and the overall view using a custom-made user interface.

In the localization experiment, the 250 abnormal images were matched with the 250 negative images in terms of size and breast density and presented in left/right pairs in three formats (original, enhanced, compressed) randomly mixed to the observers, who compared the two views, selected the suspicious one, and localized and rated abnormal finding(s) similar to the LROC test. As mentioned earlier, this setup is similar to the MAFC but it is not a true MAFC experiment because it involves many targets in different backgrounds. Nevertheless, our goal for this test was to determine the ability of the readers to identify the abnormal view from a pair, compare the result to LROC, and perform another relative comparison of the wavelet methodologies.

Our studies were approved by the institutional review board as a research study using existing medical records and exempted from individual patient consent requirements. The patient identifiers were obliterated from all images.

2.4 Data Analysis

First, the x,y coordinates selected by the readers from both tests were compared to a ground truth file to determine the number of correct and incorrect localizations. A finding was considered as a hit or correct localization, if its x,y coordinates were within ±200 pixels of those listed in the truth file. If the difference was greater than 200 pixels then the finding was considered as an incorrect localization or a miss.

The LROC program, version of 1998, was applied to the LROC data.[13] ROC and LROC fitted curves were generated in this case including estimates of the areas under these curves and their standard errors. Two performance indices were primarily considered and compared: the detection accuracy, which corresponds to the area under the ROC curve (A_{ROC}), and the localization accuracy (P_{CL}), which corresponds to the ordinate of the LROC curves.[8], [9]

For the localization experiment, performance was determined by analyzing the selections of the observers in terms of both lesions and views. Rates for "lesion hits", "lesion misses", "view hits", and "view misses" were estimated based on the correct and incorrect view selections and lesion localizations as follows: (a) the "lesion hit" rate, defined as the fraction of correctly identified abnormal views with at least one lesion correctly localized, (b) the "lesion miss" rate, defined as the fraction of correctly identified abnormal views but with none of the lesions correctly localized, (c) the "view miss" rate, defined as the fraction of negative images that were incorrectly selected as the abnormal ones. Note that the "view hit" rate, i.e., the fraction of abnormal images (benign or malignant) that were correctly selected as abnormal independent of whether the true lesion(s) was correctly localized can be determined as 1-"view miss" rate. In addition to the overall accuracy in lesion localization, the hits and misses of the observers were analyzed in terms of pathology (benign/malignant) and type of lesion (calcification cluster/mass).

3 Results

3.1 LROC Performance Indices

The results of the two that for these plots and calculations, we combined the benign and cancer cases LROC studies have been already analyzed and reported independently elsewhere.[8], [9] Figure 1 shows the ROC and LROC curves for all three readings modes, i.e, original, enhanced, and compressed mammograms for one of the three readers. Similar results were obtained from the other readers.

Tables 1-3 list the performance indices for all observers and for the three reading modes. Performance indices include the area under the ROC curve (A_z) and its standard error (SE), the area under the LROC curve, the localization accuracy (P(CL)) and its standard error. Note in one group, labeled "abnormal", and compared them to the negatives cases, "normal" group. This is different from what was previously published and focuses more on the detection than the diagnostic aspect of the studies.

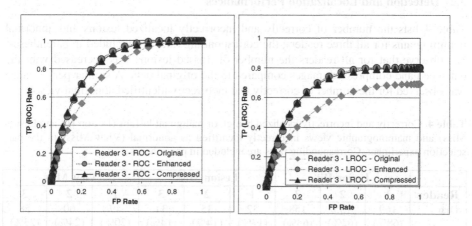

Fig. 1. Graphs for Reader 3 show fitted (a) ROC and (b) LROC curves obtained from the interpretation of original, enhanced, and compressed mammograms from patients with no findings (negative) versus mammograms from patients with benign or malignant findings. The performance indices of this reader are listed in Table 3.

Table 1. Performance indices obtained from the LROC analysis of the original data

Reader	ROC			LROC	
	A_z	SE	Area	P(CL)	SE (P(CL))
1	0.8013	0.0137	0.6027	0.7357	0.0224
2	0.7749	0.0137	0.5497	0.6964	0.0232
3	0.7718	0.0142	0.5435	0.6914	0.0249

Table 2. Performance indices obtained from the LROC analysis of the enhanced data. An average of 11% improvement was observed in localization accuracy with the enhanced images.

Reader	ROC			LROC	
	A_z	SE	Area	P(CL)	SE (P(CL))
1	0.8490	0.0128	0.6980	0.8064	0.0196
2	0.8081	0.0133	0.6163	0.7589	0.0201
3	0.8366	0.0131	0.6732	0.8016	0.0190

Table 3. Performance indices obtained from the LROC analysis of the compressed data. An average of 12% improvement was observed in localization accuracy with the compressed reconstructed images.

Reader	ROC			LROC	
	A_z	SE	Area	P(CL)	SE (P(CL))
1	0.8510	0.0128	0.7019	0.8092	0.0195
2	0.8164	0.0132	0.6328	0.7673	0.0200
3	0.8370	0.0132	0.6739	0.7971	0.0198

3.2 Detection and Localization Performances

Table 4 lists the number of correctly and incorrectly localized lesions and abnormal mammograms for all three readers; the corresponding rates are included in parentheses. We observe that for all readers the number of missed lesions was decreased with the enhanced and compressed images compared to the original data. A similar performance was observed for the number of correctly and incorrectly identified abnormal views.

Table 4. Correctly and incorrectly localized benign or malignant lesions (Lesion Hit and Lesion Miss) and mammographic views incorrectly identified as abnormal (View Miss) in the pair selection experiment. Corresponding rates are included in parentheses.

	Lesion Hit			Lesion Miss			View Miss		
Reader	1	2	3	1	2	3	1	2	3
Org	169 (68%)	155 (62%)	158 (63%)	32 (13%)	35 (14%)	34 (14%)	49 (20%)	60 (24%)	58 (23%)
Enh	197 (79%)	174 (70%)	186 (74%)	29 (12%)	39 (16%)	32 (13%)	24 (10%)	37 (15%)	32 (13%)
Comp	191 (76%)	182 (73%)	199 (80%)	21 (8%)	41 (16%)	28 (11%)	38 (15%)	27 (11%)	23 (9%)

Tables 5 and 6 break down the performance of each reader for the various types of abnormalities that were present in the mammograms, i.e., calcification clusters and masses, and pathology, i.e., benign and cancer. Both results indicate that all readers improved their localization performance with the enhanced and compressed reconstructed images. However, few differences were statistically significant.

Table 5. Number of correctly localized benign and malignant calcification clusters by each reader. Corresponding rates are included in parenheses. Note that the 250 abnormal mammographic views included a total of 193 calcification clusters (100 benign and 93 cancer).

	Calcification Clusters					
	Benign			Cancer		
Reader	1	2	3	1	2	3
Org	44 (44%)	43 (43%)	39 (39%)	44 (47%)	44 (47%)	50 (54%)
Enh	57 (57%)	48 (48%)	50 (50%)	52 (56%)	45 (48%)	52 (56%)
Comp	55 (55%)	50 (50%)	55 (55%)	48 (52%)	50 (54%)	50 (54%)

Table 6. Number of correctly localized benign and malignant masses by each reader. Corresponding rates are included in parenheses. Note that the 250 abnormal mammographic views included a total of 182 masses (98 benign and 84 cancer).

	Masses					
	Benign			Cancer		
Reader	1	2	3	1	2	3
Org	45 (46%)	36 (37%)	32 (33%)	36 (43%)	32 (38%)	37 (44%)
Enh	51 (52%)	44 (45%)	42 (43%)	37 (44%)	37 (44%)	40 (48%)
Comp	49 (50%)	48 (49%)	49 (50%)	39 (46%)	34 (35%)	45 (54%)

4 Discussion and Conclusions

Our current work focuses on issues related to the seamless integration of SFM and FFDM. This integration is seriously hindered by the lack of advanced tools and systems for the former and the significant delay in the development of such tools relative to FFDM that receives most of the attention. However, SFM is the current standard of clinical practice with millions of examinations performed worldwide. It is expected that digital will replace film in the future. Until then, however, film-based mammography clinics cannot afford to stay outside a filmless radiology department. Finding a solution to their integration should be an immediate priority.

The results of the two observer studies led to several interesting conclusions: (i) Our wavelet enhancement approach could significantly improve the detection of abnormalities in digitized softcopy mammography. The technique offers a robust and generally applicable approach independent of film digitization conditions or digitizer. Results could be further improved by modifying the algorithm to address challenging cases such as the mammograms of low breast density where the digital image quality is usually low or to better match the display medium characteristics. (ii) Our lossy wavelet compression method yielded high compression rates without compromising diagnostic performance. The mean compression rate was 59:1 for the negative mammograms, 56:1 for the benign images, and 53:1 for the cancers.[9] Such high compression rates without visual losses, and hence, without losses in diagnostic power, could offer effective solutions to the problems of display, transfer, and storage of digitized, and possibly digital mammograms. (iii) The localization experiments are valuable in understanding the observer performance. The results of both tests indicate that the true lesions are not always accurately localized by the readers and critical signals are often missed or mispositioned. Most of the benign findings are easily and automatically discarded in the review process while detection of either benign or malignant lesions is seriously limited when a single view or limited information is presented. This has a major impact on the design of validation experiments and the selection of validation methodologies.

In conclusion, the experiments presented here supported our hypothesis that wavelets hold significant advantages for digitized mammography and could bridge the gap between digitized and direct digital mammography, thus facilitating the integration of film and filmless departments. Wavelet enhancement could support softcopy reading of digitized mammograms while wavelet compression could yield visually lossless, high-rate compression of the digitized films to facilitate storage and transmission. Interestingly, the two effects may be achieved through the same algorithm as suggested by our wavelet compression technique that showed improved tumor localization similar to the enhancement process.

References

1. IEEE Trans. Med. Imaging, Special Issue on Wavelets in Medical Imaging. Unser M, Alroubi A, and Laine A. (Eds.), 2003.
2. Kallergi M, Clarke LP, Qian W, et al. Interpretation of calcifications in screen/film, digitized, and wavelet-enhanced, monitor displayed mammograms: an ROC study. *Acad Radiol* 1996;3:285-293
3. Qian W, Clarke LP, Kallergi M, Clark RA. Tree structured nonlinear filters in digital mammography. *IEEE Trans Med Imaging* 1994;13:25-36
4. Heine JJ, Kallergi M, Chetelat SM, Clarke LP. Multiresolution wavelet approach for separating the breast region from the background in high resolution digital mammography. In: Karssemeijer N, Thijssen M, Hendricks J, van Erning L, eds. *Digital Mammography: proceedings of the 4th international workshop on digital mammography*. The Netherlands, Kluwer, 1998:295-298
5. Heine JJ, Velthuizen RP. A statistical methodology for mammographic density detection. *Med Phys* 2000;27:2644-2651
6. Lucier BJ, Kallergi M, Qian W, et al. Wavelet compression and segmentation of mammographic images. J Digit Imaging 1994; 7(1):27-38.
7. Yang Z, Kallergi M, DeVore R, et al. The effect of wavelet bases on the compression of digital mammograms. IEEE Eng Med Biol 1995; 14(5):570-577.
8. Kallergi M, Heine JJ, Berman CG, Hersh MR, Romilly AP, and Clark RA. Improved interpretation of digitized mammography with wavelet processing: A localization response operating characteristic study. AJR 2004; 182:697-703.
9. Kallergi M, Lucier BJ, Berman CG, Hersh MR, Kim JJ, Szabunio MS, and Clark RA. High-Performance Wavelet Compression for Mammography: Localization Response Operating Characteristic Evaluation. Radiology 2006; 238:62-73.

10. Heine JJ, Deans SR, Cullers DK, Stauduhar R, Clarke LP. Multiresolution statistical analysis of high resolution digital mammograms. *IEEE Trans Med Imaging* 1997;16:503-515
11. Daubechies I. Ten Lectures on Wavelets. SIAM, Philadelphia, 1992.
12. Burgess AE. Comparison of receiver operating characteristic and forced choice observer performance measurement methods. Med. Phys. 1995; 22(5):643-655.
13. Swensson RG. Unified measurement of observer performance in detecting and localizing target objects on images. *Med Phys* 1996;23:1709-1725.

Evaluating the Effect of Dose on Reconstructed Image Quality in Digital Tomosynthesis

Michael P. Kempston[1], James G. Mainprize[1], and Martin J. Yaffe[1,2]

[1] Imaging Research, Sunnybrook Health Sciences Centre, 2075 Bayview Ave, Toronto, Ontario, Canada, M4N 3M5
[2] Department of Medical Biophysics, University of Toronto, Toronto, Canada

Abstract. Breast tomosynthesis has the potential to improve lesion visibility and localization compared to conventional mammography. To be clinically useful, tomosynthesis must be able to achieve high image quality at acceptable radiation doses. Tomosynthesis data sets of simple low-contrast phantoms were acquired at varying dose levels. Image quality in the reconstructed volumes was analyzed by evaluating the voxel-to-voxel signal difference to noise ratio between a simulated lesion and the surrounding "tissue". Preliminary results indicate that image quality of small lesions is limited by scatter and reconstruction artifacts. In uniform backgrounds image quality appears to be quantum-noise limited, while in more complex backgrounds the structural noise tends to dominate.

1 Introduction

Tomosynthesis is a limited-angle cone-beam CT technique that has been proposed for breast imaging, as it can potentially improve lesion visibility and localization [1, 2]. By providing tomographic images, it has the potential to improve conspicuity of lesions by reducing the problem in projection mammography of superposition of structures from the volume of the breast onto a two-dimensional image. Superposition is also frequently responsible for creating false positive results – the appearance of lesions that do not actually exist. This reduces the specificity of mammography. Our goal is to optimize breast tomosynthesis to provide improved conspicuity without delivering an unacceptably high radiation dose to the breast.

The purpose of this study is to examine image quality in reconstructed volumes under various radiation exposure schemes. This paper will discuss the development and implementation of two imaging phantoms: one with a uniform background and one with a complex background. Image quality measurements are presented as a function of radiation dose for a number of different lesion sizes.

2 Method

Tomosynthesis image acquisition was performed on a custom-built, cone-beam imaging system. Image quality was measured in terms of voxel-to-voxel signal-difference to noise ratio (SDNR) for the reconstructed volume datasets.

Susan M. Astley et al. (Eds.): IWDM 2006, LNCS 4046, pp. 490–497, 2006.

2.1 Phantom Preparation

Two imaging phantoms were designed to represent low-contrast spherical lesions in a uniform fatty background and a non-uniform, structured background. In both phantoms, the lesions were modeled using acetate beads of various diameters. The first phantom, hereafter referred to as the uniform phantom, had a background composed entirely of pure lard encased in a 9 cm diameter thin-walled cylindrical Lexan® polycarbonate container. A total of 7 beads (1.5, 2, 4, 6, 8, 10, and 12 mm) were incorporated into the uniform phantom.

The second phantom, hereafter referred to as the complex phantom, used a large sea sponge immersed in corn oil to provide a breast-realistic structured background. A total of 6 beads (1.5, 2, 4, 6, 8, and 10 mm) were embedded in the sponge, and the entire contents were encased in a 7.5 cm diameter cylindrical container of the same material as the uniform phantom.

2.2 Image Acquisition and Reconstruction

Projection images for tomosynthesis reconstruction were acquired on a custom-built tabletop system consisting of a mammographic x-ray tube (GE DMR v. 2, GE Healthcare, Milwaukee, WI) and a flat-panel imager (GE Senographe 2000D). The source-detector distance was set to 66 cm, and the phantoms were mounted such that they contacted the face of the detector. All acquisitions consisted of 11 projection images acquired at an interval of 4° using a 28kV spectrum with a rhodium anode and filter combination as well as an additional 0.4 mm of aluminum filtration. Separate image sets were acquired under several dose scenarios representing total entrance exposures ranging from 0.27 R to 0.86 R for the uniform phantom, and 0.26 R to 2.1 R for the complex phantom.

Once acquired, the images were corrected for gain and offset variations and down-sampled from a pixel resolution of 100 μm to 200 μm to facilitate reconstruction. Reconstructions were performed using a simultaneous algebraic reconstruction technique (SART) algorithm [4], implemented using software developed by our group. Reconstructed voxels were set to $200 \times 200 \times 1000$ μm^3.

Standard mammography images of both phantoms were also acquired on a Senographe 2000D (GE Healthcare) digital mammography system using the automatic optimization of parameters (AOP) setting, in which the system automatically determines the appropriate anode, filter material, kV, and mAs. For the uniform phantom, the AOP chose a Rh/Rh anode and filter, 30 kV and 97 mAs, yielding an entrance exposure of 1.2 R. For the complex phantom, the AOP chose a Rh/Rh, 29 kV and 72 mAs that produced an entrance exposure of 0.82 R.

2.3 Image Analysis

Images were obtained from the reconstructed volumes by selecting a slice parallel to the central imaging plane and through the centre of the appropriate acetate bead.

Three regions of interest (ROIs) were then selected, a principal lesion ROI and two background ROIs (a coaxial ROI located along the axis of rotation, and an off-axis ROI, located adjacent to the axis of rotation), as shown in Fig. 1. Slice images and ROIs are in identical positions for all data sets. Image quality was determined by calculating the SDNR as follows:

$$SDNR = \frac{S - S_B}{\sqrt{\sigma^2 + \sigma_B^2}},$$

(1)

where S and S_B are the pixel grey-level intensities of the lesion and background ROIs respectively and σ, σ_B are the standard deviations in these two signals. Often SDNR is defined as $(S-S_B)/\sigma_B$, however this assumes that noise is uniform in an image. In tomosynthesis slice images, the noise is expected to be non-uniform and, as such, the simpler definition of SDNR is not suitable here.

Estimates of error in SDNR values were obtained by dividing each ROI into 8 separate regions and performing the mean and standard-deviation calculations for each sub-ROI. The standard error was calculated in these sub-regions and was used as an estimate of overall measurement error.

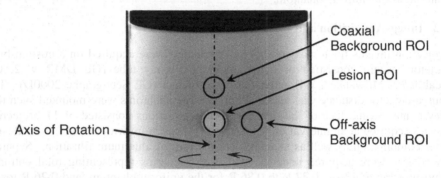

Fig. 1. Sketch of the regions of interest (ROI) placement overlaying a typical slice image

3   Results

Sample projection images and examples of reconstructed slices for the uniform phantom are provided in Fig. 2. Fig. 2b and 2c show the same reconstructed slice at two different total exposure levels (0.27 R and 2.2 R). Qualitative evaluation of the images reveals increased lesion visibility in the slice images as compared to their corresponding projection image. Additionally, increasing exposure generally appears to improve image quality. The measured signal differences (between lesion and background ROIs) for lesions in the uniform phantom are shown in Fig. 3 using the off-axis background and the coaxial background ROIs. The signal difference increases with increasing lesion size, with nearly a 4× increase from the smallest to the largest lesion.

The measured SDNR values for the uniform phantom are presented as a function of lesion diameter for each exposure level for both coaxial and off-axis ROIs in Fig. 4a and 4b, respectively. The "exposure normalized" SDNR (SDNR divided by the square root of relative exposure) is shown in Fig. 4c and 4d. Trends similar to those seen in Fig. 4 are also evident for the standard mammography image in Fig. 5.

The corresponding results for the complex phantom are shown in Fig. 6 through Fig. 8. The sponge had a number of deposits of coral and sand that, when seen as a radiograph, appeared to be surprisingly similar to microcalcifications. One such large "calcification" is seen in the slice in Fig. 6b between the two lesions, and several artifacts due to out-of-plane calcifications can also be seen in the slice (especially along the bottom of the image). Due to residual background structure the smallest lesions (2 mm and 1.5 mm) could not be located in any of the reconstructed slices (at any exposure) nor in the mammographic image.

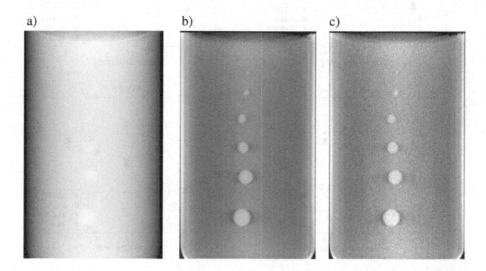

Fig. 2. (a) Sample projection of the uniform imaging phantom. (b) High exposure (2.2 R) and (c) low exposure (0.27 R) reconstructed slice image of the phantom showing increased lesion conspicuity due to improved signal uniformity in the background.

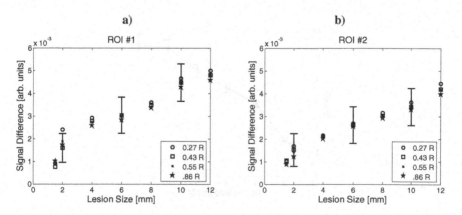

Fig. 3. Signal difference as a function of lesion size using the (a) off-axis background ROI and the (b) coaxial background ROI. Selected error bars represent the quadrature sum of the standard deviation in voxel values for the 0.43 R cases.

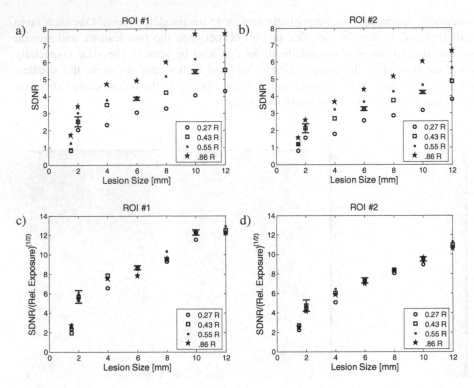

Fig. 4. SDNR and exposure-normalized SDNR in reconstructed slice images as a function of lesion size for all exposure levels using off-axis background ROIs in (a) and (c) and coaxial ROIs in (b) and (d). Selected error bars represent the standard error of repeated measurements on 8 sub-regions of the ROIs.

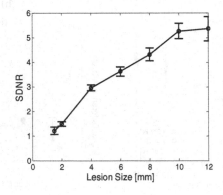

Fig. 5. SDNR as a function of lesion size for a digital mammogram acquired at 30 kV Rh/Rh and 91 mAs (1.2 R total exposure). The analysis was performed on a GE processed image (not a raw image).

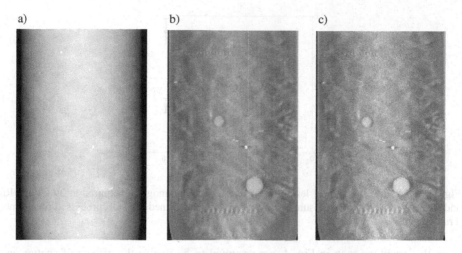

Fig. 6. (a) Sample projection of the complex imaging phantom. (b) High exposure (2.1 R) and (c) low exposure (0.26 R) reconstructed slice image of the phantom showing increased lesion conspicuity due to improved signal uniformity in the background.

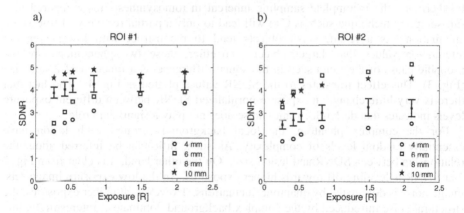

Fig. 7. SDNR in reconstructed slice images of the complex phantom as a function of total entrance exposure for all lesion sizes using (a) off-axis and (b) coaxial background ROIs. Selected error bars represent the standard error of repeated measurements on 8 sub-regions of the ROIs.

4 Discussion

Following reconstruction, the signal in each voxel represents a quantity that is directly related to the attenuation coefficient. Ideally, for a lesion in a uniform phantom, the attenuation difference between lesion and background is a constant, regardless of lesion size and exposure. In turn, it is expected that, when limited only by quantum noise, the exposure-normalized SDNR values should be constant. The departures

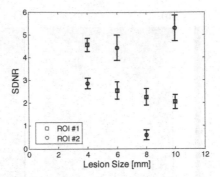

Fig. 8. SDNR as a function of lesion size for a digital mammogram acquired at 29 kV Rh/Rh and 72 mAs (0.82 R total exposure). The analysis was performed on a GE processed image (not a raw image).

from this trend, as seen in Fig. 4, are assumed to be due to the effects of scatter and incomplete spatial sampling in the reconstruction. Scatter of x-rays will tend to reduce the apparent attenuation (hence signal difference), and this effect will be more pronounced for smaller objects, which become masked by the scatter [5]. Furthermore, the incomplete sampling inherent in tomosynthesis (as compared to a full-sampling technique such as CT) will lead to only a partial recovery of true voxel attenuation. As a result, small objects tend to reconstruct with lower apparent attenuation values than larger objects. Together, these two phenomena are the probable cause of the trend seen in the signal difference as a function of lesion size (Fig. 3). This effect translates to the SDNR values plotted in Fig. 4. The fact that there is very little change in exposure-normalized SDNR between different exposure levels indicates that dark (electronic) noise does not play a significant role.

For the complex phantom, the local backgrounds around each lesion have essentially random levels of complexity. As such, little can be inferred about the relationship between SDNR and lesion size. On the other hand, it is clear from Fig. 7 that SDNR is leveling off towards higher exposures. In the low exposure image sets, image noise is dominated by quantum fluctuations. However, at higher exposures, the structural noise introduced by the complex background dominates. Interestingly, this suggests that in complex objects with non-uniform backgrounds (i.e. breast tissue), increasing the exposure beyond a certain level may have little or no benefit for tomosynthesis reconstructions. It is possible, however, that improved reconstruction techniques that suppress more of the background may benefit from higher exposures.

Preliminary analysis has shown that simple low-contrast phantoms are suitable for evaluating the effects of dose on reconstruction quality. Results, thus far, suggest that reductions in dose are feasible without unduly sacrificing image quality. To provide a more complete characterization of the dose/image quality tradeoff, it will be necessary to broaden this study to examine various acquisition parameters, including choice of x-ray spectra, angular spacing between projections, and the total number of projections acquired per data set. Additionally, optimization of reconstruction algorithms – perhaps for various levels of object complexity – remains to be explored. Finally, it would be informative to investigate further both scatter and electronic noise to gain a more complete understanding of their contribution to image quality.

References

1. Dobbins III, J.T., Godfrey, D.J.: Digital x-ray tomosynthesis: current state of the art and clinical potentials. Phys. Med. Biol. 48 (2003) R65-R106
2. Wu, T., Stewart, A., Stanton, M., et al.: Tomographic mammography using a limited number of low-dose cone-beam projection images. Med Phys 30 (2003) 365-380
3. Bloomquist, A.K., Yaffe, M.J., Pisano, E.D., et al.: Quality control for digital mammography in the ACRIN DMIST trial - Part I, Med. Phys. 33 (2006) 719-736
4. Mueller, K, Yagel, R., Wheller, J.J.: Anti-Aliased 3D Cone-Beam Reconstruction of Low-Contrast Objects with Algebraic Methods. IEEE Trans. Med. Im. 18 (1999) 519-537
5. Siewerdsen, J. H., Jaffray, D. A.: Cone-beam computed tomography with a flat-panel imager: Magnitude and effects of x-ray scatter. Med. Phys. 28 (2001) 220-231

Registration of Mammograms and Breast Tomosynthesis Images

Predrag R. Bakic[1], Frederic J.P. Richard[2], and Andrew D.A. Maidment[1]

[1] University of Pennsylvania, Philadelphia, PA
{Predrag.Bakic, Andrew.Maidment}@uphs.upenn.edu
[2] Universite Paris 5, Paris, France
Frederic.Richard@math-info.univ-paris5.fr

Abstract. Digital breast tomosynthesis is becoming a clinically attractive modality based on its potential to combine the high resolution and high contrast images, and affordability of digital mammography, with the advantages of 3D image acquisition. In order to facilitate comparison of tomosynthesis images with previous mammographic exams of the same women, there is a need for a method of registering a mammogram with a tomosynthetic image of the same breast; this is the focus of this paper. We have chosen to approach this multimodality registration problem, starting from the simpler problem of registering a mammogram and the central tomosynthesis source image. Such a registration pair represents the most similar breast images obtained from different clinical modalities. In this study of 15 pairs of mammograms and central tomosynthesis projections of the same breast, on average we were able to compensate 94 percent of the per-pixel intensity differences that existed between the two images before the registration.

1 Background

Early breast cancer detection requires identification of subtle pathological changes over time, and is often performed by comparing mammograms from previous years. Those changes can be masked by breast positioning, compression, or x-ray acquisition parameters. Similarly, multimodality breast images are acquired with different positioning, compression levels, and they also measure different material properties. An approach to compensate for the acquisition related variations is image registration, in which one image is deformed in order to match another image, based on some similarity criterion. Registration could improve the accuracy of temporal or intermodality comparison, and potentially emphasize genuine tissue alterations.

Tomosynthesis is a novel x-ray based modality for imaging 3D breast anatomy. First, a small number of projections through the compressed breast are acquired, while varying the position of the x-ray focus. By combining information from these projections one can gain information about the 3D tissue distribution. Several algorithms have been proposed, ranging from relatively simple backprojection techniques to sophisticated algebraic reconstructions [1,2]. While the limited number of projections prevents CT-like reconstruction quality, our clinical experience has

Susan M. Astley et al. (Eds.): IWDM 2006, LNCS 4046, pp. 498–503, 2006.

confirmed our ability to produce images in which a given anatomical plane is in focus while anatomical structures above and below the plane are blurred to such an extent as to be essentially removed from the image (*see Fig 2*).

Tomosynthesis is becoming a clinically attractive modality based on its potential to combine high resolution and high contrast images, and affordability of digital mammography, with the advantages of 3D breast image acquisition. In addition, there is a potential for functional imaging, in the form of contrast-enhanced tomosynthesis [3]. In order to facilitate comparison of new tomosynthesis images with previous mammographic exams of the same women, there is a need for a method of registering tomosynthetic and mammographic images, which is our focus in this paper. To the best of our knowledge, there has been no report in the literature on this specific multimodality registration problem.

In this paper we present the results of registering 15 pairs of mammograms and central tomosynthesis projections of the same breast.

2 Materials and Methods

There are two aspects to the problem of registering mammograms and tomosynthesis images: (i) Registration of a mammogram onto a tomosynthesis reconstructed volume of the same breast is a 2D-3D registration problem. (ii) Registration of an individual tomosynthesis reconstructed plane onto a mammogram is a 2D-2D problem. Such a task, however, cannot be performed by simply extending the existing mammogram registration methods, since the size and content of the breast portion within an individual reconstructed plane vary depending on the slice position. Although both images have the same physical nature, their acquisition procedures (projection vs. tomographic reconstruction) are substantially different.

As a preliminary step, in this paper we describe registration of a tomosynthesis central source projection and a medio-lateral mammogram of the same breast. The central projection is acquired in a medio-lateral (MLO) breast positioning with reduced dose and compression.

2.1 Clinical Data

At our institution, tomosynthesis source images are acquired on a Senographe 2000D (General Electric Medical Systems, Milwaukee, WI) which has been modified to allow independent motion of the x-ray tube head and removal of the anti-scatter grid. The x-ray tube can be reproducibly positioned at 9 locations, each separated by approximately $6.25°$. Each breast is compressed in an MLO position. The source images are acquired at a total dose equal to that of two MLO mammograms. Tomosynthesis breast images are reconstructed in planes parallel to detector, using a modified backprojection algorithm. To date, 51 clinical breast tomosynthesis exams have been performed under IRB review as a part of a large multimodality clinical study in our department. After informed consent, all the patients in the study were offered tomosynthesis, mammography, breast MRI, PET, and ultrasound exams. For each tomosynthesis image there is a corresponding mammogram taken on the same day by the same x-ray technologist, thus having minimal variations, which is of importance for initial testing of the registration methods.

In this study we performed registration of 15 pairs of mammograms and central tomosynthesis projections, from ten women (mean age 48.4 years; age-range 39-62 years) imaged between August 2004 and May 2005 at the Hospital of the University of Pennsylvania. Four out of these ten women had confirmed malignancies, five had findings suspicious for malignancy, and one had a benign finding. The selection criteria was that the whole breast was well visible in both the MLO mammogram and the central tomosynthesis projection. Such a criteria excluded cases of very large breasts, in which several images had to be taken to cover the whole breast in the MLO positioning. We also excluded cases with low quality of the tomosynthesis projection images, due to excessive patient motion or problems with breast positioning.

2.2 Non-rigid Registration Method

For the registration of mammograms and central tomosynthesis source images, we have used a recently developed non-rigid registration method [4]. The method focuses on matching regions of interest (ROIs) in source and target images of a registration pair, and combines intensity- and contour-based constraints. The registration task is formulated as an inverse problem of finding a geometric deformation that minimizes an energy function with free boundary conditions. The energy function includes three constraints designed (i) to provide for regularization and prevent ill-posed problems, (ii) to compensate for linear variations in image intensities, and (iii) to correct initial mapping of target image ROI onto the source image ROI.

Before the registration, the ROIs were identified as the breast regions without the pectoral muscle. The pectoral muscle area was identified as the region above the line defined by two manually selected points on the muscle contour. In this study, we registered the two images by deforming the mammogram to match the central tomosynthesis projection of the same breast. The non-rigid registration method was performed in two steps: First, an initial registration was performed, based on the contour matching only. This initial step is followed by the corrections of the differences in the pixel intensity distribution between the target and source images. Detailed description of the registration method is given in our previous publications [5]. In an evaluation using synthetic images generated with a software breast model [6], the ability of this registration method to compensate for variation in compressed breast thickness has been demonstrated [5].

In the present study of clinical images, we evaluated the registration results by the analysis of pixel intensity differences, using the percent of corrected differences as a measure of the registration performance. The percent of corrected quadratic differences, PCQD, is defined as:

$$PCQD = [\Sigma_{ij}(\Delta_{ij}^{PRE}) - \Sigma_{ij}(\Delta_{ij}^{POST})] / \Sigma_{ij}(\Delta_{ij}^{PRE}) \tag{1}$$

where Δ_{ij}^{PRE} and Δ_{ij}^{POST} represent the quadratic differences between the intensities of the pixels at position (i,j), before and after registration, respectively. $\Delta_{ij}^{P}=[(M(i,j)^{P}-CT(i,j)]^{2})$, where $M(i,j)^{P}$ represent the intensity of the pixel at postition (i,j) in the mammogram before (P=PRE) or after (P=POST) registration, and $CT(i,j)$ represent the intensity of the pixel at position (i,j) in the central tomosynthesis projection. The higher PCQD values indicate the better registration performance.

In addition, we compared the root-mean-square (RMS) differences between the mammograms and central tomosynthesis projections, computed before and after the non-rigid registration.

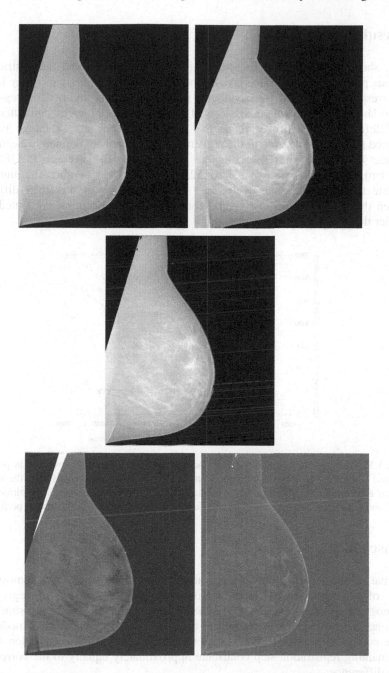

Fig. 1. The upper row shows the registration image pair: a mammogram (left) to be registered onto a tomosynthesis source image of the same breast (right). The registration result is shown in the middle row. The lower row shows the difference between the mammogram and central tomosynthesis projection, computed before (*left*) and after (*right*) the registration.

3   Results

Fig. 1. shows an example of registration of a mammogram and the central tomo-synthesis projection of the same breast. Shown are the mammogram (upper left) and the corresponding central tomosynthesis projection (upper right). The registration result is shown in the middle image as well as the difference images, computed before (lower left) and after (lower right) the registration. For all 15 image pairs we computed the PCQD measure of the registration performance (defined in Section 2.3) after the initial and after the complete registration. The average PCQD values (±standard deviations) were equal to 52±20% and 94±3%, after the initial and complete registrations, respectively. Fig. 2 shows a plot of the RMS differences between the mammograms and central tomosynthesis projections, computed before and after the non-rigid registration.

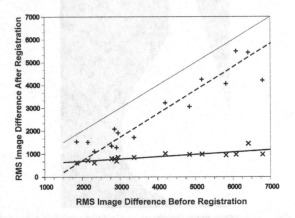

Fig. 2. RMS differences between the mammogram and the central tomosynthesis projection, computed before and after the registration. Shown are the RMS differences after the initial (+) and after the complete registration (×). The corresponding linear regressions are plotted by the dashed and bold lines, respectively. The solid unity line indicates zero registration performance.

4   Discussion

We have chosen to approach the registration of a mammogram and a tomosynthesis image of the same breast, starting from the simpler problem of registering a mammogram and the central tomosynthesis source image. Such a registration pair represents the most similar breast images obtained from different clinical modalities.

The computed average PCQD values suggest that the initial registration step and the remaining registration step contribute approximately equally to the correction of image differences.

Fig. 2 shows that after the initial registration step the difference between the registered images is proportional to image difference before the registration. After the complete registration, the image difference practically does not depend on the differences observed before the registration. In this paper, we evaluated the registration performance based on the pixel intensity differences. In future work we plan to evaluate the registration results based on the average displacements of manually or automatically extracted fiducial points.

Presently, we have considered registration of MLO mammograms with central tomosynthesis projections, since the latter are also acquired in the MLO positioning. Registration of a CC mammogram with the tomosynthesis images would require to computationally "decompress" the breast from the MLO position and "recompress" it in the CC position. Techniques allowing such transformations have been reported in the literature [7]. Novel methods could be developed by utilizing the 3D nature of tomosynthesis images.

5 Conclusions

We performed a non-rigid registration of 15 pairs of mammograms and central tomosynthesis projections acquired from ten women. The mammograms and tomosynthesis images were acquired on the same day by the same technologist, thus having minimal variations. We evaluated the registration performance by computing the percent corrected quadratic differences between the mammogram and the central tomosynthesis projection. On average we were able to compensate 94 percent of the per-pixel intensity differences that existed between the two images before the registration.

Acknowledgement

The presented work was supported by the National Cancer Institute Program Project Grant PO1 CA85484.

References

1. Niklason, L.T., Christian, B.T., Niklason, L.E., Kopans, D.B., et al.: Digital Tomosynthesis in Breast Imaging. Radiology. 205 (1997) 399-406
2. Maidment, A.D.A, Albert, M., Conant, E.F.: Three-dimensional Imaging of Breast Calcifications. In Proc. SPIE 3240 (1998) 200-208
3. Carton, A.-K., Li, J., Albert, M., Chen, S., Maidment, A.D.A.: Quantification for Contrast-enhanced Digital Breast Tomosynthesis. In Proc. SPIE 6142. (2006)
4. Richard, F.J.P., Cohen, L.: Non-rigid Image Registration with Free Boundary Constraints: Application to Mammography. Comp Vis Image Understanding 89 (2003) 166-196
5. Richard, F.J.P., Bakic, P.R., and Maidment, A.D.A.: Mammogram Registration: a Phantom-Based Evaluation of Mammographic Compression Effects. IEEE Trans Med Imag. 25 (2006) 188-197
6. Bakic, P.R., Albert, M., Brzakovic, D., Maidment, A.D.A.: Mammogram synthesis using a 3D simulation. I. Breast tissue model and image acquisition simulation. Med Phys. 29 (2002) 2131-2139
7. Kita, Y., Tohno, E., Highnam, R., Brady, M.: A CAD system for the 3D locations in mammograms. Med Image Anal 6 (2002) 267-273

Complementary Role of Computer Aided Detection in Mammography

Keiko Sugisaki[1], Hiroshi Fujita[2], Hiro Goto[1], and Hiroaki Hoshi[1]

[1] Department of Radiology, Gifu University School of Medicine, Japan
[2] Department of Intelligent Image Information, Graduate School of Medicine, Gifu University, Japan

Abstract. The experience of clinical use of breast CAD system at the hospital of Gifu University School of Medicine was reported. The CAD system was Image Checker M1000-DM available for Senographe 2000D.During February 4, 2005 to May 16, 125 cases was examined by this device and 22cases of breast cancers were found. A case was misdiagnosed by radiologist before CAD, and CAD detected the lesion. Another case was correctly detected by radiologist before CAD, but CAD could not point out the lesion. 20 remain cases were detected correctly by both radiologist and CAD. CAD was supposed to be useful for the mammographic diagnosis of breast cancer.

1 Background

In 1980 full-scale mammography was started with the introduction of CGR-Senographe 500T to the hospital of Gifu University School of Medicine. From the beginning, examination was performed with the presence of radiologists. Spot-imaging and duct graphy were performed if required based on the clinical breast examination and X-ray findings for higher-accuracy examination.

GE-Senographe DMR was introduced in 1996, and it allowed us to perform magnification spot radiography and stereotactic biopsy. Since then, one of the biplane projections was changed from ML to MLO.

Electronic medical chart was implemented with the relocation of the hospital in June, 2004, and operation of film-less mammography became an issue. There are two kinds of digital mammographic equipment; one is computed radiography using imaging plate and the other uses flat panel detector (FPD). Senographe 2000D, which was the only equipment approved by FDA at the time of planning stage of relocation, was adopted. This equipment allowed us to use Image Checker M1000-DM, computer aided diagnosis (CAD), and therefore it was applied in a clinical setting. The experience of this CAD system was discussed in this article.

2 Materials

125 cases were examined among the patients who had mammography taken at the hospital between February 4 and May 16 in 2005. The patients who had history of operations or chemotherapy for breast cancer were excluded. The ages were 17-78 years, with an average age of 51.1 years.

Susan M. Astley et al. (Eds.): IWDM 2006, LNCS 4046, pp. 504–508, 2006.

3 Method

Most of the patients who had mammography taken at the hospital were consulted by breast surgeon at first, and mammography examination was recommended based on their medical history, clinical breast examination, and ultrasound. Mammography examination was performed at the department of radiology, and both MLO and CC were taken by a radiological technician. In the meantime, medical history and the result of ultrasound were checked by a radiologist. When mammography was taken, the image was checked on 5M CRT monitor. If appropriate mammography were taken, diagnosis was given by a radiologist. After that, CAD result from Image Checker M1000-DM was referred. Further clinical breast examination by radiologist was performed, and the necessity of additional mammography, such as magnification spot radiography and duct graphy, was determined based on all information obtained. When additional mammography was required, mammography was taken by both radiologist and radiological technician. The examination was completed when appropriate additional mammography was obtained. After the examination was completed, report was prepared using reporting system by a radiologist. The prepared report was sent to an electronic medical chart and explained at the department of breast surgeon. Clinical diagnosis before CAD and CAD were compared in order to examine the clinical efficacy of CAD.

4 Results

4.1 Lesion Found

22 cases of breast cancers, 12 cases of fibroadenoma, 9 cases of cyst, and 1 case of hamartoma were found.

4.2 Number of Lesion

When lesion was found in either MLO or CC, it was considered as one lesion. When lesion was found in both MLO and CC and identified as the same lesion, it was considered as one lesion. (table1)

Table 1

number of lesions	before CAD referred	CAD
0	44	43
1	50	47
2	25	19
3	4	11
4	1	3
5	1	2

Clinical diagnosis before CAD and CAD were relatively similar. However, there were only 54 cases with the same lesion at the same region diagnosed both before CAD and CAD. There were 67 cases where lesion was found only by the diagnosis before CAD referred. On the contrary, there were 86 cases where the lesion was detected only by CAD. 22 cases were diagnosed with no abnormal finding by both diagnoses before CAD and CAD.

4.3 Detection of Breast Cancer

There was one case among 22 cases of breast cancer, which the lesion was detected only by CAD (Fig1). On the contrary, there was one case, which the lesion was pointed out only by the diagnosis before CAD (Fig2). Both of the cases were mass shadow without calcification and background was unequally highly-concentrative. These cases were an example that tumor mass was not shown clearly because of the overlap of mass shadow and mammary gland.

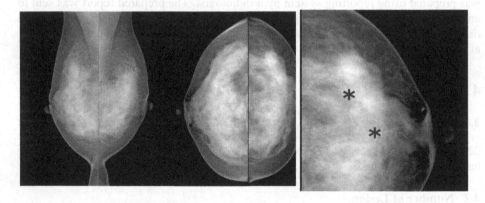

Fig. 1

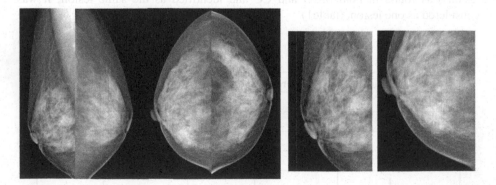

Fig. 2

4.4   Examination of the Case of Which Diagnosis Before CAD and CAD Were Mismatched

4.4.1   67cases: The Lesion Was Detected Only by Diagnosis Before CAD

The breakdown of these cases were; 46 cases of calcification, 19 cases of tumor mass, and 2 cases of tumor mass + calcification.

17cases of tumor mass out of 19 cases, which was diagnosed as BIRADS category 3, were not detected by CAD. One of them was the case of breast cancer cited above. The other cases showed clear circular tumor mass.

40 cases among the cases of calcification werc diagnosed as BIRADS category 2, but the lesion was not detected in 5 cases of BIRADS category 3. These happened due to the overlap of relatively amorphous calcification and dense breast. The other one case was the calcification of skin. 2 cases of tumor mass + calcification were calcified fibroadenoma.

4.4.2   86cases: The Lesion Was Detected Only by Diagnosis CAD

The breakdown of these cases was; 66 cases of tumor mass and 20 cases of calcification.

58 cases out of 66 cases of tumor mass were diagnosed as BIRADS category 1. Most of them were due to the overlap of breast tissue and the overlap of breast tissue with vessels. 6 cases of BIRADS category 2 were considered to be focal asymmetric density: FAD. There were 2 cases of BIRADS category 3. One was the case of breast cancer cited above, and the other was the case of FAD.

In the case of calcification, there were 13 cases of BIRADS category 1, which calcification was not found after reexamination of the region pointed out by CAD. There were 7 cases of BIRADS category 2 based on the micro round calcification, and there were no cases of BIRADS category 3, 4, 5 .

5   Discussion

Thc digitalization in the field of medical imaging is widely spreading in these days, and many facilities are operating film-less system and electronic medical chart. Senographe 2000D was set at the same time of relocation and introduction of medical chart system to the Gifu University School of Medicine. This equipment allows us to use Image Checker M1000-DM and to refer the result of CAD on the monitor easily. This is one of the superiority of digital imaging to analog imaging. Algorithm guide notes, "this equipment is used to improve the accuracy of mammography reading by pointing out the suspicious region to radiologist after mammography was read by radiologist, "[1] and it is supposed to be used at health check. The use of CAD in practical clinic was discussed in this article, but it is not necessary to distinguish practical clinic from health check in terms of improvement of film reading accuracy. CAD led us to detect the lesion in one of 22 cases of breast cancer. Even though there is only a few case obtained, the availability of CAD is shown. However, further improvement is required since it is limited to detect both tumor mass and calcification in dense breast and there are quite a few false positive.

The main aim of current breast cancer CAD is to play a supplemental role in detection of breast cancer [2]. Since CAD is developed based on diagnosis of radio- logist, diagnostic performance better than radiologist cannot be pursued. However diagnosis by radiologist is not perfect, and there seems little doubt that CAD redeems mistake of radiologist and that it is beneficial for radiologist with few experience.

6 Summary

The experience of clinical use of breast CAD system at the hospital of Gifu University School of Medicine was reported. The CAD system was Image Checker M1000-DM available for Senographe 2000D. CAD was supposed to be useful for the mammographic diagnosis of breast cancer in clinical cases.

References

[1] CAD Image Checker M1000-DM Algorithm Guide
[2] Hiroshi Fujita: The institute of image information and television engineers: 58(7), 893-897, 2004

The Refinement of Microcalcification Cluster Assessment by Joint Analysis of MLO and CC Views

Márta Altrichter and Gábor Horváth

Department of Measurement and Information Systems,
Budapest University of Technology and Economics,
P.O. Box 91, H-1521 Budapest, Hungary
grimma@sch.bme.hu, horvath@mit.bme.hu

Abstract. Most of the CAD Systems for Mammograms are composed of algorithms analysing the four X-ray images individually. It is a general experience, that algorithms in search of microcalcification clusters can obtain high sensitivity only if specificity is low. To overcome efficiency problem this paper proposes a simple algorithm to combine information of the two views (MLO/CC) of the breast. The procedure is based upon the experiences of radiologists: masses and calcifications should emerge on both views, so if no matching is found, the given object is a false positive hit. A positioning system is evolved to find corresponding regions on the two images. Calcification clusters obtained in individual images are matched in "2.5-D" provided by the positioning system. The credibility value of the hit is reassessed by the matching. The proposed approach can significantly reduce the number of false positive hits in calcification.

1 Introduction

There are several algorithms searching for microcalcification clusters on individual X-ray images [1], [2]. The main feature of these algorithms is that the positive cases are found with large probability – sensitivity is about 90-95% – but the number of false positive hits per picture is too high – 1.5-3 FP/image, specificity 0-5%.

A method is needed to decrease the number of false positive hits, which will not or will barely decrease the number of true positive ones. This paper presents a relatively simple new way of this. The method sets off from the fact that the images of calcifications and masses have to appear on both views (MLO and CC). To be more precise they must be on positions of the two views that correspond to each other. In practice a 3-D reconstruction of the breast would be needed. But the full 3-D reconstruction is impossible, because only two views of the breast are available, and because these two views are the 2-D projections of the differently compressed breast. Therefore instead of a full 3-D reconstruction we suggest a relatively simple procedure which we call "2.5-D" correspondence.

As the two main pathological abnormalities have different distinguishing features from normal tissue, their joint analysis slightly differs. During matching

Susan M. Astley et al. (Eds.): IWDM 2006, LNCS 4046, pp. 509–516, 2006.
© Springer-Verlag Berlin Heidelberg 2006

of masses the positioning system can restrict the examined picture to a region corresponding on the other view, and search within it for a mass with similar texture characteristics. On the other hand calcificated tissue and normal tissues are rather similar in texture, therefore their matching only uses the positioning system.

In this paper we focused on describing how the "2.5-D" positioning system can be built, and how it can be used to refine the assessment of a micocalcification cluster found previously by a microcalcification searching algorithm.

2   "2.5-D" Positioning System

The breast has three main control points: the pectoral muscle, the nipple and the boundary of the breast. These landmarks segment the breast to its anatomical regions.

The Cranio-Caudal and Medio-Lateral-Oblique views are two-dimensional projections of the three dimensional object. As the breast in CC view is exposed to x-ray from a different angle than in MLO, it can be assumed that a stripe will correspond on the MLO to a region taken from the CC view (this assumtion works backward as well, thus an MLO region transfered to the CC view is a stripe). The reference system is to calculate the position of this stripe. The algorithm is founded on three simple hypotheses:

1. The pectoral muscle on a CC image is the vertical axis.
2. The position of the nipple can be estimated by laying a tangent on the breast border parallel with the pectoral muscle.
3. The distance covered from the nipple perpendicular to the pectoral muscle on MLO approximately corresponds to the distance measured up on the horizontal axis from the nipple on CC.

The first step of the algorithm is to find the angle enclosed by the pectoral muscle and the horizontal axis on MLO views.

To find the angle the slightly modified method in [3] was used. First edge detection – special edge detection method: Edgeflow [4] – is made and the Region of Interest (ROI) is cut out. This ROI is the upper corner of the MLO and will contain the pectoral muscle (See Fig. 1(a).).

The second step: the iteration processing the lines in the ROI diverges from paper [3], as in this case the whole line of the pectoral muscle is not needed, just an approximation of the angle enclosed by the pectoral muscle and the horizontal axis. By cutting up the lines, and deleting improbable line segments the robustness of the algorithm is increased. (See Fig. 1.) The pseudo code is:

1. $n = 0$, $BW_0 = ROI$, $L_n =$ longest object on BW_0
2. L_n is divided to parts with uniform length along the vertical axis
3. $L\_bad_n =$ objects which enclose $< 40°$ or $> 90°$ with the horizontal axis
4. $L\_good_n = L_n - L\_bad_n$, $BW_{n+1} = BW_n - L\_bad_n$
5. if $BW_{n+1} == BW_n$ iteration stops, the pectoral muscle is the object L_good_n, else $L_{n+1} =$ longest object on BW_{n+1}, $n = n + 1$ and go to Step 2.

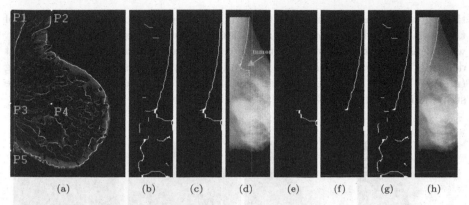

| (a) | (b) | (c) | (d) | (e) | (f) | (g) | (h) |

Fig. 1. (a) ROI selection (b) BW_0, (c) L_0, (d) $L_0 + Picture$, (e) L_bad_0, (f) L_good_1, (g) BW_1, (h) $L_1 + Picture$

After finding the angle a tangent with the same angle is laid on the breast border marking the nipple. The distances of the observed region from the tangent – u and v – are measured. The same distances are measured up on the perpendicular line to the tangent from the nipple of the other view. The two points and the angle of the pectoral muscle mark out the stripe needed for matching calcifications. (See Fig. 2.)

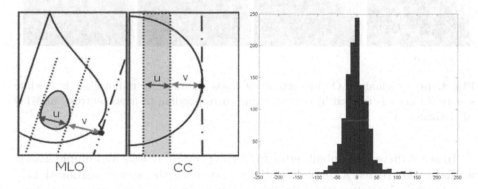

Fig. 2. The corresponding stripe on the CC of a selected region on the MLO

Fig. 3. Histogram of pixel errors, number of cases 1159

To test if the three basic hypotheses of the positioning system are correct a statistical analysis was made. 1159 cases with $400\mu/$pixel resolution (600*400 pixels) from the DDSM database [5] were selected. These cases contained only one pathological growth on each views according to the radiologists' assessments. Thus the two marks on the two views can be assumed to be the 2-D projections of the same object.

The pixel corresponding to the centroid of the growth on the MLO was determined, and the deviation of the result from the centroid of the growth on the CC was measured in pixels (See Fig. 4.). Fig. 3. shows the histogram of the deviations. There is some variance caused by wrong pectoral muscle finding, wrong radiologist assessment or the flaw of the hypotheses (because of breast deformation) for a few cases, but generally the hypotheses look to be standing (mean is around zero). To compensate the effect of variance the width of the stripe is increased by 10%.

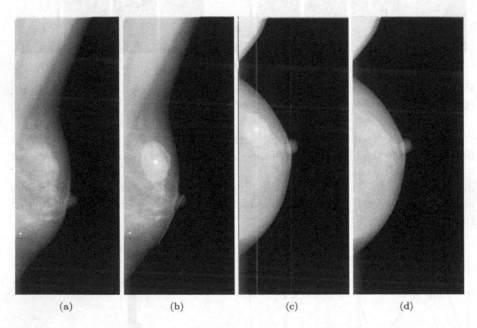

(a)   (b)   (c)   (d)

Fig. 4. (a) Original MLO (b) centroid of mass (marked by radiologist) is a white square (c) mass is marked by doctor + line corresponding to mass centroid on MLO (d) Original CC

To see if there is no inbuilt error from the pectoral muscle and nipple search, we have constructed a simple sensitivity test using the above mentioned 1159 cases and evaluation method. In the sensitivity test, a constant running from -50 to +40 was added to the pectoral muscle degree in each of the 1159 cases (90*1159 measures), the new nipple was calculated and the same deviations of pairing the centroids of radiologists' assessments were measured as in the statistical analysis (See Fig. 4.). Beside of these 90 measurement systems, an experiment on the microcalcification searching algorithm showed that the average cluster diameter is 52 pixels and the variance of the diameter is 25 pixels. On Fig. 5. we can see the percentage of the 1159 cases which are below the 27,52,77 pixel deviation plotted according to the constant change of the pectoral muscle angle. The figure shows two important facts: (a) there is no inbuilt constant error in the "2.5-D" positioning system, (b) there is quite big tolerance (around -10 to 10 degree) in finding the pectoral muscle angle.

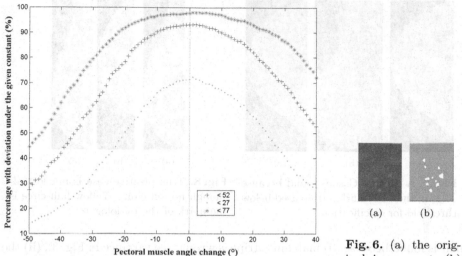

Fig. 5. The percentage of the 1159 cases which are below the constant (27,52 or 77) ploted along the error in the pectoral muscle angle imbued by the experiment

Fig. 6. (a) the original image part, (b) the calcification mask the searching algorithm provided

3 Microcalcification Cluster Matching and Reassessment

The microcalcification searching algorithm marks out suspicious regions, and provides a mask of microcacification pixels (See Fig. 6.). From the number of calcifications in the cluster, and the difference between the mean intensity of calcifications (marked by the mask) and the surrounding tissues a credibility value is assigned to each cluster: P_{calc} (Range: 0-255, 255 - highly suspicious region).

This credibility is modified by the help of the area ratio of the stripe corresponding to it and of other calcification clusters found on the other view: A_{ratio}. The new credibility is: $\hat{P}_{calc} = P_{calc} - cons_1 * (1 - A_{ratio} + cons_2)$. Fig. 8. illustrates why probability is decreased by subtracting an amount instead of simply multiplying with A_{ratio}. In this way if the microcalcification searching algorithm found the true positive cluster only on one view, but with high P_{calc}, the decreased $\hat{P}_{calc}$ is still thresholded to be a calcification. The constant $cons_2$ is to ensure, that at high correspondence the suspicion is raised.

4 Performance

The calcification matching was analyzed over 188 cases (376 pairs of mammographic images). 66 of these cases contained malignant calcifications. 1. table shows the results of the matching in a case level. Thus the 13.1% increase in specificity means that the algorithm cleared all the FP hits on the four images in those cases. The reasons for the loss of positive markers is that no matching

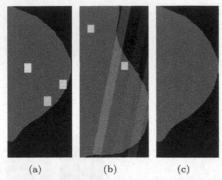

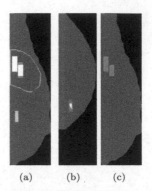

| (a) | (b) | (c) |

| (a) | (b) | (c) |

Fig. 7. A Normal Case is found because P_{calc} of the 3 FP mark is decreased below threshold for calcification

Fig. 8. True positive case is not lost although no matching. Yellow half-circe is the mark of the radiologist.

pair is found because: (i) matching stripe is wrong, see variance in Fig. 3., (ii) the lack of detected microcalcification cluster or mass in one of the views, and too small credibility for the detected one (iii) the lack of microcalcification cluster in one of the corresponding views (even radiologist could not find it).

Table 1. Table of results

	Original microcalcification algorithm	Calcifications after matching reassessment	Percentage change
Sensitivity	95.5%	92.4%	−3.1%
Specificity	0.8%	13.9%	+13.1%
FP/image	3.25 FP/image	1.57 FP/image	

5 Credibility Calculation with MLP (Multilayered Perceptron)

Currently a new method for determining the P_{calc} value is researhed. As it can be seen on Fig. 6. a calcification cluster can be described not only by the number of calcifications and intensity parameters but by area parameters (like the area of microcalcifications), by shape parameters (like the average length of the major axis of the calcifications ...), distance parameters (like the average distance between the calcifications) ...

We have acquired a 1390 true positive clusters determined by the microcalcification algorithm. These clusters are considered to be true positives as they overlap a mark of radiologists. A false positive sample set was gathered from the clusters found that did not overlap radiologists' mark. 35 parameters were determined to each cluster, out of which 13 were used as an input vector to the network. 834-834 (TP/FP) clusters were used to teach a simple MLP with Levenberg-Marquart algorithm (10 neurons in the hidden layer, -1 expected for parameters gained from a FP cluster and +1 expected for parameters gained from a TP cluster). Early stop was implemented with a testing set of 254-254 clusters. The remaining 302(TP)-284(FP) clusters were used for validation of the network.

A treshold was determined so that clusters which fall below are automatically dropped as false positive hits. 1 TP and 102 FP clusters were dropped by the network because of the treshold. The credibility values for the remaining clusters were determinded according to the distance they resulted from the treshold and the value 1. Fig. 5. shows the histogram of determined credibility values.

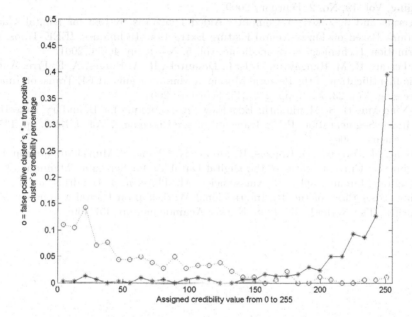

Fig. 9. The percentages of true positive and false positive cluster's credibility values

6   Conclusions

The paper proposed a relatively simple way of combining the results of microcalcification detection algorithms applied for individual X-ray breast images. The joint analysis follows the procedure of skilled radiologists: if a suspicious area can be found in one view, usually its corresponding pair should be detected in the other view of the same breast. The first results – based on a a few hundred of cases - show that using this approach the number of false positive detections can be reduced significantly while the decrease of true positive hits is relatively small.

Moreover a better method to calculate the credibility was examined using microcalcification shape information, and other features like distance as well to obtain primal P_{calc} value .

The proposed joint analysis system is still under testing. The improvement of the primal calcification searching algorithm, and the further analysis of the pairing (like drawing up a FROC curve) is needed. Also we intend to test the merging of the new credibility value assignment with the pairing, and see how the results can further change the TP/FP ratio.

References

1. Songyang Yu, Ling Guan: A CAD System for the Automatic Detection of Clustered Microcalcifications in Digitized Mammogram Films. IEEE Trans. on Medical Imaging, Vol. 19, No. 2, February 2000.
2. B. Verma and J. Zakos: A Computer-Aided Diagnosis System for Digital Mammograms Based on Fuzzy-Neural Feature Extraction Techniques. IEEE Trans. on Information Technology in Biomedicine, vol. 5. No. 1. pp. 46-54. 2001.
3. R.J. Ferrari, R. M. Rangayyan, J. E. L. Desautels, R. A. Borges, A. F. Frre: Automatic Identification of the Pectoral Muscle in Mammograms. IEEE Trans. on Image Processing, Vol. 23, No 2, pp. 232-245, February 2004.
4. Wei-Ying Ma, B. S. Manjunath: EdgeFlow: A Technique for Boundary Detection and Image Segmentation. IEEE Trans. on Image Processing, Vol. 9, No 8, pp. 1375-1388, August 2000.
5. M. Heath, K. Bowyer, D. Kopans, R. Moore, K. Chang, S. Munishkumaran and P. Kegelmeyer: Current Status of the Digital Database for Screening Mammography. In: Digital Mammography, N. Karssemeier, M. Thijssen, J. Hendriks and L. van Erning (eds.) Proc. of the 4th International Workshop on Digital Mammography, Nijmegen, The Netherlands, 1998. Kluwer Acamdemic, pp. 457-460.

The Dependence of Tomosynthesis Imaging Performance on the Number of Scan Projections

Baorui Ren, Tao Wu, Andrew Smith, Chris Ruth,
Loren Niklason, Zhenxue Jing, and Jay Stein

Hologic, Inc., 35 Crosby Drive, Bedford, Ma, 01730
bren@hologic.com

Abstract. In general, the use of more projections results in fewer tomosynthesis reconstruction artifacts. However, under a fixed dose, an excess number of projections will make the detector noise more pronounced in each of the x-ray shots and thus degrade image quality. Even in the absence of detector noise the advantages of higher projection numbers eventually have diminishing returns, making more projections unnecessary. In this study, we explore the dependence of tomosynthesis imaging performance on the number of projections, while keeping other factors fixed. We take the contrast-to-noise ratio as the figure of merit to search for the range of optimal projection number. The study is carried out through both simulations and experiments, with phantoms consisting of micro-calcification and mass objects, and a cadaver breast. The goal of this paper is to describe our methodology in general, and use a prototype tomosynthesis system as an example. The knowledge learned will help the design of future generation clinical tomosynthesis systems.

1 Background

The number of projections in a tomosynthesis scan is a very important design parameter. Because tomosynthesis is a limited angle tomographic system, objects remain visible in slices distant from their focus plane and generate what are known as shadow artifacts. In an ideal system, increasing the number of projections reduces the amplitude of the shadow artifacts. However, for a fixed total dose similar to a 2D mammogram, each projection shot in a tomosynthesis is indeed a low dose exposure. Further dividing the dose into more projection shots will adversely enhance the presence of detector noise in each exposure shot and start to reduce the detectability of features. In addition, the reduction of the shadow artifacts tend to saturate beyond certain high projection number so adding more projections becomes both unnecessary and costly in terms of data size and reconstruction time. It is of interest to develop a practical and systematic method to optimize the number of projections and derive the optimal number range under the specific design and performance parameters of each tomosynthesis system.

2 Method

Since detectability of a lesion and magnitude of shadow artifacts all relate to the contrast-to-noise ratio (CNR) of the object and its shadows, the CNR line profile along the depth Z direction through the feature and its shadows tells two things -- the peak value represents the detectability of the object at the focused slice while the values at off-peak locations represent the significance of the shadow artifacts. In this study we use the parameter of CNR as the figure of merit to study the dependence of CNR on projection number in a scan and the optimization of it. We took a prototype bread-board system as an example, and carried out both simulation and experiment to show our method, which is a two-step approach. First we investigate the dependence of peak CNR value on projection number, and then the dependence of the off-peak value and shape in the CNR profile. Images are analyzed both in the projection space and the reconstruction space. At last, we do visual evaluation of images to check the results that the CNR method suggests, and discuss advantages and limitations of the method.

2.1 Setup

The schematic of the prototype system is showed in Figure 1. It was a tabletop system with the tube scanning in the horizontal plane. The system consisted of a tungsten target x-ray tube with Al filter, and a-Se direct conversion flat panel detector of 70 μm pixel size. The detector was 24 cm by 29 cm large, and was positioned 66 cm from the focal spot. We used a 20-degree tube scan angle, 11, 15, and 21 projections per scan, and a readout rate of 1 frame/sec. The phantom of CNR study was a con-trast-detail (CD) phantom consisting of groups of micro-calcifications of 100 μm to 300 μm size and masses of 4 mm to 10 mm size, sandwiched by BR12 slabs to make certain thickness. The images were reconstructed through both backprojection (BP) and filtered backprojection (FBP) methods for comparison.

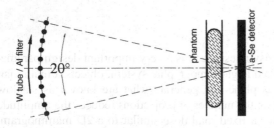
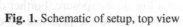
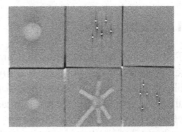

Fig. 1. Schematic of setup, top view   **Fig. 2.** ROI view of CD phantom

2.2 Dependence of the Peak CNR Value

A simplified computer model was developed to describe this prototyped tomosynthe-sis system, which consists of x-ray spectra generation, x-ray transmission through objects, and x-ray detection by detector. In particular, an analytical scattering model was adopted to simulate the scattering effect [1], together with a simplified detector noise model [2]. Simulations were carried out to evaluate the value and the dependence of CNR of typical mass and micro-calcification (uCa) objects in a breast under various conditions, e.g., dose, kVp, detector noise, and projection number. Throughout our extensive in-home studies in the past, we have done direct or indirect comparison between simulations and experiment frequently, and have thus validated the model. We have also developed optimal x-ray technique charts for phantom studies.

2.3 Dependence of the Height and Shape of the CNR Profile

The slice of interest for an object is that slice for which its image in different projections gets focused during the reconstruction's backprojection process, and further enhancement in this slice is always preferred. For all other slices, the object becomes out of focus and appears as multiple replications of itself (shadows), either connecting with each other or not. The line profile of CNR through the object and its shadows will show the significance of both in an image. We compare shapes of CNR line spread functions (LSF) from measured phantom images acquired under different projection numbers and x-ray techniques, and with different reconstruction methods.

3 Results

In this section, we show results of CNR vs. kVp curves from simulation and measurement, analyzed with projection images, and CNR profiles along slice-to-slice Z direction, analyzed with recon images. The difference between the analysis of projection and recon images is that the former one is simply a summation of all projection images together (with or without proper shift), and with no data interpolation involved, while the later one is a reconstruction process with shift and add, and with bilinear interpolation. CNR results from the two analysis methods are related but cannot be directly compared, since the interpolation is equivalent a kind of low-pass filtering that reduces image noise and improve the CNR value.

3.1 The CNR vs. kVp: From Projection Images

Fig. 3 and 4 show simulated CNR vs. kVp curves, all under constant dose of 300 mrad. The objects are 0.2 mm thick uCa and 5 mm thick mass in a 4.5 cm thick

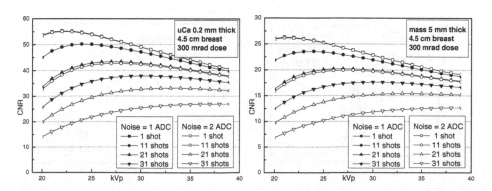

Fig. 3. Simulated CNR curves of uCa object   **Fig. 4.** Simulated CNR curves of mass object

breast. Detector noise is either 1 or 2 in ADC digital counts of our detector. The projection numbers in a scan are 1, 11, 21 and 31, respectively. Measured CNR curves of mass object in 4.5 cm thick breast under 150 mrad dose are showed in Fig. 5, with projection numbers as 11, 15, and 21, respectively. Measurements were done with the tube being stationary to the phantom and detector. CNR values were calculated from the projection image, similar to the way that simulations were carried out to generate CNR curves. The curves in Fig.5 are showed with a narrow display window, and thus the shapes should not be confused with those in Fig. 3-4, displayed in a full window.

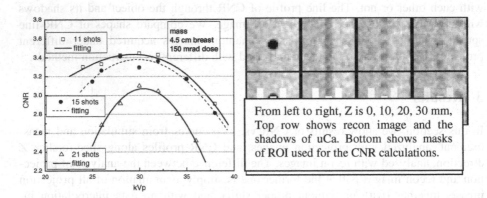

From left to right, Z is 0, 10, 20, 30 mm, Top row shows recon image and the shadows of uCa. Bottom shows masks of ROI used for the CNR calculations.

Fig. 5. Measured CNR curves of mass   **Fig. 6.** Recon images of uCa in- and out-focus

3.2 CNR vs. the Slice-to-Slice Separation Z: From Recon Images

We used reconstructed phantom images to study the CNR line spread function of uCa and mass objects. The phantom was scanned at several different kVp, dose, thickness, and all with 11, 15 and 21 projections. Images were reconstructed with both BP and FBP methods. We calculated the CNR of contrast features in each slice throughout the entire recon volume. Example in Fig. 6 shows the ROI mask selections for the

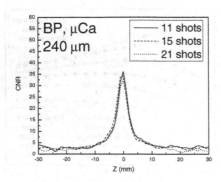

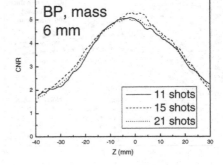

Fig. 7. CNR Z profiles of uCa of BP images   **Fig. 8.** CNR Z profiles of mass of BP images

contrast feature and its background, of both the uCa and the shadows. It also gives visual confirmation that we are indeed calculating the contrast and noise over the targeted feature region exactly throughout the entire recon volume. Subsequently CNR plots through either mass or uCa object along the Z direction are showed together to evaluate the impacts of the number of projections in a scan. In Figs. 7-10 we show results of a typical uCa and mass in 3 cm thick breast, imaged at 200 mrad, reconstructed with both the BP and the FBP methods.

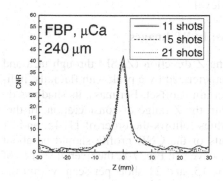

Fig. 9. CNR Z profiles of uCa of FBP images

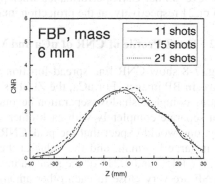

Fig. 10. CNR profiles of mass of FBP images

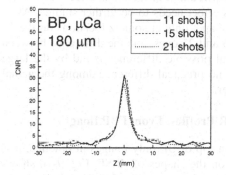

Fig. 11. CNR Z profile of a smaller sized uCa

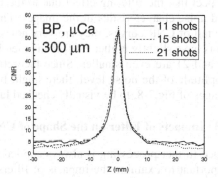

Fig. 12. CNR Z profile of a larger sized uCa

4 Discussions and Conclusions

4.1 Peak CNR and Its Dependence

Figs. 3-4 show that under given dose, detector noise and projection number, there exists optimal x-ray kVp value for a best possible CNR. Around this kVp, the change of CNR vs. kVp is very gradual. So within the optimal kVp range of a few kVp, CNR is not very sensitive to the exact kVp value. They also show that as the projection number increases, the maximum achievable CNR decreases. The larger the projection number, the more rapid the CNR degradation is. There is also a shift of the optimal kVp range toward higher values as projection number increases. For larger detector noise, the degradation in CNR can become worse while projection number is increased. Fig. 5 shows measured CNR curves at 150-mrad doses. The plots confirm that the optimal kVp range suggested by simulation, and the fact that CNR drops more rapidly for the projection number increase from 15 to 21 than from 11 to 15. The peak values of CNR of each curve are about 3.4, 3.3, and 3.1, for projection number of 11, 15, and 21, respectively. A rough estimate shows that the dose penalty would be about 6% or 18% at this dose level due to the detector noise, in order to achieve similar CNR performance when projection number is changed from the 11 to 15 or 21 respectively, at the projection image level.

4.2 The Z Profile of CNR of uCa and Mass: In BP Images

Fig. 7-8 show CNR line spread function along Z direction (ZLSF) through uCa and mass in BP images. For uCa, the ZLSF is characterized by a peak with flat tails, indicating complete shadow separation beyond certain Z-offset. For mass, its shadows do not separate completely with each other within the Z range of consideration. In theory, one would expect that the peak CNR values follows the order of 11, 15, and 21 from large to small, and the value at the tails of the CNR profile should be about $1/11^{th}$, $1/15^{th}$ and $1/21^{st}$ of the peak value. However, in Fig. 7-8, the overall shapes of ZLSF are very close to each other among 11, 15, and 21 shots per scan, within the noise magnitude of the data. For uCa, the peak CNR values seem to follow the correct order but the separations among them are very small compared to that of Fig. 5. We suspect that the filtering effect due to the interpolation process has effectively modified noise characteristics in the images. This effect needs to be further studied. As to the tail of CNR curves, they are very noisy shape, only at some z locations do the 11 shots have slightly higher CNR than other 15 and 21 ones, and the difference between 15 and 21 are even smaller. Since theoretical possible difference is hid by the large amplitude of the noise level, there might be no practical difference among the actual images of Fig.7-8, to be visually checked later.

4.3 Impacts of Filter on the Shape of CNR Profiles: From FBP Images

Since further processing is always applied on top of BP only images in practice, it is important to examine the impacts of filters on the shapes of ZLSF. Fig. 9-10 shows the ZLSF from FBP images of the same uCa and mass as Fig. 7-8. We find that the filter of FBP method has two distinct effects. For small objects (uCa), it can increase the peak CNR value as well as decrease the tail ones. The visual impact on image is that the object is greatly enhanced at in-focus slice, and the shadow is greatly suppressed at other off-focus slices. For large mass object, though it decreases the peak CNR values to some extent and reduces the contrast of the mass in the filtered image, it also reduces significantly the CNR value at the tail, making the shadow artifacts largely suppressed after filtering. This phenomenon can be explained by the filter's shape in the FBP. For a CT-type filter similar to what we used in this study, it suppresses both the high and low frequencies, and boosts the mid-range ones. In general high frequency relates mostly to the image noise while low and mid-range ones relate to the intensity of contrast. Since only the peak CNR value of uCa is increased after FBP, it suggests that sizes of uCa of this study falls in mid frequency range in Fourier domain. This finding may give us insight in designing optimal filter for FBP method.

4.4 Impacts of uCa Size on the Shape of CNR Profiles: From BP Images

In Figs. 11 and 12, we show CNR profiles of uCa of 180 μm and 300 μm sizes, in comparison the 240 μm uCa of Fig. 7, all from BP images. For the smaller 180 μm uCa, both the peak and the tail CNR values are lower than Fig. 7, as expected. The tails of CNR curves are indistinguishable among 11, 15, and 21 shots. For the larger 300 μm uCa, the tails of CNR curves are clearly separated among them, which suggest the 21 shot scan would have the least shadow artifacts. Therefore, we would emphasize here that the theoretical implication that the greater the projection number, the less the observable artifact intensity should still work under the following conditions: the uCa object has huge contrast over the background, or a very high dose is used in a scan. In both cases, the tail region of the CNR profile would separate from each other distinctly between 11-, 15, and 21 shots scans as showed by Fig. 12, since the noise in the data become relatively small. Only under such conditions, more projections could help the reduction of structure artifacts. Since the shadow's CNR is very high in this case, other nonlinear methods might be more efficient to reduce the shadow artifacts, rather than simply increasing the projection number.

4.5 Visual Comparison of Shadow Artifacts of uCa

In Fig.13, we use FBP images of uCa of two different sizes for visual examination of the artifact. The left uCa is the 240 um one shown in Fig. 7, while the right is the 300 um one in Fig. 12. Recon slices of 11, 15, and 21 shots and at z = 0, 10, 20, and 30 mm are displayed with the same background noise level for fair comparisons. For the left uCa, the shadow artifact of 11 shots is slightly worse than the 15 and 21 shots, with the later two being indistinguishable. For the right uCa, artifact of 11 shots is the worst, while that of 21 shots is the best. These image-based observations agree with previous discussions based on CNR ZLSF curves alone.

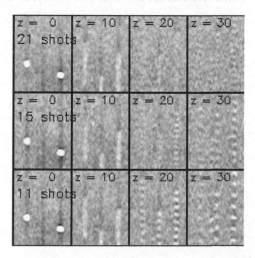

Fig. 13. Images of uCa at different z locations for 11, 15, and 21 shots. At the focused slice of Z = 0, the left uCa is 240 um one of Fig. 7, and the right is 300 um one of Fig. 12.

4.6 Advantage and Limitation of the CNR Based Method

CNR method is very simple and efficient method to evaluate the presence and the significance of artifacts in images, as shown by this paper. However in addition to the intensity, the shape and appearance of artifacts can also greatly affect the significance of its impact in an image, thus its dependence on projection numbers needs to be addressed. This is beyond the scope of the CNR based method discussed here, and will be an interesting subject for further study.

4.7 Conclusions

The study find that, [1] given a practical dose penalty tolerance limit, one can find the maximum projection number allowed for a tomosynthesis scan through simulation and measurement; [2] for small uCa, more projections makes insignificant difference in the CNR value of the shadow artifact, but for large uCa it help to reduce the shadow artifact under our test conditions. [3] for mass, more projections seems make insignificant difference in shadow artifact while the filtering of FBP will remove most of them; [4] the filtering in image reconstruction narrows down the potential benefit that more projection number would bring in term of artifact reduction thus advanced and optimal filter developed for tomosynthesis should allow scans with relative smaller projection numbers to fulfill the same task of artifact reduction.

References

1. J. M. Boone, and et al, Scatter/primary in mammography: Comprehensive results, Med. Phys., 27, p2408-2416, 2000.
2. Yorker JG, and et al, Characterization of a full-field digital mammography detector based on direct x-ray conversion in selenium, Proc. SPIE Vol. 4682, p. 21-29.

First Attempt at 3D X-Ray Visualization of DCIS (Ductal Carcinoma in Situ) Due to Refraction Contrast – In Good Relation to Pathological View

Masami Ando[1,2,3], Takao Akatsuka[4], Hiroko Bando[5], Yoshinori Chikaura[6],
Tokiko Endo[7], Eiko Hashimoto[3], Keiichi Hirano[2], Kazuyuki Hyodo[2], Shu Ichihara[8],
Anton Maksimenko[2], Chiho Ohbayashi[9], Hiroshi Sugiyama[2,3],
Ei Ueno[5], Katsuhito Yamasaki[10], and Tetsuya Yuasa[11]

[1] Institute of Science and Technology, Tokyo University of Science, Yamasaki 2641, Noda, Chiba 278-8510, Japan
[2] Photon Factory, IMSS, KEK, Oho 1-1, Tsukuba, Ibaraki 305-0801, Japan
[3] Department of Photo-Science, GUAS, Shonan, Hayama, Kanagawa 240-0193, Japan
[4] Faculty of Engineering, Yamagata University, Jonan 4-3-16, Yonezawa, Yamagata 992-8510, Japan
[5] Department of Breast-Thyroid-Endocrine Surgery, University of Tsukuba, Ibaraki 305-8573, Japan
[6] Medical Group, SPring-8, Koto 1-1-1, Mikazuki-Cho, Sayo-Gun, Hyogo 679-5198, Japan
[7] Department of Radiology, Nagoya Medical Center, National Hospital Organization, Nakaku 4-1-1, Nagoya 460-0001, Japan
[8] Department of Pathology, Nagoya Medical Center, National Hospital Organization, Nakaku 4-1-1, Nagoya 460-0001, Japan
[9] Department of Pathology, Kobe University, Kusunoki-Cho 7-5-2, Kobe, Hyogo 650-0017, Japan
[10] Institute of Genome, Kobe University, Kusunoki-Cho 7-5-2, Kobe, Hyogo 650-0017, Japan
[11] Faculty of Engineering, Yamagata University, Jonan 4-3-16, Yonezawa, Yamagata 992-8510, Japan
msm-ando@rs.noda.tus.ac.jp

Abstract. First 3D X-ray internal observation of DCIS (ductal carcinoma in-situ) is reported. Its rod shaped specimen with 3.6 mm in diameter and 4.7 mm in height was punched out to have successfully observed by using a newly made algorithm due to refraction for x-ray CT. Its data was acquired by the x-ray optics DEI (diffraction-enhanced imaging). Data of 900 projections with interval of 0.2 degrees was used at Photon Factory, KEK in Tsukuba. A reconstructed CT image may include clearly revealed ductus lactiferi, microcalcification and other structure. The voxel resolution is approximately 50 μm by the present instrumental condition. This modality could open up an x-ray pathological diagnosis.

Keywords: X-ray refraction, X-ray dark-field imaging (XDFI), DEI, breast cancer, DCIS, pathological diagnosis, clinical diagnosis, ductus lactiferi.

Susan M. Astley et al. (Eds.): IWDM 2006, LNCS 4046, pp. 525–532, 2006.
© Springer-Verlag Berlin Heidelberg 2006

1 Introduction

Mammography for early check is one of powerful screening modalities together with ultrasonography. Since the discovery of x-rays by Roentgen in 1895 all x-ray medical imaging at hospital including mammography in the world has been purely based on absorption contrast. Nevertheless limitation in their spatial resolution and contrast resolution exists in early detection. Since breast cancer is not necessarily visible with absorption contrast one may need alternative methodology of being able to visualize breast cancer with higher contrast and with higher spatial resolution.

So far a variety of imaging schemes for a phase object have been proposed [1], [2], [3], [4] (diffraction-enhanced imaging (DEI)), [5], [6], [7] and [8] (phase-interference (PIC)). Further x-ray dark-field imaging (XDFI) [9] was proposed. In order to see breast cancner following a pioneering work on imaging of breast cancer by Burattini's group [10] a trial to visualize breast cancer tissue has been performed by PCI [11], [12], DEI (diffraction-enhanced imaging) [13], [14], [15], PIC (phase-interference contrast) [16], the super magnification imaging (SMI)) [17], x-ray dark-field imaging (XDFI) [18] and XRF (x-ray fluorescence) [19].

Here we would like to propose a world first X-ray CT image that could be used for pathological diagnosis. Trial of 3D reconstruction has begun [20], [21], [22]. Maksimenko et al. have recently proposed a novel tomographic imaging protocol based on a physico-mathematically defined reconstruction algorithm [23], [24] with a paraxial-ray approximation in the domain of a geometrical optics. A satisfactory experimental result has been obtained. This has been applied to successfully visualize DCIS (ductal carcinoma in situ) with high contrast and high resolution [25].

2 Method

2.1 Mathematics

The refractive index can be described as $n = 1 - \tilde{n} + i\kappa$. κ of low atomic-number elements in soft tissue of biomedicine comprising hydrogen, carbon, nitrogen, and oxygen can not produce sufficient contrast because $\kappa \approx 0$. In case of visualizing such object with hard x-rays, for instance in clinical application, it is much more advantageous to detect variations of the propagation direction of incident x-rays using an analyzer with high angular sensitivity over conventional absorption contrast.

We start outlining the principle with the ray equation as follows:

$$d/ds\, n(r)t(r) = \nabla n(r) \tag{1}$$

where r is a spatial coordinate, $n(r)$ is a refractive index distribution, $t(r)$ is a unit tangential vector of ray propagation, and s is an arc length parameter. Executing the differentiation of LHS (light hand side),

$$n\frac{d\alpha}{ds}v + \frac{dn}{ds}t = \nabla n \tag{2}$$

$$\frac{d\tilde{n}}{ds} = \nabla\tilde{n} \cdot t \frac{d\alpha}{ds} = \nabla\tilde{n} \cdot v \tag{3}$$

$$\nabla\tilde{n}(r)\, t ds = \sum_{-\infty}^{\infty} |\nabla\tilde{n}(r_i)|cos\varphi(r_i) - \theta dq \approx 0 \tag{4}$$

$$\nabla\tilde{n}(r)\, v ds = \sum_{-\infty}^{\infty} |\nabla\tilde{n}(r_i)|sin\varphi(r_i) - \theta dq \approx \alpha(p,\theta) \tag{5}$$

where $r_i = p\ cos\theta - q\ sin\theta, p\ sin\theta + q\ cos\theta$, and $\varphi(r_i)$ is an angle between $\nabla\tilde{n}$ and the x-axis. From equations (4), (5), we obtain the following equation that is a complex-valued version of the Radon transform [26]:

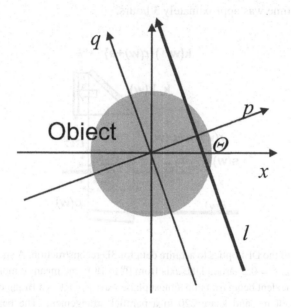

Fig. 1. Line integral projection of the 2-dimensional Radon transform

$$i\alpha(p,\theta)exp(i\theta) = \sum_{-\infty}^{\infty} |\nabla\tilde{n}(r_i)|exp(i\varphi(r_i))dq \tag{6}$$

where $r_i = p\ cos\theta - q\ sin\theta, p\ sin\theta + q\ cos\theta$, and $\varphi(r_i)$ is the angle between $\nabla\tilde{n}$ and the X-ray propagation direction. Fig. 1 shows the schematic drawing of this system.

Maksimenko et al. devised a complex-valued algorithm [23] of filtered back projection to solve the inverse problem, i.e., image recostruction from complex-valued projections that has led to the vector field $\nabla\tilde{n}$ and finally the refractive index distribution. In addition, they first succeeded experimental implementation of the algorithm to apply to reconstruct a simple structure [23] that happened to involve a small crack [24] otherwise not having been able to be visualized.

2.2 Experimental

The number of sample rotation for data acquisition in the experiment was 900. It took 200 msec ~ 1 sec for data acquisition of each frame, 2-5 seconds for data transfer to pc and 1 sec for sample rotation and additional 1 sec for stabilizing the system free from vibration due to motor. Every ten data acquisition the x-ray intensity by CCD was measured without specimen for the background subtraction. A CCD camera X-FDI 1.00:1 with air cooling type that has a view size of 8.7 mm (h) x 6.9 mm (v) was supplied by Photonic Science which is compatible with 16-bit and 1392 x 1040 pixels with pixel size of 6.3 μm x 6.6 μm. Data transfer was done by FireWire (IEEE 1394). After this series of measurement was done the angular position of the analyzer crystal was changed from either angle to continue the other series of measurement. In total the data acquisition time was approximately 3 hours.

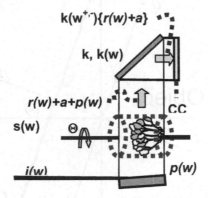

Fig. 2. Schematic of the DEI optics to acquire data for 3D reconstruction. A specimen s(w) DCIS was rotated every $\Delta \Theta = 0.2°$ around the axis from $0°$ to $180°$. mc means a monochro-collimator that converts the incident beam $i(w)$ into almost plane wave $p(w)$. k is a Bragg case analyzer. The diffracting planes of mc and k are 220 in a parallel arrangement. The beam carrying both information $r(w)$ due to refraction and a due to absorption of the sample has been analyzed by k with function of k(w). Two images both sides (+,-) of the flank of the rocking curve for each Θ in eq (6) are stored in a CCD camera.

The x-ray optics DEI [4] for 3D CT data acquisition was chosen because it has a smooth shape of both sides of the flank of the reflection curve of the angle analyzer. Extraction of information on refraction may need angularly well resolvable x-ray optics that can detect extremely small deflection angle at the order of a few times of 10^{-6} ~ 10^{-7}. Thus the X-ray optics DEI chosen is characterized by a double crystal arrangement with an asymmetric Bragg type monochro-collimator [27] that can produce highly parallel monochromatic incident X-ray onto specimen and a Bragg type angular analyzer k that can deliver the angular information from boundaries involved in the sample, as shown in Fig. 2. The angular information may include both the refraction information as well as the absorption information so that refraction component can be extracted by a mathematical procedure. each data set for a fixed angle Θ was taken at both wings of the rocking curve at $w = -0.5$ left and at $w = +0.5$ where w means the angular parameter and $w = 1$ covers the full angular range. A sample was remotely rotated with interval of $\Delta \Theta = 0.2°$. mc was asymmetrically cut Si(220) with $\alpha = 9.5$ where α is the angle between the surface and the diffracting planes. k was a symmetric Si(220) one. The energy used in the experiment was 11.7 keV. A specimen used in this experiment was a rod shaped ductal carcinoma in-situ (DCIS). Data was acquired on either flank of the rocking curve with a smooth slope.

3   Result

Thus a 3D image of the DCIS specimen was obtained [25]. A typical set of three images are shown in Fig. 3. One can easily discern calcification along each ductus lactiferi, calcification at each duct wall and some extension of calcification contrast toward outside ducts surrounding adipose tissue. The right bottom figure shows outer surface, while three others show each cross-section one shown in the right bottom figure. High contrast is seen in the center of ductus lactiferi. These areas are considered as

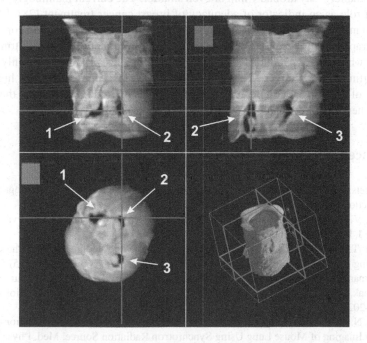

Fig. 3. Reconstructed 3D image of a DCIS is shown in the right bottom, x-z cross section in the right top, y-z cross section in the top left and the x-y cross section in the left bottom. These show three ductus lactiferi with numbers 1, 2 and 3. In almost all of them are seen microcalcification and higher contrast at each fringe and finally extension of carcinoma.

calcification. Low contrast areas are seen adjacent to calcification area. These are considered as necrotic ones. Higher contrast areas are seen surrounding outside of low contrast necrotic areas. These are considered as cancer cell layer spreading inside milk ducts. High contrast linear area or net like area are seen outside milk duct. These structures are considered as cancer cell area in interstitial tissue. Especially #3 ductus lactiferi seen in the left bottom image is almost closed. Further one can easily recognize that most of ductus lactiferis hold fringes surrounding ducts. These white structure means more electron density. Even as their extension carcinoma with irregular shape is clearly shown.

4 Discussion

Pathological diagnosis is under way so that good correlation between x-ray view and pathological view can be highly expected. Mammography is of quite significance in order to discover breast cancer at its early stage as possible; the size of the cancer which is discovered by the current technique is bigger than 5 mm. By further development of the technique described in this note the size of cancer to be able to be found out could be much smaller ~ say around 1 mm or even smaller. The current mammography has an important role as an indicator of adequacy of breast cancer treatment [28], [29]. Also magnified mammography seems far useful to recognize tumor extent than conventional mammography [30] because higher spatial resolution better than 50 μm can be expected while the conventional absorption one with less contrast can only provide with 50 μm or even larger. Then refraction based mammography has high grade potential of diagnosis compared to conventional mammography and the system proposed here could open an x-ray pathological tool.

References

1. Podurets, K. M., Somenkov, V. A. and Shil'shtein, S. Sh.: Neutron Radiography with Refraction Contrast. Physica, B156 & 157 (1989) 691-693
2. Ingal, V. N., and Beliaevskaya, E. A.: X-ray Plane-Wave Topography Observation of the Phase J. Phys. D: Appl. Phys. 28 (1995) 2314-2317
3. Davis, T. J., Gao, D. Gureyev, T. E. Stevenson, A. W. and Wilkins, S. W.: Phase-contrast Imaging of Weakly Absorbing Materials Using Hard X-rays. Nature 373 (1995) 595-598
4. Chapman, D., Thomlinson, W. Johnston, R. E., Washburn, D. Pisano, E. Gmur, N. Zhong, Z. Menk, R. Arfelli, F. Sayers, D.: Diffraction Enhanced Imaging. Phys. Me. Biol. 42 (1997) 2015-2025
5. Yagi, N. Suzuki, Y. Umetani, K. Kohmura, Y. and Yamasaki, K.: Refraction-enhanced X-ray Imaging of Mouse Lung Using Synchrotron Radiation Source. Med. Phys. 26 (1999) 2190-2193
6. Hirano, K., Maksimenko, A. Sugiyama, H. and Ando, M.: X-Ray Optics for Observing Dark-Field and Bright-Field Refraction-Contrast Images. Jpn. J. Appl. Phys. 41 (2002) L595-L598

7. Maksimenko, A., Sugiyama, H. Hirano, K. Yuasa, T. and Ando, M.: Dark-Field Imaging Using an X-Ray Asymmetric Bragg Case Transmission Analyzer Meas. Science and Technology, 15 (2004) 1251-1254

8. Momose, A.: Demonstration of phase-contrast X-ray computer tomography using an X-ray Interferometer. Nuclear Instruments and Methods in Physics Research A 352 (1995) 622-628

9. Ando, M., Sugiyama, H. Maksimenko, A. Pattanasiriwisawa, W. and Hyodo, K.: Simple X Ray Dark- and Bright- Field Imaging Using Achromatic Laue Optics. Jpn. J. Appl. Phys. 41 (2002) L1016-L1018

10. Burattini, E., Cossu, E. Maggio, C. Di. Gambaccini, M. Indovina, P. L. Marziani, M. Pocek, M. Simeoni, S. and Simonetti, G.: Mammography with Synchrotron Radiation. Radiology, 195 (1995) 239-244

11. Johnston, R.E., Washburn, D. Pisano, E. Burns, C. Thomlinson, W.C. Chapman, L.D. Arfelli, F. Gmur, N.F. Zhong, Z. and Sayers, D.: Mammographic Phantom Studies with Synchrotron Radiation. Radiology, 200 (1996) 659-663

12. Chapman, D., Pisano, E. Thomlinson, W. Zhong, Z. Johnston, R. E. Washburn, D. and Sayers, D.: Breast Disease. 10 (1998) 197

13. Michiel, M. Di., Olivo, A. Tromba, G. Arfelli, F. Bonvicini, V. Bravin, A. Cantatore, G. Castelli, E. DallaPalma, L. Longo, R. Pani, S. Pontoni, D. Poropat, P. Prest, M. Rashevsky, A. Vacchi, A. Vallazza, E.: Phase Contrast Imaging in the Field of Mammography. Medical Applications of Synchrotron Radiation, (Ando, M. & Uyama, C. eds.) Springer-Verlag, Tokyo, (1998) 78-82

14. Arfelli, F., Bonvicini, V. Bravin, A. Cantatore, G. Castelli, E. DallaPalma, L. Michiel, M. Di. Fabrizioli, M. Longo, R. Menk, R. H. Olovis, A. Pani, S. Pontoni, D. Poropat, P. Prest, M. Rashevsky, A. Ratti, M. Rigon, L. Tromba, G. Vacchi, A. Vallazza, E. and Zanconati, F.: Radiology 215 (2000) 286

15. Hasnah, M.O., Zhong, Z. Oltulu, O. Pisano, E. Johnson, R.E. Sayers, D. Thomlinson W. and Chapman, D.: Diffraction Enhanced Imaging Contrast Mechanisms in Breast Cancer Specimens. Med. Phys. 29 (2002) 2216-2221

16. Takeda, T., Wu, J. Tsuchiya, Y. Yoneyama, A. Lwin, T. T. Aiyoshi, Y. Zeniya, T. Hyodo, K. and Ueno, E.: Interferometric X-ray Imaging of Breast Cancer Specimens at 51 keV X-ray Energy. J. J. Appl. Phys. 43 (2004) 5652-5656

17. Toyofuku, F., Higashida, Y. Tokumori, K. Yoshida, A. Matsumoto, M. Ideguchi, T. Hyodo, K. Ando, M.: J. J. Med. Phys. 23, Supp.3 (2003) 127

18. Ando, M., Yamasaki, K., Toyofuku, F., Sugiyama, H., Ohbayashi, C., Li, G.., Pan, L., Jiang, X., Pattanasiriwisawa, W., Shimao, D., Hashimoto, E., Kimura, T., Tsuneyoshi, M., Ueno, E., Tokumori, K., Maksimenko, A. and Higashida, Y.: Attempt at Visualizing Breast Cancer with X-ray Dark Field Imaging. Jpn. J. Appl. Phys. 44 (2005) L528-L531

19. Ando, M., Yamasaki, K. Ohbayashi, C. Esumi, H. Li, G. Maksimenko, M. and Kawai, T.: Attempt at 2D Mapping of X-ray Fluorescence from Breast Cancer Tissue. Jpn. J. Appl. Phys. 44 (2005) L998-L1001

20. Dilmanian, F. A., Zhong, Z., Ren, B., Wu, X. Y., Chapman, D., Orion, I. and Thomlinson, W. C.: Phys. Med. Biol. 45 (1999) 933

21. Pagot E, Fielder S, Cloetens P, Bravin A, Coan P, Fezzaa K, Baruchel J, Hartwing: J Phys Med Biol 50 (2005) 709-724

22. Sera T, Uesugi K, Yagi N.: Refraction-enchanced Tomography of Mouse and Rabbit Lungs. Med. Phys. 32 (2005) 2787-2792

23. Maksimenko, A., Ando, M. Sugiyama, H. Yuasa, T.: Computed Tomographic Reconstruction Based on X-Ray Refraction Contrast Appl. Phys. Lett. 86 (2005) 124105-1~124105-3

24. Maksimenko, A., Ando, M. Sugiyama, H. Hashimoto, E.: Possibility of Computed Tomographic Reconstruction of Cracks from the X-ray Refraction Contrast. Jpn. J. Appl. Phys. 44 (2005) L633-L635

25. Ando, M., Maksimenko, A., Yuasa, T., Hashimoto, E., Yamasaki, K., Ohbayashi, C., Sugiyama, H., Hyodo, K., Kimura, T., Esumi, H., Akatsuka, T., Li, G., Xian D. and Ueno, E.: 2D and 3D Visualization of Ductal Carcinoma in situ (DCIS) due to X-Ray Refraction Contrast, Bioimages 13 (2006) 1-7

26. Kaka, A. C., and Slaney, M.: Principles of Computerized Tomographic Imaging, IEEE Press, New York (1988)

27. Kohra, K.: An Application of Asymmetric Reflection for Obtaining X-ray Beams of Extremely Narrow Angular Spread. J. Phys. Soc. Jpn. 17 (1962) 589-590

28. Sadowsky, N.L., Semine, A. Harris, J.R.: Cancer 65 (1990) 2113

29. Gluck, B.S. Dershaw, D.D. Liberman L. Deutch, B. M.: Radiology 188 (1993) 469

30. Marrow, M., Schmidt, R. Hassett, C.: Surgery 118 (1995) 621

Lossless Compression of Digital Mammograms

R. Visser, L. Oostveen, and N. Karssemeijer

National Expert and Training Centre for Breast Cancer Screening, Radboud University
Nijmegen Medical Centre, LRCB 577, P.O. Box 9101, 6500 HB Nijmegen, The Netherlands
r.visser@lrcb.umcn.nl

Abstract. The file size of images generated using digital mammography systems varies between 8 MB and 50 MB. The amount of data to be stored in digital screening programs is huge. Image compression may be helpful. In this
study 8491 digital and digitised mammography images are compressed using 14
lossless compression schemes. The results show that using lossless image compression, the total amount of data to be stored can be reduced by a factor of 1.3
to 6.9 without loss of image quality. The actual data reduction depends strongly
on the selected compression algorithm and the systems used to acquire and
process the mammograms. The JPEG-LS and JPEG 2000 algorithms, both included in the DICOM standard, prove to be promising algorithms for screening
programs because of the high compression ratios.

1 Background

For the design of the digital infrastructure for a population based breast cancer screening program, accurate data is required. The total amount of image data will have to be
known in order to determine the feasibility of archiving and communication solutions.

The amount of image data can be reduced by applying image compression. Multiple
studies on the compression of digitally stored medical images are known from literature [1,2,3,4]. From these studies it can be concluded that the achievable compression
ratio depends strongly on the image type. In these studies however, a very limited
number of digital mammography images was used. Therefore up to now there was no
reliable information on the achievable compression ratios for digital mammograms.

The purpose of this study is to quantify the possibilities for reducing the required
storage and network capacity by the usage of lossless image compression both for
digital and for digitised mammograms. This data can then be used in the planning
phase for the digitisation of screening programs for determining the required network
capacity and storage space.

2 Method

2.1 Data Set

For digital mammograms the achievable compression ratio will depend on system
properties like detector size and resolution, noise, homogeneity of the background and

Susan M. Astley et al. (Eds.): IWDM 2006, LNCS 4046, pp. 533–540, 2006.

Table 1. Number of images for each system and the specifications for the image types used

System	Detector size (cm)[1]	Pixel size (μm)	# Raw	# Proc	File size (MB)
Agfa Embrace DM1000	17.9 x 23.3	70	-[4,5]	-[4]	16.3
	23.3 x 28.7		88[5]	196	26.0
Fuji Profect CS	17.7 x 23.7	50	361[7]	361	32.0
	23.6 x 29.6		40[7]	40	53.5
GE Senograph 2000D	19.1 x 22.9[2]	100[2]	1324	1363	8.4
IMS Giotto Image MD	16.3 x 22.8	81	542	543	10.8
Kodak DirectView CR950	17.6 x 23.4	49	263	263	32.7
Lorad Selenia	17.9 x 23.3	70	234[5]	326	16.3
	23.3 x 28.7		24[5]	36	26.0
R2 ImageChecker	15.7 x 23.7[3]	100	1212	-[6]	7.1[3]
Sectra Microdose	23.9 x 26.2	49	362[7]	357	49.7
Siemens Novation DR	17.9 x 23.3	70	6[5]	5	16.3
	23.3 x 28.7		268[5]	277	26.0
			4724	3767	

[1] The *Imager Pixel Spacing* as specified in the DICOM header was used to determine the detector size.

[2] In the DICOM header of part of the GE-images the *Imager Pixel Spacing* was specified to be 94 micron, in the others it was specified to be 100 micron. The detector size was calculated using an *Imager Pixel* Spacing of 100 micron.

[3] Because the scanned films were taken from an anonimised database, the patient labels had been cut from the images. Therefore the average image width was 15.7 cm in stead of the usual 18 cm. If the images had not been anonimised the file size would have been about 8 MB.

[4] On the Agfa system at the BBNN only the full detector size is used. Therefore no images with the small detector size were available and the total amount of data stored is larger.

[5] The Agfa, Lorad and Siemens systems use equal detectors. Therefore for the unprocessed images only differences in compression ratio's due to differences in the image sizes of the collected images are to be expected.

[6] Although it would be good practise to optimise the digitised images for displaying, no processing was performed here.

[7] The unprocessed Fuji and Sectra images are usually not available, but were made available by the manufacturers specifically for this project.

the image processing performed. Also image specific factors like the size and complexity of the breast will influence compression efficiency. In order to determine the system dependency as accurate as possible, the influence of the image specific factors on the measured compression ratio must be limited as much as possible. Therefore for each manufacturer a large number of images was collected. The data set for this study contains 8491 processed and unprocessed images from 9 systems of different manufacturers (Table 1).

The Fuji and Kodak systems are CR systems, the R2 system is used for digitising analogue film, the other systems are DR systems. For the Agfa system only a limited number of unprocessed images was collected. But since this system uses the same detector as the Lorad and Siemens systems, it is to be expected that the compression results for the unprocessed images will be equal for these systems. A difference between the images from these systems is however that only for the Lorad system the option to use only part of the detector for the imaging of smaller breasts was used on a regular basis. This causes the average file size for the (uncompressed) Lorad images to be much smaller.

The digitised images used originate from an anonimised database. Because in the anonimisation process the patient information was cut from the images, these images are on average about 10% smaller than they would usually be.

2.2 Compression Algorithms

Image data can either be compressed lossless or lossy. When using lossless compression and decompression algorithms, the decompressed image will be identical to the original image. When using lossy compression the compressed image does not contain all information required to decompress the image without loss of information. For some compression algorithms the maximum deviation in pixel values after decompression can be chosen in advance of the image compression [2]. Although this allows for achieving higher compression rates by neglecting details that are barely discernable to the human eye or are not clinically relevant, in this study only lossless compression was examined. Due to the legal objections against lossy compression, extensive research on the influence of lossy image compression on the diagnostic quality of digital mammograms will be required before it can be decided if such compression could be allowed.

In this study all lossless compression algorithms currently included in the DICOM (Digital Imaging and Communications in Medicine) standard [5] are examined. Further, three commonly used or promising general compression algorithms were examined. This was done in order to check if by keeping part of the imaging chain outside the DICOM standard, substantial further data reduction could be achieved.

2.2.1 General Purpose Compression Algorithms
An extensive set of compression algorithms is available today. Some algorithms are only suitable for compressing specific types of data such as still images, video data or fax data, the others are the general purpose compression algorithms. This study uses:

- **ZLIB.** Commonly used programs like WinZip (Windows) and gzip (Unix) use the ZLIB library. This algorithm was selected because it is easily available for all common operating systems. Therefore it could be applied right away. For this study gzip version 1.3.5 (http://www.gzip.org) was used, with default settings.
- **BZIP.** The BZIP algorithm is a block sorting algorithm. It was selected because it is freely available and showed promising results in another study on the compression of medical images from several modalities[5]. For this study bzip2 version 1.0.2 (http://www.bzip.org) was used, with default settings.
- **7Z.** This algorithm was selected because it is freely available and its predecessor (UFA) showed promising results in another study on the compression of medical images from several modalities[5]. For this study 7za version 4.14 beta (http://www.7-zip.org) was used.

2.2.2 Algorithms Included in the DICOM Standard

Five lossless compression methods have been included in the DICOM standard. The advantage of using one of these algorithms is that the compressed images still are DICOM images. Therefore they are exchangeable (over a network) between DICOM systems, without the need to decompress them first. These five algorithms were all included in this study:

- **Deflated Little Endian.** This algorithm was added to the DICOM standard in May 2001 and is based on the ZLIB library. The difference with the compression method in section 2.2.1 is that in this case the zip-file header is not stored. In stead of this it has to be indicated in the DICOM header that the transfer syntax is 'Deflated Little Endian'. In this case however the DICOM header itself is not compressed. The difference between these two methods is therefore expected to be negligible. For this study the program 'dcmconv' included in the Offis DICOM Toolkit v3.5.3 (http://dicom.offis.de/dcmtk) was used for encoding and decoding of the images.
- **Run Length Encoding.** This algorithm was used originally for compressing data streams like fax data. An advantage of this algorithm is that it is extremely simple and can usually be performed in real time. This algorithm converts consecutive equal symbols into a value with a length indicator. It is especially useful for the compression of data containing many equal values like fax data (only a limited part of the data contains grey values, most of it is white). Since this algorithm does not used the 2 dimensional properties of the images, the expected compression ratios are not particularly high. The implementations used in this study for encoding and decoding are the programs 'dcmcrle' and 'dcmdrle' included in the Offis DICOM Toolkit v3.5.3 (http://dicom.offis.de/dcmtk).
- **JPEG.** This commonly used image compression algorithm was added to the DICOM standard in 1994 and can be used both for lossless and lossy image compression [6]. For the lossless version, seven settings (selection values) can be chosen. All of those were examined in this study. The implementations used in this study for encoding and decoding are the programs 'dcmcjpeg' and 'dcmdjpeg' included in the Offis DICOM Toolkit v3.5.3 (http://dicom.offis.de/dcmtk). The lossless implementation in this version of the toolkit turned out to contain bugs,

causing the compression to be lossy. By making several adjustments it was still possible to do lossless compression and determine the correct compression ratio using this software.

- **JPEG-LS.** This algorithm was included in the DICOM standard in September 2000, and was specifically developed for lossless and near-lossless compression [7]. Just the fully lossless compression scheme was examined in this study. Because implementations of the JPEG-LS algorithm are not widespread yet, a general implementation had to be used (without DICOM functionality). Therefore the compressed images had to be encapsulated in a valid DICOM header afterwards. For this study a JPEG-LS implementation by David Clunie was used (http://www.dclunie.com/jpegls.html).

- **JPEG 2000.** This algorithm was included in the DICOM standard early 2002. It is a modern compression algorithm based on wavelet technology. The JPEG 2000 standard [8] facilitates both lossless and lossy compression. It even makes it possible to make images (or parts of images) available in a resolution or quality that differs from the original, creating new possibilities for e.g. tele-radiology. In this study, just the lossless compression and decompression were examined. Like JPEG-LS, also for JPEG 2000 a general implementation without DICOM functionality had to be used. For this study the JPEG 2000 functionality in version 0.97 of the OpenJPEG library (http://www.openjpeg.org) was used.

2.2.3 Data Integrity Check

In order to guarantee that all compression algorithms used are truly lossless, all compressed images in this study have been decompressed and compared to the original images on a pixel by pixel basis.

3 Results

Table 2 shows the compression results for the seven individual selection values of the JPEG algorithm. The values for the JPEG compression in Table 3 are the compression ratios when using the most efficient selection value for each image type. From Table 3 it can be seen that for almost all image types the most efficient compression methods are JPEG-LS and JPEG 2000. Just for the processed Fuji images BZIP is more efficient. When using the JPEG algorithm (Table 2), for most image types selection value 7 is slightly more efficient than the other selection values.

The compression ratios measured for the unprocessed Agfa, Lorad and Siemens images listed in Table 3 are similar. Although these manufacturers all use the same detector, this is remarkable. All Agfa images collected and almost all Siemens images were acquired using the large detector size, while most of the Lorad images were acquired using the small detector size (Table 1). Apparently the background can not be compressed more efficiently than the area containing medical information.

Comparing the compression ratios for processed and unprocessed images in Table 3, it becomes clear that for the DR systems for most compression algorithms the compression efficiency either remains equal or increases due to image processing. For the CR systems the compression efficiency decreases due to image processing.

Table 2. Compression ratios for the seven selection values of the JPEG algorithm and the average size after compressing using the most effective compression algorithm

image type		number of images	average file size original images (MB)	compression ratio JPEG							average size after using most efficient compression algorithm (MB)
				sv1	sv2	sv3	sv4	sv5	sv6	sv7	
Agfa	raw	88	26.0	2.0	2.0	1.9	1.9	1.9	2.0	2.0	12.8
	proc	196	26.0	2.7	2.7	2.6	2.5	2.6	2.6	2.8	9.4
Fuji	raw	401	34.1	4.9	4.9	4.9	4.5	4.8	4.8	5.1	6.6
	proc	401	34.1	3.9	3.8	3.8	3.6	3.7	3.7	3.9	8.8
GE	raw	1324	8.4	3.6	3.7	3.5	3.7	3.7	3.7	3.8	2.2
	proc	1363	8.4	4.3	4.3	4.1	4.3	4.4	4.4	4.5	1.9
IMS	raw	542	10.8	3.4	3.5	3.4	3.3	3.4	3.5	3.6	3.0
	proc	543	10.8	3.4	3.4	3.4	3.2	3.3	3.3	3.5	3.1
Kodak	raw	263	32.7	3.5	3.7	3.4	3.5	3.6	3.7	3.8	8.6
	proc	263	32.7	2.8	3.0	2.8	2.8	2.8	2.9	3.0	11.0
Lorad	raw	258	17.2	2.0	2.0	2.0	1.9	2.0	2.0	2.1	8.4
	proc	362	17.2	3.2	3.1	3.1	3.1	3.1	3.1	3.2	5.4
R2 digitiser	raw	1212	7.1	2.2	2.0	2.0	2.2	2.2	2.1	2.2	3.2
Sectra	raw	362	49.7	1.8	1.8	1.7	1.8	1.8	1.9	1.9	26.7
	proc	357	49.7	4.5	4.5	4.4	4.5	4.5	4.5	4.6	10.9
Siemens	raw	274	25.8	1.9	1.9	1.9	1.8	1.8	1.8	1.9	13.5
	proc	282	25.8	4.5	4.5	4.4	4.3	4.4	4.4	4.6	5.7

Table 3. Compression ratios for all algorithms and the average size after compressing using the most effective compression algorithm

image type		number of images	average file size original images (MB)	compression ratio									average size after using most efficient compression algorithm (MB)
				not included in DICOM standard			included in DICOM standard					
				zlib	bzip2	7zip	deflated little endian	RLE	JPEG	JPEG-LS	JPEG 2000	
Agfa	raw	88	26.0	1.4	1.9	1.8	1.4	1.5	2.0	**2.2**	2.2	12.0
	proc	196	26.0	1.8	2.7	2.4	1.8	1.8	2.8	2.9	**2.9**	9.0
Fuji	raw	401	34.1	3.5	6.2	5.3	3.5	3.1	5.1	6.8	**6.9**	5.0
	proc	401	34.1	3.9	**6.0**	5.1	3.9	3.3	3.9	5.2	5.2	5.7
GE	raw	1324	8.4	2.8	4.2	3.9	2.8	3.3	3.8	**5.0**	4.9	1.7
	proc	1363	8.4	3.3	5.4	4.8	3.3	3.5	4.5	6.0	**6.0**	1.4
IMS	raw	542	10.8	2.6	3.9	3.6	2.6	3.0	3.6	**4.5**	4.4	2.4
	Proc	543	10.8	3.1	**4.5**	4.1	3.1	2.9	3.5	4.5	4.4	2.4
Kodak	raw	263	32.7	2.1	3.6	3.1	2.1	2.0	3.8	4.1	**4.2**	7.7
	proc	263	32.7	1.8	2.9	2.6	1.8	2.0	3.0	3.2	**3.2**	10.1
Lorad	raw	258	17.2	1.4	2.0	1.9	1.4	1.5	2.1	2.2	**2.2**	7.8
	proc	362	17.2	2.9	4.1	3.6	2.9	2.7	3.2	**4.2**	4.1	4.1
R2 digitiser	raw	1212	7.1	1.4	2.1	1.9	1.4	1.7	2.2	2.3	**2.3**	3.1
Sectra	raw	362	49.7	1.3	1.7	1.6	1.3	1.3	1.9	**1.9**	1.9	25.6
	proc	357	49.7	4.7	6.3	5.6	4.7	3.9	4.6	**6.5**	6.3	7.7
Siemens	raw	274	25.8	1.4	1.9	1.7	1.3	1.4	1.9	2.1	**2.1**	12.5
	proc	282	25.8	4.1	6.1	5.4	4.1	4.3	4.6	6.5	**6.5**	3.9

4 Discussion and Conclusions

The amount of (compressed) data generated depends strongly on the system, and should be taken into account when choosing one or more systems for usage within a screening program. By using lossless compression the size of mammography images can effectively be reduced. JPEG-LS and JPEG 2000 prove to be the most efficient algorithms. The choice for a specific algorithm depends among others on the required compression speed. Although not discussed in this paper, the JPEG 2000 implementation used turned out to be much slower than the JPEG-LS algorithm. This is probably caused by the complexity of the JPEG 2000 algorithm, which offers additional functionality for retrieving images or even parts of images at a lower image quality. This opens new possibilities for tele-radiologic purposes, but slows down the compression. The results of this study show that for some image types the image background can not be compressed more efficiently than the breast area. In order to improve the compression efficiency, it would make sense to homogenise the image background. For some image types the background is already homogenised by the image processing or due to the acquisition process. This may be one of the causes for the differences in achievable compression ratio found in this study. It would be interesting to see how much the compression efficiency would increase for the other images if the backgrounds are homogenised for all images in advance of compression.

References

1. A. Przelaskowski, "Compression of mammograms for medical practise", 2004 ACM Symposium on Applied Computing, 249-253, 2004.
2. D. Clunie, "Lossless Compression of Grayscale Medical Images – Effectiveness of Traditional and State of the Art Approaches" in Proc. SPIE (Medical Imaging), vol. 3980, Feb. 2000.
3. S. M. Perlmutter et al., "Image quality in lossy compressed digital mammograms", Signal Processing, vol. 59, pp. 189-210, June 1997.
4. J. Kivijärvi et al., "A comparison of lossless compression methods for medical images", Computerized Medical Imaging and Graphics, vol. 22, 323-339, 1998.
5. NEMA Standards Publication PS 3.5, Digital Imaging and Communications in Medicine (DICOM), Part 5: Data Structures and Encoding, National Electrical Manufacturers Association, 2004.
6. ISO/IS 10918-1, Digital compression and coding of continuous-tone still images: Requirements and guidelines, 1994.
7. ISO/IS 14495-1, Lossless and near-lossless compression of continuous-tone still images-baseline, 2000.
8. ISO/IS 15444-1, JPEG 2000 image coding system - Core coding system, 2002.

Capturing Microcalcification Patterns in Dense Parenchyma with Wavelet-Based Eigenimages

Nikolaos Arikidis, Spyros Skiadopoulos, Filippos Sakellaropoulos,
George Panayiotakis, and Lena Costaridou

Department of Medical Physics, School of Medicine,
University of Patras, 265 00 Patras, Greece
costarid@upatras.gr, panayiot@upatras.gr

Abstract. A method is proposed based on the combination of wavelet analysis and principal component analysis (PCA). Microcalcification (MC) candidate regions are initially labeled using area and contrast criteria. Mallat's redundant dyadic wavelet transform is used to analyze the frequency content of image patterns at horizontal and vertical directions. PCA is used to efficiently encode MC patterns in wavelet-decomposed images. Feature weights are computed from the projection of each candidate MC pattern at the wavelet-based principal components. To assess the effectiveness of the proposed method, the same analysis is carried out in original images. Candidate MC patterns are classified by means of Linear Discriminant Analysis (LDA). Free-response Receiver Operating Characteristic (FROC) curves are produced for identifying MC clusters. The highest performance is obtained when PCA is applied in wavelet decomposed images achieving 80% sensitivity at 0.5 false positives per image in a dataset with 50 subtle MC clusters in dense parenchyma.

1 Background

Mammography is currently the technique with the highest sensitivity available for early detection of breast cancer on asymptomatic women [1]. Detection of early signs of disease, such as microcalcifications (MCs), with screening mammography, is a particularly demanding task for radiologists. This is mainly attributed to the low MC contrast resolution, resulting from their small size [2]. These limitations have provided the basis for the development of Computer-Aided Detection (CAD) systems with high performance characteristics [3], [4], representing one of the most successful paradigms in medical image analysis. However, performance of such systems in case of dense tissue is challenged by the high correlation between fibroglandular tissue patches and MCs, resulting in increased false positive (FP) rate [5], [6].

One approach in CAD systems for MC detection is the use of the wavelet transform framework to analyze MCs based on their high frequency content. However, a large component of the power in a mammogram, at high spatial frequencies, is also noise, mainly originating from the inhomogeneous background of dense tissue structures, resulting in poor MC signal-to-noise ratio (SNR) [7]. Netch *et al.* [8], based on the circularly symmetric Gaussian model achieved 84% sensitivity with 1 average FP per image, using a Laplacian kernel to detect MCs as local maxima

Susan M. Astley et al. (Eds.): IWDM 2006, LNCS 4046, pp. 541–548, 2006.
© Springer-Verlag Berlin Heidelberg 2006

at different frequency bands. Strickland *et al.* [9] have shown that the average 2D gray level profile of MCs is well described by a circularly symmetric Gaussian function. Since the optimum detector of Gaussian functions is the Laplacian of Gaussian, a wavelet filter close to the Laplacian of Gaussian was used to detect significant peak responses for objects of similar shape and size as the Gaussian filter. Soft or hard thresholding was used to set the low amplitude wavelet coefficients to zero, obtaining 70% sensitivity with 1 FP per image in a varying subtlety of MC clusters. Yoshida *et al.* [10] used an undecimated wavelet transform for MC detection achieving 78% sensitivity with 0.5 average FPs per image in a dataset with subtle MCs. Drexl *et al.* [11] used the continuous wavelet transform and features based on the evolution of the wavelet coefficients across scales. At 0.5 FP per image the sensitivity achieved was approximately 85%. Qian *et al.* [12] used a tree structured wavelet transform for multiresolution decomposition and a non-linear filter for suppressing image noise, achieving 94% sensitivity with 1.6 average FP per image. The aforementioned methods have been tested in image datasets of various types of breast parenchyma including dense tissue, with the exception of Lado *et al.* [13], who has worked on dense parenchyma, yielding 2.2 FPs per image with 73% sensitivity.

The aim of this study is to efficiently encode MC patterns analyzed by combining Principal Component Analysis (PCA) and wavelet decomposition. The capability of a feature vector based on this analysis is demonstrated in a detection task of subtle MC clusters embedded in dense parenchyma. To assess the effectiveness of the proposed MC cluster encoding method, the same analysis is carried out in original images.

2 Method

2.1 Labeling of Candidate MC Regions

MCs are very small structures visible as bright spots in the mammogram because their mass attenuation coefficient is higher than any other structure in the breast. However, due to the growth of MCs, there is no absolute lower bound to their contrast. Very small MCs may have low contrast relative to their background, which is sometimes close to structure noise originating mainly from fibroglandular tissue patches.

MC candidate regions are initially labeled using contrast and area criteria. In this study, pixel contrast is measured on a local basis, exploiting wavelet analysis [14]. Specifically, pixel contrast is defined as the difference between the pixel foreground and background maps normalized by their sum. The foreground pixel map corresponds to gray level values of the original image. The background pixel map corresponds to the gray level values of a low-pass filtered image. A contrast threshold of 0.5% is selected to preserve subtle MCs in dense parenchyma and an area threshold of 1.2 mm^2 to eliminate image components, which are likely to be macrocalcifications or line structures. Breast border identification is obtained with an edge detection technique based on the magnitudes of the derivative of a Gaussian operator.

2.2 Extraction of Feature Vector

A common approach of computerized MC detection methods is based on a two-stage process utilizing image feature extraction and subsequent classification to reduce FPs.

Morphological, textural and spectral characteristics are used to access MC properties [3], [15]. The wavelet transform analyzes spectral information while preserving spatial information. PCA is applied on wavelet coefficients to provide efficient encoding of MC patterns at different frequency bands and orientations.

In this study, wavelet image decomposition is performed with Mallat's redundant dyadic wavelet transform. When the wavelet filter is selected as the second derivative of the signal smoothed at scale j, the local maxima corresponds to high curvatures [16]. Gaussian functions, like MCs, are high curvature components at both horizontal and vertical directions capable of differentiating them from line-like structures. MCs are highly correlated with the wavelet coefficients W_{2^j} at dyadic scales $j=2,3$ [10], [17], [18]. Following MC candidate region identification, local maxima of 2nd scale wavelet coefficients of these regions are used to estimate the center of MC patterns. Each MC pattern is mapped to four representations, which are the horizontal and vertical wavelet coefficients at the 2nd and 3rd dyadic scale. When the wavelet transform is combined with PCA, the wavelet coefficients at scale j are used instead of using the pixel values.

Let a MC pattern be a two-dimensional array $[v,v]$, considered as an one-dimensional vector with length $N=v \times v$. If L is the number of training MC patterns, we consider matrix $\mathbf{D}$ with L rows and N columns. Let $\mathbf{M}$ the vector of mean column values of matrix $\mathbf{D}$. A normalized matrix $\mathbf{D}'$ is constructed by subtracting the elements of $\mathbf{M}$ from the corresponding elements of each row of $\mathbf{D}$. The covariance matrix $\mathbf{C}$ of $\mathbf{D}'$ is computed:

$$\mathbf{C} = \mathbf{D}'^{\mathbf{T}} \cdot \mathbf{D}' \qquad (1)$$

where $\mathbf{D}'^{\mathbf{T}}$ is the transpose matrix of $\mathbf{D}'$ of size $N \times N$. The principal components (eigenimages) $\mathbf{A}_k$ (k: number of principal components) of $\mathbf{D}'$ are computed from the covariance matrix $\mathbf{C}$. When wavelet representations are used, the principal components $\mathbf{A}_k$, named wavelet MC eigenimages, are computed for each representation. A feature vector $\mathbf{F}_k$ is composed of the projections (weights) of the unknown wavelet decomposed pattern $\mathbf{U}$ at the wavelet-based principal components $\mathbf{A}_k$:

$$\mathbf{F}_k = \mathbf{U} \cdot \mathbf{A}_k \qquad (2)$$

Principal components characterize most of the variability of the training dataset $\mathbf{D}$ of MC patterns, by means of mean square error (MSE) minimization [19]. Unknown patterns can be differentiated by comparing their weights to those of known training classes, as proposed by Turk *et al.* [20].

The training dataset $\mathbf{D}$ used for the generation of the MC principal components consists of 41 individual subtle MC patterns, indicated by an expert radiologist. These patterns were selected from dense mammograms (density 3 and 4 of ACR BIRADS) originating from the Digital Database for Screening Mammography (DDSM).

2.3 MC Cluster Detection

Linear Discriminant Analysis (LDA) is used to classify MC patterns in three classes – individual MCs, film artifacts and fibroglandular tissue. The training dataset of the

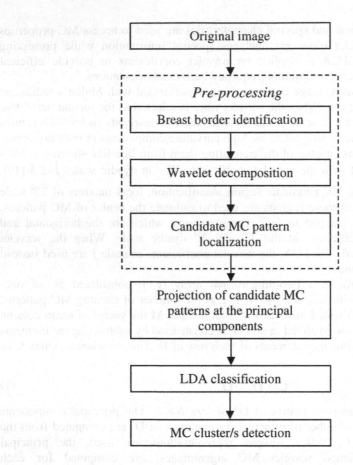

Fig. 1. MC cluster detection in wavelet-decomposed images

classifier consists of 60 MCs, 40 film artifacts and 60 fibroglandular noise patterns, as indicated by two expert radiologists. All patterns were extracted from mammographic images with subtle MCs in heterogeneously dense and extremely dense parenchyma.

The validation dataset consists of 51 dense mammograms (33 abnormal, 18 normal) containing 50 subtle MC clusters embedded in dense parenchyma, originating from the DDSM database (Howtek scanner with 12 bits pixel depth and 43.5 μm spatial resolution sub-sampled at 87 μm). The detection performance is evaluated by means of Free-response Receiver Operating Characteristic (FROC) curves, produced by varying the threshold of the estimated probability for identifying MC clusters.

A cluster is considered detected if a closed area contains three or more individual candidate MCs. Defining a disk of 1 cm in diameter around each MC pattern, a group of disks that touch or overlap forms a closed area [21]. The stages of the algorithm are provided in Fig. 1.

3 Results

The contribution of combining PCA and wavelet analysis on the efficiency of MC cluster detection is investigated (Fig. 2): (i) for different variability encodings of the training dataset (90%, 95% and 98%) and (ii) by comparing PCA carried out on wavelet-decomposed images and original images (background suppressed). When PCA is applied on original images, the resulting feature vector consists of 5, 8 and 13 principal components, while for wavelet decomposed images of 20, 28 and 36 for 90%, 95% and 98% amount of MC training variability, respectively.

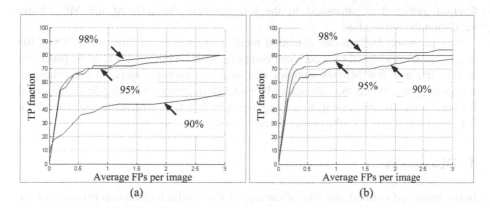

Fig. 2. FROC curves of the validation dataset for three amounts of variability encoding (90%, 95% and 98%) of the MC training dataset. PCA applied on: (a) background-suppressed images and (b) wavelet-decomposed images.

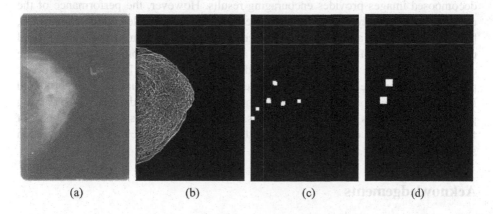

Fig. 3. Example for MC cluster identification in heterogeneously dense parenchyma (DDSM: B_3509_LEFT_CC): (a) Original image, (b) candidate MC region labeling, (c) identification of individual MC patterns using wavelet eigenimages and the LDA classifier and (d) identified clusters of MC patterns

As observed in the FROC curves, when PCA is applied on original images (Fig. 2a), the detection performance remains the same above 95% of variability encoding, requiring 8 principal components to adequately encode MC patterns. In case of applying PCA on wavelet-decomposed images (Fig. 2b), detection performance improves with increasing amount of variability encoding. At corresponding variabilities, PCA wavelet encoding outperforms PCA original encoding, especially at low variability (Fig. 2). The highest performance is achieved when PCA is applied on the wavelet-decomposed images with 98% amount of variability encoding, yielding 80% TP fraction with 0.5 average FPs per image. Thus, wavelet analysis is proven to contribute significantly in increased detection performance. The low overall TP fraction achieved is attributed to the low contrast character of the MC cluster validation dataset studied.

The proposed MC cluster detection method applied on an image of 2370x1305 pixel size, implemented on a personal computer with INTEL PENTIUM M processor at 1.3 GHz and 768 Mbytes memory size, requires approximately 73 s for the pre-processing step. When the candidate MC patterns are projected at the 36-dimensional feature vector, the processing time is approximately 8 s. A representative example of the algorithm stages for MC cluster detection is provided in Fig. 3.

4 Discussion

In the proposed method, we take advantage of the spatial localization property of the wavelet transform to encode MC pattern information and to differentiate them from film artifacts and fibrograndular noise patterns, which have the same frequency content but different patterns. Compared with other studies, with or without the application of the wavelet transform [4], [11], [21], PCA applied on wavelet-decomposed images provides encouraging results. However, the performance of the method is not directly comparable with reported MC cluster detection schemes [8], [9], [10], [11], [12], as there are differences in the composition of the datasets used regarding the type of breast parenchyma and MC clusters subtlety. Our results are only comparable to the results reported by Lado *et al.* [13], but of superior performance. For inter-comparison purposes, performance evaluation of the proposed MC cluster detection method should be expanded in a dataset with varying parenchyma densities and subtlety of MCs. These promising results are in support of further development of the proposed method into a fully automated MC detection scheme.

Acknowledgements

This work is supported by the European Social Fund (ESF), Operational Program for Educational and Vocational Training II (EPEAEK II), and particularly the Program PYTHAGORAS I (B.365.011). We also thank the staff of the Department of Radiology at the University Hospital of Patras for their contribution in this work.

References

1. Kopans, D.B.: The Positive Predictive Value of Mammography. Am. J. Roentgenol. 158 (1992) 521-526
2. Jackson, V.P., Hendrick, R.E., Feig, S.A., Kopans, D.B.: Imaging of the Radiographically Dense Breast. Radiology 188 (1993) 297-301
3. Chan, H-P., Sahiner, B., Petrick, N., Hadjiiski, L., Paquerault, S.: Computer-Aided Diagnosis of Breast Cancer. In: Costaridou L. (ed.): Medical Image Analysis Methods. Boca Raton, CRC Press, Taylor & Francis Group (2005) 1-49
4. Wei, L., Yang, Y., Nishikawa, R.M., Wernick, M.N., Edwards, A.: Relevance Vector Machine for Automatic Detection of Clustered Microcalcifications. IEEE Trans. Med. Imag. 24 (2005) 1278-1285
5. Sampat, P.M., Markey, M.K., Bovik, A.C.: Computer-Aided Detection and Diagnosis in Mammography. In: Bovik A.C. (ed.): Handbook of Image and Video Processing 2nd ed. Academic Press (2005) 1195-1217
6. Nishikawa, R.M.: Detection of Microcalcifications. In: Strickland R.N. (ed) Image-Processing Techniques for Tumor Detection. New York, Marcel Dekker Inc (2002) 131-153
7. Samei, E., Eyler, W., Baron, L.: Effects of Anatomical Structure on Signal Detection. In Beutel J., Kundel H.L., Van Meter R.L. (eds.): Handbook of Medical Imaging volume 1. Physics and Psychophysics. Bellingham, Washington: SPIE Press (2000) 655-682
8. Netsch, T., Peitgen, H.O.: Scale-Space Signatures for the Detection of Clustered Microcalcifications in Digital Mammograms. IEEE Trans. Med. Imag. 18 (1999) 774-786
9. Strickland, R.N., Hee, H.: Wavelet Transforms for Detecting Microcalcifications in Mammograms. IEEE Trans. Med. Imag. 15 (1996) 218-229
10. Yoshida, H., Doi, K., Nishikawa, R.M., Giger, M.L., Schmidt, R. A.: An Improved Computer-Assisted Diagnostic Scheme Using Wavelet Transform for Detecting Clustered Microcalcifications in Digital Mammograms. Acad. Radiol. 3 (1996) 621-627
11. Drexl, J., Heinlein, P., Schneider, W.: MammoInsight Computer Assisted Detection: Performance Study with Large Database. In: Bildverarbeitung fur die Medizin Springer 2003
12. Qian, W., Kallergi, M., Clarke, L.P., Li, H.D., Venugopal, P., Song, D., Clark R.A.: Tree Structured Wavelet Transform Segmentation of Microcalcifications in Digital Mammography. Med. Phys. 22 (1995) 1247-1254
13. Lado, M.J., Tahoces, P.G., Mendez, A.J., Souto, M., Vidal, J.J.: A Wavelet-Based Algorithm for Detecting Clustered Microcalcifications in Digital Mammograms. Med. Phys. 26 (1999) 1294-1305
14. Costaridou, L., Sakellaropoulos, P., Stefanoyiannis, A.P., Ungureanu, E., Panayiotakis, G.: Quantifying Image Quality at Breast Periphery vs Mammary Gland in Mammography Using Wavelet Analysis. Br. J. Radiol., 74 (2001) 913-919
15. Chan, H.P., Sahiner, B., Lam, K.L., Petrick, N., Helvie, M.A., Goositt, M.M., Adler, D.D.: Computerized Analysis of Mammographic Microcalcifications in Morphological and Texture Feature Spaces. Med. Phys. 25 (1998) 2007-2019
16. Mallat, S.G.: Wavelet Tour of Signal Processing. 2nd ed. San Diego. Academic Press (1999)
17. Laine, A.F., Schuler, S., Jian, F., Huda, W.: Mammographic Feature Enhancement by Multiscale Analysis. IEEE Trans. Med. Imag. 13 (1994) 725-740

18. Zhang, W., Yoshida, H., Nishikawa, R.M., Doi, K.: Optimally Weighted Wavelet Transform Based on Supervised Training for Detection of Microcalcifications in Digital Mammograms. Med. Phys. 25 (1998) 949-956
19. Van Belle, G., Fisher, L.D., Heagerty, P.J., Lumley, T.: Biostatistics: A Methodology for the Health Sciences. 2nd ed. Hoboken, New Jersey: John Wiley & Sons. Inc. (2004) 584-639
20. Turk, M., Pentland, A.: Eigenfaces for Recognition. J. Cogn. Neurosci. 3 (1991) 71-86
21. Veldkamp, W.J.H., Karssemeijer, N.: Normalization of Local Contrast in Mammograms. IEEE Trans. Med. Imag. 19 (2000) 731-738

Breast Component Adaptive Wavelet Enhancement for Soft-Copy Display of Mammograms

Spyros Skiadopoulos, Anna Karahaliou, Filippos Sakellaropoulos,
George Panayiotakis, and Lena Costaridou

Department of Medical Physics, School of Medicine,
University of Patras, 265 00 Patras, Greece
costarid@upatras.gr, panayiot@upatras.gr

Abstract. A method that performs multiresolution enhancement, adaptive to breast components, for optimal visualization of the entire breast area is presented. The method includes an edge detection step to distinguish breast area from mammogram background and employs Gaussian mixture modeling to segment breast components (uncompressed fat, fat and dense). The original image is decomposed using a redundant discrete wavelet transform and magnitude coefficients corresponding to each breast component are linearly mapped for contrast enhancement. Coefficient mapping is controlled by a gain factor provided by the parameters of the modeled breast components. The processed image is derived by reconstruction of the modified wavelet coefficients. The algorithm is compared with two enhancement methods proposed for soft-copy display, in a dataset of 68 mammograms containing lesions. The proposed method demonstrates increased performance in accentuating lesions embedded in fatty or dense parenchyma, as well as in visualization of anatomical features in the entire breast area.

1 Background

Screen film mammography is the primary imaging technique for the detection and diagnosis of breast lesions. However, the high diagnostic performance of screen film mammography is challenged by occult disease signs (microcalcifications and/or masses) due to the masking effect of dense breast parenchyma, and the over-exposure of breast periphery.

Several computer-based algorithms have been proposed to enhance subtle features of interest in digital and digitized mammograms [1], [2]. These methods can be classified according to the type of processing used (global/locally-adaptive histogram equalization, region or neighborhood adaptive enhancement and wavelet enhancement) and to target area (dense tissue and/or breast periphery).

In the advent of Full Field Digital Mammography (FFDM), it is crucial to exploit the potential of image processing algorithms in enhancing the ability of radiologists to interpret images [1], [2]. To be eligible, candidate methods should also fulfill functionality requirements of robustness and computational speed for soft-copy display.

Susan M. Astley et al. (Eds.): IWDM 2006, LNCS 4046, pp. 549–556, 2006.

In this study, an automated wavelet-based enhancement method is proposed adaptive to breast components. For this purpose we adopted the rationale of the Mixture Model Intensity Windowing (MMIW) technique [3], in order to derive linear mapping functions of wavelet coefficients for breast components. The method is demonstrated by means of a preference study including two additional image enhancement methods proposed for soft-copy display, in a pilot dataset containing lesions (masses and/or microcalcifications-MCs).

2   Method

2.1   Breast Border Identification

The breast border is identified using an edge detection technique which is performed in the following four steps:

i)   The mean value of grey levels is calculated in the most homogenous rectangular region (164x164pixels) of the mammogram background (over-exposed area of the film). The most homogenous region is defined by means of quantitative criteria including the minimum grey level value and standard deviation.

ii) The gradient magnitude of the image is calculated using a derivative of Gaussian operator.

iii) An initial breast edge point is defined by the location of maximum gradient magnitude along a line passing horizontally through the center of a breast. Final acceptance of this point to the breast edge is subject to fulfillment of a similarity criterion of its rectangular neighborhood mean grey level value similar to that of the homogenous region of the mammogram background ($\pm 0.2\%$).

iv) The rest of breast edge points are progressively defined by identifying adjacent points that fulfill the same two criteria.

2.2   Breast Components Segmentation

Segmentation of the three breast components (uncompressed fat-UF, fat-F and dense-D) is performed using Gaussian Mixture Modeling [4], [5]. Specifically, the breast area is modeled by a linear combination of k weighted Gaussian distributions (a mixture of Gaussians) given by:

$$f_k(x) = \sum_{j=1}^{k} \pi_j \varphi(x; \theta_j) \tag{1}$$

with:

$$\sum_{j=1}^{k} \pi_j = 1 \tag{2}$$

where π_j are the mixing weights ($\pi_j \geq 0$, for $j=1,2,...k$), $k=3$ components and $\varphi(x;\theta_j)$ the 1-dimensional Gaussian probability density function, corresponding to each breast component, parameterized by its mean m and variance σ^2, is given by:

$$\varphi(x;\theta) = \frac{1}{(2\pi\sigma^2)^{\frac{1}{2}}} \exp\left\{-\frac{(x-m)^2}{2\sigma^2}\right\},$$

(3)

where $\theta=(m, \sigma^2)$.

The parameters of each Gaussian (x,θ) are iteratively determined by the Expectation Maximization (EM) algorithm [6], which maximizes the log-likelihood of the data representing the distribution. Specifically, a training set $X_n=\{x_1,x_2,...,x_n\}$ of the independent and identically distributed pixels $x_i \in R^1$ (image) is assumed to be sampled from eq. (1). The task is to estimate the parameters of the mixture that maximize the log-likelihood:

$$L = \frac{1}{n}\sum_{i=1}^{n}\log f_k(x_i)$$

(4)

Fig. 1 is an indicative example of mammographic component modeling using the mixture of three Gaussians.

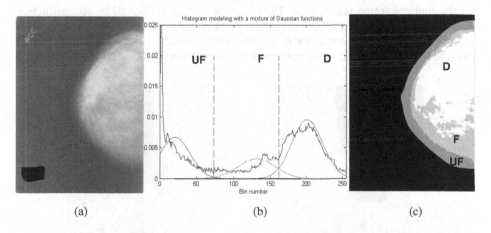

| | | |
| (a) | (b) | (c) |

Fig. 1. (a) Original mammogram. (b) Histogram of the breast area along with the mixture of Gaussians. Dashed lines indicate the intercept points of the Gaussian functions. (c) Segmented mammographic components. To visualize segmentations, every pixel has been grey level coded to reflect the component to which it has been assigned.

2.3 Component-Adaptive Wavelet Enhancement

A fast, biorthogonal, Redundant Discrete Wavelet Transform (RDWT) [7] is utilized to obtain a multiresolution representation of the original image. The wavelet used in RDWT is quadratic spline function with compact support and is the first derivative of a Gaussian-like smoothing function [7]. Use of RDWT as a basis for contrast enhancement is beneficial due to shift-invariance and lack of aliasing. The algorithm is implemented using a filter bank algorithm, called "algorithme à trous" [8], which does not involve subsampling. The image is decomposed into a multiresolution hierarchy of subband images, at the first four resolution scales (s =1-4), consisting of a coarse approximation image and a set of wavelet detail images. The wavelet magnitude coefficients, corresponding to each breast component are linearly mapped to accomplish contrast enhancement. Coefficient mapping of each breast component is controlled by a gain factor (GF) provided by the parameters of the corresponding Gaussian distribution, previously determined by the EM algorithm. Specifically, linear mapping of the multiscale gradients (magnitude coefficients) of each breast component (k) can be mathematically expressed by:

$$M(k)_s^e(m,n) = GF(k)_s M(k)_s(m,n), \qquad k = 1,2,3 \qquad (5)$$

where $M(k)_s(m,n)$ and $M(k)_s^e(m,n)$ are the initial and enhanced gradient magnitude values at position (m,n) and $GF(k)_s > 1$ is the gain factor given by:

$$GF(k)_s = (GL_{max} - GL_{min})/(I_{max} - I_{min}) \qquad (6)$$

where GL_{min} and GL_{max} are the minimum and maximum gray level values of the entire breast area, respectively, while I_{min} and I_{max} are the intercept points of the corresponding Gaussian function of the kth breast component with its neighboring Gaussian functions, provided by the EM algorithm. The gain factor is kept constant for the four resolution scales used. The processed image is derived by reconstruction of the modified wavelet coefficients of all breast components. Fig. 2 is an application example of the component adaptive wavelet enhancement. Lower and upper arrows indicate a MC cluster and a circumscribed mass containing MC cluster, respectively.

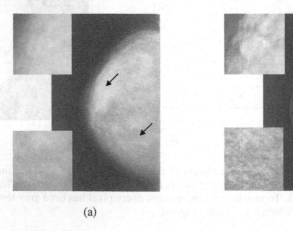

(a)   (b)

Fig. 2. (a) Original mammogram. (b) Processed image. Arrows indicate lesions also presented in magnified regions of interest.

2.4 Quantitative Performance Evaluation Metrics

An initial quantitative performance evaluation of this method was performed, using 30 normal mammographic images, originating from the DDSM database [9], with embedded simulated masses [10], [11]. Contrast and noise measurements were carried out in the region of the simulated mass. In order to assess the effect of the gain factor (*GF*) on image quality, images were processed with varying percentages of the gain factor (60%, 80%, 100%, 120% and 140%). The following quantitative metrics were used:

(a) Contrast improvement index (*CII*) defined as C_{prod}/C_{orig}, where contrast C is provided by $(x_M-x_B)/(x_M+x_B)$, where x is the mean gray level value of pixels located in the simulated mass (*M*) and in mass background (*B*) defined by an area of 10 pixels radius around the mass.
(b) Noise amplification index (*NAI*) measured as $\sigma_{prod}/\sigma_{orig}$, where σ is a noise estimation within the mass, proposed by Rank *et al.* [12].
(c) Contrast-to-noise ratio index (*CNRI*) defined as *CII/NAI*.

2.5 Preference Study

Performance evaluation was carried out using a dataset of 68 mammographic images originating from the DDSM database [9]. Mammograms selected, contain lesions (50 MC clusters and 36 masses) and correspond to all density categories according to ACR BIRADS^{TM} lexicon (density 1: 12, density 2: 20, density 3: 24, density 4: 12).

The proposed method was compared with two image enhancement algorithms proposed for soft-copy display; the Contrast Limited Adaptive Histogram Equalization (CLAHE) method [13] and a Spatially Adaptive Wavelet-based (SAW) enhancement method [14], [15]. Methods' performance was evaluated by means of a preference study. Two experienced radiologists ranked the performance of each original and the corresponding processed images of the sample (from 1=best to 4=worst) with respect to contrast and morphological (MC cluster criteria: number, shape, size, density; mass criteria: center, contour, shape, size) characteristics of lesions as well as overall visualization of anatomical features (periphery: nipple, areola, skin, veins and Cooper's ligaments; dense and fatty tissue).

2.6 Visualization Tool

An image visualization tool, developed in our department [16], was used for implementation of segmentation, enhancement and performance evaluation procedures. This tool is domain-specific to medical imaging. In addition to conventional visualization operations, it provides global and adaptive wavelet functionality [17].

3 Results

Fig. 3 provides average values of *CII*, *NAI* and *CNRI* measured on images, with simulated masses, processed by the proposed enhancement method by successively altering the gain factor.

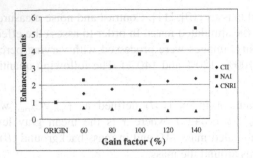

Fig. 3. Average values of contrast improvement index (*CII*), noise amplification index (*NAI*) and contrast-to-noise ratio index (*CNRI*) for different gain factors of enhancement

As expected, increase of the gain factor results in increase of both *CII* and *NAI*. However, the increase of *NAI* is more rapid compared to the increase of *CII*, resulting in decreased *CNRI* of the processed images.

The average rank obtained from the two radiologists, for original and the three image enhancement methods with respect to (a) contrast and (b) morphology of lesions (MC clusters and masses) is provided in Fig. 4. Fig. 5 provides methods' performance with respect to overall visualization of anatomical features. A low rank indicates a high preference.

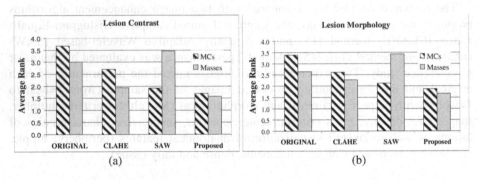

Fig. 4. Average rank for original and the three image enhancement methods with respect to (a) contrast and (b) morphology of lesions (MCs and masses)

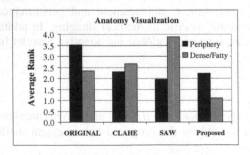

Fig. 5. Average rank for original and the three image enhancement methods with respect to visualization of anatomical features (periphery, dense/fatty tissue)

4 Discussion

According to the preference study, the proposed method has shown promising results in enhancing visibility of lesions against dense parenchymal background and enhancing visibility of low-density (fat) regions of the breast.

As observed, all methods outperform original images with respect to visualization of lesions' contrast and morphology. The proposed method demonstrates the highest performance in both lesion types. The SAW method fails in visualizing masses efficiently, since it only enhances masses' border but losing information from masses' interior. The CLAHE method had the lowest preference in visualizing MC clusters due to morphology distortion and suboptimal contrast enhancement in case of MCs located in dense breast parenchyma.

Concerning visualization of anatomical features, the proposed method demonstrates the highest preference. Due to the linear mapping of the wavelet coefficients the method does not cause overenhancement of normal tissue structures and provides an image comparable in appearance to the standard screen-film mammograms that radiologists are acquainted with. Furthermore, no artifacts are observed in the boundaries of the reconstructed breast components. However, the method, in some cases, fails in enhancing breast periphery (uncompressed fat). This is attributed to the suboptimal performance of the breast border identification method used. Refinement of the proposed method should include improvement of breast border identification, and segmentation of pectoral muscle to deal with mediolateral oblique mammograms.

The SAW method fails in depicting fatty and dense tissue, which can not even be distinguished. On the contrary, it demonstrates the highest performance in visualizing anatomical features located in breast periphery due to its edge enhancement character. The CLAHE method does not distinguish dense from fatty tissue as well. Specifically, it seems to bias mammographic density category, since fatty tissue regions in original images are depicted as dense tissue regions in processed images.

Noise amplification (*NAI*) associated with the proposed method, according to the quantitative performance evaluation metrics, did not influence radiologists' assessment who ranked the method as the most preferred. A noise reduction stage [14], [15] will be considered in future implementations. Performance evaluation of the method should be expanded in lesion detection and characterization tasks, augmentation of the dataset and comparison with additional image processing algorithms.

Acknowledgements

This work is supported by the European Social Fund (ESF), Operational Program for Educational and Vocational Training II (EPEAEK II), and particularly the Program PYTHAGORAS I (B.365.011). We also thank the staff of the Department of Radiology at the University Hospital of Patras for their contribution in this work.

References

1. Pisano, E.D., Cole, E.B., Hemminger, B.M. et al.: Image Processing Algorithms for Digital Mammography: A Pictorial Essay. RadioGraphics 20 (2000) 1479-1491
2. Sivaramakrishna, R., Obuchowski, N.A., Chilcote, W.A., Cardenosa, G., Powell, K.A.: Comparing the Performance of Mammographic Enhancement Algorithms: A Preference Study. Am. J. Roentgenol. 175 (2000) 45-51
3. Aylward, S.R., Hemminger, B.M., Pisano, E.D.: Mixture Modeling for Digital Mammogram Display and Analysis. In: Karssemeijer, N., Thijssen, M., Hendriks, J., van Erning, A. (eds.): Digital Mammography Nijmegen. Dordrecht, the Netherlands: Kluwer Academic (1998) 305-312
4. McLachlan, G.J., Basford, K.E.: Mixture Models. New York, Marcel Dekker, Inc. (1988)
5. Ferrari, R.J., Rangayyan, R.M., Borges, R.A., Frere, A.F.: Segmentation of the Fibro-glandular Disc in Mammograms via Gaussian Mixture Modeling. Med. Biol. Eng. Comput. 42 (2004) 378-387
6. Dempster, A.P., Laird, N.M., Rubin, D.B.: Maximum Likelihood from Incomplete Data via the EM algorithm. Journal of Royal Statistical Society Series B, 39 (1977) 1-38
7. Mallat S., Zhong S.: Characterization of Signals from Multiscale Edges. IEEE Trans. Pat. Anal. Machine Intell. 14 (1992) 710-732
8. Shensa, M. J.: The Discrete Wavelet Transform: Wedding the "à trous" and Mallat algorithms. IEEE Trans. Signal Proc. 40 (1992) 2464-2482
9. Heath, M., Bowyer, K., Kopans, D., Moore, R., Kegelmeyer, P.: The Digital Database for Screening Mammography. Proceedings of the 5th Int. Workshop on Digital Mammography, Toronto, Canada, (2000) 212–218.
10. Skiadopoulos, S., Costaridou, L., Kalogeropoulou, C.P., Likaki, E., Livos, L., Panayiotakis, G.: Simulating the Mammographic Appearance of Circumscribed Lesions. Eur. Radiol. 13 (2003) 1137-47
11. Costaridou, L., Skiadopoulos, S., Sakellaropoulos, P., Likaki, E., Kalogeropoulou, C.P., Panayiotakis, G.: Evaluating the Effect of a Wavelet Enhancement Method in Characterization of Simulated Lesions Embedded in Dense Breast Parenchyma. Eur. Radiol. 15 (2005) 1615-22
12. Rank, K., Lendl, M., Unbehauen, R.: Estimation of Image Noise Variance. *IEEE Proc. Vis. Image Signal Proc.* **146 (1999)** 80–84
13. Pisano, E.D., Zong, S., Hemminger, B.M., et al.: Contrast Limited Adaptive Histogram Equalization Image Processing to Improve the Detection of Simulated Spiculations in Dense Mammograms. J. Digit. Imaging 11 (1998) 193-200
14. Sakellaropoulos, P., Costaridou, L., Panayiotakis, G.: A Wavelet-based Spatially Adaptive Method for Mammographic Contrast Enhancement. Phys. Med. Biol. 48 (2003) 787-803
15. Costaridou, L., Sakellaropoulos, P., Skiadopoulos, S., Panayiotakis, G.: Locally Adaptive Wavelet Contrast Enhancement. In: Costaridou, L. (ed.): Medical Image Analysis Methods. Boca Raton, Taylor & Francis Group LLC, CRC Press (2005) 225-257
16. Sakellaropoulos, P., Costaridou, L., Panayiotakis, G.: An Image Visualization Tool in Mammography. Med. Inform. 24 (1999) 53– 73
17. Sakellaropoulos, P., Costaridou, L., Panayiotakis, G.: Using Component Technologies for Web Based Wavelet Enhanced Mammographic Image Visualization. Med. Inform. 25 (2000) 171-181

Using Wavelet-Based Features to Identify Masses in Dense Breast Parenchyma

Filippos Sakellaropoulos, Spyros Skiadopoulos, Anna Karahaliou,
Lena Costaridou, and George Panayiotakis

Department of Medical Physics, School of Medicine,
University of Patras, 265 00 Patras, Greece
panayiot@upatras.gr, costarid@upatras.gr

Abstract. Automated detection of masses on mammograms is challenged by the presence of dense breast parenchyma. The aim of this study is to investigate the feasibility of wavelet-based feature analysis in identifying spiculated and circumscribed masses in dense breast parenchyma. The method includes an edge detection step for breast border identification and employs Gaussian mixture modeling for dense parenchyma labeling. Subsequently, wavelet decomposition is performed and intensity as well as orientation features are extracted from approximation and detail subimages, respectively. Logistic regression analysis (LRA) is employed to differentiate spiculated and circumscribed masses from normal dense parenchyma. The proposed method is tested in 90 dense mammograms containing spiculated masses (30), circumscribed masses (30) and normal parenchyma (30). Free-response receiver operating characteristic (FROC) analysis is used to evaluate the performance of the method, achieving 83.3% sensitivity at 1.5 and 1.8 false positives per image for identifying spiculated and circumscribed masses, respectively.

1 Background

Computer-Aided Detection (CAD) is one of the promising approaches for improving mass detection sensitivity in mammography [1]. Various image features in combination with classification methods have been proposed for automated mass detection [2]. Kegelmeyer *et al.* [3] have introduced edge orientation features based on local edge orientation histogram analysis as well as Laws' texture energy measures to identify spiculated mass containing areas. Karssemeijer *et al.* [4], [5] detected spiculated masses employing orientation features based on three directional second-order Gaussian derivatives. Wei *et al.* [6], [7] proposed multiresolution texture analysis extracted from spatial Gray Level Dependence Matrices (GLDM) for differentiation of masses from normal tissue. Liu *et al.* [8] extended mass edge orientation analysis with a multiresolution scheme for the detection of spiculated masses. Petrick *et al* [9] and Kobatake *et al.* [10] have utilized a combination of boundary (morphological) and texture features (GLDM analysis) to identify and segment the extent of masses, respectively. Zwiggelaar *et al.* [11] introduced area patterns using principal component and factor analyses for differentiating areas

Susan M. Astley et al. (Eds.): IWDM 2006, LNCS 4046, pp. 557–564, 2006.

containing masses from normal tissue. Chang *et al.* [12] and Baydush *et al.* [13] applied knowledge-based approaches for discriminating masses from normal tissue.

The performance of the aforementioned mass detection methods is characterized by high sensitivity (84-96%) and is challenged by the high number of false positive detections per image (1.0-4.4), especially in case of dense parenchyma (3.7-8.4) [14], [15], [16].

The aim of this study is to investigate the feasibility of wavelet-based features in identifying spiculated and circumscribed masses in dense breast parenchyma. A set of intensity and gradient-orientation multiresolution features are investigated, in combination with Logistic Regression Analysis (LRA) as classification scheme for differentiating masses from dense breast parenchyma.

2 Method

The steps of the proposed mass identification method are provided in Fig. 1. For each mammogram, the breast border is identified using an edge detection technique based on magnitudes calculated from the derivative of a Gaussian operator. Gaussian mixture modeling is then employed for segmenting the three breast components (uncompressed fat, fat and dense parenchyma) and labeling the dense parenchyma [17]. Following, wavelet decomposition is performed and multiresolution features are extracted for each pixel of dense parenchyma. These features are used as inputs in a trained logistic regression classifier (Fig. 2). Probability images are generated and

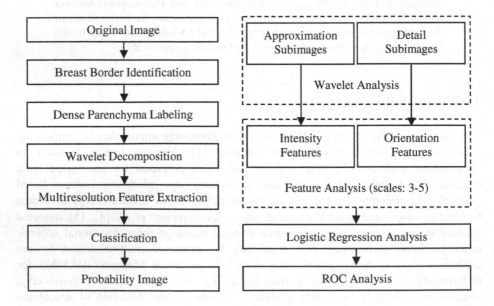

Fig. 1. Flow chart of the proposed method for breast mass identification

Fig. 2. Steps for classifier training in differentiating breast masses from normal dense parenchyma

Free-response Receiver Operating Characteristic (FROC) analysis is performed for evaluation of the proposed method.

2.1 Wavelet and Feature Analysis

In this study, a fast, biorthogonal, Redundant Discrete Wavelet Transform (RDWT) is utilized to obtain a multiresolution representation of the original image. It is based on a family of wavelet functions $\psi_{2^k}(x)$ with compact support, which are first-order derivatives of corresponding Gaussian-like spline functions $\theta_{2^k}(x)$. The algorithm is implemented using a filter bank algorithm, called "algorithme à trous", which does not involve subsampling. The discrete wavelet transform is a uniform sampling of the wavelet transform series, discretized over the scale parameter s at dyadic scales 2^k [18], [19]. The RDWT is calculated up to a coarse dyadic scale K. Therefore, the original image is decomposed into a multiresolution hierarchy of subband images, consisting of a coarse approximation image $S_{2^K} f$ and a set of wavelet images $\left(W_{2^k}^1 f(m,n), W_{2^j}^2 f(m,n) \right)_{1 \le k \le K}$, which provide the details that are available in $S_1 f$ (original) but have disappeared in $S_{2^K} f$. All subband images have the same number of pixels as the original, thus the representation is highly redundant. The RDWT computes the multiscale gradient vector. Coefficient subband images are proportional to the sampled horizontal and vertical components of the multiscale gradient vector, and thus they are related to local contrast [20]. The magnitude-orientation representation of the gradient vector, in the discrete case, is given by:

$$M_{2^k}(m,n) = \sqrt{\left| W_{2^k}^1(m,n) \right|^2 + \left| W_{2^k}^2(m,n) \right|^2} \ , \ A_{2^k}(m,n) = \arctan\left(\frac{W_{2^k}^2(m,n)}{W_{2^k}^1(m,n)} \right) \quad (1)$$

To extract significant information from masses three resolution scales ($k=3,4,5$) were selected to be analyzed, as masses reside in coarse scales, in contrast to microcalcifications which reside in fine scales (2nd and 3rd) [21]. Specifically, for capturing intensity variations of masses, four intensity features were calculated from the low-frequency band (approximation subimage) of the three resolution levels for each pixel: Mean value (*MEAN*), Standard Deviation (*STDE*), Skewness (*SKEW*) and Kurtosis (*KURT*).

In addition, to capture significant information from mass edges, three gradient-orientation features were calculated from the high-frequency band (detail subimage):

- Standard Deviation of Folded Gradient-Orientation (*SDFO*) [8]:

$$\sigma_{2^k}^{\gamma}(i,j) = \sqrt{\frac{1}{N-1} \sum_{(m,n) \in W} \left(\gamma_{2^k}(m,n) - \overline{\gamma_{2^k}(i,j)} \right)^2} \quad (2)$$

where the folded gradient-orientation $\gamma(i,j)$ for position (i,j) is defined as:

$$\gamma_{2^k}(i,j) = \begin{cases} A_{2^k}(i,j) + \pi, & if \ \overline{A^+_{2^k}(i,j)} - A_{2^k}(i,j) > \dfrac{\pi}{2} \ and \ KP \geq QL \\ A_{2^k}(i,j) - \pi, & if \ A_{2^k}(i,j) - \overline{A^-_{2^k}(i,j)} > \dfrac{\pi}{2} \ and \ KP < QL \\ A_{2^k}(i,j), & otherwise \end{cases} \tag{3}$$

where

$$\overline{A^+_{2^k}(i,j)} = \frac{1}{KP}\left(\sum_{A_{2^k}(m,n) \geq 0} A_{2^k}(m,n) \right), \qquad \overline{A^-_{2^k}(i,j)} = \frac{1}{QL}\left(\sum_{A_{2^k}(m,n) \leq 0} A_{2^k}(m,n) \right) \tag{4}$$

are the mean values of positive and negative gradient orientations within a window W, respectively. KP and QL are the number of positive and negative gradient orientations within W, respectively.

- Orientations' Coherence (measure of degree of anisotropy) (*COHE*) [22,23]:

$$C_{2^k}(i,j) = M_{2^k}(i,j) \frac{\displaystyle\sum_{(m,n) \in W} M_{2^k}(m,n)\left|\cos(A_{2^k}(i,j) - \cos(A_{2^k}(m,n)\right|}{\displaystyle\sum_{(m,n) \in W} M_{2^k}(m,n)} \tag{5}$$

where $M_{2^k}(i,j)$ and $A_{2^k}(i,j)$ denote magnitude and orientation of position (i,j) at scale k, respectively.

- Orientations' Entropy (*ENTR*) [23]:

$$E_{2^k}(i,j) = \sum_{(m,n) \in W} A_{2^k}(m,n) \cdot \log\left(A_{2^k}(m,n)\right) \tag{6}$$

A total of 21 features (= 7 features x 3 scales) were extracted for each dense label.

2.2 Performance Evaluation

For training the classifier the aforementioned multiresolution features were extracted from regions of interest (ROIs) containing normal dense parenchyma and masses embedded in dense parenchyma. ROIs were selected from mammograms corresponding to dense parenchyma originating from the Digital Database for Screening Mammography (DDSM), with an image visualization tool developed in our department [24]. The training dataset consists of 166 ROIs, 60 ROIs containing spiculated masses, 40 ROIs containing circumscribed masses and 66 ROIs of normal dense tissue. The mean size (longest dimension) was 19 mm (range: 7-49 mm) and 12 mm (range: 6-31 mm) for spiculated and circumscribed masses, respectively. Histogram of mass subtlety (from 1=subtle to 5=obvious), according to DDSM database, is provided in Fig. 3.

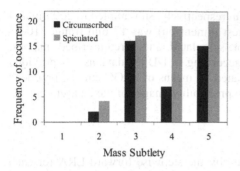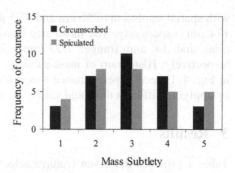

Fig. 3. Histogram of subtlety for spiculated and circumscribed masses of the training dataset

Fig. 4. Histogram of subtlety for spiculated and circumscribed masses of the validation dataset

Stepwise forward LRA was employed to determine the optimal subset of features differentiating masses from normal dense parenchyma. The area under Receiver Operating Characteristic (ROC) curve (A_z) was used as a feature performance metric. To study the effect of mass type (spiculated and circumscribed) in classification accuracy, separate logistic regression models were constructed for two differentiation tasks: (a) spiculated masses from normal dense tissue (S-N) and (b) circumscribed masses from normal dense tissue (C-N).

The two models were constructed in the form of *logit(p)* values:

$$\log it(p) = \log_e\left(\frac{\Pr ob(Y = y_2)}{\Pr ob(Y = y_1)}\right) = \beta_0 + \sum_{s=1}^{n} \beta_s X_s \tag{7}$$

where X_s are the independent variables (features), Y is the binary dependent variable, which has two possible values, y_1 (*0*: normal) and y_2 (*1*: mass), β_o is the intercept and β_s are the logistic regression coefficients. From these *logit(p)* values, the estimated probability *(p)* of the presence of a mass can be obtained from:

$$p = \frac{\exp(\log it(p))}{1 + \exp(\log it(p))} \tag{8}$$

The half-half training and testing methodology was applied for each task and the classification performance was evaluated by means of ROC curves, in terms of A_z area and standard error (Fig. 2).

The multiresolution features, selected by the stepwise forward LRA for the two models constructed, were used for classifying the labeled dense parenchyma and generating the probability image (Fig. 1). The overall performance of the proposed mass identification method in the two differentiation tasks (spiculated masses vs. normal dense tissue and circumscribed mass vs. normal dense tissue) was tested in a validation dataset of 90 dense mammograms originating from the DDSM, other than those used in training the classifier. Specifically, mammographic images corresponding to heterogeneously dense or extremely dense tissue (density 3 and 4, according to BIRADS lexicon) were selected (30 of normal dense parenchyma, 30 containing subtle spiculated masses and 30 containing subtle circumscribed masses). Images have been digitized with Lumisys or Howtek scanner, at 12 bits pixel depth with spatial resolution of 50 μm and 43.5 μm respectively, subsampled to 200 μm and 174 μm respectively. The mean size (longest dimension) was 17 mm (range: 10-38 mm) and 14 mm (range: 7-23 mm) for spiculated and circumscribed masses, respectively. Histogram of mass subtlety, according to DDSM database, is provided in Fig. 4. Detection performance was evaluated by means of FROC curves, produced by applying different threshold values in the probability images of the dataset.

3 Results

Table 1 provides the seven features selected by the stepwise forward LRA for each logistic regression model constructed. As observed, different features were selected for each differentiation task. The ROC curves produced from models for the two differentiation tasks are presented in Fig. 5. The A_z values are 0.956±0.033 and 0.932±0.036 for the S-N and C-N training datasets, respectively. In Fig. 6, FROC curves for the two differentiation tasks are provided. Overall performance of the proposed method achieves sensitivity of 83.3% at 1.5 and 1.8 false positives per image for identifying spiculated and circumscribed masses, respectively.

Table 1. Features – scales selected by the stepwise forward LRA for the two logistic regression models and the corresponding A_z values achieved

	Spiculated *vs.* Normal model		Circumscribed *vs.* Normal model	
a/a	Feature Added	A_z	Feature Added	A_z
1	SKEW - 5	0.835	COHE - 3	0.860
2	ENTR - 4	0.868	STFO - 3	0.864
3	STDE - 3	0.886	ENTR - 3	0.899
4	STFO - 5	0.923	KURT - 5	0.909
5	KURT - 5	0.938	SKEW - 5	0.917
6	COHE - 4	0.947	SKEW - 4	0.930
7	SKEW - 4	0.956	COHE - 5	0.932

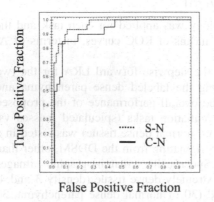

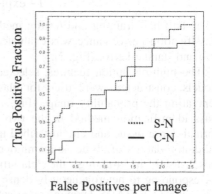

Fig. 5. ROC curves for differentiating masses from normal dense parenchyma

Fig. 6. FROC curves for identifying spiculated and circumscribed masses

4 Discussion

These preliminary results suggest that intensity and orientation features extracted from the coefficients of an overcomplete wavelet transform in combination with LRA can provide a successful classification scheme for differentiation of spiculated and circumscribed masses from dense breast parenchyma, as proven by ROC and FROC analyses. Higher performance is achieved in the detection of spiculated masses, as the orientation features are more sensitive in the presence of spiculations.

The performance of the proposed mass identification method is not directly comparable with all other reported mass detection schemes, due to the composition of the dataset used regarding the type of breast parenchyma [3], [4], [6], [8]. The results of the proposed method is comparable with and of superior performance of those reported for dense breast parenchyma [14], [15], [16], although there are differences in the datasets used regarding mammograms and mass subtlety. Future efforts will be focused on implementation of additional multiresolution features and use of other wavelet transform and classification schemes.

Acknowledgements

This work is supported by the European Social Fund (ESF), Operational Program for Educational and Vocational Training II (EPEAEK II), and particularly the Program PYTHAGORAS I (B.365.011). We also thank the staff of the Department of Radiology at the University Hospital of Patras for their contribution in this work.

References

1. Chan, H-P., Sahiner, B., Petrick, N., Hadjiiski, L., Paquerault, S.: Computer-Aided Diagnosis of Breast Cancer. In: Costaridou L. (ed): Medical Image Analysis Methods. Boca Raton, CRC Press, Taylor & Francis Group (2005) 1-49
2. Sampat, P.M., Markey, M.K., Bovik, A.C.: Computer-Aided Detection and Diagnosis in Mammography. In: Bovik A.C. (ed) Handbook of Image and Video Processing 2nd ed. Academic Press (2005) 1195-1217
3. Kegelmeyer, J., Pruneda, J.M, Bourland, P.D, Hillis, A., Riggs, M.W., Nipper, M.L.: Computer-Aided Mammographic Screening for Spiculated Lesions. Radiology 191 (1994) 331-337
4. Karssemeijer, N., te Brake, G.M.: Detection of Stellate Distortions in Mammograms. IEEE Trans. Med. Imag. 15 (1996) 611-619
5. te Brake, G.M., Karssemeijer, N., Hendricks, J.H.C.L.: Automated Detection of Breast Carcinomas Not Detected in a Screening Program. Radiology 207 (1998) 465-471
6. Wei, D., Chan, H-P., Helvie, M.A., Sahiner, B., Petrick, N., Adler, D.D., Goodsitt, M.M.: Classification of Mass and Normal Breast Tissue on Digital Mammograms: Multiresolution Texture Analysis. Med. Phys. 22 (1995) 1501-1513

564   F. Sakellaropoulos et al.

7. Wei, D., Chan, H-P., Petrick, N., Sahiner, B., Helvie, M.A., Adler, D.D., Goodsitt M.M.: False-Positive Reduction Technique for Detection of Masses on Digital Mammograms: Global and Local Multiresolution Texture Analysis. Med. Phys. 24 (1997) 903-914
8. Liu, S., Babbs, C.F., Delp, E.J.: Multiresolution Detection of Spiculated Lesions in Digital Mammograms. IEEE Trans. Image Proc. 10 (2001) 874-884
9. Petrick, N., Chan, H-P, Wei, D., Sahiner, B., Helvie, M.A, Adler, D.D.: Automated Detection of Breast Masses on Mammograms Using Adaptive Contrast Enhancement and Texture Classification. Med. Phys. 23 (1996) 1685-1696
10. Kobatake, H., Murakami, M., Takeo, H., Nawano, S.: Computerized Detection of Malignant Tumors on Digital Mammograms. IEEE Trans. Med. Imag. 18 (1999) 369-378
11. Zwiggelaar, R., Parr, T.C., Schumm, J.E., Hutt, I.W., Taylor, C.J., Astley, S.M., Boggis, C.R.M.: Model-based Detection of Spiculated Lesions in Mammograms. Med. Image Anal. 3 (1999) 39-62
12. Chang, Y.-H., Hardesty, L.A., Hakim, C.M., Chang, T.S., Zheng, B., Good, W.F., Gur, D.: Knowledge-based Computer-Aided Detection of Masses on Digitized Mammograms: A Preliminary Assessment. Med Phys. 28 (2001) 455-461
13. Baydush, A.H., Catarious, D.M., Abbey, C.K., Floyd, C.E.: Computer Aided Detection of Masses in Mammography Using Subregion Hotteling Observers. Med. Phys. 30 (2003) 1781-1787
14. Ho, W.T., Lam, P.W.T.: Clinical Performance of Computer-Assisted Detection (CAD) System in Detecting Carcinoma in Breast of Different Densities. Clin. Radiol. 58 (2003) 133-136
15. Li, L., Zheng, Y., Zhang, L., Clark, A.: False-Positive Reduction in CAD Mass Detection Using a Competitive Classification Strategy. Med. Phys. 28 (2001) 250-258
16. Tourassi, G.D, Vargas-Voracek, R., Catarious, D.M, Floyd, C.E.: Computer-Assisted Detection of Mammographic Masses: A Template Matching Scheme Based on Mutual Information. Med. Phys. 30 (2003) 2123-2130
17. Aylward, S.R., Hemminger, B.M., Pisano, E.D.: Mixture Modeling for Digital Mammogram Display and Analysis. In: Karssemeijer N., Thijssen M., Hendriks J., van Erning, A. (eds.): Digital Mammography Nijmegen. Dordrecht, the Netherlands: Kluwer Academic (1998) 305-312
18. Sakellaropoulos, P., Costaridou, L., Panayiotakis, G.: A Wavelet-based Spatially Adaptive Method for Mammographic Contrast Enhancement. Phys. Med. Biol. 48 (2003) 787-803
19. Costaridou, L., Sakellaropoulos, P., Skiadopoulos, S., Panayiotakis, G.: Locally Adaptive Wavelet Contrast Enhancement. In: Costaridou, L. (ed.): Medical Image Analysis Methods. Taylor & Francis Group LCC, CRC Press, Boca Raton, FL (2005) 225-270.
20. Costaridou, L., Sakellaropoulos, P., Stefanoyiannis, A., Ungureanu, E., Panayiotakis, G.: Quantifying Image Quality at Breast Periphery vs. Mammary Gland in Mammography Using Wavelet Analysis. Br. J. Radiol. 74 (2001) 913-919
21. Yoshida, H., Doi, K., Nishikawa, R.M., Giger, M.L., Schmidt, R.A.: An Improved Computer-Assisted Diagnostic Scheme Using Wavelet Transform for Detecting Clustered Microcalcifications in Digital Mammograms. Acad. Radiol. 3 (1996) 621-627
22. Chang, C-M., Laine, A.: Coherence of Multiscale Features for Enhancement of Digital Mammograms. IEEE Trans. Med. Imag. 3 (1999) 32-46
23. Mudigonda, N.R., Rangayyan, R.M., Desautels, L.J.E.: Detection of Breast Masses in Mammograms by Density Slicing and Texture Flow-Field Analysis. IEEE Trans. Med. Imag. 20 (2001) 1215-1227
24. Sakellaropoulos, P., Costaridou, L., Panayiotakis, G.: An Image Visualization Tool in Mammography. Med. Inform. 24 (1999) 53-73

Leveraging the Digital Mammography Image Screening Trial (DMIST) Data for the Evaluation of Computer-Aided Detection (CAD) Devices: A Proposal

Nicholas Petrick, Kyle J. Myers, Sophie Paquerault, Frank W. Samuelson, Brandon D. Gallas, and Robert F. Wagner

U.S. Food and Drug Administration, Center for Devices and Radiological Health, Rockville, MD 20852
{nicholas.petrick, kyle.myers, sophie.paquerault, frank.samuelson, brandon.gallas, robert.wagner}@fda.hhs.gov

Abstract. The availability of the large dataset of screen/film and full-field digital mammograms acquired through the Digital Mammography Imaging Screening Trial (DMIST) presents an extraordinary opportunity for the assessment of CAD devices. The National Cancer Institute and the National Institute of Biomedical Imaging and Bioengineering at the U.S. National Institutes of Health have engaged FDA scientists in the development of a plan to leverage this imaging resource to benchmark the performance of current CAD systems. In this talk, we will present an initial proposal for utilizing the DMIST data to quantitatively assess current CAD systems. It is our goal to engage the IWDM community and other interested groups in the development of a consensus on acceptable study designs for this purpose.

1 Background

A variety of computer-assist devices have been approved by the U.S. Food and Drug Administration (FDA) as aids to a mammographer in the detection of breast cancer. These devices were originally approved for screen/film mammography on the basis of a study design that demonstrated the potential for computer-aided detection (CAD) systems to identify missed cancers without the systems producing a substantial increase in the number of patients recalled for additional procedures [1]. Some of these initial screen/film approvals were later extended for application with select full-field digital mammography (FFDM) systems. The FDA approval studies performed by most of the CAD manufacturers were modest in their scope because of a limited patient population, their focus on screen/film mammography and the retrospective nature of the study design.

1.1 Recent Studies of Breast CAD

A recent prospective study by Gur, *et al.* on the benefits of mammographic CAD in an academic clinical radiology practice concluded that the introduction of CAD in their clinical practice was not associated with statistically significant changes in recall or breast cancer detection rates [2]. Similar results were reported for both the entire

Susan M. Astley et al. (Eds.): IWDM 2006, LNCS 4046, pp. 565–568, 2006.
© Springer-Verlag Berlin Heidelberg 2006

group of 24 radiologists who participated in the study and the subset of radiologists who interpreted the highest volume of mammograms. While the conclusions of this study are limited to patients in the University of Pittsburgh system, screen/film mammography and one mammographic CAD device, they strongly suggest that additional studies to benchmark and evaluate the adjunctive benefit of CAD would be of practical value to the public at large.

Even fewer studies, and none with a large diverse patient population, have been conducted to benchmark and evaluate the adjunctive benefit of mammographic CAD with FFDM. The Blue Cross Blue Shield Technical Evaluation Center (TEC) recently conducted a MEDLINE literature search addressing the question as to whether the use of CAD can improve the sensitivity and specificity of FFDM [3]. A prior assessment of CAD in screen/film mammography conducted by the TEC concluded that evidence is available to support the conclusion that CAD improves the accuracy of screen/film mammography by increasing the true-positive rate without a disproportionate increase in the recalls compared with single-reader radiologist interpretation. For CAD as an adjunct to FFDM, the search yielded no high-quality articles in peer-reviewed journals assessing this combination. Therefore, the TEC concluded that "until results from better studies focusing on the use of CAD with FFDM become available, the benefits of CAD with FFDM cannot be determined." This conclusion again supports the need for additional studies to benchmark and evaluate the adjunctive benefit of CAD when combined with FFDM.

1.2 Digital Mammography Imaging Screening Trial

The American College of Radiology Imaging Network (ACRIN), under the direction of Etta Pisano, M.D., conducted the Digital Mammography Imaging Screening Trial (DMIST) [4, 5]. Funding for the trial was provided by the NIH National Cancer Institute and the total cost was on the order of $30 million. The primary goal of this large population-based trial was to compare the diagnostic accuracy of digital and screen/film mammography in a breast cancer screening population of asymptomatic women [5]. The trial was designed to measure small but potentially clinically important differences in diagnostic accuracy between digital and screen/film mammography in the overall population of asymptomatic women and in particular subgroups of denser breasted women where digital mammography might be expected to have an improved diagnostic ability [4].

The DMIST trial collected both digital and screen/film mammograms, in random order, from 49,528 women at 33 sites in the United States and Canada. Five digital mammography systems were utilized in the trial. These systems included the SenoScan (Fischer Imaging), the Computed Radiography for Mammography (Fuji), the Senographe 2000D (General Electric), the Lorad/Trex Digital Mammography System (Hologic) and the Selenia Full Field Digital Mammography System (Hologic) [5]. The screen/film and digital mammograms were each read independently by different radiologists with each reader rating patients using both a seven-point malignancy scale and a Breast Imaging Reporting and Data System (BI-RADS) [6] classification. All relevant information was available for 42,760 of these women, including 335 women subsequently identified as having breast cancer. Breast cancer status was based on the results of a breast biopsy within 15 months after the screening study or by a follow-up mammogram at one year.

The results from the trial showed that the diagnostic accuracy of digital and screen/film mammography were similar in terms of area under the fitted receiver operating characteristic curve (A_Z). However, the accuracy of digital mammography was significantly higher than that of screen/film mammography among women under the age of 50 years ($\Delta A_Z=0.15$; $p=0.002$), women with heterogeneously dense or extremely dense breasts on mammography ($\Delta A_Z=0.11$; $p=0.003$), and premenopausal or perimenopausal women ($\Delta A_Z=0.15$; $p=0.002$) [4].

2 Method

The National Cancer Institute and the National Institute of Biomedical Imaging and Bioengineering at the U.S. National Institutes of Health have engaged FDA scientists' participation in the development of a plan to leverage this imaging data to address other important public health issues. Breast CAD was identified as an area of significant interest because of CAD's potential for improving breast cancer screening, the lack of population-based studies evaluating breast CAD in a general setting, and the conflicting performance results for commercial breast CAD that have been reported in the literature [1, 2]. In addition, no significant information is available to the radiology community either benchmarking current CAD algorithms in combination with screen/film or digital mammography systems or studying the influence of CAD on overall breast cancer screening in a large and diverse patient population.

As a start to understanding the public health implication of breast CAD, we will present an initial proposal for utilizing the DMIST data to quantitatively assess current CAD systems. In particular, we will outline a proposal for benckmarking the current performance of breast CAD for screen/film and a select set of digital mammography systems. This will include details on plans for digitizing screen/film mammograms, establishing truth on the location, extent, and type of lesions visible in the mammograms, and a plan for statistically evaluating and comparing the different algorithms.

3 Discussion

It is our goal to engage the participation of the IWDM community in the development of a consensus on acceptable study designs for benchmarking CAD performance and to start the process of systematically understanding the public health benefits of breast CAD. This presentation and discussion is the first in potentially a series of discussions toward development of a consensus among NIH, FDA, ACRIN, DMIST, industry, academia, advocacy groups and the public at large on how to leverage this and other medical image resources. The DMIST data were acquired at great cost, signifying a resource unlikely to ever be duplicated. This is an ideal time to initiate a discussion on how best to make use of this tremendous image resource to improve public health through the accurate assessment of the performance of CAD devices in the early detection of breast cancer.

References

1. Warren Burhenne LJ, Wood SA, D'Orsi CJ, et al.: Potential contribution of computer-aided detection to the sensitivity of screening mammography. Radiology. 215 (2000) 554-562
2. Gur D, Sumkin JH, Rockette HE, et al.: Changes in breast cancer detection and mammography recall rates after the introduction of a computer-aided detection system. Journal of the National Cancer Institute. 96 (2004) 185-190
3. Computer-Aided Detection With Full-Field Digital Mammography. http://www.bcbs.com/tec/tecinpress/08.html. Last Access: April 7, 2006, (2006)
4. Pisano ED, Gatsonis C, Hendrick E, et al.: Diagnostic performance of digital versus film mammography for breast-cancer screening. New England Journal of Medicine. 353 (2005) 1773-1783
5. Pisano ED, Gatsonis CA, Yaffe MJ, et al.: American College of Radiology Imaging Network digital mammographic imaging screening trial: objectives and methodology. Radiology. 236 (2005) 404-412
6. Breast Imaging Reporting and Data System (BI-RADS), 4th ed. American College of Radiology Reston, VA (2003)

Comparison of Computerized Image Analyses for Digitized Screen-Film Mammograms and Full-Field Digital Mammography Images

Hui Li, Maryellen L. Giger, Yading Yuan, Li Lan, Kenji Suzuki, Andrew Jamieson, Laura Yarusso, Robert M. Nishikawa, and Charlene Sennett

Department of Radiology and Committee on Medical Physics, The University of Chicago, Chicago, IL 60637 USA
m-giger@uchicago.edu

Abstract. We have developed computerized methods for the analysis of mammo-graphic lesions in order to aid in the diagnosis of breast cancer. Our automatic methods include the extraction of the lesion from the breast paren-chyma, the characterization of the lesion features in terms of mathematical des-criptors, and the merging of these lesion features into an estimate of the probability of malignancy. Our initial development was performed on digitized screen film mammograms. We report our progress here in converting our methods for use with images from full-field digital mammography (FFDM). It is apparent from our initial comparisons on CAD for SFM_D and FFDM that the overall concepts and image analysis techniques are similar, however reoptimization for a particular lesion segmentation or a particular mammo-graphic imaging system are warranted.

1 Introduction

We have developed computerized methods for the analysis of mammographic lesions in order to aid in the diagnosis of breast cancer [1-9]. The automatic methods include the extraction of the lesion from the breast parenchyma, the characterization of the lesion features in terms of mathematical descriptors, and the merging of these lesion features into an estimate of the probability of malignancy. Our initial development was performed on digitized screen film mammograms (SFM_D; 0.1 mm pixel size). We report our progress here in converting our methods for use with images from full-field digital mammography (FFDM).

2 Databases

Our digitized screen/film mammographic (SFM_D) database and our FFDM database currently arise from different cases. Thus, comparison of image analysis results between SFM_D and FFDM is not directly possible. However, conclusions can be drawn by the analysis of trends seen in the data. The SFM_D database includes screen/film mammograms digitized to 0.1 mm pixel size and 10-bit quantization. The FFDM database includes images from a GE Senographe 2000D.

Susan M. Astley et al. (Eds.): IWDM 2006, LNCS 4046, pp. 569–575, 2006.
© Springer-Verlag Berlin Heidelberg 2006

3 Lesion Segmentation

We continue to investigate methods with which to extract the lesion (margin) from the parenchymal background in a mammographic image. These methods have included a region growing technique [1,2], a radial gradient index technique (RGI) [3], and an active contour snake method [9]. In the region growing method, the lesion image undergoes histogram equalization followed by gray level thresholding. By monitoring the size and shape of the evolving contour with each incremented gray level threshold step, a lesion contour is automatically selected at an abrupt transition from high circularity to low circularity, and from small size to larger size. In the RGI method, a Gaussian constraint function is applied to the image data in order to suppress the influence of distant pixels. From a series of potential contours obtained by thresholding, the contour whose margin yields the maximum RGI value is chosen as the one that best delineates the lesion. The RGI value corresponds to the average proportion of the gradients in the radially outward direction. The snake method involves a two-stage segmentation that uses an active contour algorithm to minimize an energy function based on the homogeneities inside and outside of the evolving contour. The minimization algorithm solves, by the level set method, the Euler-Lagrange equation that describes the contour evolution. Prior to the application of the active contour algorithm, the RGI-based segmentation method is applied to yield an initial contour closer to the lesion margin location in a computationally efficient manner. This initial RGI segmentation also estimates an effective background, for subsequent use in the active contour approach, by using the values of the image within a given radius of the initial contour.

Our evaluation of the three methods on SFM_D and FFDM included only images on which human-delineated lesion margins had been obtained. Performance was determined based on an overlap measure [3], where the overlap was calculated by the ratio of the areas within the intersection of the human-delineated margin contour (Rad. A) and the computer-determined margin contour to the union of the two areas. The results are presented in terms of percent of lesion images accurately segmented at a given threshold cutoff (e.g. at a threshold cutoff of 0.4 as shown in Table 1). It is apparent from Table 1 and Figure 1 that, overall, the two-stage active contour snake method is the most promising for both the SFM_D and FFDM databases.

Table 1. Percent of lesion images accurately segmented at an overlap threshold cutoff of 0.4 for the **SFM_D and FFDM databases** and the three segmentation methods

SFM_D Database	Total Cases	Total Images	Region growing	RGI	Snake
Malignant	55	96	74.0%	66.7%	86.7%
Benign	29	51	76.5%	90.2%	88.2%
Total	84	147	74.8%	74.8%	87.1%

FFDM Database	Total Cases	Total Images	Region growing	RGI	Snake
Malignant	148	412	66.0%	66.7%	75.7%
Benign	139	327	72.5%	81.0%	85.6%
Total	287	739	68.9%	73.1%	80.1%

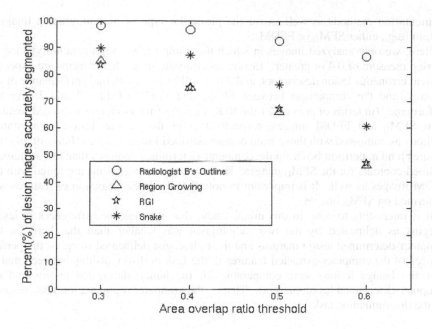

Fig. 1. The percent of SFM$_D$ lesion images correctly segmented at different overlap cutoffs using Radiologist A manually-delineated margins as "truth"

For both the SFM$_D$ and FFDM segmentation analyses, the same breast radiologist (C.S.) manually outlined the lesion margin as the segmentation "truth" – Rad. A. For the SFM$_D$, we also had human-delineated lesion margins from another radiologist and the percent of lesion images accurately segmented at an overlap threshold cutoff of 0.4 by the other radiologist, in comparison with the first, was 96.6%. This indicates that the radiologists highly agreed on the lesion margins.

4   Computer-Extracted Lesion Features

In our computerized image analyses for aiding in the discrimination between malignant and benign lesions, we automatically extract various mathematical descriptors (features) of the lesions. In our past studies [8], four general features were selected for use in our intelligent workstation: (a) "margin sharpness" as the magnitude of the gradient along the margin of the lesion, (b) "texture" as determined from the standard deviation of the average gradient within the lesion, (c) "spiculation" as determined from the full width at half maximum of the normalized edge-gradient distribution relative to the radial direction, and (d) "radial gradient index" that corresponds to the average proportion of the gradients in the radially outward direction and thus contains shape information. In this initial study, we extracted these same four features from the images in the two databases and determined the performance of each in the task of distinguishing between malignant and benign lesions using ROC analysis [10,11]. It should be noted that eventually we will optimize the feature selection for the different segmentation methods as well as for the particular type of mammographic imaging system (e.g., either SFM_D or FFDM).

Here, we only analyzed images in which the computerized segmentation yielded an overlap measure of 0.4 or greater. Erroneous computer-extracted margins are expected to yield erroneous lesion descriptors, and thus would mask the actual performance of the features, and the comparison between SFM_D and FFDM. Tables 2 and 3 give the performance (in terms of area under the ROC curve) of the computer-extracted features from SFM_D and FFDM images, respectively, for the various lesion segmentation methods as compared with those from human-outlined lesion margins. Interestingly, the features tend to perform better on the computer-determined contours than on the human-outlined contours for the SFM_D images. However, promising results are found with the FFDM images as well. It is important to note that the initial selection of features was performed on SFM_D images.

It is interesting to note, in this initial study, that although the differences in lesion margins as delineated by the two radiologists was smaller than that between the computer-determined lesion margins and the radiologist-delineated margins, the performances of the computer-extracted features in the task of distinguishing between malignant and benign lesions were comparable for the human-delineated lesions and the computer-determined lesion margins. That is, the computer segmentation was adequate for the discrimination task.

Table 2. Performance (in terms of area under the ROC curve) of computer-extracted features from **SFM_D images** for the various lesion segmentation methods as compared with those from human-outlined lesion margins (Rad. A). Also included is a comparison of feature performances obtained from segmented lesions by two different radiologists (Rad. A and Rad. B).

	Rad. A	Region Growing	p value
Margin Sharpness	0.54	0.57	0.59
Texture	0.55	0.59	0.25
Spiculation	0.71	0.74	0.76
RGI	0.78	0.75	0.41
	Rad. A	RGI	p value
Margin Sharpness	0.55	0.67	0.02
Texture	0.55	0.64	0.01
Spiculation	0.69	0.69	0.92
RGI	0.75	0.68	0.20
	Rad. A	Snake	p value
Margin Sharpness	0.57	0.67	0.04
Texture	0.54	0.56	0.33
Spiculation	0.71	0.67	0.80
RGI	0.77	0.75	0.56
	Rad. A	Rad. B	p value
Margin Sharpness	0.51	0.62	<0.001
Texture	0.56	0.56	0.92
Spiculation	0.73	0.67	0.16
RGI	0.80	0.73	0.003

Table 3. Performance (in terms of area under the ROC curve) of computer-extracted features from **FFDM images** for the various lesion segmentation methods as compared with those from human-outlined lesion margins

	Rad. A	Region Growing	p value
Margin Sharpness	0.51	0.61	<0.0001
Texture	0.61	0.70	<0.0001
Spiculation	0.71	0.69	0.29
RGI	0.72	0.66	0.003
	Rad. A	RGI	p value
Margin Sharpness	0.51	0.58	<0.001
Texture	0.59	0.63	0.003
Spiculation	0.69	0.65	0.05
RGI	0.71	0.62	<0.0001
	Rad. A	Snake	p value
Margin Sharpness	0.51	0.57	0.18
Texture	0.60	0.67	<0.0001
Spiculation	0.69	0.65	0.13
RGI	0.71	0.63	<0.0001

5   Comparison to Physical Imaging Properties

We are currently relating these performance variations to differences in the physical image quality between the SFM_D and FFDM systems. (see Table 4) From our evaluation of the physical image quality for the two systems, we have found that the SFM_D exhibits, as compared to FFDM, higher spatial resolution, increased noise, and higher contrast, as measured by the modulation transfer functions (MTF), the noise Wiener spectra, and the characteristic curves, respectively. Note that, in this pilot study, the gradient-based computer-extracted features such as margin sharpness, spiculation, and RGI performed better on SFM_D – being the system with the superior spatial resolution. Also, the texture-based features performed better on FFDM – being the system with the lower noise and the better contrast.

Table 4. Performance (in terms of area under the ROC curve) of computer-extracted features from **SFM_D and FFDM images** obtained with the snake lesion segmentation method

	SFM_D	FFDM
Margin Sharpness	0.67	0.57
Texture	0.56	0.67
Spiculation	0.67	0.65
RGI	0.75	0.63

6 Summary

It is apparent from this initial comparison study for CAD for SFM$_D$ and FFDM that the overall concepts and image analysis techniques are expected to be similar, however re-optimization for a particular lesion segmentation or a particular mammographic imaging system are warranted. Our analysis was performed on actual clinical cases, and thus our results are expected to be translated to the clinical arena. It is also important to note that only individual computer-extracted features were analysed for this paper. As we have shown in the past, we expect that by merging the features, a significant improvement in discrimination performance will be achieved [2,5-8].

A limitation of our initial study is that the databases for SFM$_D$ and FFDM came from different cases. In the future, we hope to obtain a database of both SFM$_D$ and FFDM from the same set of women. Cases from the recent DMIST trial of FFDM vs. SFM would satisfy this criterion.

Acknowledgements

The authors are thankful to the late Carl J. Vyborny for earlier contributions to this research. This research is supported in parts by USPHS Grant CA89452. M. L. Giger, L. Lan, and R. M. Nishikawa are shareholders in R2 Technology, Inc. (Sunnyvale, CA) and receive royalties and research funding from R2. It is the policy of the University of Chicago that investigators disclose publicly actual or potential significant financial interests that may appear to be affected by the research activities.

References

1. Huo, Z., Giger, M.L., Vyborny, C.J., Bick, U., Lu, P., Wolverton, D.E., Schmidt, R.A.: Analysis of spiculation in the computerized classification of mammographic masses. Med. Phys. 22 (1995) 1569-1579
2. Huo, Z., Giger, M.L., Vyborny, C.J., Wolverton, D.E., Schmidt, R.A., Doi, K.: Automated computerized classification of malignant and benign mass lesions on digitized mammograms. Acad. Radiol. 5 (1998) 155-168
3. Kupinski, M.A., Giger, M.L.: Automated seeded lesion segmentation on digital mammograms. IEEE Trans. Med. Imaging 17 (1998) 510-517
4. Kupinski, M.A., Giger, M.L.: Feature selection with limited datasets. Med. Phys. 26 (1999) 2176-2182
5. Huo, Z., Giger, M.L., Vyborny, C.J., Wolverton, D.E., Metz, C.E.: Computerized classification of benign and malignant masses on digitized mammograms: a robustness study. Acad. Radiol. 7 (2000) 1077-1084
6. Huo, Z., Giger, M.L., Vyborny, C.J.: Computerized analysis of multiple-mammographic views: Potential usefulness of special view mammograms in computer-aided diagnosis. IEEE Trans. Med. Imaging 20 (2001) 1285-1292
7. Huo, Z., Giger, M.L., Vyborny, C.J., Metz, C.E.: Effectiveness of CAD in the diagnosis of breast cancer: An observer study on an independent database of mammograms. Radiology 224 (2002) 560-568

8. Horsch, K., Giger, M.L., Vyborny, C.J., Lan, L., Mendelson, E., Hendrick, R.E.: Multi-modality computer-aided diagnosis for the classification of breast lesions: Observer study results on an independent dataset. Radiology (in press) (2006)
9. Yuan, Y., Giger, M.L., Suzuki, K., Li, H., Jamieson, A.R.: A two-stage method for lesion segmentation on digital mammograms. Proc. SPIE Med. Imaging (in press) (2006)
10. Metz, C.E.: ROC methodology in radiologic imaging. Invest. Radiol. 21 (1986) 720-733
11. Metz, C.E.: Some practical issues of experimental design and data analysis in radiological ROC studies, Invest. Radiol. 24 (1989) 234-245

Comparison Between CRT and LCD Displays for Full-Field-Digital-Mammography (FFDM) Interpretation

Chiara Del Frate[*], Alexia Bestagno, Viviana Londero, Raffaella Pozzi Mucelli, Valerio Salomoni, and Massimo Bazzocchi

Insitute of Radiology, University of Udine, Italy

Abstract. Purpose: To evaluate efficacy and diagnostic accuracy of BARCO LCD 5Mpixel displays, compared to BARCO CRT 5Mpixel displays in full-field-digital-mammography (FFDM) interpretation.

Material and Methods: FFDM mammograms obtained by 100 patients, were analyzed by three independent radiologists experienced in breast imaging, using two different CRT and LCD displays. All cases were selected by a fourth radiologist in order to cover several possible ages and types of breast. Half of cases were negative and half were positive for malignancy, proven by percutaneous biopsy. Readers were blinded to history of patients, ultrasound examination and biopsy results. To minimize recall bias, an interval of at least 30 days between interpretations of each case on two different monitors was chosen. Each reader evaluated cases classifying them according the ACR BIRADS categories. Moreover, they assigned a rate (0-100) corresponding to the Probability of Malignancy (POM) of each case classified into BIRADS categories 3 to 5. Finally, they assigned a rate (0-100) corresponding to reading confidence.

Analysis included ROC curves of POM for each doctor and for pooled data, sensitivity and specificity for the BIRADS≥3 and BIRADS≥4 thresholds for each doctor and for pooled data, and finally main results of "Multireader-Multicase ROC Analysis Of Variance". For each analysis a comparison was made between the two monitors.

Results: No statistical significance was seen between the two displays regarding POM, sensitivity and specificity, nor for single reader either for pooled data.

Conclusions: This study provides a reasonable assurance that the examined CRT and LCD display systems are comparable for FFDM interpretation.

1 Background

Several trials demonstrated that Full-Field Digital Mammography (FFDM) is at least comparable to analogic mammography in the detection rate of cancers (1-3). At the same time, it is well known that the analysis of digital mammograms cannot be performed on printed images but requires high resolution monitors (5 MegaPixels),

---

[*] Corresponding author. E-mail address is chiara.delfrate@med.uniud.it

Susan M. Astley et al. (Eds.): IWDM 2006, LNCS 4046, pp. 576–584, 2006.
© Springer-Verlag Berlin Heidelberg 2006

dedicated to mammography (3-5). Actually, two different technologies for monitors are available: the commonly used Cathode Ray Tube (CRT) monitors and the more recently introduced Liquid Crystal Display (LCD) monitors. The two technologies have different characteristics and both present advantage and disadvantage. It is not still clear which of the two should be used in clinical practice (6, 7).

The purpose of our study was to evaluate efficacy and diagnostic accuracy of BARCO LCD 5Mpixel displays, compared to BARCO CRT 5Mpixel displays in full-field-digital-mammography (FFDM) interpretation.

2 Material and Methods

Three radiologists, experienced in breast imaging, with respectively 9, 8 and 3 years of experience, reviewed 100 cases of FFDM, using BARCO CRT monitors (MammoMeDis HD, model V9600123) and BARCO LCD monitors (Coronis 5MP Mammo, Model V9600800). The characteristics of the two different monitors are summarized in Table 1. All digital mammograms were obtained with FFDM unit GIOTTO IMAGE MD (IMS – Bologna, Italy).

Table 1. Characteristics of CRT and LCD Monitors

Characteristics	CRT	LCD
Dimension	304mm x 380 mm	337mm x 422mm
Contrast	>2000 :1	>700 :1
Matrix	2048 x 2560	2048 x 2560
Refresh Rate (Frequency)	76 Hz	50 Hz
Viewing angle	± 135°	± 25°
Luminance	400 cd/m2	600 cd/m2
Luminance Uniformity	>90%	>90%
Ambient light	< 10 LUX	< 10 LUX

3 Patient's Selection

The 100 cases were selected by a forth radiologist, experienced in breast imaging, in order to cover several possible ages (range 40-83 years, mean 53.5 years) and a great variety of breasts, considering particularly different possible densities. 40% of cases consisted of biopsy-proved malignancies while 60% of cases were negative or with benign findings, with at least one year follow-up. The fourth radiologist anonimized all cases and presented them randomly to the three readers, on CRT monitors and LCD ones. Only the fourth radiologist was aware of the results of histology.

4 Imaging Interpretation

To make the conditions as reproducible as possible, ambient light was always in the limit and the angle with which the doctors were positioned in front of the LCD was into the limits (position of the eyes approximately in the middle of the LCD at a distance of approximately 30/40 cm).

Each examination was independently interpreted by the three radiologists. To minimize recall bias, an interval of at least 30 days between interpretations of the same case on the two different monitors was planned. The images were evaluated randomly, observing at the same moment both breasts, in the two views (CC and MLO). No prior films, patient histories or any other demographic information accompanied the interpretation of either modality.

ACR BIRADS categories, reported in Table 2, was used to assess findings for each modality.

Table 2. ACR BIRADS categories

ACR BIRADS Category	Findings
0	Needs further evaluation
1	Normal
2	Abnormal – benign
3	Abnormal – probably benign
4	Suspicious for cancer
5	Highly suspicious for cancer

Besides this, each radiologist assigned a rate (on a scale from 0 to 100) corresponding to the Probability of Malignancy (**POM**) of each case classified into BI-RADS categories **3**, **4** or **5** and was required to give a location for each finding. Finally, each radiologist was required to define the rate of confidence for the presence of the abnormality.

5 Statistical Analysis

Sensitivity and specificity were calculated for each reader and each monitor. Moreover,

ROC curves were created:

- the trapezoidal ROC curves of the probability of malignancy for each doctor;
- the trapezoidal ROC curves of the probability of malignancy for the pooled data;
- the sensitivity and specificity for the BIRADS≥3 and BIRADS≥4 thresholds for each doctor;
- the sensitivity and specificity for the BIRADS≥3 and BIRADS≥4 thresholds for the pooled data;
- the main results of the "Multireader-Multicase ROC Analysis Of Variance Using Gaussian Distribution" performed with the LABMRMC application (see for details).

6 Results

6.1 Reader 1

As regards Reader 1, we obtained the following results.

The specificity and sensitivity analysis was performed for the BIRADS≥3 and BIRADS≥4 thresholds (Table 4)

Table 3

	Sensitivity for BIRADS≥3 (95% C. I.)	Specificity for BIRADS≥3 (95% C. I.)	Sensitivity for BIRADS≥4 (95% C. I.)	Specificity for BIRADS≥4 (95% C. I.)
CRT	0.816 (0.657 to 0.922)	0.847 (0.730 to 0.928)	0.605 (0.434 to 0.759)	0.966 (0.883 to 0.995)
LCD	0.789 (0.627 to 0.904)	0.898 (0.792 to 0.961)	0.421 (0.263 to 0.592)	0.966 (0.883 to 0.995)

The ROC curves obtained from the Probability Of Malignancy (POM) are shown in Figure 1 and the data reported in Table 4.

Table 4

	Trapezoidal area under the ROC curve for POM	Standard Error	95% Confidence Interval
CRT	0.861	0.042	0.776 to 0.923
LCD	0.857	0.042	0.772 to 0.920
CRT-LCD	0.004	0.035	-0.065 to 0.073

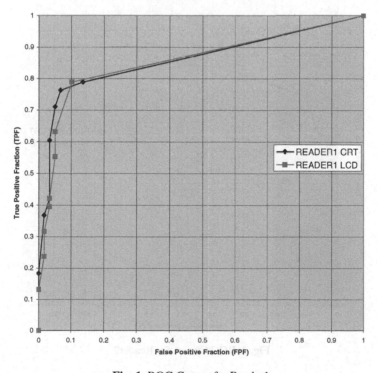

Fig. 1. ROC Curves for Reader1

6.2 Reader 2

As regards Reader 2, we obtained the following results.

The specificity and sensitivity analysis was performed for the BIRADS≥3 and BIRADS≥4 thresholds (Table 5).

Table 5

	Sensitivity for BIRADS≥3 (95% C. I.)	Specificity for BIRADS≥3 (95% C. I.)	Sensitivity for BIRADS≥4 (95% C. I.)	Specificity for BIRADS≥4 (95% C. I.)
CRT	0.658 (0.486 to 0.804)	0.898 (0.792 to 0.961)	0.474 (0.310 to 0.642)	0.966 (0.883 to 0.995)
LCD	0.658 (0.486 to 0.804)	0.881 (0.771 to 0.951)	0.526 (0.358 to 0.690)	0.966 (0.883 to 0.995)

The ROC curves obtained from the Probability Of Malignancy (POM) are shown in Figure 2 and the data reported in Table 6.

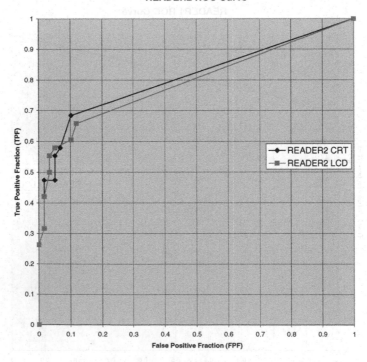

Fig. 2. ROC Curves for Reader2

Table 6

	Trapezoidal area under the ROC curve for POM	Standard Error	95% Confidence Interval
CRT	0.808	0.048	0.716 to 0.881
LCD	0. 794	0.049	0.700 to 0.869
CRT-LCD	0.015	0.037	-0.058 to 0.087

6.3   Reader 3

As regards Reader 3, we obtained the following results.

The specificity and sensitivity analysis was performed for the BIRADS≥3 and BIRADS≥4 thresholds (Table 7).

The ROC curves obtained from the Probability Of Malignancy (POM) are shown in Figure 3 and the data reported in Table 8.

Table 7

	Sensitivity for BIRADS≥3 (95% C. I.)	Specificity for BIRADS≥3 (95% C. I.)	Sensitivity for BIRADS≥4 (95% C. I.)	Specificity for BIRADS≥4 (95% C. I.)
CRT	0.789 (0.627 to 0.904)	0.831 (0.710 to 0.915)	0.421 (0.263 to 0.592)	0.983 (0.909 to 0.997)
LCD	0.763 (0.598 to 0.885)	0.831 (0.710 to 0.915)	0.579 (0.408 to 0.737)	0.966 (0.883 to 0.995)

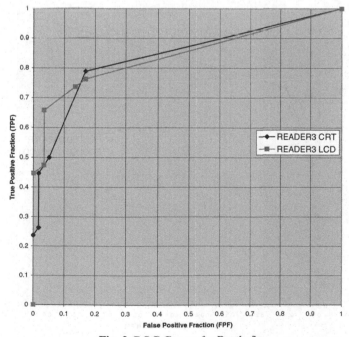

Fig. 3. ROC Curves for Reader3

Table 8

	Trapezoidal area under the ROC curve for POM	Standard Error	95% Confidence Interval
CRT	0.840	0.044	0.751 to 0.906
LCD	0.844	0.044	0.756 to 0.910
CRT-LCD	-0.004	0.033	-0.060 to 0.068

7   Pooled Data

As regards the pooled data, we obtained the following results.

The specificity and sensitivity analysis was performed for the BIRADS≥3 and BIRADS≥4 thresholds (Table 9).

The ROC curves obtained from the Probability Of Malignancy (POM) are shown in Figure 4 and the data reported in Table 10.

Table 9

	Sensitivity for BIRADS≥3 (95% C. I.)	Specificity for BIRADS≥3 (95% C. I.)	Sensitivity for BIRADS≥4 (95% C. I.)	Specificity for BIRADS≥4 (95% C. I.)
CRT	0.754 (0.665 to 0.830)	0.859 (0.799 to 0.906)	0.500 (0.405 to 0.595)	0.972 (0.935 to 0.991)
LCD	0.737 (0.646 to 0.815)	0.870 (0.811 to 0.916)	0.509 (0.413 to 0.604)	0.966 (0.928 to 0.987)

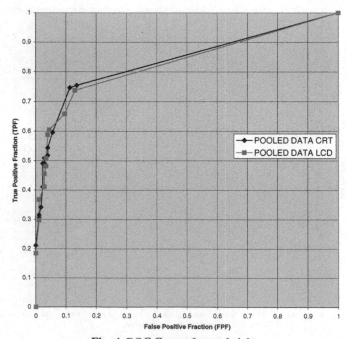

Fig. 4. ROC Curves for pooled data

Table 10

	Trapezoidal area under the ROC curve for POM	Standard Error	95% Confidence Interval
CRT	0.838	0.026	0.791 to 0.879
LCD	0.830	0.026	0.782 to 0.871
CRT-LCD	0.008	0.020	-0.031 to 0.048

8 Multireader-Multicases Analysis

The multireader-multicase analysis performed with LABMRMC gave the following results (Table 11-14).

Table 11. Standard Errors And 95% Confidence Interval For MRMC Analyses

	Area found by LABMRMC	Standard Error	95% Confidence Interval
CRT	0.9107	0.0292	N.A.
LCD	0.8974	0.0340	N.A.
CRT-LCD	0.0133	0.0318	-0.0498 to 0.0764

Table 12. Reader Means

	Area found by LABMRMC
READER1	0.9332
READER2	0.8917
READER3	0.8871

Table 13. Monitor Type Means

	Area found by LABMRMC
CRT	0.9107
LCD	0.8974

Table 14. Reader Means For Each Monitor Type

	CRT	LCD
READER1	0.9275	0.9389
READER2	0.9050	0.8785
READER3	0.8994	0.8747

9 Conclusions

The following conclusions can be drawn from the results presented in the previous chapter:

- For each reader the difference of the area under the trapezoidal ROC curves for CRT and LCD is not significant because the value 0.0 is included in the 95% confidence interval of the difference of the two areas.

- For the pooled data, the difference of the area under the trapezoidal ROC curves for CRT and LCD is not significant because the value 0.0 is included in the 95% confidence interval of the difference of the two areas.
- For each reader and for each sensitivity and specificity threshold, the 95% confidence intervals for CRT and LCD overlap, so there are no significant differences in sensitivity and specificity.
- For the pooled data, for each sensitivity and specificity threshold, the 95% confidence intervals for CRT and LCD overlap, so there are no significant differences in sensitivity and specificity.
- As regards the multireader-multicases analysis performed by the LABMRMC application, we can see that there are no significant differences between CRT and LCD since the value 0.0 is included in the 95% confidence interval of the difference of the two areas.

From all these conclusions, we can state that this study showed no significant differences between the clinical performances on mammography images of CRT and LCD monitors.

References

1. Lewin JM, Hendrick RE, D'Orsi CJ, et al. Clinical comparison of full-field digital mammography and screen-film mammography for detection of breast cancer. Am J Roentgenol 2002; 179: 671-677.
2. Skaane P, Young K, Skjennald A. Population-based mammography screening: comparison of screen-film and full-field digital mammography with soft-copy reading – Oslo I Study. Radiology 2003; 229: 877-884.
3. Skaane P, Skjennald A. Breast Imaging. Screen-film mammography versus full-field digital mammography with soft-copy reading: randomized trial in a population-based screening program – Oslo II Study. Radiology 2004; 232: 197-204.
4. Mahadevappa M. AAPM/RSNA Physics tutorial for residents. Digital Mammography: an overview. Radiographics 2004; 24: 1747-1760
5. Suryanarayanan S, Karellas A, Vedantham S, Ved H, Baker SP, D'Orsi CJ. Flat-panel digital mammography system: contrast – detail comparison between screen-film radiographs and hard-copy images. Radiology 2002; 225: 801-807.
6. Samei E. AAPM/RSNA Physics tutorial for residents: Technological and psychophysical considerations for digital mammographic displays. RadioGraphics 2005; 25: 491-501.
7. Badano A. AAPM/RSNA Tutorial on equipment selection: PACS equipment overview. Display systems. RadioGraphics 2004; 24: 879-889.

A Harmonized Quality Control Program for Digital Mammography

Martin Yaffe, Gordon Mawdsley, and Aili Bloomquist

Imaging/Bioengineering Research, Sunnybrook Health Sciences Centre
and Department of Medical Biophysics, University of Toronto
Room S657, 2075 Bayview Avenue, Toronto, ON, Can M4N 3M5
Martin.yaffe@swri.ca

Abstract. Digital mammography is rapidly becoming a mature imaging modality. To maintain high quality in mammography, a routine quality control program is necessary to detect drifting or degradation of system performance over time. The American College of Radiology is developing a quality control program which will apply to all types of full-field digital mammography equipment, and provide effective and more efficient validation of performance. In the DMIST trial, there were no failures for many of the QC tests during the 24 months imaging was performed. When systems failed, they generally did so suddenly, rather than through gradual deterioration of performance. A recommended set of tests is presented, which can be used to ensure that full-field digital mammography (FFDM) systems are functioning correctly, and consistently producing mammograms of excellent image quality.

Keywords: Digital mammography, quality control, image quality.

1 Introduction

Digital mammography is an evolving imaging modality, quickly moving into regular clinical use with over 1300 full-field digital mammography (FFDM) units accredited in the US in March 2006, and the expectation of rapid acceptance of photostimulable phosphor systems. There are now a number of systems and technologies available on the market. Current US (MQSA) regulations [1] require that sites follow the quality control (QC) procedures described by the individual manufacturers of the FFDM systems, which has resulted in discordance among the various QC protocols. To ensure that image quality is optimal and to support an effective accreditation program; routine QC, standard physics evaluation methods and acceptance test practices that are independent of the manufacturer are required.

The American College of Radiology (ACR) has established a subcommittee to develop a harmonized QC program for digital mammography. The goals of this program are:

1) to provide as much as possible, a uniform set of tests that can be used across the range of commercial digital mammography systems that will be used clinically,
2) to effectively test those aspects of imaging performance that are relevant to diagnostic image quality and safety,

Susan M. Astley et al. (Eds.): IWDM 2006, LNCS 4046, pp. 585–592, 2006.

3) to streamline the program to make it as efficient as possible, thereby eliminating unnecessary costs and labour, and

4) as much as possible to keep these tests similar or familiar to those currently performed by technologists and medical physicists who carry out QC in screen-film mammography (SFM) [2].

In the DMIST trial [3],[4] the QC program was designed to be as comprehensive as possible, with tests which could be applied generically among the different FFDM systems. Because little was known regarding the expected modes or frequencies of equipment failure, a test schedule was designed with more frequent evaluations than that required for SFM systems.

For a QC program to be practical and able to be followed by all facilities, some pragmatic decisions about the usefulness of individual tests and scope and extent of site survey testing must be made. In DMIST, the testing process was quite time consuming and while it generated information that was relevant to the characterization of digital systems, most of the information was of limited use for QC purposes. If one test can act as a surrogate for a number of others (offering high sensitivity, but possibly low selectivity), that test should be used in the QC program, and only if the system fails that test, should more selective diagnostic tests be performed outside of the QC program.

Historically, for SFM, x-ray generator technology was rather simple and fluctuations in the quantity or quality of X rays produced were not uncommon, and x-ray output was quite likely to drift over time, having an impact on image quality or radiation dose received by the breast. Modern x-ray generators used in digital systems, employ high frequency technology and extensive feedback and control systems, ensuring that their performance is stable and well regulated. Furthermore, modern radiographic equipment performs internal self-tests and has interlocks that prevent exposures being initiated when problems are detected.

The availability of image data in digital form provides opportunities for improvement of QC testing and allows for the introduction of objective and quantitative tests as well as more sophisticated measurements that are not practical for analogue systems. An additional benefit of harmonized tests is that cross-vendor validation of system compatibility is possible.

2 DMIST Recommendations for Testing

The tests used in DMIST were categorized into the evaluation of three areas: 1) the performance of the image acquisition system, 2) the dose and image quality, or 3) the image display system. For the ACR program, the physicist performs an annual equipment evaluation, which establishes that the equipment is performing at the expected level, and provides baseline target values that must be met by the technologist tests. The technologist performs routine tests to detect problems that may interfere with interpretation.

2.1 Tests Eliminated

DMIST results indicated that several tests currently required for SFM were of limited utility and should be eliminated from the program. These include:

Evaluation of imaging plate fogging on CR Systems. There was no evidence of problems due to fogging, even on the narrowest display window setting.

kV accuracy and reproducibility. Modern x-ray generators used in digital mammography are highly stable and once calibrated, seldom drift. A service engineer should verify kV calibration at installation and when the generator is serviced. A precise measurement of HVL can be used as an assessment of beam quality.

X-ray linearity, output rate and reproducibility. All current mammographic x-ray sources easily meet the requirement for output rate and the generators are extremely stable. Image noise tests will provide a surrogate test for problems related to linearity and/or reproducibility.

Detector linearity and reproducibility. Detector characteristics were found not to vary. Problems with linearity will manifest as a change in signal measurements from the technologist's weekly uniform phantom image (i.e. shift of measured mean pixel values or S-numbers). Unacceptable deviations could automatically trigger a warning message, prompting investigation of whether the deviation arose from the x-ray generation system or from the detector.

Focal spot. The focal spot is not the limiting factor affecting spatial resolution. A test of overall system MTF is more objective and more useful.

Routine imaging of the Mammography Accreditation Phantom. In DMIST, there were almost no phantom image failures and those that occurred were mainly a result of problems that could easily be detected through other means. The current screen-film mammography accreditation phantom is not discriminative enough to be appropriate for quality control of digital mammography systems. On the other hand, if the phantom test was made more challenging by changing the pass thresholds for detection of the internal structures, the failure rate increases rapidly, even for systems that are operating according to their design.

Routine printing of the Mammography Accreditation Phantom image. In DMIST, there was no benefit found to printing the phantom image.

While subjective phantom tests are appealing, they tend to be unreliable indicators of system performance, as it is very difficult both to replicate the critical tasks in breast imaging and to evaluate phantom images in a consistent manner both within and between observers.

2.2 Test Devices

The three recommendations regarding test devices are:

1) A uniform flat phantom with a 1 mm deep flat-bottomed well and reference target objects should be used to verify that artifacts are minimal and permit a measurement of the signal-difference-to-noise ratio (SDNR). We believe that this will be the best practical indicator of image quality and equipment performance. The reference objects are structures that can be viewed to aid in setting display levels for evaluating image artifacts.

2) For measurement of MTF, a 25 mm medium-contrast square with sharp edges should be used, to record the edge-spread function, from which the MTF can be calculated [5]. The pattern should be positioned at the level of the upper surface of the standard breast. The test would be facilitated by the provision of validated software,

accessible from the workstation of the system, and having a user-friendly interface for both the physicist and the technologist.

3) The TG18 QC and TG18 LN patterns [6] with appropriate format for the individual FFDM acquisition systems should be used for evaluation of soft and hard copy displays, with a simplified set of tests performed.

2.3 X-Ray Production and Physical Safety

In most QC programs, measurable parameters of the x-ray production system and basic dosimetry are emphasized. The following tests are recommended:

Unit evaluation performed in a thorough manner annually by the physicist and in an abbreviated manner monthly by the technologist ensures that all **locks, detents, angulation indicators, breast thickness** indication, maximum **compression force, mechanical support devices** for the X-ray tube and **breast support assembly** are operating properly and that the **DICOM header** information is correct. The unit evaluation verifies the overall safety of the equipment

Collimation and alignment including a measure of **tissue excluded** at the chest wall evaluated annually ensures patient and operator safety.

Tube output measurement by the physicist annually monitors the tube x-ray output over a range of clinically relevant settings of kV, x-ray target and beam filter, providing an overall performance check and the data necessary for computing estimated mean glandular dose.

HVL measurement annually by the physicist assures that the half-value layer of the x-ray beam is adequate to minimize breast dose, while not so high that contrast is lost in the resultant image. This ensures that the x-ray beam quality is consistent with the target, filter and kV selected; and enables the calculation of mean glandular dose. We recommend that HVL specification tables should be provided by the manufacturer for each model of digital mammographic unit to facilitate dose calculations and to allow verification of correct HVL. These tables should specify the expected HVL under typical target/filter/kV combinations for clinical use. After initial testing, if the HVL is compliant with the manufacturer's specification, the measured value should be adopted as the reference value and changes from that value tracked.

2.4 Dose and Image Quality

Since image quality and dose are inversely related, it is important to ensure that the system is operating in an optimum manner when initially evaluated, and maintains that level of operation throughout the year. The following set of tests attempts to maintain and track performance.

Uniform phantom. A phantom should be imaged weekly by the technologist with signal and **SDNR** measurements made to track consistent behavior of the imaging chain.

Artifacts should be analyzed by the physicist annually. The technologist should test for artifacts weekly. The use of a uniform phantom image for the detection of artifacts is probably the most effective test for the maintenance of high quality imaging.

Noise levels and noise power spectrum. This test should be performed upon acceptance testing of the unit, and after servicing of the detector or digitization subsystems.

Effective system modulation transfer function (MTF) should be measured annually, and after service to the detector, tube, bucky or CR plate reader. The MTF of the system in the magnification configuration should also be measured. For systems with moving parts (scanning systems or CR), it is recommended that in addition, MTF be tested monthly by the technologist. To facilitate use by the technologist, software for the calculation of MTF should be available that incorporates the pass criteria and communicates the pass/fail result clearly to the user.

Thickness tracking should be evaluated at least annually by the physicist. A thickness tracking test incorporating an SDNR measure is useful, but more experience is necessary to establish recommended ranges of SDNR for different thicknesses.

Geometric distortion should be evaluated annually, and after service to the detector assembly for machines with moving parts (e.g., systems with mechanical scanning and CR systems, which employ a laser scanner).

Entrance exposure and mean glandular dose for a "standard" breast (approximately 4.2-cm compressed breast thickness—50% adipose, 50% fibroglandular composition) should be measured annually, to permit calculation of the mean glandular dose (MGD), which should not exceed 3 mGy per view. If the MGD is displayed for an image, or reported in the DICOM header, that value should match the value calculated by the physicist to within 15%.

Image detector ghosting evaluation should be performed on all types of systems at acceptance testing and upon replacement of the detector. This test evaluates the severity of any residual artifact due to previously exposed images. In this measurement, a ghost or residual image is induced in a manner similar to what would occur in clinical operation, and the results are quantified. As detector technology matures this test may no longer be required.

2.5 Display

The interface of the FFDM acquisition system to the diagnostician through the physician review station is probably the most important link in the digital mammography chain. The digital display devices, both softcopy and hardcopy are analogous to the processor and viewboxes used in SFM in that they are a major source of variability in imaging performance., Picture archiving and communications systems (PACS) are now an integral part of the imaging process, and the ability to display images acquired by multiple devices produced by different vendors is essential. If there are multiple locations where primary diagnosis is performed, all of those devices must meet the same standards. The test images should emulate (i.e. have the same format, number of bits and Presentation State) the images produced by each model of digital mammography unit in the facility, or which might be interpreted at that workstation. The workstation should be evaluated under typical operating conditions. It is essential that cross-vendor compatibility be verified by the physicist before images from one vendor can be interpreted on another vendor's workstation.

This includes any specialized software considered to be important for proper viewing of such images.

2.5.1 Monitor Evaluation

It is recommended that digital test patterns be displayed on every soft copy workstation used for diagnosis. Subjective tests of spatial resolution, contrast, and artifacts should be carried out and quantitative measurements of brightness in test areas in the pattern should be made.

The complete TG18 test program for monitors is extensive and provides excellent tools for the laboratory environment. Flat panel and LCD monitors will require a different testing protocol than that used for CRT monitors, and we expect that TG-18 will evolve to meet these requirements. For practical clinical field testing, an abbreviated version of that program is probably adequate. This should include qualitative evaluation of the TG18 QC pattern and a reduced set of spatial resolution measurements.

Overall display quality – The TG18-QC test pattern should be displayed on all primary medical display devices used to interpret digital mammograms. The physicist should perform a comprehensive evaluation of the test pattern annually. The technologist should verify that the image has no artifacts, and that the 0-5% and 95-100% contrast patterns are visible.

The technologist should visually check the **luminance response of the soft copy display** for correct calibration by examining the contrast of the TG-18 QC test pattern at least weekly. The luminance response of monitors should be measured by a physicist at least annually using the TG18 protocol. The auto-calibration software and self-monitoring features that are now often supplied with newer monitors should make maintaining correct monitor calibration less onerous; however, it is important to verify luminance with an independent photometer in case the one attached to the unit becomes inaccurate. Conformance with the DICOM grey scale display function (GSDF) [7] should ensure that the luminance response is perceptually linear and that images are displayed consistently, however, not all manufacturers workstations are calibrated according to the GSDF.

Laser printer evaluation should be performed annually on all printers used to print digital mammograms. Printing of the TG18-QC pattern should be done from the review workstation, so that any image transformations performed during the image transfer and printing processes are included. Further experience is needed to determine a reasonable criterion for determining acceptable conformance to the GSDF. The technologist should visually inspect the printed test pattern quarterly to ensure that the printed image quality is acceptable. In addition, a uniform image should be printed monthly to verify that artefacts are minimal.

Printer sensitometry should be performed by the technologist daily, for printers with wet processing, and monthly for printers with dry processing for which the stability is greater. The optical density of the mid-density step and density difference should be within 0.15 OD units of their target values. The measured base plus fog should be no more than 0.03 OD units above the target value.

Softcopy viewing conditions assessment assures that the ambient light levels incident on the review work station monitors do not degrade the quality of the clinical images. The ambient room illuminance falling on the monitor must be measured by a medical physicist at least annually or when lighting changes are made. Because the light incident on the monitor degrades the perceived contrast in displayed images, diffuse light incident on the present generation of monitors should be no greater than 10Lux and this level should be maintained the same as it was when the monitor was calibrated to the GDSF. No specular reflections should appear on the monitor screen. The ambient light level recommendations and protocols in AAPM TG-18 report should be followed. A daily room lighting checklist should be available to the technologists which provide them guidance in reviewing the lighting conditions in the room.

Evaluation of the viewbox luminance and illuminance of the reading room Is also important where hard copy digital images are interpreted or previous SFM examinations are compared to current images. To comply with the DICOM GSDF, the calibration of the film printer must be done with knowledge of the luminance of the viewboxes on which the resulting films will be interpreted and the ambient illuminance, as these affect the perceived luminance levels in the resulting films. Therefore, once a printer is correctly calibrated, it becomes important to ensure that viewing conditions do not change significantly. For workstations, the minimization of extraneous light is also very important. Daily, the technologist should verify that lighting conditions in the reading room are acceptable and the physicist should measure viewbox luminance and reading room illuminance annually.

3 Conclusions

Review of the physics QC data from the DMIST program suggests that certain currently-performed tests, primarily tests on the x-ray generator function, appear to be of very little value in FFDM.

For practical purposes, there must always be compromises between the time required to perform tests, and the degree of characterization of the system that is achieved. Digital imaging systems lend themselves to quantitative, automated testing procedures which are self-logging. We recommend that these testing procedures be implemented to as great an extent as practical. This will contribute to high compliance in QC testing while reducing the impact on both cost and the time of valuable personnel.

Test procedures have been modified based on the DMIST experience. There is still a need to further improve and streamline test procedures for the display monitors.

We believe that these recommendations will provide a useful framework for definition of a QC program for FFDM. Without question, recommended QC procedures will evolve along with the systems, and with our increasing understanding of FFDM. It will be necessary to modify the tests, their frequency and pass/fail criteria as more experience is gained in the field, and as the technology matures. We are optimistic that a more generalized and less labour-intensive harmonized QC program can be developed based on this knowledge.

References

1. MSQA. Mammography Quality Standards Act Regulations 21 CFR PART 900—Mammography (2002)
2. Hendrick R. E. et al., *American College of Radiology (ACR) Mammography Quality Control Manual for Radiologists, Medical Physicists and Technologists*, American College of Radiology, Reston, VA (1999)
3. Bloomquist A.K. et al., "Quality Control for Digital Mammography in the ACRIN DMIST Trial: Part I", Med. Phys. **33**, 719-736 (2006)
4. Yaffe M. J. et al., "Quality Control for Digital Mammography: Part II, Recommendations from the ACRIN DMIST Trial", Med. Phys. **33**, 737-752 (2006)
5. Fujita H. et. al, "A simple method for determining the modulation transfer function in digital radiography", IEEE Trans. Med. Imaging **11**, 34-39 (1992)
6. Samei, E. et al, *Assessment of Display Performance for Medical Imaging Systems*, American Association of Physicists in Medicine, Task Group 18. Medical Physics **32**, 1205-1225 (2005)
7. National Electrical Manufacturer's Association, *Digital Imaging and Communications in Medicine (DICOM) Part 14: Grayscale Standard Display Function*, PS 3.14-2004, National Electrical Manufacturer's Association, Rosslyn, VA (2004)

Contrast Threshold of 4 Full Field Digital Mammography Systems Using Different Measurement Methods

A.-K. Carton[1], H. Bosmans[1], C. Vanongeval[1], G. Souverijns[2], G. Marchal[1],
J. Jacobs[1], D. Vandenbroucke[3], H. Pauwels[1], and K. Nijs[1]

[1] Radiology, University Hospital Gasthuisberg, B-Leuven
[2] Virga-Jesse, B-Hasselt
[3] Agfa, B-Mortsel

Abstract. We compared three conspicuity tests applied to four full field digital mammography (FFDM) systems. The tests included: 1) the calculation of noise equivalent quanta (NEQ); 2) contrast-detail analysis with the CDMAM 3.4 phantom and 3) evaluation of the detectability of (simulated) microcalcifications with specific well-known dimensions in mastectomy images. For each contrast-resolution test method, the exposure, processing and viewing conditions were identical. As a result, the only variable for a given test was the physical performance of the detector. The three test methods each rank the detectors in the same order. The flat-panel detector ranked the best overall, the dual-sided read-out storage phosphor detector ranked second and the single-sided-read-out storage phosphor detectors with 50 μm and 100 μm pixel sizes ranked similarly and were inferior to the other 2 detectors.

1 Purpose

Digital mammographic detectors need both high spatial resolution and excellent contrast. These characteristics can be measured in several, very different, ways and ultimately determine the contrast threshold visibility for various object sizes. In the present study, we have applied three test methods that assess efficacy in different ways: 1) the calculation of noise equivalent quanta (NEQ) [1]; 2) a contrast threshold detectability study using a contrast-detail phantom [2]; and 3) a detectability study of (simulated) microcalcifications on a mammographic background [3,4]. The first and second methods are generally accepted tests used by medical physicists.

2 Material and Methods

The four detectors encompassed an amorphous-selenium based detector (the Embrace DM1000 of Agfa, (acronym: DM1000)) and three storage phosphor detectors (the FCR 5000MA of Fuji (acronym: FCR), the Embrace CR of Agfa with pixel size 100μm (acronym: Emb100) and a non-commercially available CR detector of Agfa with pixel size 50μm (acronym: Emb50)). The FCR has the unique feature of a double-sided readout of the plates with a pixel size of 50μm. The Emb100 and the Emb50 make use of the same storage phosphor plates by Agfa. They were read-out

Susan M. Astley et al. (Eds.): IWDM 2006, LNCS 4046, pp. 593–600, 2006.
© Springer-Verlag Berlin Heidelberg 2006

with the same single-sided reader but with a pixel size of 100µm (Emb100) and 50µm (Emb50). The FCR, Emb50 and Emb100 images were acquired with a M-IV Platinum mammography unit (Lorad, Danburry, CT). The DM1000 detector is integrated in a mammography x-ray system of identical make and model using a similar x-ray generator, anode and filter combinations. The only difference of this system is the linear moving grid, whereas the M-IV Platinum mammography unit (used for the CR plates) has a cellular grid.

2.1 NEQ

The horizontal and vertical NEQs [1] were derived from the measured pre-sampled modulation transfer functions (MTF) [5] and normalized noise power spectra (NNPS) [6] as follows:

$$NEQ(\omega) = \frac{MTF^2(\omega)}{NNPS(\omega)}$$

where ω is the spatial frequency. The MTFs were calculated from images of a 5cm by 5cm, 30µm thick Pb-edge laminated between two 20mm thick PMMA slabs. The NNPS were computed from images of a 40mm thick homogeneous PMMA slab. The exposures were made at 28 kVp (nominal) and Mo/Mo. We used 64mAs for the FCR, Emb50 and Emb100 and 55mAs for the DM1000. The computations were performed in the raw data; i.e. linear with exposure. Errors on the NEQs were computed from the propagation of the absolute errors calculated for the MTF and NNPS.

2.2 Contrast-Resolution from CDMAM 3.4

The CDMAM 3.4 [2] sandwiched between two 20mm thick PMMA slabs was exposed at 26 kVp, Mo/Mo and 160mAs for the FCR, Emb50 and Emb100 and 129mAs for the DM1000. Repeated exposures were acquired with each detector. The raw image data were square-root compressed. The window width and level were optimized and set identical for all images. The images were printed with a high resolution (508 ppi – 8 bits) Mammoray 4500 Drystar printer (Agfa, Mortsel, Belgium). All images were viewed by 7 experienced medical physicists in a darkened room on the same view box. The use of a magnifying glass was encouraged and a minimum viewing time of 15' was imposed. Contrast-detail curves averaged over all 7 observers and 2 images per detector were plotted for the four detectors. The fractional standard deviation SE_t on the average threshold contrast was calculated using the equation given by Swets and Pickett [7]:

$$SE_t = \left(\frac{S_c^2}{n} + \frac{S_b^2}{l} + \frac{S_w^2}{nml} \right)^{1/2}$$

In this equation S_c^2 is the fractional case sample variance, S_b^2 is the fractional between-observer variance and S_w^2 is the fractional within-observer variance. The number of replica images for each detector is n, the number of observers is l and the number of times an image is read is m. S_w^2 was calculated from the rereading (3x) by three observers of the first case-sample of each detector. SE_t was calculated with $n=2$, $l=7$ and $m=1$.

2.3 Contrast-Resolution from Simulated Microcalcifications in Real Mammographic Backgrounds

Five mastectomies with compressed thickness between 38mm and 49mm were exposed at 25kVp, Mo/Mo and clinical exposures. The unprocessed image data were transferred to a workstation where they were made linearly proportional to dose.

Each image had a random set of microcalcifications embedded using a previously described method [3, 4]: Each image was multiplied by a software phantom which consisted of multiple simulated microcalcifications.

- The template for each simulated microcalcifications was derived from the x-ray images of real microcalcifications. These images were acquired with an Agfa prototype CR plate with 100μm pixels and a magnification of 2. The images were spatially filtered to simulate an ideally sharp detector (MTF=1 to the Nyquist frequency) and then filtered again for the MTF of the system under consideration. Finally, the templates of the microcalcifications were adjusted for the difference in pixel size of the four detectors.

- Five equivalent diameter groups (>300-400μm, >400-500μm,>500-600μm, >600-700μm, >700-800μm) and four aluminium equivalent thickness groups (>0-200μm, >200-400μm,>400-600μm, >600-800μm), calculated for the ideally sharp detector, were used. This made 20 aluminium equivalent thickness/diameter groups. We simulated 30 microcalcifications for each group. All microcalcification templates were used more than once. In total we inserted 600 simulated microcalcifications into the mastectomy images of each detector.

Each software phantom had 0 to 14 microcalcifications randomly distributed in 2cmx2cm frames. They were embedded in regions with constant breast thickness (i.e. constant system noise) [8]. Various background types were used. We had to add separately the simulated microcalcifications to the mastectomy images for each of the four detectors. In order to have microcalcifications with exactly the same anatomic background structure we used a translation, rotation and scaling algorithm to align the objects to the backgrounds.

The raw image data were square-root compressed and the clinical processing protocol of Agfa, namely MUSICA (24), was applied. This processing algorithm was developed for general radiology. The window/level, Look Up Table (LUT) and MUSICA parameters were selected as appropriate for an average image by an experienced mammographic technologist.

The experiments were performed on softcopy. The softcopy display system included a MGD 521M monitor (Barco, Kortrijk, Belgium) with a Barco 5MP2 AURA display card, run on a Dell Precision 530 computer.

The images were fully randomly presented to three experienced radiologists (R1, R2 and R3). They were asked to indicate the locations of the microcalcifications by mouse clicks on the locations they thought contained the microcalcifications. They rated their confidence using four response categories. There was no limit on reading time and reading distance. Zoom functions were available and the window/level was adjustable.

For comparison of the observer performance, FROC analysis [9] was performed on the scores collected for each reader and each detector. The average TP ratings versus the average numbers of false positives (FP) per image were calculated for each score and each observer. For each data point, we estimated the errors in the means using a bootstrap procedure with replacement [10].

3 Results

Figure 1 illustrates the horizontal and vertical NEQs for the DM1000, FCR, Emb50 and Emb100. The horizontal and vertical NEQ of the DM1000 are for all frequencies significantly higher than the horizontal and vertical NEQs of the FCR, Emb50 and Emb100. Up to 5lp/mm, the horizontal and vertical NEQ of the FCR are significantly higher than the horizontal and vertical NEQs of the Emb50 and Emb100. The horizontal and vertical NEQs of the Emb50 and Emb100 are very similar.

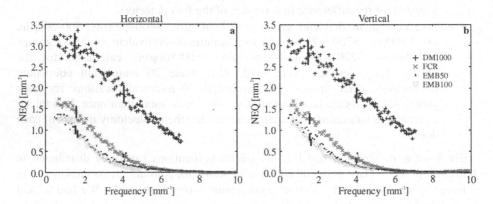

Fig. 1. Horizontal (a) and vertical (b) NEQs of the DM1000, FCR, Emb50 and Emb100 at a similar radiation quality. Error bars represent the standard deviations in the mean from five exposures.

Figure 2 a, b and c show the contrast-detail curves, averaged over the 7 observers and the 2 samples per system for the small diameter, medium diameter and large diameter groups. The fractional standard error SE_t in average threshold contrast among the 7 observers, 2 samples for each system and one reading per image is equal to 0.123. For the smallest disk diameters (except 0.06 mm), the DM1000 outperforms the FCR, the Emb50 and the Emb100 (Figure 2 a). The FCR ranks second but is not significantly lower than the DM1000 for the smallest disks. The Emb50 and Emb100 rank third and fourth; performance is not significantly different. The DM1000 is

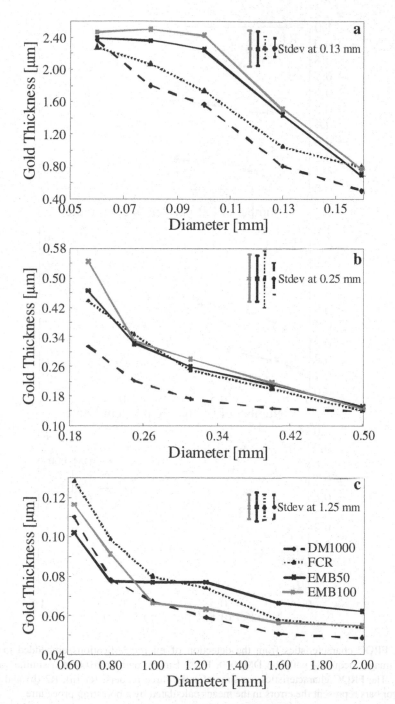

Fig. 2. Contrast-detail curves of the DM1000, FCR, Emb50 and Emb100 for 3 diameter classes of the gold disks. The curves are averaged over 7 observers, 2 replicate images sampled for each system and one reading of a given film. Standard errors are shown.

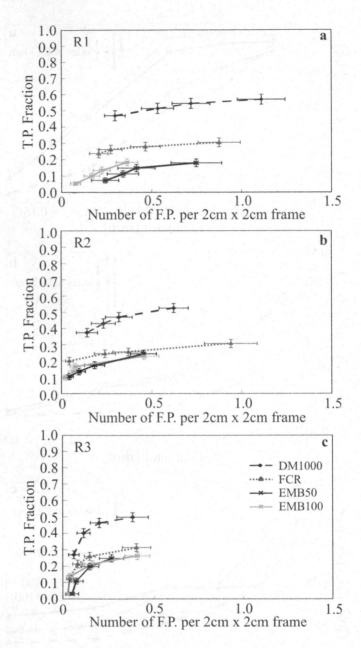

Fig. 3. FROC characteristics from the detection of microcalcifications embedded in maste-ctomy images acquired with the DM1000, FCR, Emb50 and Emb100 at a similar radiation quality. The FROC characteristics are shownfor the three readers, R1 (a), R2 (b) and R3 (c). The error bars represent the errors in the means calculated by a bootstrap procedure.

significantly superior to the Emb50 and Emb100 for the smallest diameters. The DM1000 performs significantly better than the FCR, Emb50 and Emb100 for the medium diameter disks (except 0.50 mm). The FCR, Emb50 and Emb100 perform very similarly for medium diameters (Figure 2 b). Overall, the threshold contrasts for the DM1000 appear lower for the largest gold disks, but no significant differences between the four imaging systems exist (Figure 2 c).

Figure 3 shows the FROC curves of the three radiologists R1, R2, and R3 for the DM1000, FCR, Emb50 and Emb100. The three radiologists perform very similarly for the DM1000, FCR and Emb100; the standard errors in the means overlap. For the Emb50, R1 is inferior to R2 and R3. Figure 3 demonstrates that the DM1000 is significantly superior for all readers. The average FROC curves of the FCR rank second. However the performance of the FCR is not significantly different from the Emb50 and Emb100. The average FROC curves for the Emb50 and Emb100 are ranked similarly by R2 and R3. The average FROC curve of the Emb100 is higher than the Emb50 for R1.

4   Conclusion and Discussion

We have illustrated that the three different methods for assessment of different contrast resolution (NEQ, contrast visibility from CDMAM and detectability of simulated microcalcifications) result in the same ranking of the four detectors. We believe that this work supports the use of NEQ in comparing clinical system performance. This study also suggests that we can quantitatively determine how various physical parameters impact on the detectability of simulated microcal-cifications. This has the potential to allow more rapid assessment of observer perfor-mance to new image processing methods of new image systems.

Acknowledgements

We thank Fuji Medical Systems for providing the raw Fuji images. We are very grateful to Kristien Smans, Tom Deprez, Frank Rogge and Kris Govaerts for partici-pating in the readout of the CDMAM 3.4 images. Andrew D.A. Maidment is greatly acknowledged for the interesting suggestions. Ann Similon is greatly acknowledged for all practical help with the acquisitions of the mastectomies.

References

1. "Medical Imaging - The Assessment of Image Quality", ICRU Report 54, April 1996.
2. User Manual CDMAM 3.4, Artinis, Medical Systems B.V.
3. Carton, A.-K., Bosmans, H., Vanongeval, C., Souverijns, G., Rogge, F., Van Steen, A., Marchal, G.: Development and validation of a simulation procedure to study the visibility of microcalcifications in digital mammograms, Med. Phys. 30 , August 2003, 2234-2240.
4. Carton, A.-K., Bosmans, H., Vandenbroucke, D., Souverijns, G., Van Ongeval, C., Dragusin, O.: "Quantification of Al-equivalent thickness of just visible micro calcifications in full field digital mammograms", Med.Phys. 31, July 2004, 2165-2176.

5. Samei, E., Flynn, M. J., and Reimann, D. A.: A method for measuring the presampled MTF of digital radiographic systems using an edge test device, Med. Phys. 25, 102-113 (1998).
6. Dobbins III, J. T.: "Image Quality Metrics for Digital Systems" Chapter 3 in *Hanbook of Medical Imaging, Volume 1. Physics and Psychophysics*, SPIE 2000.
7. Swets, J.A. and Pickett, R..M.: *Evaluation of diagnostic systems: Methods from signal detection theory*, (Academic, New york, 1982)
8. Burgess, A.E.: "Mammographic structure: Data preparation and spatial statistics analysis", Medical Imaging 1999: Image Processing, K. Hanson (ed.), Vol.3661, 642-653, SPIE, Bellingham WA 1999.
9. Chakraborty, D. P.: "The FROC, AFROC and DROC variants of the ROC Analysis", Chapter 16 in *Handbook of medical imaging, Physics and Psychophysics* Vol. 1,Edited by J. Beutel, H.L. Kundel, R.L. Van Metter (SPIE, Bellingham, WA, 2000).
10. Efron, B.: *The Jacknife, the Bootstrap and Other Resampling Plans*, (SIAM, Philadelphia, Pennsylvania, 1982).
11. The European Protocol for the Quality Control of the physical and technical aspects of mammography screening: Addendum on Digital Mammography, November 2003.

The Use of Multi-scale Monogenic Signal on Structure Orientation Identification and Segmentation

Xiao-Bo Pan[1], Michael Brady[2], Ralph Highnam[1], and Jérôme Declerck[1]

[1] Siemens Molecular Imaging Limited, Oxford, UK
[2] University of Oxford, Oxford, UK
bo.pan@mirada-solutions.com

Abstract. A method of extracting salient image features in mammograms at multiple scales using the monogenic signal is presented. The derived local phase provides structure information (such as edge, ridge etc.) while the local amplitude encodes the local brightness and contrast information. Together with the simultaneously computed orientation, these three pieces of information can be used for mammogram segmentation including locating the inner breast edge which is important for quantitative breast density assessment. Due to the contrast invariant property of the local phase, the algorithm proves to be very reliable on an extensive datasets of images obtained from various sources and digitized by different scanners.

1 Background

Medical image processing often involves identifying structures of several different types (edge – of a mass, or of the breast, ridge – e.g. ducts, etc.) as a basis for segmentation in complex images such as mammograms, and a great deal of effort has been expended on making those algorithms scale, intensity and contrast invariant.

When dealing with digitized mammograms, due to variations in X-ray acquisition protocols, breast density and digitizing scanners, there can be large differences in both the image intensity range and contrast. This poses a considerable challenge to developing fully automated algorithms without prior knowledge about the scanner and imaging protocol. In this paper, we describe a novel segmentation algorithm which can effectively handle mammogram images from various sources and which are digitized using different scanners.

It is well known that a 1D signal can be split into local amplitude and local phase using the analytic signal, in which the local phase provides the structural information and the local amplitude encodes the brightness and contrast information [1-3]. The split into these two independent and complementary kinds of information makes the local phase brightness and contrast invariant. The monogenic signal, introduced by Felsberg et al [4], is an extension of the analytic signal to 2D/3D/4D, where, in the case of 2D images, three pieces of information are extracted: the local amplitude, local phase, and local (image) orientation.

We have developed a multi-scale strategy to apply the monogenic signal to images, and extract distinct structure, orientation and contrast information. This information is of interest for a range of applications (e.g. mass detection, breast density quantification,

Susan M. Astley et al. (Eds.): IWDM 2006, LNCS 4046, pp. 601–608, 2006.

detection of curvilinear structures or the pectoral muscle boundary), and particularly for differentiation of structures in an image. In this paper we demonstrate its utility in segmenting a range of structures in the same mammogram such as the film area, the breast and the inner breast edge.

Many methods have been developed for mammogram segmentation and these have been based on the intensity histogram [5], the intensity gradient [6-8], polynomial modeling [9, 10], or active contours [11, 12]. Many of these methods require manually adjustment of parameters, inevitably limiting the range of images that the algorithm can be applied to automatically, that is, without supervision or intervention.

Our method aims to solve the problem automatically and deals with the following difficulties: varying brightness and contrast; the skin-air breast boundary, which has low contrast to background, and sometimes has been cut off due to limited sensitivity of the digitizer; the background intensity and noise, which vary considerably; the images obtained from various scanners (CCD and laser based): CCD based scanners (e.g. Canon) are usually noisier and less sensitive than laser based scanners (e.g. Lumisys, Array, DBA).

2 Method

The method essentially relies on the exploitation of properties of the monogenic signal extracted from the image. In this section, we recall some of these properties and explain how they were exploited to create an application specific algorithm for mammogram segmentation.

2.1 Definition of Local Amplitude, Local Phase and Local Orientation

Hilbert transform, 1D analytic signal
To extract the structure and local amplitude information of a 1D signal f(x), the is convolved with its   Hilbert transform $f_H(x) = h(x) \otimes f(x)$, where the transfer function of Hilbert transform is defined as [1]:

$$H(\omega) = i\,\text{sign}(\omega) = i \;(\omega > 0)\,,\, 0\;(\omega = 0),\; -i\;(\omega < 0) \tag{1}$$

And *h(x)* is the spatial representation of the frequency representation *H(ω)*. The analytic signal is formed as $f_A(x) = f(x) - i f_H(x)$. The local amplitude *A(x)* and the local phase *φ(x)* are derived from f$_A$(x) as:

$$A(x) = \|f_A(x)\| = \sqrt{f^2(x) + f_H^{\,2}(x)} \tag{2}$$

$$\varphi(x) = arg(f_A(x)) = \arctan 2(f_H(x), f(x)),\; \varphi(x) \in [-\pi, \pi) \tag{1}$$

2D Monogenic signal
In the 2D case, Felsberg and Sommer used the Riesz transform to extend the Hilbert transform to 2D or arbitrarily higher dimensions. The Riesz transform in 2D is defined as:

$$H_1(\omega_1,\omega_2) = i\omega_1 / \sqrt{\omega_1^2 + \omega_2^2}, \quad H_2(\omega_1,\omega_2) = i\omega_2 / \sqrt{\omega_1^2 + \omega_2^2} \tag{4}$$

Let $h_1(x_1,x_2)$ and $h_2(x_1,x_2)$ be the spatial representation of the Riesz transforms. The monogenic signal is a 3D vector formed by the signal with its Riesz transform. The local features are derived from f_M:

$$f_M(x_1,x_2) = (f(x_1,x_2),(h_1 \otimes f)(x_1,x_2),(h_2 \otimes f)(x_1,x_2)) \tag{5}$$

The *local amplitude*: $A_f(x_1,x_2) = \sqrt{f^2 + (h_1 \otimes f)^2 + (h_2 \otimes f)^2} \tag{6}$

The *local phase*: $\varphi(x_1,x_2) = \mathrm{acos}(f(x_1,x_2)/A_f(x_1,x_2))$, $\varphi \in [0,\pi)$ \tag{7}$

The *local orientation*: $\theta(x_1,x_2) = \mathrm{atan2}(h_2 \otimes f, h_1 \otimes f)$, $\theta \in [-\pi,\pi)$ \tag{8}$

2.2 Structure and Scale

Idealized signal structures can be detected by the local phase [2]: $\varphi=0$ (ridge), $\pi/2$ (up step), π (valley), $-\pi/2$ (down step). An example of a simple, noise-free 1D signal is shown in **Fig. 1**, the structure points are marked with *, and have unique phase values, regardless of the signal intensity and contrast.

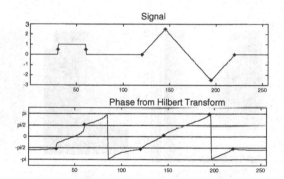

Fig. 1. Signal and its phase, showing the relationship of the structure and phase. Sudden changes of phase at abscissas ~85 and ~195 are wrap from π to $-\pi$.

Scale Space Analysis Using Quadrature Filters
The local amplitude and local phase can be derived at multiple scales by filtering the signal with bandpass filters in a selected frequency range. The bandpass filters need to be analytical, which is equivalent to having quadrature pairs of filters. One such that has been used frequently, and is used in our examples, is the log-Gabor filter [1-3]. The log Gabor function is defined in the frequency domain by:

$$G(\omega) = e^{-(\log(\omega/\omega_0))^2/(2(\log(\kappa/\omega_0))^2)}, \text{ if } \omega>0, \text{ and zero otherwise} \tag{9}$$

where ω_0 is the filter's centre frequency. The term κ / ω_0 is held constant. A κ / ω_0 value of 0.74, 0.55, 0.41 results in a filter bandwidth of approximately one, two or three octaves, respectively. With the band pass filtering, the monogenic signal is defined as following in 2D:

$$f_M(x_1, x_2) = ((g \otimes f), (h_1 \otimes g \otimes f), (h_2 \otimes g \otimes f))(x_1, x_2). \tag{10}$$

2.3 Phase, Orientation, and Amplitude

Fig. 2 a, b, c, d show the original image, the phase, orientation and amplitude obtained from the filter response of a monogenic filter at a global scale. With a fixed threshold $\pi/2$, two principal structures can be separated: the phase $< \pi/2$ area includes most of the breast and label regions (**Fig. 2e**); whereas the phase $\geq \pi/2$ area includes the dark background region (**Fig. 2f**). The separation edge (phase $= \pi/2$) near the breast boundary corresponds to where the intensity changes rapidly, which is approximately where the breast begins to leave the compression plates. We call this the inner breast edge, and it turns out to be a crucial structure in estimating breast density [13]. The actual breast boundary is always in the background region (**Fig. 2f**).

Next we need to refine the segmentation to separate the off-film, label and breast areas from the area defined by [phase $< \pi/2$], and we need to find the breast boundary from the area [phase $\geq \pi/2$]. To do this, we use the phase computed at a local scale, and we define the neighbourhood of the breast boundary using the local orientation information. Within this neighbourhood area, we compute a phase threshold corresponding to the breast

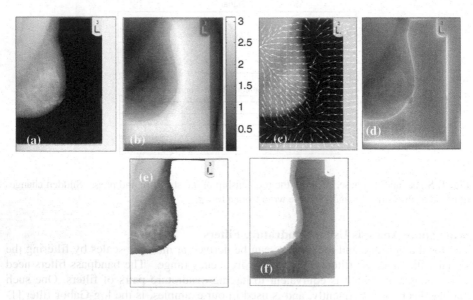

Fig. 2. (a) Original image. (b) Phase. (c) Orientation vector on the original image. (d) Amplitude. (e) Phase $< \pi/2$ region, with original image superimposed on it. (f) Phase $> \pi/2$ region.

boundary, based on the local amplitude. By using the structure information encoded in the phase image at different scales, we overcome the image variation problem introduced by different digitizers.

Off-Film Area

The off-film area is an almost constant white (occasionally black) region around the film generated at the digitizing stage. We can detect this region using a local phase (phase2) at a finer scale (a log-Gabor filter of bandwidth 3 octaves and a centre frequency equal to 1/45) (**Fig. 3**a). Using a fixed threshold (phase2 > $\pi/2$) the off-film area is identified as the outer dark region (**Fig. 3**b). The off-film region often overlaps with bright labels or patient information regions. To distinguish such regions, we assume that the off-film area consists of vertical and horizontal strips at the boundary of the film, detected by vertical and horizontal line fitting, and that what is left are regions that correspond to labels. If required, refinements can be made to accommodate slightly angled films. **Fig. 3**c shows the detected bright off-film area.

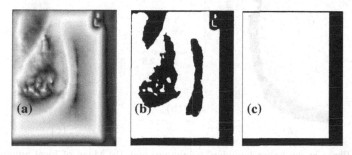

Fig. 3. (a) phase2 at fine scale. (b) phase2 > $\pi/2$.(c) Detected bright off-film region.

Neighbourhood of Breast Boundary

Fig. 4a illustrates that the local orientation around the breast boundary and the inner breast edge is very similar. Based on this observation, we define a neighbourhood area outside the inner breast edge, in which lies the breast boundary (**Fig. 4**b). This neighbourhood not only defines the area where we compute the local amplitude curve versus phase, to generate the threshold for the breast boundary, but also limits the area in which we apply the threshold, thus improving both reliability and accuracy.

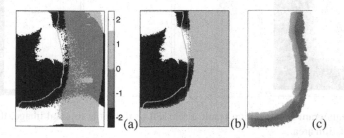

Fig. 4. (a) Local orientation in 4 orientation bands. (b) Selected regions contain the inner breast edge and breast boundary. (c) Breast boundary neighbourhood.

We group the orientation image into four kinds of regions, where the orientation in each region is one of the following groups: -pi ↔ -pi/2, -pi/2 ↔ 0, 0 ↔ pi/2, pi/2 ↔ pi. All regions that contain the breast inner edge are selected. Holes in selected regions are filled. The neighbourhood is then defined within the selected region over the pixels whose phase is greater than $\pi/2$.

Threshold for the Breast Boundary

Observe in **Fig. 5**a that the phase value is very similar at the breast boundary. We determine a phase threshold for the breast boundary by using the mean of local amplitude against phase in the neighborhood area (**Fig. 5**b). The local amplitude is expected to attain a maximum value at the breast boundary. For this reason, we look for the phase in the range of (pi/2 ↔ pi) with the maximum mean local amplitude to be the threshold. The segmented breast boundary is plotted in **Fig. 5**c.

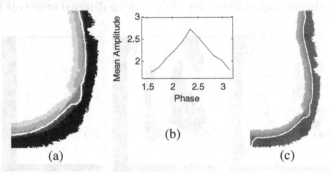

(a)   (b)   (c)

Fig. 5. (a) Phase in the breast boundary neighbourhood. (b) Mean of local amplitude against phase (c) Resulting estimated breast boundary.

3 Results

Fig. 6 shows a typical segmentation result. Images are: the original image, the segmented breast region, the label region, and off-film region.

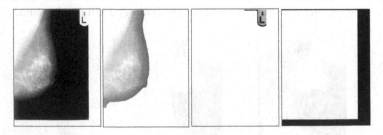

Fig. 6. Mammogram segmentation result. From left to right, the original image, the breast, the label, the off-film area.

Stability and Accuracy

This segmentation algorithm has been tested on 3880 mammogram images digitized using a Canon scanner, and 840 mammograms digitized using a Lumisys scanner with no failures as assessed visually by an expert in mammographic image processing (148 extreme cases of large, partially captured breast image are detected and removed from the first study) [14]. The algorithm performed similarly well (as judged by the same expert) on several hundred samples of mammogram images digitized by Array scanners and a small sample of images from Howtek.

The accuracy of the segmentation was tested using 100 images which were manually segmented by an expert researcher. The manual segmentation was made by connecting line segments between points selected by the expert. The average distance between the selection points is around 1-2cm (depending on the area), which means that the accuracy of the manual segmentation be within a couple of pixels (<1mm). **Fig. 7** shows the regions segmented manually and automatically. Two measures were used for evaluation: i) the averaged distance between the automatic and manually generated breast boundary. The mean absolute value is 1.88 mm, and ii) the percentage of the difference of breast area against the manually segmented breast area is 3.23%.

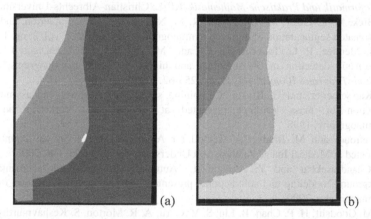

(a)   (b)

Fig. 7. Segmentation accuracy test. (a) Manually segmented regions. (b) Automatically segmentation regions. Differences can be noticed in the inferior part of the thorax.

4 Discussion

Using the feature sets generated by the monogenic signal has proved to be very successful for segmentation of mammograms. The stable inner breast edge identified in this way has improved considerably the performance of a breast density quantification algorithm. We believe that the fundamental reason for this is that the local phase and orientations at multiple scales captures the structure of the object, encodes neighbourhood information and that they are salient measures. Segmentation based on these scale selected features is contrast and brightness invariant and so they should be more robust, flexible and stable than algorithms that rely entirely upon brightness or upon gradient measures. This method applies to 2D/3D data, and can be extended to multiple dimensions, for example to 4D spatiotemporal data.

Acknowledgments

Part of this work was funded by the EU MammoGrid Project (Information Societies Project, EU contract IST-2001-37614).

References

[1] S. Mallat and S. Mallat, *A Wavelet Tour of Signal Processing*. New York: Academic, 1998.
[2] M. C. Morrone and R. A. Owens, "Feature detection from local energy," *Pattern Recognition Letters*, vol. 6, pp. 303-313, 1987.
[3] P. Kovesi, "Invariant Measures of Image Features from Phase Information," *Videre: Journal of Computing Vision Research*, vol. 1, 1999.
[4] M. Felsberg, "Low-Level Image Processing with the Structure Multivector," in *Institut fur Informatik und Praktische Mathematik*. KIEL: Christian-Albrechts-Universitat, 2002.
[5] U. Bick, M. L. Giger, R. A. Schmidt, R. M. Nishikawa, D. E. Wolverton, and K. Doi, "Automated segmentation of digitized mammograms," *Acad Radiol*, vol. 2, pp. 1-9, 1995.
[6] A. J. Mendez, P. G. Tahoces, M. J. Lado, M. Souto, J. L. Correa, and J. J. Vidal, "Automatic detection of breast border and nipple in digital mammograms," *Comput Methods Programs Biomed*, vol. 49, pp. 253-62, 1996.
[7] N. Karssemeijer and G. Brake, "Combining single view features and asymmetry for detection of mass lesions," presented at International Workshop on Digital Mammography, 1998.
[8] S. Petroudi and M. Brady, "A Method for Automatic Breast Border Segmentation," presented at Medical Image Analysis and Understanding, Sheffield, UK, 2003.
[9] R. Chandrasekhar and Y. Attikiouzel, "Automatic breast border segmentation by background modeling and subtraction," presented at International Workshop on Digital Mammography, 2000.
[10] M. M. Goodsitt, H. P. Chan, B. Liu, S. V. Guru, A. R. Morton, S. Keshavmurthy, and N. Petrick, "Classification of compressed breast shapes for the design of equalization filters in x-ray mammography," *Med Phys*, vol. 25, pp. 937-48, 1998.
[11] T. Ojala, J. Nappi, and O. Nevalainen, "Accurate segmentation of the breast region from digitized mammograms," *Comput Med Imaging Graph*, vol. 25, pp. 47-59, 2001.
[12] R. J. Ferrari, R. M. Rangayyan, J. E. Desautels, R. A. Borges, and A. F. Frere, "Identification of the breast boundary in mammograms using active contour models," *Med Biol Eng Comput*, vol. 42, pp. 201-8, 2004.
[13] R. Highnam, X. Pan, J. M. Brady, B. Ancelin, K. Dixon, R. Warren, and M. Jeffreys, "SMF As a Reprocucible Estimation Of Breast Density," presented at IWDM, 2004.
[14] M. Jeffreys, R. Warren, R. Highnam, and S. G. Davey, "Initial experience of using an automated volumetric measure of breast density: the standard mammogram form (SMF)," *British Journal of Radiology*, 2006.

Breast Density Segmentation Using Texture

Styliani Petroudi and Michael Brady

Wolfson Medical Vision Laboratory, Oxford University, Oxford,
OX2 7DD, United Kingdom
{styliani, jmb}@robots.ox.ac.uk

Abstract. This paper describes an algorithm to segment mammographic images into regions corresponding to different densities. The breast parenchymal segmentation uses information extracted for statistical texture based classification which is in turn incorporated in multivector Markov Random Fields. Such segmentation is key to developing quantitative mammographic analysis. The algorithm's performance is evaluated quantitatively and qualitatively and the results show the feasibility of segmenting different mammographic densities.

1 Introduction

Breast parenchymal density refers to the prevalence of fibroglandular tissue in the breast as it appears on a mammogram. Many studies have stressed the importance of breast density and it has been shown that breast density is an important factor in the development and risk of breast cancer [1]. The findings are intuitively appealing, since breast cancer mostly arises from the epithelial lining of the ductal/lobular glands. Segmentation of the mammogram into different mammographic densities is useful for risk assessment, quantitative evaluation of density changes, mammogram matching, region enhancement etc. However segmentation of the breast to even a simple fatty and non-fatty set of regions is much more difficult than it appears due to the large differences in parenchymal type appearances and the variability of image acquisition and acquisition parameters.

A small number of articles have suggested ways to segment the mammographic breast parenchyma. Miller and Astley [2] were the first to attempt to automatically identify regions in the breast corresponding to adipose and fibroglandular tissue, and they showed that texture analysis forms a good basis for automatically classifying breast tissue. For their classification, they investigated granulometry techniques (grey-level opening operations) and Laws' texture energies (filtering with a small set of masks depicting certain features such as lines and spots). However, their process failed on dense tissue that was relatively uniform. This may have been due to the low resolution of the images in the database that was used, and/or the size of the neighbourhoods used for processing. Zwiggelaar et al. [3] investigated the use of an Expectation-Maximisation algorithm on grey-level values and texture feature vectors (comprised of the difference in grey-level from the four closest neighbours) for mammogram segmentation. The results are shown on an undefined number of classes that can be as low as 3, - including the

Susan M. Astley et al. (Eds.): IWDM 2006, LNCS 4046, pp. 609–615, 2006.

pectoral muscle. Comparison of the proportion of dense tissue with an estimate provided by a radiologist looking at the image showed agreement of 67%.

All mammograms, normal or abnormal, from either young or an older woman, are textured: the texture of a region being a visual expression of its anatomical make up. Texture often remains largely invariant even to relatively large anatomical changes. This leads directly to the idea of segmenting each mammogram into texture regions for which the texture is deemed homogeneous for use in mammogram analysis. The success of the statistical based texture classification framework for breast pattern classification [4] motivated the investigation of textons and texture for a more local segmentation ro classification of the breast area. This paper presents a method for segmenting a mammogram into different densities using texture based statistical modelling.

2 Method

The segmentation algorithm presented in this paper uses textons in a Hidden Markov Random Field (HMRF) framework to achieve breast tissue/density segmentation. Textons (texture primitives) [4], are defined as the centres of the clustered filter responses achieved via convolution with a filter bank followed by nearest neighbour matching. First, we construct a texton dictionary by processing a large number of segmented mammograms and then aggregating and clustering the filter responses using K-means analysis. Given the texton dictionary, each image pixel in the breast region is assigned a label by the texton which lies closest to it in the filter space. It is considered that pixels from similar tissue have similar texture properties as texture often remains largely invariant even to relatively large anatomical changes such as involution and use of HRT.

MRF theory provides a convenient and consistent way of modelling. Context-dependent entities such as image pixels, corresponding vectors and correlated features by characterising mutual influences among such entities using conditional MRF distributions. A MRF is a collection of random variables which are defined on a finite lattice, either regular or irregular and where each variable interacts with some subgroup of that lattice termed its neighbourhood [5]. The MRF framework used is an extension of MRFs from scalar intensity images (2-D) to vector images [6]. The algorithm includes Pseudo Likelihood for parameter estimation. We developed the extension in order to enable MRFs to be used for feature vector image segmentation, and to incorporate estimation of all the parameters. The multi-vector Gaussian Hidden Markov Random Fields (GHMRFs) based on the texton feature vectors incorporate both contextual and spatial neighbourhood information. The multi-vector image representation which is achieved using the filter bank [7] results in a segmentation which is superior to the segmentation of corresponding scalar images [8]. The tissue segmentation is achieved as the result of applying the Iterated Conditional Modes (ICM) algorithm proposed by Besag [9] followed by Expectation - Maximisation (EM) and Pseudo Likelihood evaluation for estimating the unknown needed model parameters until the resulting segmented images converge. An initialisation of probabilistic moments is incorporated into a Gaussian probability model for each density class. The class labels are assumed to follow a Gibbs distribution [10] and the energy function is a sum of potentials taken from a multilevel logistic model for MRFs. The segmentation is obtained via maximisation of the posterior probability distribution function. The number of textons used, as well as the size of the neighbourhood, was based on observations in the literature [11], [3].

A number of pre and post processing steps are needed for the HMRF vector image segmentation algorithm to better approximate the radiologist's segmentation. Initially, the entire breast region is segmented [12] and processed so that each pixel is represented by its corresponding texton. Every new mammogram is represented by its texture feature vector representation. The tissue segmentation algorithm is initialised by assigning to each multi-vector pixel of the vector image the label of the texton that lies closest to it using a Euclidean distance measure. To implement the HMRF based vector image segmentation, the mean vector and the covariance matrix associated with each texton present in the initial segmentation are calculated. These statistical moments enable the textons present, to adjust accordingly with every mammogram and to provide the information needed for starting the HMRF based segmentation.

The result of the segmentation is a mammogram segmented into regions of different density/texture. However, due to the use of a large number of texture classes some density classes are represented by more than one label. To reduce the number of density classes, some labels are combined to give the same category classification. This classification is done in a supervised training manner, according to an expert radiologist's ground truth. This final categorisation takes place after the HMRF algorithm has converged.

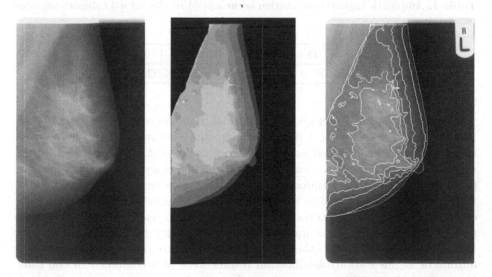

Fig. 1. Application of the texture based HMRF vector image segmentation algorithm. (a) The original mammogram. (b) The mammogram after the HMRF segmentation. (c) The automatic segmentation boundaries over the original mammogram.

3   Results

The goal of the segmentation algorithm is to see if texture could separate different densities (as described by Wolfe [13] for the different breast patterns) in the breast (adipose, glandular, *etc.*) according to what the radiologist perceived as different density region while viewing a mammogram. The segmentation results demonstrate anatomically plausible breast density segmentation. According to the radiologist evaluation, the segmentation results into regions with the following appearances of density and texture: fat tissue corresponding to the breast edge, purely adipose tissue, adipose tissue with some apparent structures (curvilinear structures, or strands of fibrous tissue), relatively dense tissue with some apparent structure that may also include more lucent areas (fibrotic stromal tissue, glandular tissue), dense tissue with an apparent texture structure (not homogeneous), and highly dense tissue (homogeneous) [14]. An example is shown in Figure 1. The results show a strong correspondence between the different textures and the radiologists perception of the different density areas in the breast.

Results are also shown in Figure 2. In the segmentation images resulting from the presented algorithm the darker the colour, the lower the corresponding density of the identified texture. The figure includes the automatic segmentation classification along with the segmentation provided by the radiologist. The images are evaluated qualitatively and quantitatively (where the radiologist's segmentation/classification is available).

Table 1. Automatic region segmentation accuracy(%) results for a 3 category segmentation

Segmentation	Dense	Fatty	Breast Edge
Accuracy(%)	96.7%, $\sigma = 3.4\%$	93.8%, $\sigma = 2.9\%$	92.8%, $\sigma = 4.2\%$

The algorithm was evaluated on 32 normal mammograms collected and digitised for the "Screen" project [15]. For the qualitative evaluation of the segmentation, a highly experienced breast screening radiologist was asked to rate the segmentation in one of four categories: very satisfactory, satisfactory, good or poor. 28 out of the 32 mammograms' segmentations were rated as very satisfactory while 3 were rated as satisfactory and 1 as good. For the quantitative evaluation of the algorithm the manual segmentation results were combined to provide a three class segmentation: dense tissue, fatty tissue and breast edge tissue, in keeping with the other works in the literature [16]. The corresponding automatic segmentation/classification results were also combined in the same three classes to facilitate comparison. The results are presented in Table 1. The segmentation accuracy (%) is modified to the percentage of the area of intersection of the automatically segmented region with the manually segmented region, over the area of their union. This definition provides a conservative estimate of the accuracy in order to account for cases where the automatically segmented region overestimates or underestimates the actual region.

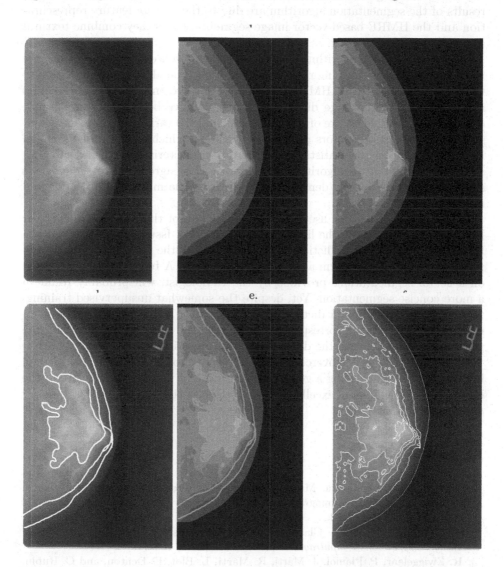

Fig. 2. Application of the texture based HMRF vector image segmentation algorithm on a mammogram belonging to Wolfe class P1 and comparison with the radiologist's ground truth segmentation. (a) The original mammogram. (b) The mammogram after one iteration of the HMRF algorithm. (c) The mammogram after the HMRF segmentation. (d) The mammograms with the segmentation from the radiologist. (e) The radiologist's segmentation overlapped on the results of the automatic HMRF segmentation algorithm. (f) The automatic segmentation boundaries over the original mammogram.

4   Discussion – Conclusions

We have presented a method for segmenting the breast to areas of different density which investigates the use of texture statistical modelling and MRFs. The results of the segmentation algorithm are due to the texture feature representation and the HMRF based vector image segmentation as they combine textural and structural information.

The segmentation algorithm allows for segmentation of the different texture regions in the breast for a more localised analysis. The algorithm combines texture feature vectors with HMRFs, providing a representation that overcomes issues relating to the large differences in appearance between mammograms, due to the projective nature of mammograms and the variability of image acquisition. Texture based vectors provide the basis on which a probabilistic model is built both upon the statistical and spatial characteristics of the vector images. The results of the algorithm demonstrate close agreement to radiologist's segmentation and texture/density interpretation. The method is objective and reproducible.

The number of textons used, as well as the size of the neighbourhood, was based on observations in the literature ([11], [2], [3]). Issues relating the chosen filtering to get the texton dictionary, the influence of the number of textons and the neighbourhood size form a basis for future work. A texton dictionary based on a set of segmentations provided by the radiologist, will probably result in a more concise segmentation. Yet, despite the somewhat unsupervised training, the choices for the texton dictionary as well as the neighbourhood, the algorithm achieves a strong correspondence between the different textures and the radiologists perception of the different density areas in the breast.

The presented method overcomes difficulties due to the image acquisition and breast variability achieving a good representation of texture and density in the breast, thus providing an excellent base for density risk assessment, asymmetry detection and matching.

References

1. J. Heine and P. Malhotra. Mammographic tissue, breast cancer risk, serial image analysis and digital mammography. part 1. tissue and related risk factors. *Academic Radioly*, 9:298–316, 2002.
2. P. Miller and S. Astley. Classification of breast tissue by texture and analysis. *Image and Vision Computing*, 10:277–282, 1992.
3. R. Zwiggelaar, P. Planiol, J. Marti, R. Marti, L. Blot, E. Denton, and C. Rubin. EM texture segmentation of mammographic images. In H. Peitgen, editor, *International Workshop on Digital Mammography*, pages 223–227, Bremen, Germany, 2002. Springer.
4. S. Petroudi, T. Kadir, and M. Brady. Automatic classification of mammographic parenchymal patterns: A statistical approach. In *Proceedings of EMBC, International Conference on Engineering in Medicine and Biology*, pages 798–801. IEEE, 2003.

5. P. Brault and A. Mohammad-Djafari. Bayesian segmentation and motion estimation in video sequences using a markov-potts model. In *Proceedings of WSEAS Conference on Applied Mathematics 2004*, 2004.
6. Y. Zhang, M. Brady, and S. Smith. Segmentation of brain MR images through a hidden markov random field model and the expectation maximization algorithm. *IEEE Trans. Med. Imag.*, 20(1):45–57, 2001.
7. M. Varma and A. Zisserman. Classifying images of materials: Achieving viewpoint and illumination independence. In *Proceedings of the European Conference on Computer Vision, Copenhagen, Denmark*, pages 255–271, 2002.
8. J. K. Fwu and P. M. Djuric. Unsupervised vector image segmentation by a tree structure-icm algorithm. *IEEE Trans. Med. Imag.*, 15(6):871–880, 1996.
9. J. Besag. On the statistical analysis of dirty pictures. *Journal of the Royal Statistical Society, Series B (Methodological)*, 48(3):259–302, 1986.
10. J. Besag. Spatial interaction and the statistical analysis of lattice systems. *Journal of the Royal Statistical Society, Series B*, 36(2):192–236, 1974.
11. M.G. Linguraru, K. Marias, and J.M. Brady. Temporal mass detection. In *International Workshop on Digital Mammography*, 2002.
12. S. Petroudi and M. Brady. Breast segmentation. In *Seventh International Workshop on Digital Mammography*. Medical Physics Publishing, 2004.
13. J.N. Wolfe. Breast parenchymal patterns and their changes with age. *Radiology*, 121:545–552, 1976.
14. N. Vujovic and D. Brzakovic. Establishing correspondence between control points in pairs of mammographic images. *IEEE Transactions on Image Processing*, 6(10):1388–1399, 1997.
15. C.J.G. Evertsz, A. Bodicker, S. Bohnenkamp, D. Dechow, C. Beck, H.-O. Peitgen, L. Berger, U. Weber, H. Jurgens, C.L. Hendriks, N. Karssemeijer, and M. Brady. Soft-copy reading environment for screening mammography - screen. In M. Yaffe, editor, *Fifth International Workshop in Digital Mammogrphy*, pages 566–572, 2000.
16. P. Miller and S. Astley. Automated detection of mammographic asymmetry using anatomical features. *International Journal of Pattern Recognition and Artificial Intelligence*, 7(6):1461–1476, 1993.

Texture Based Mammogram Classification and Segmentation

Yang Can Gong, Michael Brady, and Styliani Petroudi

Wolfson Medical Vision Laboratory
Robotics Research Group
University of Oxford, Oxford, UK
{yangcan, jmb, styliani}@robots.ox.ac.uk

Abstract. Several studies have showed that increased mammographic density is an important risk factor for breast cancer. Dense tissue often appears as textured regions in mammograms, so density and texture estimation are inextricably linked. It has been demonstrated that texture classes can be learned, and that subsequently textures can be classified using the joint distribution of intensity values over extremely compact neighbourhoods. Motivated by the success of texture classification, we propose an fully automated scheme for mammogram texture classification and segmentation. The classification method first has a training step to model the joint distribution for each breast density class. Subsequently, a statistical comparison is used to determine the class label for new images. Inspired by the classification, we combine the so-called image patch method with a HMRF(Hidden Markov Random Field) to achieve mammogram segmentation.

1 Introduction

Many studies have stressed the importance of breast density, which has been shown to be an important factor in breast cancer risk [Byng et al., 1996], [Saftlas and Szklo, 1987], [Oza and Boyd, 1993]. Wolfe was the first to study the relationship between breast patterns and risk. He proposed four breast density classes: N1, P1, P2 and NY, which represent respectively: normal breast tissue, fatty tissue, dense tissue and very dense tissue. N1 and P1 are considered low risk whereas P2 and NY are high risk classes. Later, the American College of Radiologists suggested a modification, known as the BI-RADS classification [American College of Radiology,1998]. BI-RADS generally follows Wolfe, and so in this paper, we use Wolfe Patterns, though it should be understood that our approach can be adapted straightforwardly to other classifications (BI-RADS, SCC). The goal of this paper is to use the image patch method to classify mammograms and to segment the breast into different regions, each representing a different tissue type – both based on the Wolfe classification. The idea of a texture is intuitively familiar. For the past 40 years, researchers have analysed textures in terms of what have been called "textons", which may be thought of as the

Susan M. Astley et al. (Eds.): IWDM 2006, LNCS 4046, pp. 616–625, 2006.

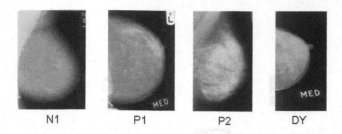

N1   P1   P2   DY

Fig. 1. Example mammograms of Wolfe Pattern

basic building blocks of a texture, i.e., a texture can be conceptualised as a suitable geometric and statistical repetition of its textons. Numerous definitions have been proposed to make precise the concept of texture and texton, and for deriving textons automatically from images. In one recent proposal, a texton was defined by Leung and Malik as a cluster centre in a suitable filter response space [Leung and Malik, 2001]. This motivated us to explore how textons could be adapted to the mammogram density evaluation.

2 Method

2.1 A Statistical Model for Breast Classification

The aim in this section is to assign a single Wolfe class to each mammogram. A set of 200 mammograms were chosen randomly from the Oxford Database, collected and digitised for the "Screen" project [Evertsz et al., 2000b], [Evertsz et al., 2000a]. The background, pectoral muscle and labels are removed using Petroudi's method [Petroudi and Brady 2001], and the mammogram pixel values are normalized to be in the range 0 to 1. 20 mammograms were then chosen randomly from each Wolfe Pattern class as the training set.

The classifier is divided into two stages: a training stage in which statistical distribution models of texture classes are learnt from training examples; and a subsequent classification stage where test images (none of the training images are subsequently used for testing) are classified by comparing their distributions to the learnt models. In the *training stage*, for each pixel of the training image, the raw pixel intensities of a $N * N$ square neighbourhood around that point are taken and row reordered to form a vector in an N^2 dimensional feature space. These "image patch" vectors are then aggregated over images from the same texture class and clustered together, and exemplars (textons) chosen via K-means clustering [Duda et al., 2001]. Finally, all the textons learnt from the (four, in this case) different classes are brought together to form a single texton dictionary. The choice of clustering each density class separately was made so that important texture primitives can be learnt from each class. In the case of mammograms, five textons are chosen from each class – greedy

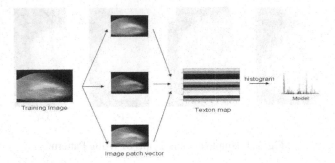

Fig. 2. Generating the corresponding model for selected training images. The image patch vector at each pixel is a 8-vector (3*3 patch excluding the central pixel), and clustering those vectors gives centres, which is what we called textons.

algorithm experiments demonstrated that five textons per class suffices to extract all the important features from mammograms.

To characterize each class, the model is learnt for a particular training image by labeling each pixel with its closest texton in the feature space. The model is the normalized frequency histogram of pixel texton labellings, i.e. an n-vector of texton probabilities for the image, where n is the number of textons. Each texture class is represented by a number of models corresponding to training images of that class. (Figure 2) Once the models for each class are generated as showed above, a nearest neighbour classifier is applied and the χ^2 statistic[Press et al., 1992] defined by:

$$\chi^2\left(P_{Model}, P_{Novel}\right) = \sum_i \frac{\left(P_{Novel} - P_{Model_i}\right)^2}{P_{Novel} - P_{Model_i}}.$$

2.2 Image Patch Method for Mammogram Segmentation

The success of assigning a single Wolfe classification to each mammogram motivated our investigation of using textons for breast segmentation. The texture of a region in a mammogram is a visual expression of its anatomical distribution. The algorithm we have developed is based on texton features, as above, and a particular segmentation algorithm, namely a HMRF(hidden Markov random field)[Marroquin, 2003], which propagates information acquired at each pixel to its surroundings, since textures occupy extended regions. Recall that a mammogram is represented as a textured vector (image patch vector) image. Evidently, the segmentation algorithm should be based both on the spatial and statistical information in the image. The spatial coherence of texture can be modelled in a number of ways. Markov random field (MRF) theory provides a convenient and consistent way to model context-dependent entities such as image pixels and correlated features. The statistical property is modelled using vector textons in our approach. A MRF is a collection of random variables which are defined on a finite lattice, either regular or irregular, and where each variable interacts with some subgroup of that lattice termed its neighbourhood [Brault and Mohammad-Djafari, 2004]. The MRF presented here is an extension of the conventional MRF, since it is based on feature vectors at each pixel.

Initialization. Using a similar process to that described in the previous section, several textons can be extracted. It turns out that in practice, some of the textons are rather similar, and so a greedy algorithm is used to eliminate such similarity. The mammogram to be segmented is then converted into a vector image, and, for each pixel, we assign the closest texton as its label. This yields an initial segmentation. As we can see from the figure below, the dense region of the mammogram is highlighted in both segmentation initialization images. Note that at this point each pixel is treated independently. We now use the HMRF to generate the final segmentation.

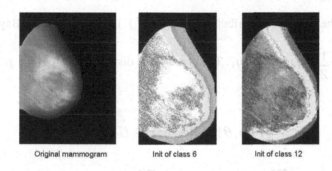

Original mammogram   Init of class 6   Init of class 12

Fig. 3. Initialization of the mammogram using 6 and 12 classes

HMRF(hidden markov random field). Marroquin proposed a novel HMRF framework which differs from the traditional MRF. Instead of altering the currently favoured class label for each pixel at each iteration, Marroquin's method maintains for each pixel an additional hidden field p, which encodes at each iteration the probability that the pixel belongs to the various classes, and which is a Markov random vector field generated with distribution $P(p) = \dfrac{1}{K}\exp[-\sum_C W_C(p)]$, where K is a normalizing constant, C are the cliques of a given neighbourhood system, W_C are given potential functions, and where each vector $p(r)$ takes values on the M-vector simplex S_M :

$$S_M = \{u \in \Re^M : \sum_{k=1}^{M} u_k = 1, u_k \geq 0, k = 1,...,M\}.$$

The key idea in Marroquin's method is that at each iteration, at each pixel, the values of the probabilities of membership of each class are updated. Finally, the maximum a posteriori class is chosen for each pixel. Hence the prior for f is: $P_f(f) = \int_{S_M^N} P(f \mid p) dP(p)$, and a potential function with 2-point neighbourhood system is used:

$$W_{rs}(p(r), p(s)) = \lambda \mid p(r) - p(s) \mid^2 = \lambda \sum_{k=1}^{M} (p_k(r) - p_k(s))^2$$

where λ is a positive parameter, and $< r, s >$ are neighbouring sites in L with a certain clique C. The posterior distribution $P(p, \theta \mid I)$ is obtained from Bayes rule as:

$P(p, \theta \mid I) = \frac{1}{Z} P(I \mid p, \theta) P_\theta(\theta)$. The conditional distribution $P(I(r) \mid p, \theta)$ may be obtained:

$$P(p, \theta \mid I) = \frac{1}{Z} \exp[-U(p, \theta)]$$

with $U(p, \theta) = -\sum_{r \in L} \log(v(r) \cdot p(r)) + \sum_C W_C(p) - \log P_\theta(\theta)$, where we consider cliques of size 4 and potentials as described above.

Now the segmentation problem is simplified to the following two steps:

1. Find the MAP estimators p^*, θ^* for p, θ:

$$p^*, \theta^* = \arg \max_{p \in S_N^M, \theta} P(p, \theta \mid I)$$

2. Find f^* as the maximizer of $P(f \mid p = p^*, \theta^*, I)$.

The first step is equivalent to the minimization of $U(p, \theta)$ subject to the constraints: $p(r) \in S_M$, for all $r \in L$, and the second step simply consists of finding the mode for each discrete measure $p^*(r)$ in a decoupled way: $f^* = \arg \max_k p_k^*(r)$.

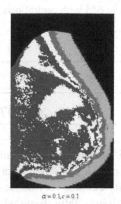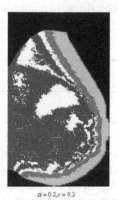

$\alpha = 0.1, c = 0.1$ $\alpha = 0.2, c = 0.2$

Fig. 4. Segmentation results after 50 iterations from mammogram in figure 3, with different noise parameter settings

3   Implementation Details and Results

As in the previous section, a set of 200 mammograms were chosen randomly from the Oxford Database, collected and digitised for the "Screen" project [Evertsz et al., 2000b], [Evertsz et al., 2000a]. The background, pectoral muscle and labels were removed using Petroudi's method[Petroudi and Brady 2001], and the mammogram pixel values were normalized to lie in the range 0 to 1. Twenty mammograms were then chosen randomly from each Wolfe Pattern class as the training set. To construct the texton library for classification and for segmentation, the 20 images for each Wolfe class were pooled and clustered via the K-means algorithm. K = 7 textons are learnt from each of the 4 Wolfe classes using 20 models per class. To evaluate the algorithm, 43 randomly chosen mammograms from the Screen project were used. The table below shows the classification result under this setup.

Table 1. Breast classification result with patch size 3*3

	N1	P1	P2	DY
Accuracy	91.4%	80.9	85.7%	90.3%
Low & High	95.7%		95.6%	

By altering the size of the patch, we get a different result (see table 2). Increasing the number of patch size can result in slower computation in training step. 5*5 patch size with the central pixel left out is slightly better than 3*3 patch.

Table 2. Classification result with patch size 5*5 with central pixel left out

	N1	P1	P2	DY
Accuracy	92.3%	80.9	83.2%	95%
Low & High	96%		97%	

To evaluate the segmentation algorithm, 15 images from the same database were compared with an experienced breast-specialist radiologist's hand-drawn segmentation. The breast can be segmented into different density classes: very dense tissue, dense with structures (fibrotic stromal tissue and glandular tissue), fatty tissue which represents the fatty background of the mammogram (Wolfe's normal breast pattern), and fatty breast edge [Linguraru et al., 2002]. Typical segmentation results are shown in figure 5 and 6.

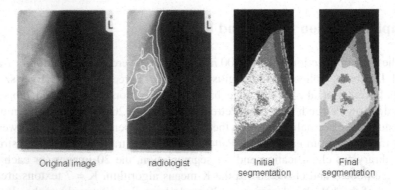

Original image   radiologist   Initial   Final
                                          segmentation   segmentation

Fig. 5. Segmentation using texture image patch method and HMRF

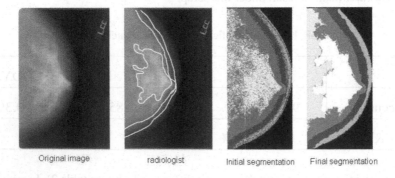

Original image   radiologist   Initial segmentation   Final segmentation

Fig. 6. Image segmentation compared with the radiologists' ground truth, the image is from Wolfe class P2

We next evaluate, for each class, our segmentation result with that of the radiologist,. This is computed for each density class k as the percentage of the intersection area of the manually selected area and the automatically generated area over their union:

$$t_k = \frac{T_k \cap R_k}{T_k \cup R_k}$$

Where T_k is the region of class k using the automatic segmentation, and R_k is the region of class k in the radiologist's hand-drawn segmentation. The Table below shows the resulting accuracy.

Table 3. The accuracy over 16 test images, 4 from each Wolf class, σ is the variance

Segmenta-tion Accuracy (%)	Dense	Dense with structures	Fatty	Fatty edge
	97%, $\sigma = 2.7\%$	95.7%, $\sigma = 2\%$	91.9%, $\sigma = 2\%$	97.2%, $\sigma = 3.6\%$

Changing the texton size and neighbourhood constants will slightly affect the segmentation result. However, the represented texture based mammogram segmentation algorithm can effectively segment the breast into different tissue classes. The presented breast density segmentation algorithm has been evaluated using 30 different mammograms spanning the 4 Wolfe classes. The method works robustly and the computation time (including training) is very fast – 100 iteration for each image is good enough to reach a steady segmentation -- although the result depends on the parameters chosen. Different texton numbers and neighbourhood cliques may alter the segmentation slightly, but from our experiments, 3 textons per Wolfe class leads the best segmentation.

We note that the classification accuracy is particularly high on Wolfe class N1 and DY, but slightly lower on P1 and P2. By looking at the distribution of (the five) different texton classes from the segmentation result, we can analyse the model for each class in terms of the percentage contribution it makes.

We can see from the above figure that class N1 and DY are clearly distinguished from the others. However, class P1 and P2 are, as expected, quite similar to each other. Further, P2 differs from P1 mostly in terms of the percentage of the texton class 4, which represents the dense part of the breast. Most of the P2 models have a relatively higher percentage of the texton class 4 than P1. We believe that by looking at more training images, we can generate a more precise boundary of P1 and P2 class.

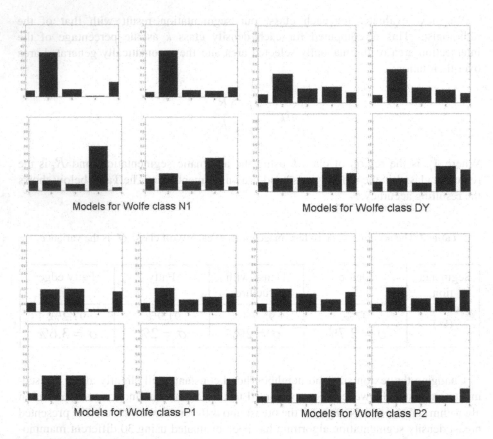

Fig. 7. Wolfe models. These models are extracted with texton size 3*3 and 5 texton classes. Four probability plot per class represented above are collected from class models, which corresponds to different model types of each class. Texton class 2 and 4 correspond to dense and dense with structures.

References

1. Varma, M., *Statistical Approaches to Texture Classification.* 2004.
2. Boyd, N.F., et al., *Quantitative classification of mammographic densities and breast cancer risk: results from the Canadian National Breast Screening Study.* J Natl Cancer Inst, 1995. **87**(9): p. 670-5.
3. Saftlas, A.F. and M. Szklo, *Mammographic parenchymal patterns and breast cancer risk.* Epidemiol Review, 1987. **9**: p. 146-174.
4. Oza, M. and N.F. Boyd, ***Mammographic parenchymal patterns: a marker of breast cancer risk.*** Epidemiol review, 1993. **15**: p. 196-208.
5. Wolfe, J.N., *Breast parenchymal patterns and their changes with age.* Radiology, 1976a. **121**: p. 545–552.

6. Leung, T. and J. Malik, *Representing and Recognizing the Visual Appearance of Materials using Three-dimensional Textons*. International Journal of Computer Vision, 2001. **43**(1): p. 29-44.
7. Evertsz, C.J.G., et al., *Soft-copy reading environment for screening mammography - screen*. Fifth International Workshop in Digital Mammogrphy, 2000. **566-572**.
8. Petroudi, S. and M. Brady., *An automated algorithm for breast background segmentation*. Medical Imaging Understanding and Analysis, 2003a: p. 181-184.
9. Duda, R.O. and P.E. Hart, *Pattern Classificaton and Scene Analysis*. Wiley, 1973.
10. Brault, P. and A. Mohammad-Djafari, *Bayesian segmentation and motion estimation in video sequences using a markov-potts model*. Proceedings of WSEAS Conference on Applied Mathematics 2004, 2004.
11. Evertsz, C.J.G., et al., *Highthroughput soft-copy reading system for digital mammography in nationwide european screening mammography programs: Requirements and first solutions*. Proceedings of the Radiographic Society of North America,, 2000.
12. Petroudi, S. and M. Brady, *Automatic nipple detection on mammograms*. Medical Image Computing and Computer-Assisted Intervention, 2003: p. 971-972.
13. Jose L. Marroquin, Edgar Arce Santana and Salvador Botello, Hidden Markov Measure Field Models for Image Segmentation. IEEE Pattern Analysis and Machine Intelligence, November 2003 (Vol. 25, No. 11) pp. 1380-1387.

Mammographic Risk Assessment Based on Anatomical Linear Structures

Edward M. Hadley[1], Erika R.E. Denton[2], and Reyer Zwiggelaar[1]

[1] Department of Computer Science, University of Wales,
Aberystwyth, UK
emh05@aber.ac.uk, rrz@aber.ac.uk
[2] Department of Radiology, Norfolk and
Norwich University Hospital, UK

Abstract. Mammographic risk assessment is concerned with the probability of a woman developing breast cancer. Recently, it has been suggested that the density of linear structures is related to risk. For 321 images from the MIAS database, a measure of line strength was obtained for each pixel using the Line Operator method. The proportion of pixels with line strength above a threshold level was calculated for each image and the results categorised by Tabar pattern, Boyd SCC class and BI-RADS class. The results indicated a significant difference between Boyd classes 1–3 (low risk) and classes 4–6 (high risk), and between most Tabar patterns and BIRADS classes.

1 Background

Mammographic risk assessment is concerned with estimating the probability of women developing breast cancer. Risk assessment is a rapidly developing area of research and aims to improve the likelihood of the early detection of breast cancer. Breast density is an important indicator of mammographic risk [1] and the best predictor of mammographic sensitivity [2]. However, more recently, it has been suggested that the distribution of linear structures is also correlated with mammographic risk [3, 4, 5]. So far it is not entirely clear if it is just the density of linear structures (either by percentage area or volume) or if the distribution of the linear structures plays a role as well.

Tabar et al. have proposed a mammographic risk assessment model based on four structural components, where the relative proportions of each component is linked to the risk of developing breast cancer [3, 4, 5]. One of the four structural components is linear density. The main purpose of this work is to investigate if automatic methods can be used to correlate the density of linear structures to mammographic risk classification metrics.

Three classification models are used: Tabar patterns [5], Boyd SCC classes [6] and Breast Imaging Reporting and Data System (BIRADS) classes [7]. Tabar's classification consists of five *patterns*, where patterns I–III represent a low risk of developing breast cancer, and patterns IV–V indicate a higher risk. Screening tests have shown that cancer prevalence in women with patterns IV-V is approximately twice that in women with patterns I-III [5]. The Boyd SCC model

Susan M. Astley et al. (Eds.): IWDM 2006, LNCS 4046, pp. 626–633, 2006.

consists of a scale of six classes where class 1 indicates the lowest risk and class 6 indicates the highest risk. Finally, the BIRADS classification uses a scale of four classes, where class 1 represents a low risk and class 4 represents a high risk.

2 Method

Three hundred and twenty-one mammographic images from the Mammographic Image Analysis Society (MIAS) database were classified according to Tabar patterns [5], Boyd SCC [6] and BIRADS classes [7] by an expert radiologist. Example images of low, moderate and high risk mammograms are shown in Fig. 1 (a).

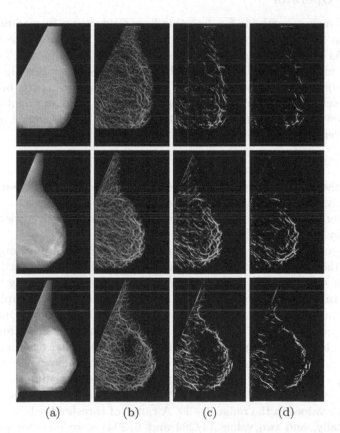

(a)   (b)   (c)   (d)

Fig. 1. The top row shows a mammogram of Boyd SCC class 1/Tabar pattern II/BIRADS class 1 (low risk), the middle row shows a mammogram of Boyd SCC class 3/Tabar pattern III/BIRADS class 2 (moderate risk) and the bottom row shows a mammogram of Boyd SCC class 6/Tabar pattern IV/BIRADS class 3 (high risk). The images in column (a) show the original mammograms, column (b) shows the results after processing with the line operator, and columns (c) and (d) show the results after thresholding at 4/204 and 6/204 respectively. The lines in (b), (c) and (d) have been enhanced for viewing.

The images were processed using Dixon and Taylor's line operator method [8, 9] (see Sect. 2.1), producing a measurement of line strength at each pixel. The multi-scale line operator has been shown to be more effective at detecting linear structures in mammographic images than other methods [9].

Figure 1 (b) shows examples of low, moderate and high risk mammograms following processing with the line operator.

The relative proportion of pixels with line strength values above a range of thresholds was calculated for each image. Figure 1 (c, d) shows examples of the resultant images after thresholding. Subsequently, the results were analysed for differences between images of each Tabar pattern, Boyd SCC class and BIRADS class.

2.1 Line Operator

A study of various methods for detecting linear structures in mammograms [9] showed that Dixon and Taylor's line operator [8] is more accurate than other methods. As such, the line operator was used in our experiments. The method produces a measure of line strength and orientation for each pixel in an image.

The line orientation is determined by calculating the mean pixel brightness of a line of pixels running through the target pixel at a range of orientations. The orientation with the largest mean brightness is taken to be the line orientation. The line strength, S, is then given by

$$S = (L - N), \tag{1}$$

where L is the mean brightness of the line of pixels, and N is the mean brightness of a similarly orientated square of pixels.

Our experiment used a line length of five pixels and twelve orientations as suggested by earlier work [9].

A multi-scale approach was used in order to detect lines of a range of thicknesses and the resultant images were combined to produce line strength values for pixels at the original scale. Scaling of the images was achieved firstly by blurring the image using a 3x3 Gaussian kernel and subsequently by subsampling to provide a resultant image of half the width and height of the original. Our approach comprised processing with the line operator at three scales, since this appeared to produce the most reasonable output for the images under examination.

Finally, the pixel line strengths were thresholded to remove background texture. Using a line length of 5, the measures of line strength fall in the theoretical range of $0 - 204$, however the results showed that most (if not all) pixels had line strength values in the range $0 - 30$. A range of threshold values were chosen experimentally, and two values (4/204 and 6/204) were used for our analysis as they removed most background noise whilst maintaining most of the linear structure information (see Fig. 1 (c, d)).

3   Results

The relative linear structure density for the various Tabar patterns, Boyd SCC classes and BIRADS classes are shown in Figs. 2, 3 and 4 respectively. These

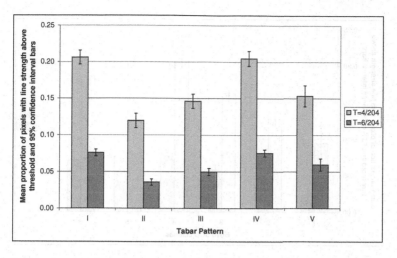

Fig. 2. Graph showing the mean proportion of pixels with line strengths above each threshold T and 95% confidence intervals for images of each **Tabar** pattern

Table 1. The p-values obtained by Mann-Whitney tests on each combination of **Tabar** patterns for each threshold T. Results not significant at $\alpha = 0.05$ are shaded.

Tabar	II	III	IV	V
I	0.0000	0.0000	0.7938	0.0000
II		0.0003	0.0000	0.0002
III			0.0000	0.3597
IV				0.0000

$$T = 4/204$$

Tabar	II	III	IV	V
I	0.0000	0.0000	0.9069	0.0059
II		0.0001	0.0000	0.0000
III			0.0000	0.0336
IV				0.0050

$$T = 6/204$$

graphs provide an overview of the difference between the patterns and classes, and for more detailed analysis, Mann-Whitney tests were performed on each pair of Tabar patterns, Boyd SCC and BIRADS classes. These are shown in Tables 1, 2 and 3 respectively. Parametric tests, such as analysis of variance (ANOVA) tests were not used because the test data did not fulfill the necessary assumptions, however the relatively small number of classes made pairwise Mann-Whitney tests possible.

The Mann-Whitney test results provide an indication as to whether there was a statistically significant difference between two classes of images in our data set. A significant difference would mean that it is possible to reliably distinguish between different classes of images.

As mentioned, two threshold values were used in our analysis (4/204 and 6/204). This is to demonstrate the effects of varying the threshold level and thus including more or less of the linear structure information.

The results of the analysis by Tabar pattern (see Fig. 2, Table 1) demonstrate the ability to reliably distinguish between patterns II–III (low risk) and patterns IV–V (high risk) at a threshold of 6/204, with low risk pattern I being indistinguishable from high risk pattern IV. The results at a threshold of 4/204

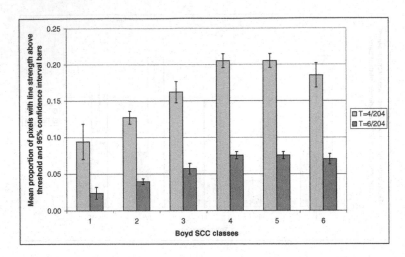

Fig. 3. Graph showing the mean proportion of pixels with line strengths above each threshold T and 95% confidence intervals for images of each **Boyd SCC** class

Table 2. The p-values obtained by Mann-Whitney tests on each combination of **Boyd SCC** classes at each threshold T. Results not significant at $\alpha = 0.05$ are shaded.

Boyd	2	3	4	5	6
1	0.0332	0.0023	0.0001	0.0001	0.0008
2		0.0002	0.0000	0.0000	0.0000
3			0.0000	0.0000	0.0362
4				0.6693	0.0287
5					0.0833

$$T = 4/204$$

Boyd	2	3	4	5	6
1	0.0155	0.0009	0.0001	0.0000	0.0004
2		0.0001	0.0000	0.0000	0.0000
3			0.0000	0.0000	0.0031
4				0.7621	0.4828
5					0.6612

$$T = 6/204$$

are less promising, since the low risk pattern III becomes indistinguishable from high risk pattern V.

The results of the analysis by Boyd SCC class (see Fig. 3, Table 2) differ somewhat, and it is clear that the proposed method is able to distinguish between classes 1–3 and classes 4–6 and both thresholds, with a general trend through classes 1–4/5 indicating that a greater linear density is indicative of a greater risk. The three lower risk classes are each distinguishable from all other classes, whilst the three higher risk classes are distinguishable from the three lower risk

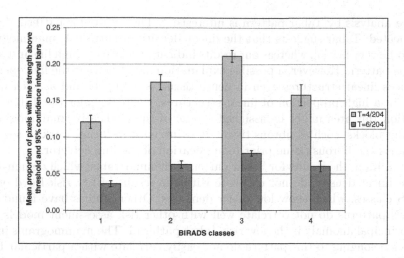

Fig. 4. Graph showing the mean proportion of pixels with line strengths above each threshold T and 95% confidence intervals for images of each **BIRADS** class

Table 3. The p-values obtained by Mann-Whitney tests on each combination of **BI-RADS** classes at each threshold T. Results not significant at $\alpha = 0.05$ are shaded.

BIRADS	2	3	4	BIRADS	2	3	4
1	0.0000	0.0000	0.000	1	0.0000	0.0000	0.000
2		0.0000	0.0771	2		0.0000	0.8636
3			0.0000	3			0.0002

$$T = 4/204 \qquad\qquad T = 6/204$$

classes, but are indistinguishable from one another at $T = 6/204$. At $T = 4/204$ classes 4 and 6 become distinguishable from one another.

Results from the analysis by BIRADS class (see Fig. 4, Table 3) demonstrate the ability to distinguish the low risk class 1 from all other classes, and the higher risk class 3 from all other classes. However, it is not possible to distinguish the lower risk class 2 from the higher risk class 4. The trend shown here differs from the analysis by Boyd class; here the highest risk class 4 indicates a markedly lower average linear density than the moderately high risk class 3 and a similar density to the lower risk class 2. Whilst Boyd class 6 does show a slightly lower linear density than class 5, it is much less marked. This is reflected in the Mann-Whitney tests.

4   Discussion and Conclusions

Whilst the proposed approach is simplistic, the results are promising and the analysis by Boyd SCC class demonstrates a clear ability to automatically distinguish between lower risk mammograms (classes 1–3) and higher risk mammograms (classes 4–6).

The analysis by Tabar pattern is interesting. The results for pattern V were unexpected. Tabar suggests that the linear density in pattern V mammograms should be very low [5], whereas our results indicate a relatively high linear density for this pattern. However, a possible explanation might be that the line operator enhances linear structures even in dense tissue (see Fig. 1) and as such might result in a high proportion of linear structures, whereas under the Tabar classification this area might be assigned to one of the alternative mammographic building blocks, such as fibrous tissue. It is intended in future work to segment and mask the fibrous tissue prior to application of the line detector.

In addition, the results for Tabar pattern I mammograms, which demonstrate a high linear density, do not correlate with the results of low risk Boyd or BI-RADS classes, which show low linear densities. Other studies have found that Tabar's patterns do not correlate well with other risk assessment models [10]. The principal anomaly is the low risk Tabar pattern I. The mammograms in our test set belonging to this pattern do not easily correlate with a particular Boyd classification, instead being spread amongst Boyd classes 2-5, with the majority seeming to belong to the high risk classes 4-5[10].

The analysis by BIRADS class are also less promising than the analysis by Boyd class, since it is not currently possible to distinguish between the low risk class 2 and the high risk class 4. We see in the analysis by Boyd class that the highest class (6) shows a slightly lower linear density than the classes immediately below it. At a threshold of 6/204 this decline is only slight and there is no significant difference between the linear densities of classes 4–6 (see Table 2). The density of class 6 is also significantly higher than all three of the low risk classes. The decline is accentuated when a threshold of 4/204 is taken, where we see a significant difference between classes 4 and 6. This indicates a dependence on the threshold value and part of our future work will include an investigation in to a more principled approach to determine the threshold.

Similarly, the highest risk BIRADS class (4) is indistinguishable at either threshold from the low risk class 2 based on this method, but is significantly lower than class 3. The trend seen in the results by Boyd class is also present in the BIRADS results. Owing to a lack of distinction between BIRADS classes 2 and 4, we are unable to make a reliable estimate on the BIRADS scale, and further information will be necessary to achieve this. It is possible that a distinction may be achievable by applying the proposed method at a wider variety of scales, or alternatively additional data may be necessary, such as information relating to the distribution of the linear structures.

In summary, the proposed approach is promising but simplistic in that it considers only the density of linear structures and does not take in to account information relating to their distribution. Since several risk assessment models are based on the parenchymal patterns in the breast [1, 3, 5], it is intended for further work to investigate whether the distribution of linear structures in addition to their density is related to mammographic risk, and whether this information can be used to improve risk assessment classification.

References

1. Wolfe, J.N.: Risk for breast cancer development determined by mammographic parenchymal pattern. Cancer **37**(5) (1976) 2486–2492
2. Kolb, T.M., Lichy, J., Newhouse, J.H.: Comparison of the performance of screening mammography, physical examination, and breast us and evaluation of factors that influence them: An analysis of 27,825 patient evaluations. Radiology **225**(1) (2002) 165–175
3. Tabar, L., Dean, P.B.: Mammographic parenchymal patterns. risk indicator for breast cancer? Journal of the American Medical Association **247**(2) (1982) 185–189
4. Gram, I.T., Funkhouser, E., Tabar, L.: The Tabar classification of mammographic parenchymal patterns. European Journal of Radiology **24**(2) (1997) 131–136
5. Tabar, L., Tot, T., Dean, P.B.: Breast Cancer - The Art and Science of Early Detection with Mammography. Georg Thieme Verlag, Stuttgart (2005)
6. Boyd, N.F., Byng, J.W., Jong, R.A., Fishell, E.K., Little, L.E., Miller, A.B., Lockwood, G.A., Tritchler, D.L., Yaffe, M.J.: Quantitative classification of mammographic densities and breast cancer risk: results from the Canadian National Breast Screening Study. Journal of the National Cancer Institute **87** (1995) 670–675
7. American College of Radiology: Illustrated Breast Imaging Reporting and Data System. 3rd edn. American College of Radiology (1998)
8. Dixon, R.N., Taylor, C.J.: Automated asbestos fibre counting. Institute of Physics Conference Series **44** (1979) 178–185
9. Zwiggelaar, R., Astley, S.M., Boggis, C.R.M., Taylor, C.J.: Linear structures in mammographic images: Detection and classification. IEEE Transactions on Medical Imaging **23**(9) (2004) 1077–1086
10. Muhimmah, I., Oliver, A., Denton, E.R.E., Pont, J., Perez, E., Zwiggelaar, R.: Comparison between wolfe, boyd, bi-rads and tabar based mammographic risk assessment. Lecture Notes in Computer Science **this volume** (2006)

Comparison of Methods for Classification of Breast Ductal Branching Patterns

Predrag R. Bakic[1], Despina Kontos[2], Vasileios Megalooikonomou[2],
Mark A. Rosen[1], and Andrew D.A. Maidment[1]

[1] Department of Radiology, University of Pennsylvania,
3400 Spruce St., Philadelphia, PA USA 19104
{Predrag.Bakic, RosenMar, Andrew.Maidment}@uphs.upenn.edu
[2] Computer and Information Sciences Department, Temple University,
1805 N.Broad St., Philadelphia PA USA 19122
{DKontos, Vasilis}@temple.edu

Abstract. Topological properties of the breast ductal network have shown the potential for classifying clinical breast images with and without radiological findings. In this paper, we review three methods for the description and classification of breast ductal topology. The methods are based on ramification matrices and symbolic representation via string encoding signatures. The performance of these methods has been compared using clinical x-ray and MR images of breast ductal networks. We observed the accuracy of the classification between the ductal trees segmented from the x-ray galactograms with radiological findings and normal cases in the range of 0.86-0.91%. The accuracy of the classification of the ductal trees segmented from the MR autogalactograms was observed in the range of 0.5-0.89%.

1 Background

The vast majority of breast cancers originate from the epithelial tissue of breast ducts. Due to low radiographic contrast, ducts are barely visible in mammograms. However, the breast ducts contribute to the complexity of the parenchymal pattern, which has been used in computer algorithms for early cancer detection and cancer risk estimation [1].

Breast ductal branching patterns have been previously analyzed by manually tracing ductal trees from galactograms, 2D x-ray images of contrast-enhanced ducts. That preliminary analysis, performed using ramification matrices (R matrices), was applied to classify galactograms with radiological findings and normal cases (i.e., no radiographic findings) [2]. More recently, the analysis has been extended to include other descriptors of ductal topology [3,4]. This paper compares three methods for describing and classifying breast ductal topology. The performance of these methods is compared using breast ductal networks as visualized in clinical x-ray and MR images.

2 Methods

In this section, we describe methods to acquire clinical images of the ductal network and to extract ductal topology descriptors from clinical images.

Susan M. Astley et al. (Eds.): IWDM 2006, LNCS 4046, pp. 634–641, 2006.

2.1 Data Acquisition

We have traced ductal topology in clinical x-ray galactograms and magnetic resonance (MR) autogalactograms (see Fig. 1). Galactograms are x-ray images of the breast, in which a small amount of contrast material has been injected into a nipple opening leading to a ductal lobe (subtree). The ductal subtrees have been segmented manually.

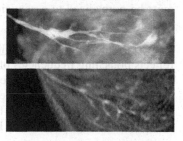

Autogalactograms refer to breast MR images of women in which portions of their ductal network enhanced due to the presence of protein or blood in the ducts [5]. The enhanced portions of the ductal tree were segmented in MR slices acquired with a 3D GRASS pulse-sequence [5]. A semi-automated region growing algorithm was used for segmentation. The 3D ductal topology was manually reconstructed from the segmented portions in each slice.

Fig. 1. Breast ductal network visualized in a galactogram (top) or an autogalactogram (bottom)

In this project we analyzed 22 clinical x-ray galactograms obtained retrospectively from 14 women (mean age 49.2 years, range 29–75 years), examined at the Thomas Jefferson University Breast Imaging Center, Philadelphia, PA, during the period of June 1994 through January 2001. Of these, seven women (13 images) had radiological findings corresponding to benign abnormalities, and eight women (12 images) had no findings; no malignant cases were available.

We also analyzed nine clinical autogalactograms obtained retrospectively from eight women (mean age 53.1 years; range 40-72 years), who had their breast MR studies at the Hospital of the University of Pennsylvania between June 2000 and April 2005. The five of eight women had radiological findings (four benign and one malignant; the latter with two identifiable ductal subtrees) and three cases were normal.

2.2 Description of Ductal Topology

R matrices. Elements of R matrices represent probabilities of branching at different levels of a ductal tree, computed following the Strahler labeling of individual ducts (see Fig. 2) [6]. Each R-matrix element $r_{k,j}$ can be expressed as [2]:

$$r_{k,j} = b_{k,j} / a_k, \tag{1}$$

where a_k is the total number of branches at the same level of the tree (those branches are identified by label k) and $b_{k,j}$ is the number of branches with label k, where the child branches are labeled k and j. The lateral branching is identified by labels $j{\neq}k$, while $j{=}k$ identifies bifurcation into child branches of the same order. The method for R matrix estimation from ductal trees has been described previously [7]. The R matrices estimated from clinical images have been used to realistically generate synthetic ductal network [8]. In addition, such estimated branching probabilities have been used for classification of galactograms with radiological findings and normal cases [2]. In this paper, we have extended that classification approach to include MR autogalactograms.

String encoding based descriptors. Another approach to represent the branching topology of the ductal network is to apply string encoding techniques. These techniques transform the initial ductal tree to a corresponding string signature. Further analysis is applied to these characterization signatures to investigate the properties of the branching topology. To avoid the problem of tree isomorphism, the ductal trees must be normalized to a canonical form [9]. The next step is to label the nodes (or branches) of the tree.

Prüfer encoding and tf-idf weighting. *Prüfer* encoding is a tree encoding scheme that reflects branching frequencies of the tree nodes [3]. This encoding constructs a unique string representation for each tree-like structure. The algorithm visits each node of the tree following an in-order traversal and depth-first search. During this process the encoding string is constructed; for each non-root node, the label of its parent is used to represent it. Fig. 2 shows the Prüfer encoding string for a sample labeled tree.

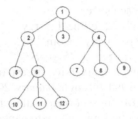

Fig. 2. An example of a labeled rooted tree. The corresponding: *Prüfer* encoding representation {*1 2 2 6 6 6 1 1 4 4 4*}, DFSE representation {*1 2 5 6 10 11 12 3 4 7 8 9*}.

The *tf-idf* weighting text mining technique can be further applied to the Prüfer encoding signatures to assign a significance weight to each string term (i.e., node label) and construct corresponding vectors of significance weights for each ductal tree. The cosine similarity metric can be applied to the tf-idf vectors in order to perform classification of the initial ductal trees [3].

Depth-first encoding and fractal dimension. *Depth-first string encoding* (DFSE) is a straightforward encoding scheme that constructs a string representation for a tree by visiting each node following an in-order depth-first traversal. During this process each node is represented in the string by its label. Fig. 2 shows the DFSE for a sample labeled tree.

These DFSE signatures can be used for investigating the fractal properties of the ductal branching topology [4]. The *regularization dimension* [10] of the signatures is computed, which detects self-similar properties of the signature by looking into the scaling behavior of the lengths of less and less regularized versions of the string encoding representation. Classification is performed by thresholding the fractal dimension values. The performance can be assessed by ROC analysis [4].

Fig. 3 illustrates computation of the classification features for the three methods of ductal topology description, applied to the clinical galactogram from Fig. 1.

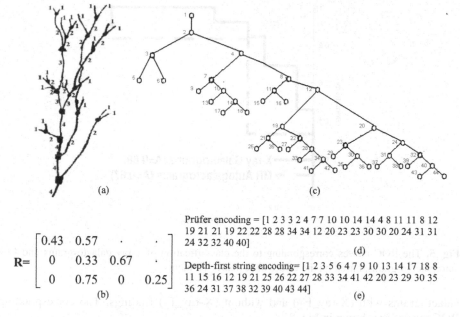

$$R = \begin{bmatrix} 0.43 & 0.57 & \cdot & \cdot \\ 0 & 0.33 & 0.67 & \cdot \\ 0 & 0.75 & 0 & 0.25 \end{bmatrix}$$

(b)

Prüfer encoding = [1 2 3 3 2 4 7 7 10 10 14 14 4 8 11 11 8 12
19 21 21 19 22 22 28 28 34 34 12 20 23 23 30 30 20 24 31 31
24 32 32 40 40]

(d)

Depth-first string encoding= [1 2 3 5 6 4 7 9 10 13 14 17 18 8
11 15 16 12 19 21 25 26 22 27 28 33 34 41 42 20 23 29 30 35
36 24 31 37 38 32 39 40 43 44]

(e)

Fig. 3. An example of (a) manually traced ductal tree, (b) the corresponding R matrix, (c) the canonical form the tree labeled in a breadth-first manner, and the corresponding (d) Prüfer- and (e) Depth-first string encoded signatures. We computed tf-idf weighted vector and regularization dimension based on the signatures in (d) and (e), respectively.

3   Results

<u>R matrices.</u> Fig. 4 shows the range of values of the R matrix element used as the classification feature. The feature values were averaged separately over the auto-galactograms with (MR_F+) and without (MR_F-) findings, and over the

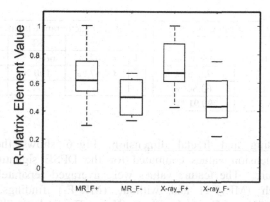

Fig. 4. Box-whisker plots of R-matrix based feature values used for classification of ductal trees. The whiskers indicate maximum and minimum feature values and the box indicates 25-, 50-, and 75-percentile values.

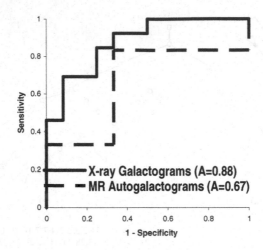

Fig. 5. The ROC curves corresponding to the class-ification of x-ray galacto-grams and MR auto galacto-grams, based on the values of R-matrix elements

galactograms with (X-ray_F+) and without (X-ray_F-) findings. The corresponding ROC curves are shown in Fig. 5.

Prüfer encoding and tf-idf weighting. Table 1 lists the accuracies of classifying x-ray galactograms and MR autogalactograms, based on the string representations computed using the Prüfer encoding and the tf-idf weighting. Leave-one-out k-nearest neighbor classification was performed based on the cosine similarity metric. The maximum accuracy was observed for x-ray galactograms at $k=4$. As there were only three MR autogalactograms with radiological findings, we were restricted to $k \leq 2$.

Table 1. Comparative x-ray galactogram and MR autogalactogram classification accuracies for Prüfer string encoding, assuming leave-one out k-nearest neighbor classifier based on cosine similarity

	Galactogram Classification Accuracy				Autogalactogram Classification Accuracy		
k	NF	RF	Total	k	NF	RF	Total
1	80 %	41.67 %	59.09 %	1	66.67 %	66.67 %	66.67 %
2	80 %	66.67 %	72.73 %	2	66.67 %	100 %	**88.89 %**
3	80 %	50 %	63.64 %	--	--	--	--
4	100 %	83.3 %	**90.91 %**				

Depth-first encoding and fractal dimension. Fig. 6 shows the range of the regularization dimension values computed for the DFSE signatures, used as the classification feature. The feature values were averaged separately over the auto-galactograms with (MR_F+) and without (MR_F-) findings, and over the galactograms with (X-ray_F+) and without (X-ray_F-) findings. The corresponding ROC curves are shown in Fig. 7. Fig. 7 shows also the ROC curve obtained after

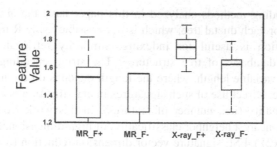

Fig. 6. Box-whisker plots of fractal based regularization dimension values used for classification of ductal trees. The whiskers indicate maximum and minimum feature values and the box indicates 25-, 50-, and 75-percentile values.

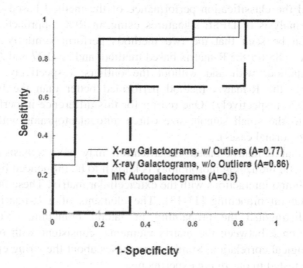

Fig. 7. The ROC curves corresponding to the class-ification of x-ray galacto-grams and MR auto galacto-grams, based on the regular-ization dimension values

removing two x-ray galactograms, whose regularization dimension values were identified as statistical outliers [4]. The two images were removed from the set of galactograms with radiological findings.

4 Discussion

The three methods for describing breast ductal topology compared are inherently different. The R-matrix method is based on the probabilistic nature of R matrices. Elements of an R matrix represent probabilities of branching at various levels of the ductal tree. Thus, a single matrix could be used to describe a family of the trees, with characteristic topological properties. We used this feature to generate synthetic ductal networks with realistic topological properties [8].

The string encoding methods analyzed in this paper have the ability to generate unique signature for each ductal tree, which is not possible using R matrices. Such a unique representation is useful for indexing, similarity retrieval, and similarity searches in large databases of tree structures. The string encoding signatures are usually vectors of variable length, where the length depends on the number of nodes in the analyzed tree. Direct use of such signatures in classification is a problem due to the high-dimensionality (i.e., number of features). In this work we considered two solutions: (1) the k-nearest neighbor classification of high-dimensional tf-idf weighted Prüfer strings and (2) DFSE signature vector dimension reduction by fractal analysis. Table 1 shows that relatively high classification accuracy (90.91% for x-ray galactograms and 88.89% for MR autogalactograms) was achieved using tf-idf weighted Prüfer strings signatures and k-nearest neighborhood classifier. This classification performance however, depends on the available sample size.

We evaluated the classification performance of the method based on R matrices and the fractal analysis of DFSE signatures using an ROC approach. Figs. 5 and 7 show that it can be seen that the two methods perform similarly for the x-ray galactograms; A=0.88 for the R-matrix based method, and A=0.77 and A=0.86 for the fractal based method, with and without the outliers, respectively. For the MR autogalactograms, the R-matrix method performed better than the fractal method (A=0.67 vs A=0.5, respectively). One reason for this difference in performance may be attributable to the small sample size (three autogalactograms with radiological findings and five normal cases).

We believe that R-matrix based classification may have a basis in the ductal biology. The ductal branching morphology is known to be influenced by variations in hormonal stimuli and interactions with the extracellular matrix. These factors alter the probability of lateral branching [11-13]. The elements of a R-matrix are able to quantify and distinguish the probability of lateral branching. We observed a significant difference between the matrix elements, consistent with our hypothesis about their biological correlation. Similar hypotheses about the string encoding based methods will be tested in our future experiments.

5 Conclusions

Classification results have been obtained using the three methods of description of the breast ductal branching topology. The methods were applied on two sets of ductal trees, extracted from clinical x-ray galactograms and MR autogalactograms. The R-matrices offer a higher-level representation of the tree branching topology. We hypothesize that such a representation may be related to the biological nature of breast pathology. On the other hand, string encoding based descriptors introduce a transformation of the tree topology from the 2D or 3D image space to the 1D signal (signature) space. A number of 1D signal processing methods could be then applied. Such methods could be advantageous for indexing and similarity retrieval in large databases of tree-like structures.

Acknowledgement

The work was funded by the Toshiba America Medical Systems Inc./Radiological Society of North America Research Seed Grant SD0329, by the National Cancer Institute Program Project Grant PO1 CA85484, and by the National Science Foundation under grant IIS-0237921. The authors are grateful to Catherine Piccoli, M.D. and Andrea Frangos, M.S. from Thomas Jefferson University, Philadelphia, PA, for providing anonymized x-ray galactographic images.

References

1. Li, H., Giger, M.L., Huo, Z., Olopade, O.I., Lan, L., Weber, B., Bonta, I.: Computerized analysis of mammographic parenchymal patterns for assessing breast cancer risk: effect of ROI size and location. Med. Phys. 31 (2004) 549-555
2. Bakic, P.R., Albert, M., Maidment, A.D.A.: Classification of Galactograms with Ramification Matrices: Preliminary Results. Acad Radiol. 10 (2003) 198-204
3. Megalooikonomou, V., Kontos, D., Danglemaier, J., Javadi, A., Bakic, P.R., Maidment, A.D.A.: A Representation and Classification Scheme for Tree-like Structures in Medical Images: An Application on Branching Pattern Analysis of Ductal Trees in X-ray Galactograms. In Proc. SPIE. 6144 (2006) 488-496
4. Kontos. D, Megalooikonomou, V., Javadi, A., Bakic, P.R., Maidment, A.D.A.: Classification of Galactograms using Fractal Properties of the Breast Ductal Network. In Proc. 3rd IEEE International Symposium on Biomedical Imaging. 2006 ISBI (2006)
5. Bakic, P.R., Rosen M.A., Maidment A.D.A.: Comparison of breast ductal branching pattern classification using x-ray galactograms and MR autogalactograms. In Proc. SPIE 6144 (2006) 707-716
6. Strahler, A.N.: Hypsometric area-altitude analysis of erosional topography. Bull. Geol. Soc. Am. 63 (1952) 1117–1142
7. Viennot, X.G., Eyrolles, G., Janey, N., Arques, D.: Combinatorial analysis of ramified patterns and computer imagery of trees. Comput. Graph. 23 (1989) 31–40
8. Bakic, P.R., Albert, M., Brzakovic, D., Maidment, A.D.A.: Mammogram synthesis using a 3-D simulation. III. Modeling and evaluation of the breast ductal network. Med. Phys. 30 (2003) 1914-1925
9. Chi, Y, Yang, Y, Muntz, R.: Canonical forms for labeled trees and their applications in frequent subtree mining. Knowledge and Info Systems 8 (2005) 203-234
10. Roueff, F., Vehel, J.L.: A regularization approach to fractional dimension estimation," in Proc. of Fractals 98, Malta, 1998.
11. Fata, J.E., Werb, Z., Bissell, M.J.: Regulation of mammary gland branching morphogenesis by the extracellular matrix and its remodeling enzymes. Breast Cancer Research 6 (2004) 1-11
12. Robinson, G.W., Hennighausen, L., Johnson, P.F.: Side-branching in the mammary gland: the progesterone-Wnt connection. Genes & Devel 14 (2000) 889-894
13. Sternlicht, M.D., Key stages in mammary gland development: The cues that regulate ductal branching morphogenesis. Breast Cancer Research 8 (2006) 201-211

Validation of Graph Theoretic Segmentation of the Pectoral Muscle

Fei Ma[1], Mariusz Bajger[1], John P. Slavotinek[2], and Murk J. Bottema[1]

[1] Flinders University, Adelaide SA 5001, Australia
murkb@infoeng.flinders.edu.au
[2] Flinders Medical Centre, Bedford Park SA 5042, Australia

Abstract. Two graph theoretic methods are used in conjunction with active contours to segment the pectoral muscle in 82 screening mammograms. To validate the method, the boundaries are also marked by four radiologists with different levels of experience in mammography. The simultaneous truth and performance level estimation (STAPLE) method is used to estimate the true boundary and to estimate the sensitivity and specificity of the segmentation schemes. The performance of one of the two algorithms is found not differ significantly from radiologists.

1 Introduction

In order to develop or compare algorithms for segmentation, it is necessary to estimate the level of accuracy by some criterion. Often, the best available method is to ask a radiologist or other expert to segment the image manually and use the resulting boundaries as the true boundaries. The difficulty is that boundaries drawn by different experts usually do not agree. Such validation problems are ubiquitous in medical image analysis.

Recently, a method was devised for estimating the true boundary given a set of boundaries drawn by experts. The method, called simultaneous truth and performance level estimation (STAPLE) [1] is based on the expectation-maximization (EM) algorithm. The method also provides estimates of the performance of segmentation algorithms in terms of sensitivity and specificity.

Here we report on the use of STAPLE to estimate the performance of two segmentation algorithms based on graph theory, the adaptive pyramid (AP) algorithm [2] and the minimum spanning tree algorithm (MST) [3]. These algorithms were used to find the pectoral muscle in screening mammograms.

The pectoral muscle is only of marginal clinical interest. However, for automatic detection of breast cancer using computers, the pectoral muscle represents a region where the intensity statistics are likely be quite different from the rest of the image. Hence it is convenient to identify this region in order to apply different processing steps or to ignore it entirely. The pectoral muscle is also a significant landmark for use in automated image registration. Finally, in developing new methods for segmenting mammograms, or medical images in general, identifying the pectoral muscle is a convenient initial test.

Thus neither the objective of the study (the detection of the pectoral muscle) nor the method (STAPLE) directly improve clinical detection of breast cancer.

Susan M. Astley et al. (Eds.): IWDM 2006, LNCS 4046, pp. 642–649, 2006.

Both the task and the method are aimed at improving studies on computer-aided detection of breast cancer.

2   Graph Theoretic Segmentation and Active Contours

A graph, $G = (V, E)$ consists of a set of vertices, V, and a set of edges, E. An edge, $e \in E$, consists of pair of vertices, $e = (v_i, v_j)$, where $v_i, v_j \in V$. In the case of image segmentation, V is the set of pixels and E determines which pixels are viewed as being associated. In this setting, image segmentation is equivalent to finding (disjoint) subgraphs of G.

2.1   AP Algorithm

The AP algorithm builds sequences of ever smaller graphs. This sequence of graphs is often pictured as a pyramid with the original full graph forming the base of the pyramid and successive graphs forming smaller and smaller layers above. At the base level, the graph consists of V_0, the set of all pixels in the image, and E is such that every pixel is joined to its immediate eight neighbors. A vertex survives to the next level if it is more representative of its immediate neighborhood than are its neighbors. If two pixels are connected by an edge, then both are not allowed to survive to the next level. Also, for every pixel, at least one of the pixels to which it is connected survives to the next level. Two surviving pixels are connected in the next level if the regions they represent in the previous level have similar mean intensity but not otherwise. If a surviving pixel does not represent a region in the previous level similar to other surviving pixels, this surviving pixel is called a root. Passing back down the layers of graphs, root pixels identify a subset of V that is accepted as a region of the image [2],[4].

2.2   MST Algorithm

The MST algorithm starts with the graph such that V is the set of all pixels and E is the empty set. However, there is a set of candidate edges E_c consisting of all edges that join pixels to other pixels in small neighborhood. All the edges in E_c are assigned an edge weight that measures how well the two pixels comprising the edge match according to a pre-defined criterion. These candidate edges are ordered by increasing edge weight.

Starting with the edge with smallest weight, each edge is considered for inclusion in the final graph. An edge is accepted if the two vertices are in disjoint components of the current graph and the edge weight is small compared to the internal variation within the two components. Once all the candidate edges in E_c have been considered, V together with all the accepted edges is the final graph. The disjoint subgraphs of the final graph form the segmentation [3],[5].

2.3   Active Contour

The AP and MST algorithms were generally found to identify the pectoral muscle in terms of general location and shape. However, the edges of the components identified as the pectoral muscle were found to be locally irregular and ragged. In order to take advantage of the known smooth and slowly varying nature of pectoral muscle boundaries, the AP and MST results were used to initialize a simple active contour scheme.

The coordinates forming the pectoral muscle boundary in a screening mammogram can be described as a single value function of the vertical axis. Thus the coordinates are of the form $(g(y), y)$. Accordingly, points on the contour may be modeled as moving only in the horizontal direction. The active contour model consists of an internal energy given by

$$E_{in,i} = a_1 V'(v_i) + a_2 V''(v_i) \tag{1}$$

and the external energy given by

$$E_{ex,i} = -|I_x(v_i)| / \max_I(I_x), \tag{2}$$

where $V = v_1, v_2, \ldots, v_c$ denotes the sequence of vertices comprising the current contour, $V'(v_i)$ and $V''(v_i)$ denote the first and second derivatives of V along the contour, a_1 and a_2 are constants, I is the image, and I_x is the spatial derivative of I in the horizontal direction [4], [5].

3   The STAPLE Algorithm

Suppose R raters have performed a segmentation of an image I. The raters may be experts, non-experts, or computer algorithms. Let N denote the number of pixels in the image and let D denote a matrix of size $N \times R$ such that $D(i,r) = 1$ if rater r assigned pixel i to the region in question (the pectoral muscle in our case) and $D(i,r) = 0$ otherwise. Let T denote the unknown binary vector of length N that indicates the true segmentation. Let p_r and q_r denote the sensitivity and specificity resulting from a segmentation and let p and q denote the column vectors $p = (p_1, p_2, \ldots, p_R)^t$ and $q = (q_1, q_2, \ldots, q_R)^t$. The objective is to determine $\hat{p}$ and $\hat{q}$ defined by

$$(\hat{p}, \hat{q}) = \arg\max_{p,q} \ln f(D, T | p, q), \tag{3}$$

where $f(D, T | p, q)$ is the probability mass function.

Solving (3) is difficult because T is not known. Hence the expectation maximization (EM) algorithm is used. First, initial guesses for $\hat{p}$ and $\hat{q}$ are used to estimate the true segmentation, T. This is the E step. Second, updated estimates $\hat{p}$ and $\hat{q}$ are found by solving the maximization problem in Equation 3. This is the M step. These steps are iterated to convergence [1]. The algorithm produces estimates of $\hat{p}$ and $\hat{q}$ and the most likely "true" boundary based on T.

4   Methods

Initially, 84 images from the Mammographic Image Analysis Society data base (Mini-MIAS) were selected for this study. These particular images were chosen because one expert drawn boundary of the pectoral muscle was available for each of these images from previous work by Ferrari et al. [6]. In addition, a radiologist from our group with expertise in mammogrpahy (JPS) and two radiologists with minimal experience in mammography were asked to draw boundaries of the pectoral muscle independently for these images, resulting in a total of four human drawn boundaries per image. The positioning of the breast in two of the images (mdb098 and mdb109) was such that the pectoral muscle did not appear in the image and so the study was conducted using the remaining 82 images.

To implement the STAPLE algorithm, it is necessary to specify the prior probability of the true segmentation and to set initial values for $\hat{p}$ and $\hat{q}$. Let $f(T_i)$ denote the prior probability that pixel i is part of the region being segmented. This function is unknown and must be assigned. In the case of the pectoral muscle in a screening mammogram, this function may be assigned based on prior understanding of image. Assuming a left breast (with the obvious changes for a right breast) the pectoral muscle appears in the top left corner of the image. If $c(r)$ is the column index marking the true boundary in row r, then $T_i = 1$ for $i < r$ and $T_i = 0$ for $i > r$. The true column index $c(r)$ is not known but can be estimated by

$$\hat{c}(r) = \frac{1}{R} \sum_{j=1}^{R} c_j(r),$$

where $c_j(r)$ is the column index for the boundary drawn by rater j in row r. Since $\hat{c}(r)$ is an estimate, the prior probabilities were not assigned strictly as 1 on the left and 0 on the right. Instead the probabilities were assigned in row r as

$$f_r(c) = \frac{1}{1 + e^{\alpha(c - \hat{c}(r))}},$$

for a constant α determined by experimentation.

The boundaries drawn by the two radiologists with expertise in mammography were assigned as expert raters. The boundaries drawn by the two radiologist without expertise in mammography and the boundaries found by the algorithms were assigned as non-expert raters. Expert raters were assigned the initial sensitivity and specificity as $\hat{p} = \hat{q} = 1 - \epsilon$ and non-expert raters were assigned $\hat{p} = \hat{q} = \epsilon$ for a small number ϵ.

Initial experiments were conducted to determine sensible values for α and ϵ. Segmentation results were largely insensitive to ϵ over a large range and insensitive to α for $\alpha > .1$. For very small values of α, $\hat{p}$ and $\hat{q}$ converged to zero for some images. The values $\alpha = 1$ and $\epsilon = .001$ provided plausible values for $\hat{p}$ and $\hat{q}$ as well as plausible "true" boundaries (Fig. 1) and were adopted for the main study.

In all images, convergence was achieved in about ten iterations of the EM algorithm.

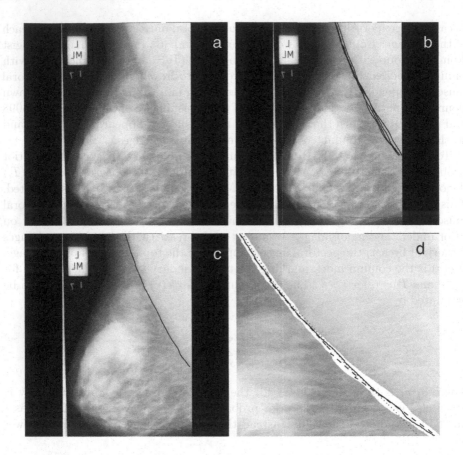

Fig. 1. (a) Image mdb115. (b) Boundaries of the pectoral muscle drawn by four radiologists. (c) Estimate of the true boundary produced by STAPLE. (d) The pectoral muscle region. The white band shows the range of human drawn boundaries in (b), ·- STAPLE true boundary as in (c), - - AP algorithm, ··· MST algorithm.

5   Results

The STAPLE algorithm provided a sensitivity score p_i and a specificity score q_i for rater i, $i = 1, 2, \ldots, 6$ (four radiologist and the two algorithms) for each of the 82 images. The performance of each rater for each image was taken to be the value $s_i = p_i + q_i$. Note that $s = 2$ for a perfect rater. The distributions of s scores for each rater over the 82 images was computed (Fig. 2).

The following null hypotheses were tested: $s_i = s_j$ for $i \neq j$. Since all the raters considered the same set of images, analysis of paired data was used. Thus for each pair of raters i and j, $i \neq j$, the value $d_{ij} = s_i - s_j$ was computed and the probability that $d_{ij} \neq 0$ by chance alone was estimated (Table 1).

The difference in performance between the MST algorithm and any one of the radiologists cannot be attributed to chance alone. However, the hypotheses that the AP algorithm performs the same as radiologists cannot be rejected.

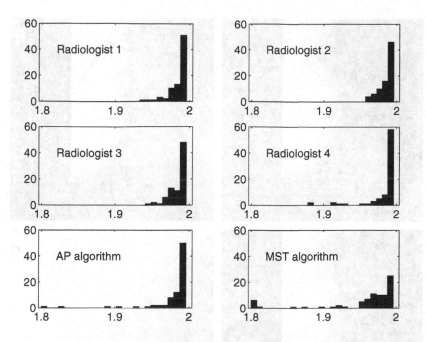

Fig. 2. Histograms of s for four radiologists and the two algorithms AP and MST

Table 1. Probability that the observed difference of performance scores, d_{ij}, is due to chance alone for all combinations of raters. R_1 and R_2 are radiologists with experience in mammography, R_3 and R_4 are radiologist with little experience in mammography, AP and MST are the algorithms discussed in the paper.

	R_1	R_2	R_3	R_4	AP	MST
R_1	-	0.8521	0.8568	0.3745	0.1206	0.0001
R_2	0.8521	-	0.4236	0.2397	0.1142	0.0001
R_3	0.8568	0.4236	-	0.3814	0.1366	0.0001
R_4	0.3745	0.2397	0.3814	-	0.2843	0.0003
AP	0.1206	0.1142	0.1366	0.2843	-	0.0000
MST	0.0001	0.0001	0.0001	0.0003	0.0000	-

6 Discussion and Conclusion

The table shows that the performance of the AP algorithm is not statistically different from radiologists. Previous work [4] showed that the AP algorithm performed about as well as an algorithm based on Gabor filters [6]. Accordingly, it seems that the current best algorithms for detecting the pectoral muscle are approaching the natural limit for this task. Further improvements will be difficult to distinguish from variation among radiologists.

The comments in the previous paragraph apply to performance over a large numbers of images. The statistics do not reflect the fact that there are still

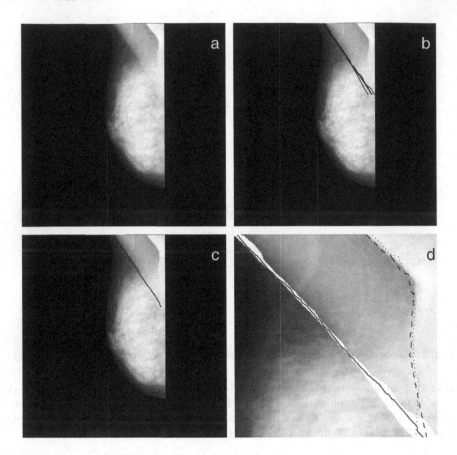

Fig. 3. (a) Image mdb039 showing a skin fold. (b) Boundaries of the pectoral muscle drawn by four radiologists. (c) Estimate of the true boundary produced by STAPLE. (d) The pectoral muscle region. The white band shows the range of human drawn boundaries in (b), - STAPLE true boundary as in (c), - - AP algorithm, ··· MST algorithm. In this example, the algorithms were completely fooled by the skin fold.

systematic differences between algorithms and radiologists on small subsets of images. In the case of the AP algorithm, there are two images for which the s value is conspicuously lower than any radiologist (Fig. 2) . The two images corresponding to these low s values are both examples of skin folds in the mammogram. A skin fold can superficially mimic pectoral muscle boundaries (Fig. 3).

An experienced radiologist can easily distinguish between skin folds and the true pectoral muscle but, as is the case with many tasks of cognition, this is not easy to duplicate automatically. In some cases, the AP and MST algorithms found the correct pectoral muscle boundary even if there was a skin fold, but failed in other cases. This issue should not be important. In many screening programs, images with skin folds are routinely rejected as being of insufficient technical quality. Thus the only obvious differences between the AP algorithm and radiologists appears on images that probably should not be considered by humans or computers.

Acknowledgement

The authors would like to thank R. J. Ferrari and R. M. Rangayyan for providing one set of the expert drawn pectoral muscle boundaries. Thanks also to Leigh Mosel and Ramon Pathi for drawing one set of boundaries each.

References

1. Warfield, S.K., Zou, K.J., Wells, W.M.: Simultaneous truth and performance level estimation (staple): An algorithm for the validation of image segmentation. IEEE Trans. Med. Imag. **23** (2004) 903–921
2. Jolion, J., Montanvert, A.: The adaptive pyramid: A framework for 2d image analysis. Computer Vision, Graphics, and Image Processing **55** (1992) 339–348
3. Felzenszwalb, P.F., Huttenlocher, D.P.: Efficient graph-based image segmentation. Int. Jour. Computer Vision **59** (2004) 167–181
4. Ma, F., Bajger, M., Bottema, M.J.: Extracting the pectoral muscle in screening mammograms using a graph pyramid. In Lovel, B.C., Meader, A.J., eds.: Workshop Proceedings, APRS Workshop on Digital Image Computing (WDIC2005), University of Queensland (2005) 39–42
5. Bajger, M., Ma, F., Bottema, M.J.: Minimum spanning trees and active contours for identification of the pectoral muscle in screening mammograms. In Lovel, B.C., Meader, A.J., Ourselin, S., Caelli, T., eds.: Proceedings of Digital Image Computing: Techniques and Technology (DICTA2005), IEEE (2005)
6. Ferrari, R.J., Rangayyan, R.M., Desautels, J.E.L., Borges, R.A., Frère, A.F.: Automatic identification of the pectoral muscle in mammograms. IEEE Trans. Med. Im. **23** (2004) 232–245

Author Index

Lecture Notes in Computer Science

For information about Vols. 1–3964

please contact your bookseller or Springer

Vol. 4007: C. Àlvarez, M. Serna (Eds.), Experimental Algorithms. XI, 329 pages. 2006.

Vol. 4006: L.M. Pinho, M. González Harbour (Eds.), Reliable Software Technologies – Ada-Europe 2006. XII, 241 pages. 2006.

Vol. 4005: G. Lugosi, H.U. Simon (Eds.), Learning Theory. XI, 656 pages. 2006. (Sublibrary LNAI).

Vol. 4004: S. Vaudenay (Ed.), Advances in Cryptology - EUROCRYPT 2006. XIV, 613 pages. 2006.

Vol. 4003: Y. Koucheryavy, J. Harju, V.B. Iversen (Eds.), Next Generation Teletraffic and Wired/Wireless Advanced Networking. XVI, 582 pages. 2006.

Vol. 4001: E. Dubois, K. Pohl (Eds.), Advanced Information Systems Engineering. XVI, 560 pages. 2006.

Vol. 3999: C. Kop, G. Fliedl, H.C. Mayr, E. Métais (Eds.), Natural Language Processing and Information Systems. XIII, 227 pages. 2006.

Vol. 3998: T. Calamoneri, I. Finocchi, G.F. Italiano (Eds.), Algorithms and Complexity. XII, 394 pages. 2006.

Vol. 3997: W. Grieskamp, C. Weise (Eds.), Formal Approaches to Software Testing. XII, 219 pages. 2006.

Vol. 3996: A. Keller, J.-P. Martin-Flatin (Eds.), Self-Managed Networks, Systems, and Services. X, 185 pages. 2006.

Vol. 3995: G. Müller (Ed.), Emerging Trends in Information and Communication Security. XX, 524 pages. 2006.

Vol. 3994: V.N. Alexandrov, G.D. van Albada, P.M.A. Sloot, J. Dongarra (Eds.), Computational Science – ICCS 2006, Part IV. XXXV, 1096 pages. 2006.

Vol. 3993: V.N. Alexandrov, G.D. van Albada, P.M.A. Sloot, J. Dongarra (Eds.), Computational Science – ICCS 2006, Part III. XXXVI, 1136 pages. 2006.

Vol. 3992: V.N. Alexandrov, G.D. van Albada, P.M.A. Sloot, J. Dongarra (Eds.), Computational Science – ICCS 2006, Part II. XXXV, 1122 pages. 2006.

Vol. 3991: V.N. Alexandrov, G.D. van Albada, P.M.A. Sloot, J. Dongarra (Eds.), Computational Science – ICCS 2006, Part I. LXXXI, 1096 pages. 2006.

Vol. 3990: J. C. Beck, B.M. Smith (Eds.), Integration of AI and OR Techniques in Constraint Programming for Combinatorial Optimization Problems. X, 301 pages. 2006.

Vol. 3989: J. Zhou, M. Yung, F. Bao, Applied Cryptography and Network Security. XIV, 488 pages. 2006.

Vol. 3988: A. Beckmann, U. Berger, B. Löwe, J.V. Tucker (Eds.), Logical Apporaches to Computational Barriers. XV, 608 pages. 2006.

Vol. 3987: M. Hazas, J. Krumm, T. Strang (Eds.), Location- and Context-Awareness. X, 289 pages. 2006.

Vol. 3986: K. Stølen, W.H. Winsborough, F. Martinelli, F. Massacci (Eds.), Trust Management. XIV, 474 pages. 2006.

Vol. 3984: M. Gavrilova, O. Gervasi, V. Kumar, C.J. K. Tan, D. Taniar, A. Laganà, Y. Mun, H. Choo (Eds.), Computational Science and Its Applications - ICCSA 2006, Part V. XXV, 1045 pages. 2006.

Vol. 3983: M. Gavrilova, O. Gervasi, V. Kumar, C.J. K. Tan, D. Taniar, A. Laganà, Y. Mun, H. Choo (Eds.), Computational Science and Its Applications - ICCSA 2006, Part IV. XXVI, 1191 pages. 2006.

Vol. 3982: M. Gavrilova, O. Gervasi, V. Kumar, C.J. K. Tan, D. Taniar, A. Laganà, Y. Mun, H. Choo (Eds.), Computational Science and Its Applications - ICCSA 2006, Part III. XXV, 1243 pages. 2006.

Vol. 3981: M. Gavrilova, O. Gervasi, V. Kumar, C.J. K. Tan, D. Taniar, A. Laganà, Y. Mun, H. Choo (Eds.), Computational Science and Its Applications - ICCSA 2006, Part II. XXVI, 1255 pages. 2006.

Vol. 3980: M. Gavrilova, O. Gervasi, V. Kumar, C.J. K. Tan, D. Taniar, A. Laganà, Y. Mun, H. Choo (Eds.), Computational Science and Its Applications - ICCSA 2006, Part I. LXXV, 1199 pages. 2006.

Vol. 3979: T.S. Huang, N. Sebe, M.S. Lew, V. Pavlović, M. Kölsch, A. Galata, B. Kisačanin (Eds.), Computer Vision in Human-Computer Interaction. XII, 121 pages. 2006.

Vol. 3978: B. Hnich, M. Carlsson, F. Fages, F. Rossi (Eds.), Recent Advances in Constraints. VIII, 179 pages. 2006. (Sublibrary LNAI).

Vol. 3977: N. Fuhr, M. Lalmas, S. Malik, G. Kazai (Eds.), Advances in XML Information Retrieval and Evaluation. XII, 556 pages. 2006.

Vol. 3976: F. Boavida, T. Plagemann, B. Stiller, C. Westphal, E. Monteiro (Eds.), NETWORKING 2006. Networking Technologies, Services, and Protocols; Performance of Computer and Communication Networks; Mobile and Wireless Communications Systems. XXVI, 1276 pages. 2006.

Vol. 3975: S. Mehrotra, D.D. Zeng, H. Chen, B. Thuraisingham, F.-Y. Wang (Eds.), Intelligence and Security Informatics. XXII, 772 pages. 2006.

Vol. 3973: J. Wang, Z. Yi, J.M. Zurada, B.-L. Lu, H. Yin (Eds.), Advances in Neural Networks - ISNN 2006, Part III. XXIX, 1402 pages. 2006.

Vol. 3972: J. Wang, Z. Yi, J.M. Zurada, B.-L. Lu, H. Yin (Eds.), Advances in Neural Networks - ISNN 2006, Part II. XXVII, 1444 pages. 2006.

Vol. 3971: J. Wang, Z. Yi, J.M. Zurada, B.-L. Lu, H. Yin (Eds.), Advances in Neural Networks - ISNN 2006, Part I. LXVII, 1442 pages. 2006.

Vol. 3970: T. Braun, G. Carle, S. Fahmy, Y. Koucheryavy (Eds.), Wired/Wireless Internet Communications. XIV, 350 pages. 2006.

Vol. 3969: Ø. Ytrehus (Ed.), Coding and Cryptography. XI, 443 pages. 2006.

Vol. 3968: K.P. Fishkin, B. Schiele, P. Nixon, A. Quigley (Eds.), Pervasive Computing. XV, 402 pages. 2006.

Vol. 3967: D. Grigoriev, J. Harrison, E.A. Hirsch (Eds.), Computer Science – Theory and Applications. XVI, 684 pages. 2006.

Vol. 3966: Q. Wang, D. Pfahl, D.M. Raffo, P. Wernick (Eds.), Software Process Change. XIV, 356 pages. 2006.

Vol. 3965: M. Bernardo, A. Cimatti (Eds.), Formal Methods for Hardware Verification. VII, 243 pages. 2006.